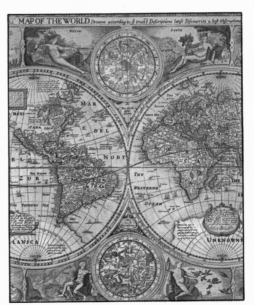

Perioperative Patient Care
The Nursing Perspective

Perioperative Patient Care

The Nursing Perspective

Julia A. Kneedler, R.N., Ed.D.

Director Staff Development
Porter Memorial Hospital
Denver, Colorado

Gwen H. Dodge, R.N., M.S.

Nurse Consultant, Education Design
Denver, Colorado

Blackwell Scientific Publications, Inc.
Boston Oxford London Edinburgh Melbourne

To avoid the stereotypical use of pronouns, (i.e., the doctor and patient always being "he," the nurse always being "she"), we have alternated the use of pronouns between chapters. In one chapter, the anonymous doctor, nurse, and patient are referred to as "he," and in the next they are referred to as "she."

Blackwell Scientific Publications
Editorial offices at:
52 Beacon Street, Boston 02108, USA
Osney Mead, Oxford OX2 0EL, England
8 John Street, London WC1N 2ES, England
9 Forrest Road, Edinburgh EH1 2QH, Scotland
99 Barry Street, Carlton, Victoria 3053, Australia

Distributors:

USA
  Blackwell Mosby Book Distributors
  11830 Westline Industrial Drive
  St. Louis, Missouri 63141

Canada
  Blackwell Mosby Book Distributors
  120 Melford Drive
  Scarborough, Ontario, M1B 2X4

Australia
  Blackwell Scientific Book Distributors, Pty., Ltd.
  31 Advantage Road
  Highett, Victoria 3190

Outside North America and Australia
  Blackwell Scientific Publications Ltd.
  Osney Mead
  Oxford OX2 0EL
  England

Library of Congress Cataloging in Publication Data

Kneedler, Julia A., 1938–
  Perioperative patient care.

  Includes index.
  1. Surgical nursing. I. Dodge, Gwen H.,
1928–   . II. Title. [DNLM: 1. Surgical
nursing—Methods. WY 161 P445]
RD99.K57 1983   610.73'67   83-3875
  ISBN 0-86542-010-6

1 2 3 4 5 6 7 8 9

This book is dedicated to the members of
the Association of Operating Room Nurses
who have a commitment to excellence in
the practice of perioperative nursing.

Contents

Foreword

Anyone reading this book will have to agree that that branch of nursing concerned only with the operating room no longer exists. The phrase operating room nursing is replaced by the term perioperative nursing and the use of this new name is a conscious attempt to change the conception of this field of nursing and to promote a truly professional practice.

Thoughts that this branch of nursing is "technical," "mechanical," a "physician's assistant role," or "just not nursing," are dispelled by this book. Perioperative nursing is presented with all its complexities as a professional and specialized field of nursing. The authors describe and stress the rights of patients and the corresponding responsibilities of the nurse, thereby depicting the social contract of professional nursing practice.

The intellectual, clinical decision-making nature of nursing is described as part of every nurse-patient encounter. Autonomy within the scope of perioperative nursing and the profession's role in regulating that practice are clear. One additional characteristic of the professional nature of perioperative nursing, namely a practice that generates from a distinct knowledge base, is presented by these authors. In addition to being an encyclopedia of perioperative nursing, this book delivers a message on the nature of professional nursing in the 1980's. It is a valuable contribution to the literature.

To label this book incredible is an understatement. The authors have combined in one volume an intensive and extensive presentation of both the art and the science of nursing relevant to the practice of perioperative nursing. The authors deal with the entire scope of perioperative nursing from a perspective that emphasizes psychosocial factors to the same degree as physiological and environmental factors. They have been successful in conveying the need to approach all types of patient cues with equal concern and rigor.

It is obvious that the authors have the experience and academic backgrounds relevant to perioperative nursing. The ease with which they move from the abstract to the concrete, with enough intermediate steps that the novice can track the logical flow, is impressive. Only experts in the field could have such command of both the art and the science. Only truly seasoned, knowledgeable nurses would be able to conceptualize the scope of practice and present nursing actions and the nuances of practice in the detailed manner of these authors.

This book is a valuable contribution to the nursing literature. It will serve as a useful guide for those in practice; as a text for those entering this field of practice; and a helpful reference for those concerned with the scope and complexity of nursing practice.

Carol A. Lindeman, RN, PhD, FAAN
Dean, School of Nursing
The Oregon Health Sciences University

Preface

This text presents a fresh, innovative approach to the care of patients having surgery. Its intent is to show the progression of the patient from admission for surgery until discharge from the postanesthesia area. Integrated throughout are the roles and functions of the nurse while caring for the patient. Equal emphasis is given to professional and technical responsibilities.

Nursing's role in the health care matrix is constantly adapting to society's expectation, scientific and medical advancement, and social change. It is imperative that a nursing resource such as this text operationalize the new concept associated with the term "perioperative" as applied to patient care and nursing activities. A complete understanding of the concept of perioperative patient care accompanied by a blueprint is given to assist nurses as they strive to fulfill their expanding responsibilities to surgical patients. The content will add to the theory base in nursing and provide a framework for further exploration of concepts underlying the perioperative role. Associated with such a purpose is the intent to furnish a reference point for investigative research to validate the role as described in the text.

This text has been written specifically with the practicing registered nurse in mind. Prior to this publication little has been written for this group of nurses who desperately seek material to guide them in developing their unique role in caring for the perioperative patient. Because students of nursing have limited exposure during their formal education, it is hoped that nursing faculty will use this text as an adjunct to curriculum content. It will furnish the novice with a wealth of information about providing care to the surgical patient through the use of the nursing process and implementation of perioperative standards of practice. Other members of the health care team will find this text useful in increasing their understanding of the patient's surgical experience. Team members will also be able to grasp professional nurses' perioperative functions as well as how they interrelate as members of a team whose primary goal is to return patients to their highest level of wellness.

The book comprises five parts. Part I lays the groundwork for the entire book. It includes a philosophical discussion of the nurse's approach to perioperative care, an historical background of operating room nursing, and an explanation of the perioperative role.

Parts II, III, IV, and V encompass the four components of the nursing process—assessment, planning, implementation, and evaluation. Each component is defined in the first chapter of its respective part along with an

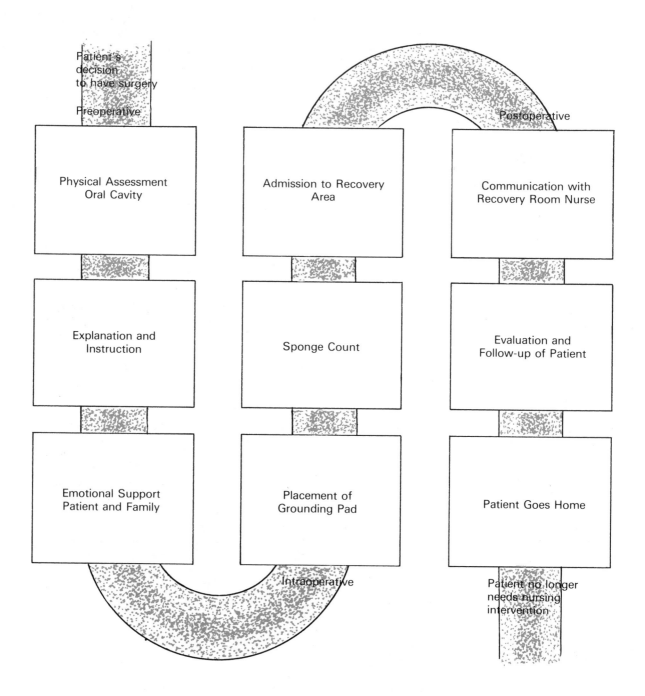

Patient's
decision
to have surgery

Preoperative

Physical Assessment
Oral Cavity

Explanation and
Instruction

Emotional Support
Patient and Family

Admission to Recovery
Area

Sponge Count

Placement of
Grounding Pad

Intraoperative

Postoperative

Communication with
Recovery Room Nurse

Evaluation and
Follow-up of Patient

Patient Goes Home

Patient no longer
needs nursing
intervention

explanation of the *Standards of Perioperative Nursing Practice* that are applicable to the nursing process component.

Collecting psychological and physiological data and formulating a nursing diagnosis make up the chapters in Part II, "Assessing the Perioperative Patient." Part III, "Planning Perioperative Patient Care," forces the nurse to look at patient goals. Six of the chapters are based on goals that are common to all patients having surgery and toward which nursing care is directed. Part IV, "Implementing Perioperative Patient Care," deals with nursing actions performed by the nurse, beginning with transporting the patient to the operating room and ending with immediate postoperative care in the postanesthesia room. Evaluating the extent to which patient goals were met and measuring the effectiveness of nursing care

are the subjects of the two chapters in Part V, "Evaluating Perioperative Patient Care."

Readers of this textbook, whether nurses, students, faculty or other members of the health care team can readily visualize the organizational framework used to present the content. There are two major focuses throughout—the surgical patient and the professional nurse who provides some or all of the nursing care for the patient during the surgical experience.

The organizational framework is fully depicted in Chapter 3, "Perioperative Patient Care: A Dynamic New Focus." We have used a framework based on the needs and experiences of the patient having surgery. The text follows the patient through all phases of surgical intervention as the nurse applies the nursing process through implementation of standards of

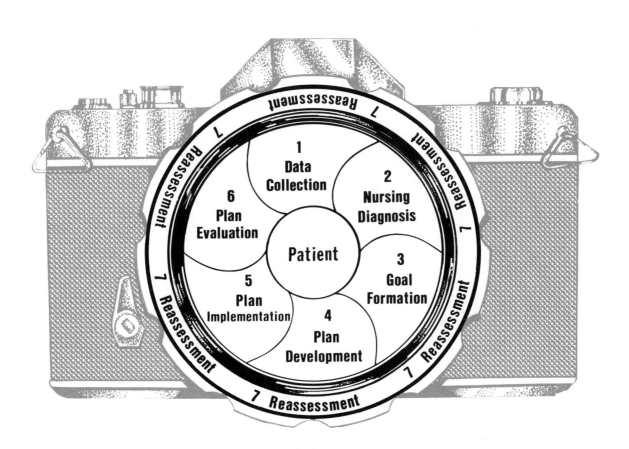

practice. (See diagram on page xii.) Intervention begins with the decision to have surgery and ends when the patient no longer needs nursing care associated with surgery. The three phases are preoperative, intraoperative, and postoperative. The preoperative phase commences when the patient makes the decision to have surgery and ends when the patient is transferred to the operating room. The intraoperative phase begins when the patient is transferred to the operating room and ends when the patient is admitted to the recovery room. The postoperative phase commences with admission to the recovery room and ends when the patient is discharged from the hospital.

The camera lens used as the graphic design for each chapter represents the dual focus of the text. (See diagram on previous page.) Because a camera lens enables one to change focal points without phasing out an image entirely, it was chosen as the model to provide continuity throughout the text. Overall, the focal point or center of the lens is the patient, even though some chapters have deliberately focused on the nurse.

The nursing process is the framework the nurse uses in providing care. The standards of care and the nursing process are represented as the various lens settings that permit a sharper focus on one image without eliminating the central focus. Throughout the text the reader is visually reminded of the predominant standard or standards that are specific to that chapter. We have made every attempt to present material in a manner that is practical when absorbed by the reader.

We truly believe the *Standards of Perioperative Care* are guides to practice and should be used daily. To reinforce this belief, a true patient situation is used throughout. This patient had a left hemiglossectomy, left hemimandibulectomy, and a temporary tracheostomy. The patient situation starts in Chapter 5, which details his assessment, and ends with evaluation of his care in Chapter 26. A patient care plan is included in appropriate chapters to illustrate application of content.

Acknowledgments

The skeleton of the perioperative patient care concept described in this text was conceived during two intense evenings in 1976 when we were staff employees in the Education Department of the Association of Operating Room Nurses. A number of association members and nurses in the general nursing community put the meat on the bones and so made the concept workable. Their contributions are a matter of historical record. However, it was the dozens of practitioners performing patient care in the operating room who made the concept a living reality. Fired with the true pioneer spirit, a commitment to quality surgical patient care and an enthusiasm for a broader professional focus, they sallied forth to put the concept into practice. They welcomed the challenge and responded to it. Although individual recognition is not possible here, the authors salute those early advocates and acknowledge the credit they so richly deserve. Without them, the concept would have been just another idea.

Our gratitude to the writers who contributed to the manuscript is profound. Although the material of specific contributing authors has not been credited directly due to editorial considerations, their expertise was essential for a book of this nature. Many of them are nurses practicing perioperative patient care and all of them are busy people. For some, the translation of their expertise into the written word was an arduous and time-consuming task they undertook with some trepidation. We hope their experience positively reinforces their own professional images and was growth producing. For those to whom writing was easier, we acknowledge the responsibility a commitment of this kind requires and the sacrifice of personal time involved. We extend our deepest appreciation for each and every effort.

We are especially indebted to our editors in Colorado who reviewed the manuscript for consistency and content omissions, suggested organizational revisions, burned the midnight oil, and suffered through some of our early drafts. They kept us on track when we wandered and made sure the writing level corresponded with the target audience's level of understanding. They were also involved in the planning, coordination, and production of some of the graphics used in the text. Without them, our task would have been insurmountable. Their expertise made it possible.

Jack Milne of Denver and his wife, Florence, were our photographic models for the surgical patient and his family pictured throughout the book. Their concentration on what was being discussed or was supposed to be happening produced photographs of remarkable realism.

Mr. Milne's ability to identify with the patient role contributed a great deal to the effectiveness of our planning. Lilly Goeringer is a nurse in perioperative patient care who portrayed that role in the photographs. Aside from her photogenic quality, she practices what she modeled and was therefore an effective catalyst in creating the realistic atmosphere for the photographic sessions. Our other nurse models were Anita Snyder and Cyndy Yanick. Judith Pfister coordinated our photographic sessions and attended to the technical accuracy of the shots. She also took a few of the pictures. Two of the contributing authors, June Persson and Mark Phippen, with their colleagues' assistance, produced or obtained photographs to illustrate their material.

The patient situation used to illustrate application of content throughout the book was a real one. Although some alteration in certain data was made, we are indebted to Mr. Ralph Pfister who let us share his surgical experiences with the readers and gave us permission to access his hospital records for that purpose.

Porter Memorial Hospital, Denver, Colorado, granted permission for us to use its operating room suite for photographs as well as some of its forms and materials. Staff at the hospital critiqued some of the content for accuracy and currency. No institution could have been more supportive or caring.

Steve Nazario, medical illustrater for Porter Hospital, produced several of the graphics. Charles Pfister was responsible for the drawings depicting the standards-camera model. His ability to draw from a verbal description is uncanny.

Sue Olson typed most of the initial drafts and the publisher's draft of the manuscript. As in times past, we have cause to appreciate not only her exceptional ability to make sense from obscure directions and illegible scratching but also her ability to produce under pressure. As always, her performance was superb. Connie Atkins and Vicky Bath helped with some of the drafts of chapters and with the extensive early correspondence.

Last, but certainly not least, we acknowledge the support of our Education Design colleagues, Judith Pfister and Carol Alexander, who not only wrote for the book but who listened to our numerous frustrations, soothed ruffled feelings, sorted and filed, located lost papers, worked over and around us, tolerated the organized disorganization of the office, and generally kept us sane during the most intensive period of work. To them, our friends, and family we say—thank you for being there when we needed you and for giving us the time to do what had to be done.

Julia A. Kneedler
Gwen H. Dodge
September 1982

List of Contributors

Each chapter is the result of the work of many hands. While individual chapters are not credited to specific persons, all of the following, together, prepared this book.

CAROL J. ALEXANDER, R.N., M.S.
Nurse Consultant
Denver, CO

CAROL J. APPLEGEET, R.N., B.S.N.
Surgical Services Manager
Surgical Center of Indiana
Jeffersonville, IN

GWEN H. DODGE, R.N., M.S.
Nurse Consultant, Education Design
Denver, CO

CAROL G. ELLIOTT, C.R.N.A., M.A.
Chairman—Department of Nurse Anesthesia
University of Kansas
School of Allied Health
Kansas City, KS

CHARLENE FOSTER, C.R.N.A., M.N., M.A.E.
Staff Nurse Anesthetist
Eastside Group Health Hospital
Redmond, WA

JULIA S. GARNER, R.N., M.N.
Nurse Consultant—Hospital Infections Program
Center for Infectious Diseases—Centers for Disease Control
Atlanta, GA

LILLIAN S. GOERINGER, R.N., B.S.
Perioperative Nurse Level III
Porter Memorial Hospital
Denver, CO

DARLENE A. HARDER, R.N., M.S.N.
Director, Health Services
Sunny Acres Villa
Thornton, CO

PATRICIA ROBERTSON HERCULES, R.N., M.S.
Assistant Director of Nursing—Operating Rooms
The Methodist Hospital
Houston, TX

ANITA E. JENSEN, R.N.
Head Nurse, Recovery Room
Porter Memorial Hospital
Denver, CO

JULIA A. KNEEDLER, R.N., Ed.D.
Director Staff Development
Porter Memorial Hospital
Denver, CO

ROSE MARIE McWILLIAMS, R.N., M.A., (Ph.D. Candidate)
Associate Professor/Assistant Director of Nursing Services
University Hospital, University of Colorado Health Sciences Center
Denver, CO

LINDA ROONEY PAJANK, R.N., B.S.N.
Perioperative Nurse
Porter Memorial Hospital
Denver, CO

ANNETTE PARSONS, R.N., M.S., C.N.O.R.
Coordinator Perioperative Services
Mercy Medical Center
Denver, CO

JUNE C. PERSSON, R.N., B.S.N.
Director of Sterile Processing and Distribution
Saint Agnes Medical Center
Fresno, CA

JUDITH I. PFISTER, R.N., B.S.
Nurse Consultant
Education Design
Denver, CO

MARK L. PHIPPEN, R.N., M.N.
Captain, Army Nurse Corps
Instructor
U.S. Army Academy of Health Sciences
Fort Sam Houston
San Antonio, TX

HAZEL V. RICE, R.N., M.S., Ed.S.
Associate Chairman
Southern College of Seventh-Day Adventists
Orlando, FL

JANET K. SCHULTZ, R.N., M.S.N.
Manager Operating Room Systems
American V. Mueller
Division of American Hospital Supply Corporation
Chicago, IL

ELAINE A. THOMSON, R.N., B.S.N., C.N.O.R.
Administrative Supervisor
Neurosensory Operating Rooms
The Methodist Hospital
Houston, TX

LINDA TOLLERUD, R.N.
Head Nurse
Ambulatory Surgery
The Methodist Hospital
Houston, TX

CYNTHIA YANICK, R.N.
Instructor Staff Development Operating Room
Porter Memorial Hospital
Denver, CO

I

Perioperative
Patient Care

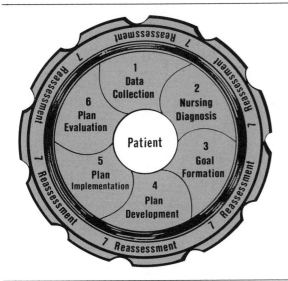

Philosophical approaches are reflected in nursing care focused on the patient.

A Philosophical Approach to Perioperative Nursing

The nursing process of an operating room nurse reflects both her general philosophy of nursing as well as her beliefs about perioperative nursing. A philosophy is the general beliefs, concepts, and attitudes of an individual or group. It reflects the values and general understanding of reality based on reasoning. Nursing as a profession has a philosophical basis, and nurses as individuals have philosophies.

Some nurses may be uncomfortable with the intellectual connotation of the word *philosophy*. But whether or not they recognize it as such, all nurses have a philosophy of nursing based on their personal beliefs, values, and attitudes acquired through their professional education. These are then shaped and redefined almost daily by nursing practice and life experiences.

Beliefs about nursing formed while still a student nurse or recent graduate, or even before, will change as a nurse gains experience and begins to put theory into practice. Interaction with colleagues and patients, professional practice, and continuing education all constantly reaffirm or reshape each nurse's personal philosophy. A personal philosophy helps give meaning to the nurse's practice and provides a rational basis for her actions.

For the nurse who intends to practice perioperative nursing, an examination of the ideological base for the role will demonstrate its values and concepts. With only superficial comprehension of the role, there is danger that the role of the nurse in the operating room (OR) will remain what it was in the past—a skilled manipulation of equipment and supplies in the operating room environment. The contemporary role of the perioperative nurse is patient oriented—not environmental or physician oriented.

Examining the philosophical foundations and acquiring concrete awareness of her philosophy have tangible benefits for the nurse. A philosophy is helpful in several ways. It helps define the major beliefs held by an individual or institution. It establishes a direction for action. It determines the level or quality of care and is the reference point for development of practice and policies.

Writing a philosophy down helps clarify the concepts underlying nursing practice as well as values and beliefs. A written philosophy need not be lengthy, but should cover the basic components. Once written, a philosophy should not be shelved. It is a working tool, providing guidance for practice and professional behavior.

As a statement of the major beliefs and values of an individual or institution, a philosophy makes short, clear statements that are action oriented. Take, for example, the statement: "Human beings are holistic individuals with physical, intellectual, emotional, and spiritual needs." The statement covers a number of separate but related beliefs. These beliefs may direct the nurse's behavior or provide direction for an institutional nursing service. The nurse, for example, who believes in the patient as a whole person with a broad spectrum of needs will attempt to help a patient meet his intellectual, emotional, and spiritual needs as well as the immediate physical needs of his illness. The nursing service that holds this belief will provide staffing and time for nurses to meet patient needs.

A philosophy establishes direction for action both for the individual and institution. For the nurse, a philosophy guides short- and long-term planning and career decisions. A nurse who views the patient holistically would be frustrated in a work environment that did not permit time for caring about individual patient needs and would soon seek other employment. On the other hand, if a nurse is aware of the philosophy of an institution, it is easier to predict the success or failure of plans and activities. A nursing service based on a centralized administrative philosophy, for example, would probably not be receptive to a proposal for a decentralized management plan for the surgical services.

The Perioperative Perspective of the Patient

The perioperative role of nurses caring for surgical patients is not new but is a natural extension of the operating room nurse's traditional role. Before the advent of anesthesia and antiseptic technique, surgery was performed only under dire circumstances, and the specialty of operating room nursing did not exist. Nurses assisted in the operating room and also cared for patients preoperatively and postoperatively. As surgery became safer and more common in the late 1800s, nurses began to specialize in intraoperative patient care, often losing personal contact with patients. Such specialization was instigated by physician specialization in surgery as well as an expanding knowledge of asepsis and its application in the field of surgical therapy. A surgeon's demand for the skilled surgical nurse and the nurse's assumption of responsibility for managing the operating room environment confined her to the operating room. Nurses rarely left the surgical suite to communicate with conscious patients. Premedicated patients were often unaware that professional nurses were involved with their care during surgery. To them, nurses were their surgeon's helpers with faces hidden behind masks. At the same time, nurses concerned themselves with equipment, supplies, and meeting surgeons' needs rather than with meeting patient needs.

The perioperative patient care concept has made that limited technical role obsolete. The perioperative role is a new philosophical direction. Nursing has changed so much that the surgical patient's needs can no longer be met by the generalist nurse from the surgical unit. According to the American College of Surgeons, 45.2 percent of short-stay hospital patients have had surgery, yet nurses who work on surgical units may have a limited knowledge of what transpires in the operating room and the effects of intraoperative occurrences on patients. To resolve this, nursing roles have been realigned to meet obligations to surgical patients. Nurses from the operating room come to patient care units to gather information important to intraoperative nursing and assist patients through instruction. After surgery, they return to evaluate their planning and the effects of implementation. They have opened lines of communication with unit nurses so these nurses are better informed about intraoperative events and their effects on patients.

The well-being of the patient is the primary concern of all nurses. Nursing consists essentially of a service directed toward alleviation of existing or anticipated health problems so an individual may attain a state of optimum wellness relative to her particular condition. The concept of the patient's optimum well-being does not necessarily imply that the patient is restored to health. In the extreme, it may mean that the nurse assists the patient to achieve a peaceful, natural death. In certain instances, the psychological comfort of human contact may be more important than any material or psychological comforts provided by technology.

Perioperative nurses recognize that a patient's needs are not likely to be satisfied by being connected to the latest machine or by a nurse's understanding of the newest surgical procedure. They realize that the patient may need personal contact, help in coping with her fears and anxiety, and explanations other than those provided by the surgeon and anesthetist. They acknowledge their professional and legal accountability for making nursing judgments and decisions within the area of their nursing expertise for the optimum well-being of the surgical patient.

For the perioperative nurse, the patient is an individual—not a disease, a symptom, or a case. She has interdependent physiological, psychological, and social needs and is capable of rational, mature behavior.

Nurses have not always had such positive views of patients. A strong concept of Western civilization has been that human beings are naturally bad. They are born that way and the aim of designated mentors is to force them into the paths of righteous or good behavior. Education has been based on the idea that children need strong discipline by a righteous teacher. In health care, physicians and nurses replaced the authoritarian teacher, and the patient assumed the role of the ignorant schoolchild. Patients were expected to obey these authorities without question. Much of the authoritarian behavior of nurses stems from this theory of human nature. Such behavior may annoy or antagonize contemporary patients, producing uncooperative responses or encouraging childish rather than adult responses.

Health care professionals are now influenced by more modern theories of human nature that portray each person as aspiring or evolving. The adaptation model of human nature, based on the theories of Charles Darwin and Sigmund Freud, shows human beings continually adapting to an ever changing physical and social environment. Calista Roy's adaptation model of nursing uses this framework. Abraham Maslow's hierarchy of human needs is based on the idea of striving human beings whose basic needs for physiological essentials, safety, and belonging must be partially met before they can look toward satisfying self-esteem needs. Once esteem needs are met to some degree, each person aspires to achieve self-actualization or her own potential (1).

Maslow's theory of motivation has been influential in health care. Nurses are aware that the patient's physiological and psychological needs must be met, not just her gallbladder removed or cancerous tumor excised. Maslow's theory has come to be a widely accepted basis for contemporary nursing practice.

Perioperative nurses consider patients as individuals because treating a patient in such a way is beneficial to her well-being. The assessment phase of the diagnostic process in nursing is important not only to acquire a data base for health problem identification but also to reduce the patient's anxiety by providing information. By listening to the patient's concerns and answering her questions, the nurse shows respect for the patient and reaffirms her self-worth.

In the operating room, the nurse continues to treat the patient as an individual. Special needs will have been identified by preoperative assessment data. If the patient is extremely heavy, the necessary special equipment for the patient's safety and comfort will be immediately at hand. In addition, the nurse acts as a patient advocate in the operating room when the patient is incapacitated. For instance, the nurse makes certain the Mayo stand is not resting on the patient's toes or reminds assistants not to lean on the patient's chest. Or in some situations, if the surgeon must make an intraoperative decision, the nurse's opinion of the patient's preference, based on preoperative assessment data, may be sought.

The perioperative nurse's view of the patient as a rational and mature individual recognizes and encourages the patient's ability to learn because her cooperation is necessary for her health. In most cases, the patient is internally motivated because she understands how this benefits her. Through learning, the patient assumes a responsibility for her own health care. Maturity is recognized by involving a patient in planning her care and giving her the freedom to make choices when feasible.

Professional nursing in the United States reflects American beliefs in optimal health, cleanliness, individualism, and technology. Nursing in other cultures may incorporate other values. A recent visit to the Soviet Union made it possible to superficially compare nursing philosophy between the U.S.S.R. and the United States as it is reflected in social values. In the United States, primary emphasis is on individual health. Society's health is secondary. U.S. citizens tend to believe that what is good for the individual benefits society at large. The U.S. health care system is based on the free enterprise system with the federal government assuming responsibility for the health of all citizens in such areas, for example, as pre-

venting importation of disease from abroad. In contrast, the Soviet Union emphasizes the overall good of society first and acknowledges individual health needs to the extent that they have a bearing on the overall productiveness of society. For example, the dental health of individual Soviet citizens is important because people with dental problems are likely to be poorly nourished and prone to other unhealthy conditions, and productivity therefore suffers. The Soviet health care system is free for all intents and purposes. It is centrally administered by the Soviet government, which sets policy and devises the means for implementing policy. In the United States, nurses focus on meeting health needs of individuals, devoting time and attention to individual problems, concerns, and comfort. In the U.S.S.R., the individual comfort needs of hospitalized patients are met by family members. Nurses control patient activities in health care centers through rigid enforcement of rules and doctors' treatment orders. The rules are there to benefit everybody, and exceptions are infrequently permitted. Even children are expected to tolerate assaults on their persons in the name of diagnosis and treatment without crying or complaining. Soviet nurses seem little inclined to dwell on individual responses to health problems.

The Perioperative Perspective of the Nurse

The perioperative role is patient-oriented nursing, benefiting both patients and nurses. For the nurse the role emphasizes the professional, intellectual, and human aspects of nursing and increases responsibility to the patient and her family. The patient benefits from direct communication with the perioperative nurse as well as from individualized care. Because the nurse sees the role as significant and gains greater personal satisfaction, better nursing care may be given, which also directly benefits the patient.

As a specialty, perioperative patient care is based on general definitions and concepts of nursing. Nursing has been and still is predominantly a women's profession. Nurses are still expected to demonstrate so-called feminine characteristics. They are expected to be caring and compassionate and even self-sacrificing. With the women's movement and the shifting role of women in society, the women and men entering the profession bring to it different characteristics. These nurses are no longer willing to simply carry out medically related activities. They clearly see the independent functions of nursing as well as the different focus nursing has in contast to medicine. Perioperative nursing reflects this perspective. Although perioperative nurses perform medically related activities during surgical procedures, they also give direct nursing care in collaboration with physicians and other health care personnel.

As professionals, nurses have become more assertive. Although they still value the caring characteristics of nursing, they expect to be fairly compensated for their work and acknowledged for their professional nursing skills. For both men and women in nursing, the challenge is not to discard what might be considered feminine—the caring and compassion —but to combine these characteristics with a professional knowledge-based nursing.

Defining nursing is not easy. There are almost as many definitions of nursing as there are nurses. Lack of a commonly accepted definition of nursing is one of the profession's problems identified in the *Study of Credentialing in Nursing: A New Approach* (2). One of the first definitions of nursing is Florence Nightingale's. In *Notes on Nursing: What It Is and What It Is Not*, she wrote that the knowledge of nursing was "how to put the constitution in such a state as that it will have no disease, or that it can recover from disease" (3:1). It was her belief that health nursing involved "charge of the personal health of somebody, whether child or invalid" (3:1). However, she distinguishes in this work between the nursing provided by women in general and the trained nurse. Nightingale describes nursing as an art with a specific body of knowledge. According to another of her writings, nursing consists of two types: the "art of nursing proper," involving direct care to the sick, and health nursing

for the purpose of keeping people healthy. "Nursing proper is therefore to help the patient suffering from disease to live—just as health nursing is to keep or put the constitution of the healthy child or human being in such a state as to have no disease" (4:26). This two-pronged belief of nursing as care of the sick and the healthy persists in modern definitions.

A current definition of nursing by the American Nurses' Association is published in *Nursing: A Social Policy Statement*. Here nursing is defined as "the diagnosis and treatment of human responses to actual or potential health problems" (5:9).

In developing the perioperative role concept, the Association of Operating Room Nurses Task Force, composed of operating room nurses and other nursing leaders, used Rozella Schlotfeldt's definition in which she holds that nursing is an independent, autonomous, self-regulating profession with the primary function that of helping each person attain his highest level of general health. Further, she believes the practice of nursing focuses

on assessing people's health status, assets, and deviations from health, and on helping people to regain health, and the well or near-well to maintain or attain health through selective application of nursing science and the use of available nursing strategies (6:769).

This statement provides a framework for the perioperative role.

A common theme in all these definitions is that nursing addresses health-related human responses; that is, nursing focuses on the reactions of individuals or groups to actual or potential health problems. In so doing nurses diagnose and treat these responses. If, for instance, the perioperative nurse observes signs of anxiety in a patient, she will endeavor to discover the threat to the patient's safety causing the anxiety and plan strategies for helping the patient cope, if appropriate.

All the definitions fail to acknowledge that there are certain health problems that nurses are qualified and licensed to treat. Such problems include self-care limitations, impaired functioning in areas such as rest and sleep, and strains related to birth, death, growth, and development.

Nurses use a set of concepts to guide general decisions about what to assess and diagnose, how to intervene, and what to evaluate. This set, in nursing language, is called a conceptual framework. The perioperative role is based on the nursing process. This four-step process of assessment, planning, implementation, and evaluation of outcomes is an adaptation of problem-solving theory and widely used in nursing practice. Structured on the nursing process, this book will go through the nursing process as it applies to perioperative nursing. In the perioperative role, intellectual activities predominate over technical skills. Although technical skills will always be important in the operating room, technical mastery most often is necessary for tasks that can be delegated to less prepared personnel. Nurses functioning in the perioperative role must value and consciously carry out activities that require intellectual skills and professional preparation. Professional nursing education prepares practitioners for arriving at nursing diagnoses, making data-based decisions, and evaluating outcomes related to patient health care problems. The nurse who devotes time to technical functions while patient health needs are unmet is wasting professional expertise. This nurse is not fulfilling professional accountability to patients.

Nurses should be able to ascertain what activities the professional nurse alone can accomplish and concentrate attention in that direction, assigning others to nonprofessional personnel. The nurse demonstrating proficiency and expertise in cleaning and caring for general surgical instruments only makes the nonprofessional person wonder why a professional nurse is needed in the operating room. For too long, nurses have believed and acted as if they personally had to do everything in the operating room—or elsewhere—otherwise it would not be done properly or safely. The perioperative role is not for nurses who prefer technical to professional activities. Nurses who do not have the inclination, warmth, and skill to work directly with patients have no place in a role emphasizing those qualities.

Perioperative nursing requires a strong philosophical belief that the role is a nursing role in a specialized area. Nurses are nurses before they engage in any of the other roles they are occasionally called upon to fulfill. Although the perioperative nurse may need to perform tasks in the role of surgeon's assistant, epidemiologist, or mechanic, these roles are only transitory. Perioperative nurses must see themselves first as nurses before they see themselves as specialists. What influences nursing affects them; what concerns nursing should also concern nurses in a specialist nursing role.

Recognition of the professional activities inherent in the perioperative role and the desire to fulfill them sometimes require commitment in the face of opposition. As nurses from the operating room have expanded their activities to include nursing diagnosis and patient outcome evaluation, they have encountered some opposition from nursing colleagues and physicians who see the role as encroaching on their territory. Administrators have argued that perioperative nursing requires more time—an expensive commodity in a cost-conscious era.

Introducing the perioperative role may require carefully planned strategies. A planning committee may be helpful. Through good communication and documentation by published research findings, nursing colleagues in other areas as well as physicians can be shown that perioperative nursing assessment and postoperative evaluation do not in any way detract from the roles of other health care professionals, but complement them in ways meaningful to the patient. Nurses functioning in the perioperative role must recognize the limits of their role and refrain from infringing on other's roles. It is the surgeon's legal responsibility, for instance, to explain to the patient the location, direction, and length of the incision through which the surgical procedure will be performed, just as it is the anesthesiologist's responsibility to discuss the anesthetic agent and its administration. Administrators may need to be persuaded of the value of quality patient care in attracting patients and surgeons to the hospital and the merit of better communication with patients in preventing complaints and even lawsuits.

Although nurses from the operating room have sometimes met with opposition in implementing the perioperative role, they have also been welcomed with enthusiasm as they have moved into the mainstream of nursing. Nursing colleagues in the past have judged nurses from the operating room as technicians rather than professional nurses. But as perioperative nurses have come to the units to care for patients and demonstrated their knowledge of the nursing process, they have shown colleagues that they are practicing professional nursing. As they interact with nurses on patient care units and in other areas of the hospital, they are recognized as professional peers.

Code for Nurses

Nursing ethics are an integral part of any nursing philosophy and perioperative patient care. Professional behavior of nurses is guided by the American Nurses' Association *Code for Nurses* (see Fig. 1.1). Ethics is a system of moral principles—the rights and wrongs of human behavior and the underlying values. These principles prescribe generally how reasonable human beings should behave in relation to other human beings. Professional ethics are the rules of conduct expected of practitioners to whom society entrusts certain functions. Professional ethics presupposes the presence of a moral value system of rightful behavior upon which professional rules of conduct can be built. The *Code for Nurses* addresses the professional duties of nursing. Constantly reviewed, the *Code* remains current and applicable to nursing practice as nursing adjusts to social and technological change.

In the first and principle statement, the *Code* establishes the basic responsibility of all nurses to provide services with respect for the human

Figure 1.1. Code for Nurses. *Copyright* © *by the American Nurses' Association, 1976. Reprinted with permission of the American Nurses' Association.*

Preamble

The *Code for Nurses* is based on a belief about the nature of individuals, nursing, health, and society. Recipients and providers of nursing services are viewed as individuals and groups who possess basic rights and responsibilities, and whose values and circumstances command respect at all times. Nursing encompasses the promotion and restoration of health, the prevention of illness, and the alleviation of suffering. The statements of the *Code* and their interpretation provide guidance for conduct and relationships in carrying out nursing responsibilities consistent with the ethical obligations of the profession and quality in nursing care.

Code for Nurses

1. The nurse provides services with respect for human dignity and the uniqueness of the client unrestricted by considerations of social or economic status, personal attributes, or the nature of health problems.
2. The nurse safeguards the client's right to privacy by judiciously protecting information of a confidential nature.
3. The nurse acts to safeguard the client and the public when health care and safety are affected by the incompetent, unethical, or illegal practice of any person.
4. The nurse assumes responsibility and accountability for individual nursing judgments and actions.
5. The nurse maintains competence in nursing.
6. The nurse exercises informed judgment and uses individual competence and qualifications as criteria in seeking consultation, accepting responsibilities, and delegating nursing activities to others.
7. The nurse participates in activities that contribute to the ongoing development of the profession's body of knowledge.
8. The nurse participates in the profession's efforts to implement and improve standards of nursing.
9. The nurse participates in the profession's efforts to establish and maintain conditions of employment conducive to high quality health care.
10. The nurse participates in the profession's efforts to protect the public from misinformation and misrepresentation and to maintain the integrity of nursing.
11. The nurse collaborates with members of the health professions and other citizens in promoting community and national efforts to meet the health needs of the public.

dignity of the patient regardless of social or economic status, personal attributes, or the nature of the health problems. This is an absolute duty, and there can be no moral justification for any exception. To act otherwise is failure to act as a professional nurse.

Inherent in this statement, however, is the nurse's right to refuse to participate in the management of health problems or procedures that she holds to be morally wrong. In exercising this right, the nurse must give sufficient warning that a certain treatment or procedure constitutes a moral conflict. This may be established at time of employment. Also, adequate and competent nursing care must be available for the patient. These two conditions imply that the patient's right to care supersedes the nurse's right to refuse care for a patient. Consider the following situation: On emergency call, a nurse is called in for a cesarean section on a 30-year-old woman with a footling presentation. One of the infant's legs has been delivered, but the other is crossed upon the upper abdomen, and the obstetrician cannot grasp the ankle and straighten the leg to deliver the infant vaginally. The infant is showing signs of distress. While the nurse is setting up for the procedure, the physician informs the nurse that she also intends to perform a tubal ligation at the patient's request. Since the nurse is opposed to any form of birth control on moral grounds, she does not want to participate in the procedure. But there is no other nurse available who has the necessary knowledge and skills to provide nursing care. The nurse in this situation cannot refuse to participate in the patient's care because any delay would further compromise the infant and could endanger the mother's life. Under no circumstances is it permissible to abandon the patient.

The first three statements of the *Code* outline the nurse's obligation to protect patient rights and safety. The patient's right to control what is done to her person is also addressed in the first statement. The right to privacy, spoken to in the second statement, requires constant vigilance. In the operating room these rights are protected by preventing unnecessary exposure of the patient and excluding all but essential personnel from the room. Patient records are of course confidential, but the patient's privacy is also considered in conversations that might be overheard or when posting surgical schedules.

There is research to indicate that some generally anesthetized patients are able to recall conversations between surgical team members (7:1). Discussion of anatomical characteristics of patients, off-color jokes, and other non-health-problem-related comments might be remembered by any patient as being applicable to her and considered a violation of the privacy right.

Under the third statement, the nurse acts as an advocate to protect the patient from any incompetent, unethical, or illegal practice. Especially in the operating room, where the patient is unable to defend her person, this is an important nursing responsibility. The nurse has the responsibility to bring any substandard or improper care of which she is aware to the attention of the person involved. If corrective measures are not taken, the next highest person in the chain of command must be informed. In a 1981 lawsuit that involved a surgeon removing nineteen feet of a patient's small bowel through a perforated uterus, the operating room nurses were asked whether they should have stopped the surgeon. They believed they could question the surgeon if their observations clearly indicated something was wrong, but they could not stop him or interrupt the procedure (8:992). The nurses were found liable by the court. The decision was based on the testimony of expert witnesses who stated that professional ethics and hospital procedure demand that nurses stop a doctor's action if in their judgment it is incorrect. (The decision is being appealed.) The nurse has a responsibility to act if aware of negligence, and failure to do so constitutes negligence on the nurse's part if harm is sustained by the patient. Nurses have encountered hostility and resistance from physicians, administrators, and their nursing peers when they have raised questions about patient care or the competency of care-givers. At least one state, Oregon, has passed a law protecting nurses and others who report questionable practice. Hospitals should also have written policies and procedures for reporting substandard or questionable practice.

The next three statements of the *Code* address the nurse's qualifications in giving patient care. The fourth statement concerns the nurse's responsibility and accountability for nursing judgments and actions. Perioperative nurses comply with this principle, for example, by documenting care in the patient's record, completing incident reports, making nursing diagnoses based on facts, and performing postoperative evaluations. They also participate in hospital or departmental quality assurance programs and peer review processes for measuring the effectiveness of care and correcting deficiencies.

The fifth statement obligates the nurse to maintain competency in nursing. Although the merits of mandatory continuing education for nursing license renewal are debatable, most nurses believe continuing education is essential for maintaining competency. They regularly attend workshops, seminars, courses, and national meetings to update their knowledge and skills. Accountability for continued competency is evidenced by the number of nurses who voluntarily seek certification as a generalist or specialist.

The sixth statement encourages the nurse to use expert judgment and awareness of her own competence and qualifications in accepting responsibility, seeking help, and delegating nursing activities to others. Nurses in the operating room, for instance, are sometimes asked to staff the postanesthetic recovery room. If the nurse lacks knowledge and skills in caring for patients recovering from anesthesia, the assignment should not be accepted until the needed education has been acquired. Nurses also should exercise judgment in delegating nursing activities to nonprofessionals. Although technicians have been well accepted in the operating room in the scrub position, their training prepares them only to perform technical tasks, not professional functions. In perioperative patient care, the professional nurse performs supervisory functions, circulating duties, and other activities that require professional nurs-

ing education and skills. These activities include data collection from patients, making nursing diagnoses, developing patient care plans, and evaluating patient care. Delegation of professional responsibilities to personnel who are not qualified to meet them is ethically wrong and in several states illegal.

Although the last five statements in the *Code* refer to the nurse's responsibility to the profession and society, many nurses overlook these obligations. All nurses benefit from the activities of professional organizations. Yet of the more than 1 million working nurses, only about 160,000 belong to the American Nurses' Association (ANA). The Association of Operating Room Nurses (AORN) has estimated that about 50 percent of nurses working in the operating room belong to it. Statement number seven of the *Code* indicates that nurses should contribute to the profession's body of knowledge. This means the nurse has an obligation to conduct or participate in nursing research, to write for publication, or to develop speaking skills so knowledge may be shared with colleagues. Development and testing of nursing diagnoses are a professional arena likely to profit from perioperative nurse involvement. Designing workshops and acting as a preceptor in the perioperative role are other activities.

The eighth statement refers to the nurse's obligation to implement and improve standards of nursing. ANA and AORN have jointly published standards for perioperative nursing, and AORN has published a number of recommended technical practices. Nevertheless some nurses resist using the standards, preferring to rely on ritualistic practice—"the-way-its-always-been-done" type of practice. But most nurses welcome the opportunity to base their practice on generally accepted standards and research findings.

ANA has been active for many years in upgrading the economic and general welfare of nurses. Through its state associations, it now represents approximately 100,000 (9) nurses in collective bargaining units working toward conditions of employment conducive to high-quality health care, as mandated in the ninth statement. ANA also is deeply involved in national health care legislation and, through its Washington office, monitors federal government activities of concern to nurses and nursing. Constituent state associations carry on these activities at the state level. Although not registered as a union and not involved in collective bargaining, AORN has supported the registered nurse as supervisor and circulator in the operating room when regulatory agencies have attempted to downgrade these positions. AORN members participated in these efforts by writing letters to agencies, members of Congress, and newspapers.

The nurse also has an obligation to participate in the profession's efforts, as stated in the tenth proposition, to protect the public from misinformation and misrepresentation. Because nurses teach and provide information about health care, they are cautioned against endorsing or implying endorsement of any commercial products or services in advertising through public media. Intentional or implied endorsement of a product or service by a nurse in public advertising may be interpreted by the public as professional approval. Nursing is also frequently misrepresented in public media (10, 11). Nurses are working to correct the false image and establish in the public's mind a truly professional image of nursing.

Nurses are expected to have concerns about society's health in general. The final statement of the *Code* speaks to the nurse's obligation to work with other health care professionals and citizens to support community and national efforts to meet health care needs of the public. The nurse's concern should go beyond individual patients to include participation in local or national health goals. Nurses carry out this obligation by volunteering their services for hypertension, cancer, and other screening programs, blood and United Way contribution drives, and health fairs. They act as first-aid counselors for scout troops and teach Red Cross lifesaving classes. They are active in promoting public awareness of health problems, such as multiple sclerosis and sudden infant death syndrome, through participation in voluntary health groups. Nurses have also become increasingly aware and active politically in recent years.

The *Code* provides a framework for making ethical decisions as well as a yardstick for measuring ethical conduct. Since it is impossible to address all the situations in which nurses may need to make ethical decisions, the *Code* considers in general the major ethical issues confronting nurses. Representing the moral values held by the profession, the *Code* indicates to both nurses and the public the responsibilities and expectations required by the profession. It is the profession's response to the trust invested by society in nursing. For amplification of the *Code* see *The Code for Nurses with Interpretative Statements* (12) and *Perspectives on the Code for Nurses* (13).

Although the *Code* is not a legally binding document, in malpractice cases it is cited as the standard of conduct for the profession. Some of its values have been incorporated into nursing practice acts or rules and regulations governing the practice of nursing. Most nurses comply voluntarily with the *Code's* precepts. Failure to abide by its principles erodes the public trust, threatening nursing's control over professional matters and affairs.

Ideals Versus Reality

The ideals nurses acquire in school sometimes are threatened when they begin to practice. They may find their philosophy of nursing conflicts with that of their employer. And they find that society's expectation for health care cannot always be met.

Making the transition from the educational setting to the practice setting can be difficult. Basic education provides the nurse with facts, principles, values, and beliefs. These are obtained through contact with faculty, student peers, and practicing nurses as well as through nursing courses. The type of education a nurse receives influences her philosophy of nursing. Associate degree programs are geared to produce nurses proficient in technical and clinical skills. A four-year program is designed to prepare nurses with greater depth in understanding a patient's physiological and psychosocial responses. But regardless of basic preparation, moving into the work setting will shake and test each nurse's ideals. Ideals may survive and grow stronger or they may be abandoned.

Nurses talk about reality shock. Later they talk about burnout. Many become disillusioned and leave nursing. Baccalaureate nurses feel they have wasted expensive college educations when their knowledge is denigrated by physicians and even other nurses. Many nurses are frustrated when they are unable to practice the nursing they learned in school. During a student's clinical experience, for example, she may have cared for one or two surgical patients at a time. Her learning experience with these patients probably allowed adequate opportunity to diagnose their health problems, write care plans, and evaluate care. But now that she is in practice, life is much more hectic. She is so busy managing the care of many patients, she can only spend a brief time with each patient, completing a minimal assessment.

As a result of different educational and personal backgrounds, nurses vary in their philosophies. In the operating room, some nurses are patient oriented, while others are more concerned with technical aspects of care. For instance, a common problem for surgical patients is anxiety. The patient-oriented nurse learns ways to help the patient cope with anxiety and, as part of her philosophy of practice, helps the patient alleviate her anxiety. A technically oriented nurse might not have the skills to recognize the problem, particularly if the patient has disguised it, or might not feel capable of helping the patient.

A hospital's philosophy may also influence how nursing is practiced. In cost-pressured hospitals, the quality of patient care may suffer. This is not only frustrating, but it presents a moral dilemma for nurses who cannot, because of staffing and time, meet their own standards of patient care. A hospital might discourage perioperative nursing care because it requires additional staffing. But if a hospital's philosophy is oriented to a high level of patient care, it might see preoperative assessment by a nurse from the operating room as an important component of patient care.

A hospital's philosophy will also dictate the proportion of professional nurses to patients and the ratio of nurses to paraprofessionals. If a hospital believes in the best individual care for patients, it will have a higher number of professional nurses to patients and a low number of paraprofessionals. Standards of care will be identified and enforced in the operating room where patient care is given a high priority, there will be a high proportion of nurses to technicians. In purchasing, nurses and physicians will participate in decisions about supplies and equipment. Patient safety will be more important than cost alone.

While hospital philosophy affects nursing practice, nurses also influence hospital philosophy. Nurses are gaining stronger representation in hospital management, where they can make the importance of their philosophy of care known. They are serving on committees and interacting with administrators and physicians. Through collective bargaining, nurses are negotiating contracts that establish working conditions with sufficient staffing to provide good nursing care. Although at one time nurses saw themselves as powerless against administrators and physicians, they are now realizing their importance in the hospital structure and are being more assertive in working toward what they believe is important to patient care.

Costs of Care

Nurses may feel that they are caught in the dilemma of society's expectations for health care and its decreasing ability to pay for it. One of society's basic beliefs is that everyone is entitled to health care regardless of ability to pay. Health care is one of the primary social needs of any society. The World Health Organization has adopted the goal of "health care for all by the year 2000." Many countries have instituted national health insurance or socialized medicine as the way to provide health care for all its citizens. But the United States, despite its wealth and sophisticated medical technology, is seeing a widening gap between health care for those who can afford it and those who cannot. Recently, a burn patient was turned away from more than 40 medical centers because he had no insurance and no way to pay for his care. In the past, hospitals were able to absorb costs of indigent patients through charges to private patients, or local agencies paid the bills. Then with the Great Society of the 1960s, Medicare and Medicaid were enacted to pay for health care of the elderly and the poor. National health insurance was a goal. Everyone would have equal access to health care regardless of ability to pay.

That was the ideal, but now we face the reality. Health care costs have risen so drastically that they are now a drain on the national economy. According to federal government figures, in 1960, health care costs were $27 billion, 5.3 percent of the gross national product. In 1980, these costs increased tenfold to $275 billion, 9.6 percent of the gross national product. The causes are multiple. Medicare and Medicaid as well as tax incentives for private medical insurance are blamed. Since most health care costs are paid by insurers, the consumer is not cost-conscious. Lawsuits and availability of high technology encourage expensive diagnostic testing, which can then be followed by sophisticated care such as that offered in intensive care units.

Paying for and providing access to health care is one of our most critical social problems. The government, private insurers, and the health care industry are looking for ways to solve the problem. Like the causes, the solutions will also be multiple. It seems unlikely, however, that we will be able to return to the past. Cost containment and cost-consciousness will be one of the constraints on health care. People may be willing to accept a lower level of care. One poll indicated that 54 percent of the respondents were willing to accept cheaper and more limited insurance coverage. The implication is that they might be willing to consult with a nurse practitioner rather than a physician; that they might be willing to go to a clinic rather than to a private office. Ambulatory surgery will continue to be used for many surgical procedures, while hospital-stay surgery will decrease.

A nurse's philosophy has to be strong to give her direction as she experiences society's demands, her profession's and patients' expectations, and her demands on herself. Her philosophy will continue to grow as she learns and gains experience, but its base will be the values and beliefs acquired early in her life. As she gains in nursing practice experience, a nurse's philosophy of nursing practice will be strengthened, or if necessary, even changed. Her experience will either verify her beliefs or indicate where they need to be reexamined. A philosophy gives strength and support to a nurse's practice.

References

1. Maslow, Abraham H. *Motivation and Personality*, New York: Harper and Row, 1954.
2. American Nurses' Association. *Study of Credentialing in Nursing: A New Approach.* Kansas City: ANA, 1979.
3. Nightingale, Florence. *Notes on Nursing: What It Is and What It Is Not.* London: Harrison and Sons, 1859.
4. Nightingale, Florence. "Sick nursing and health nursing." In Isabel Hampton, ed. *Nursing the Sick 1893.* New York: McGraw-Hill, 1949.
5. American Nurses' Association. *Nursing: A Social Policy Statement.* Kansas City: ANA, 1980.
6. Schlotfeldt, Rozella M. "Planning for progress." *Nurs Outlook* 21:766–769, 1973.
7. Guerra, Frank, and Aldrete, Antonio J., eds. *Emotional and Psychological Responses to Anesthesia and Surgery.* New York: Grune and Stratton, 1980.
8. Cushing, Maureen. "A matter of judgment." *Am J Nurs* 82(6):992, 1982.
9. American Nurses' Association. Nurse Staff Member, Labor Relations Department, ANA, July, 1982.
10. Kalisch, Philip, and Kalisch, Beatrice. "Nurses on prime-time television." *Am J Nurs* 82(2):262–270, 1982.
11. Kalisch, Philip, and Kalisch, Beatrice. "The image of the nurse in motion pictures." *Am J Nurs* 82(4):605–611, 1982.
12. American Nurses' Association. *The Code for Nurses with Interpretative Statements.* Kansas City: ANA, 1976.
13. American Nurses Association. *Perspectives on the Code for Nurses.* Kansas City: ANA, 1978.

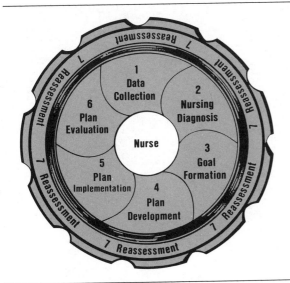

History of operating room nursing evolves into perioperative nursing.

Origins of Operating Room Nursing

The specialty of operating room nursing emerged in the late 1880s as surgery increased and as surgeons recognized the important assistance nurses provided. Before this time, nurses had been shadow figures in the operating room who handed and wrung out sponges and kept the operating theater "fresh," according to Eva C. E. Luckes. An English nurse in the late nineteenth century, Luckes added, "Nurses are not there to *see* the operation . . . but to make their presence realized by the perfectly quiet way in which all wants are foreseen or supplied" (1:122). Care of the patient and preparation of the operating room were not considered nursing responsibilities until later.

At first, the nurse's most important function was to hand sponges to the surgeon. Wringing out sponges was one of the chief duties of American OR nurses in the late 1880s (see Fig. 2.1). Instrument care was not a duty, but Luckes did advise nurses, "It is well for you to notice them as you have the opportunity. They should be covered with a towel, that the patient may be spared the sight of them" (1:121–122).

Early Surgery

In the mid-nineteenth century, surgery was a new specialty making some remarkable ad-

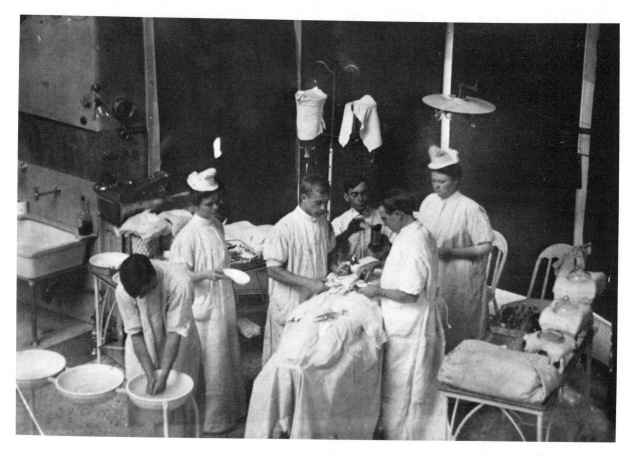

Figure 2.1. During the early years of surgery, nurses came from patient care units to perform technical tasks needed by surgeons. They donned coverups to protect uniforms and wore nursing caps. Surgery was performed without gloves, and hands were cleansed by washing in an antiseptic solution. Anesthesia consisted of open-drop ether or chloroform administered through a gauze-covered, cone-shaped mask. Windows in every operating room provided natural daylight for surgical visibility and could be opened on warm days for air circulation. Upon completion of the operation, the same nurses accompanied the patient back to the surgical ward, providing care until discharge. One junior nurse or nursing student was left behind to clean the room and equipment. There might be one highly skilled nurse permanently assigned to the operating room to supervise tasks performed by transient nurses and to prepare sponges, linen, instruments, pans, and sutures needed in the future. Photograph c. 1890–1900, courtesy of Porter Memorial Hospital Audiovisual Department, Denver.

vances. Although surgeons had an adequate knowledge of surgical anatomy and physiology, surgical mortality was high. "Pain, hemorrhage, infection, and gangrene were rife in the hospital wards, and mortality from surgical instruments was as high as ninety and even one hundred percent" (2:16–17). Concepts of antisepsis were vague, and many surgeons thought infections in surgical wounds should be encouraged. Surgeons were also careless, frequently operating in their street clothes, using

the same instruments on patient after patient, and only washing their hands *after* surgery. In fairness to the surgeons and hospitals of this era, their cities and towns were also unsanitary and dirty, and personal hygiene was poor. Accident victims frequently arrived at hospitals for surgery with an infection already started.

As a result, surgery was usually performed as a last resort. Most operations were limited to "the removal of superficial tumors of various sorts, drainage of infection, traumatic surgery, removal of stone in the bladder, and operations about the head and face . . . operations upon the contents of the peritoneal and pleural cavity were practically unknown" (3:79).

Antiseptic techniques and anesthesia changed the course of surgery and the role of the operating room nurse. Antisepsis and, later, asepsis dramatically reduced surgical mortality from infection. And if antisepsis made surgery safe, anesthesia not only made it painless, but also made it possible for the surgeon to perform longer procedures. Gradually, surgery became a means to improve and prolong life instead of a last resort. Most important for operating room nurses, "Lister's revolutionary discovery of the value of antisepsis in surgery . . . made it absolutely necessary that nurses should be of such an intellectual calibre and development as would permit them to be trained in the prevention of infection through absolute cleanliness" (4:125).

As surgery became more complex and demanding, nurses acquired new and broader responsibilities. For example, the Scottish physician Joseph Bell (c. 1888) required nurses to prepare patients, instruments, table sponges, dressings, and the patient's bed. He suggested that nurses prepare checklists of the instruments they used. Because nurses in the operating room had new responsibilities, Bell said they needed "very special training . . . for certain important surgical cases and operations. You must try to get this from the senior staff nurses, from the residents, and even a few most precious hints from the acting surgeon" (5).

Early Training Programs and Nursing Education

General training programs for nurses were first established in hospitals, using the model developed by Florence Nightingale in England. In 1873, three Nightingale schools were opened in the United States: Bellevue in New York City, the Connecticut Training School in New Haven, and the Massachusetts General Hospital Training School in Boston. These schools were among the first to change the existing American concept of nursing as a subservient and menial profession. They were established to improve the care of the sick and to educate nurses. These goals, plus Nightingale's belief that nursing schools should be controlled and run by qualified nursing staff, ruffled many physicians' feathers. Others criticized the Nightingale programs for overtraining nurses.

Today, when we look back on nurses training programs of the late 1800s and early 1900s, these concerns seem unnecessary. The early Nightingale programs were usually only a year long, with student nurses committed to another year's employment with the hospital upon completion of the program. Curriculum was dictated by services offered by the hospital. There were no real classes, few formal lectures, and faculty did not follow standards or use curriculum guides. Instruction was usually carried out at the patient's bedside, where daily nursing functions were conducted at the same time. There was a variety of instructors—physicians, staff nurses, and other nursing students. Student nurses also took on housekeeping and cooking chores at their hospital, and during their first year of training, student nurses were generally paid—sometimes $4 to $10 a month (6)!

Operating room nursing education began at Massachusetts General Hospital in 1876 when student nurses were first allowed in the operating room for clinical instruction (6). By the 1880s, many hospitals were integrating specialty instruction, such as operating room nursing, into their nurses' training. By the early 1900s, student nurses were regularly placed in operating rooms for daily clinical experience, and it would be safe to say that nurses' training programs generally identified specific content for preparing OR nurses. For example, the National League of Nursing Education incorporated a section on operating room technique into its standard curriculum in 1919. The content included the nurse's duties in relation to equipment, the sterilizing room, the instrument and supply room, preparation of dressings and supplies, and duties during surgery (6).

Clinical experience in the operating room could vary widely. For example, a student nurse could be required to prepare surgical patients and operating rooms.

She sterilized supplies and made sterile salt solutions . . . The gas pipe railing around the rising rows of wooden seats in the amphitheatre had to be wiped with carbolic and the seats were damp dusted with bichloride of mercury. She had already soaked towels and bandages in bichloride the night before and hung them to dry. She had to consider the needs of the anesthetist and be prepared to handle instruments or sponges. Natural sea sponges were prepared for use in the operation after sand and shell were beaten from them. Boric acid crystals were used in the abdominal cavity, packing was iodized gauze. The pupil nurse would spend the whole day in the operating room, which was air-tight as could be and her dinner was brought in on a tray (6:80).

Students were also required to know the properties and uses of anesthetics, to hold the patient's jaw and sponge out mucus during anesthetization, and to administer artificial respiration if necessary.

Emergence of OR Nursing as a Specialty

The actual specialty of operating room nursing emerged in 1888 at Johns Hopkins Hospital in Baltimore, partly the result of an attempt to pacify two feuding nurses. A graduate of Bellevue Hospital School of Nursing, Isabel Hampton came to Johns Hopkins in 1889 as its director of nursing. She was also charged with organizing a school of nursing for the hospital. Caroline Hampton (no relation to Isabel) arrived in 1889 as head nurse of the hospital's surgical division. There is disagreement about what happened next.

One report says that "an intense animosity" existed between the two nurses because Caroline, a Southerner, disliked taking orders from Isabel, a Canadian. Hopkins' chief of surgery, William S. Halsted, appointed Caroline operating room supervisor to relieve some of the tension that existed between the two women (7:276). A second version has Isabel appointing Caroline head nurse of the surgical wards in an attempt to relieve an apparent shortage of nurses. However, there are those who believe

the appointment was made "to limit Caroline Hampton's activities to the operating room" (8:60).

In 1894, Hunter Robb, an associate in gynecology at Johns Hopkins, suggested that a team be used in the hospital's operating rooms. His recommendation that a surgeon, the head nurse, a second nurse, and five assistant surgeons be present at every surgery was quickly adopted. The head nurse became the scrub nurse; the second nurse performed "all duties which involve the handling of any articles which have not been rendered aseptic" and watched for "any opportunity to be of service to the surgeon and his assistants" (9:160–161). By the turn of the century, the operating room team concept was being used in hospitals throughout the United States, and nurses became permanent and necessary members of every surgical team.

The specialty of operating room nursing had evolved: operating room technique had become a recognized part of nursing education curricula, and operating room nurses had become integral members of the operating room team. All this was accomplished during the last 50 years of the nineteenth century. The twentieth century would see operating room nursing's growth and refinement.

It took two world wars to project nursing in general into a position of national interest and importance. Operating room nursing naturally benefited from this national attention. By the end of the Spanish-American War in 1900, Dr. Anita Newcomb McGee saw a critical need to organize and improve health care delivery in the armed forces. Hospital corpsmen had been trained to care for the sick and wounded, but in wartime, there were too few corpsmen and too little time to train them. McGee proposed that fully accredited graduate nurses be enlisted for military nursing service. Within 10 years, the fledgling Army Nurse Corps had 233 regular nurses and 170 reserve nurses (7:344).

During World War I, nurses' roles were primarily limited to caring for the sick and wounded recuperating at base and auxiliary hospitals. About 10,000 nurses served overseas. Because most nurses were women, none were stationed at field hospitals, which were on or near the front. Goodnow writes, "Most wounds were from shrapnel, a few were from bombs, still fewer from bullets. Wounds of the head and face were common and terrible" (10:99–100). Most surgeons took a somewhat conservative approach to surgery because of the serious threat of infection. Wounds were generally stabilized, and the patient sent to a base hospital for further treatment. Most patients arrived at the base hospital with an infection raging—not because of poor surgical or medical treatment but because of the poor hygienic atmosphere in the trenches. Goodnow adds, however, that "dental and plastic surgery was perfected; the Carrel-Dakin treatment for infected wounds was developed. All these new methods needed expert nurses" (10:99–100).

The global nature of World War II created new roles and responsibilities for women and for nurses in particular. Nurses in the armed forces as well as those serving in volunteer agencies such as the Red Cross found themselves working at the battlefront, in prisoner-of-war camps, and in the midst of air, land, and sea attacks. In the face of personnel shortages, both military and civilian nurses were required to take on new administrative roles and expand their nursing functions in many areas. The operating room team, including the operating room nurse, performed in a variety of environments and conditions. With the development of sulfa and penicillin and the subsequent reduction in postoperative infection, wartime surgery became more aggressive. Larger, more specialized teams were required to handle heavier surgical loads, and operating room nurses were required to perform a wider range of duties. In fact, an operating room nurse's responsibilities frequently included anesthesia, asepsis, and sanitation; preparation of the surgical patient, instruments, and the operating area; supervision of other OR personnel; and under special circumstances, surgical assistance.

Nurses returning from military service wanted to retain many of these new responsibilities in civilian hospitals and operating rooms. By the late 1940s, operating room nurses managed the care of patients in the operating room

and assisted surgeons. Many OR nurses also believed it was time to organize the members of their specialty to pool professional knowledge and exchange new ideas. In January 1949, 17 operating room supervisors in the New York City area met to discuss forming an independent association of operating room nurses. A month later, officers and a board of directors were elected from a group of 56 staff and administrative operating room nurses. These nurses appointed a committee to work with the American Nurses' Association (ANA) and the National League for Nursing (NLN) in forming an independent organization solely for operating room nurses.

Formation of AORN

The first national conference of the Association of Operating Room Nurses (AORN) was held in 1954. At this meeting, ANA and NLN officers joined AORN members to look at the question posed by the association: "Where do we belong?" (among nursing organizations). Although the panel discussion was inconclusive, the program led to an agreement to explore the issue further. By 1956, AORN's officers and board of directors felt the association was ready for "a special affiliation with ANA permitting it to hold an annual national meeting and develop the specialty of nursing in the operating room" (11:146). ANA disagreed and countered the board's proposal, stating that its programs already met OR nurses' needs. Nevertheless, the association's board of directors presented the plan to the House of Delegates at the association's fourth annual meeting in 1956. The plan was enthusiastically accepted, a constitution and bylaws adopted, and officers and a board of directors elected. Edith Dee Hall, a driving force behind the advancement of operating room nursing who strongly promoted the idea of an independent OR nursing organization, was appointed executive secretary. Her New York City apartment became the association's first national headquarters.

By 1960, organized groups or chapters of operating room nurses existed throughout the

United States. The primary purpose of the newly formed association was to exchange ideas, gain new knowledge, and explore methods of improving nursing care of patients undergoing surgery. At first, the association's goals were (11:142):

1. To stimulate operating room nurses in other parts of the country to form similar groups
2. To be a specific group to pool and share nursing knowledge and technology
3. To provide the surgical patient with optimum care through a broad educational program
4. To make a body of knowledge available to operating room nurses
5. To motivate experienced operating room nurses to share their expertise with others
6. To be an association for the benefit of all professional operating room nurses

AORN faced one of its first great challenges in the early 1960s. The nature of nursing education was changing, with increasing emphasis placed on the college- or baccalaureate-prepared nurse. The focus of nursing education was shifting from hospital-based programs, which offered student nurses maximum experience in the operating room, to four-year college programs that stressed a broader psychosocial approach to patient care. In these programs, operating room nursing was sometimes overlooked as less patient-oriented and more technical in practice. Concerned for the future of professional nurses, the association adopted the statement, "Definition and objectives for clinical practice of professional operating room nursing," in 1969. It was AORN's first attempt at defining nursing care in the operating room.

AORN was concerned with the nature of operating room practice, the means for improving that practice, standards for practice, and the appropriate education for operating room nurses. The 1969 statement provided guidelines for nursing educators and administrators who wanted to incorporate concepts of OR nursing into their curriculum or daily patient care. Operating room staff nurses could use the statement in developing a professional role that included providing nursing care to their patients before, during, and after surgery.

Further clarification of the operating room nurse's role was required in the 1970s. Nurses in other specialties based their practice around the nursing process: they assessed their patient's physical and emotional needs and then planned, implemented, and evaluated the care they performed in terms of these needs. Nurses argued that the nursing process could not be applied in the operating room. They also said that nursing in general had outgrown the "handmaiden" image that OR nurses seemed to retain. Still other health professionals suggested that nursing care was no longer necessary in the operating room since nonnursing personnel, such as operating room technicians, had been trained to perform scrub and other duties previously performed by nurses.

These challenges prompted delegates at the association's 1973 Congress to approve the statement, "The necessity for the registered nurse in the operating room." The statement showed that professionals with a nurse's training and background were necessary for the optimum care of surgical patients. Unlike OR nurses, personnel trained to only carry out certain technical duties could not adequately care for the patient physically and emotionally. The statement also maintained that operating room nurses used the nursing process in their care of surgical patients; they assessed the needs of patients coming to surgery; planned and implemented preoperative, intraoperative, and postoperative care to meet these needs; and then documented their care. This statement would lay some of the groundwork for the group of operating room nurses who were working to create the concept of perioperative nursing.

Many AORN members believed that more was needed to keep their specialty vital. By the end of 1975, *Standards of Nursing Practice: OR* (12) was published jointly by the association and ANA. The association encouraged nurses to either use the standards in their daily practice or incorporate them into the existing operating room procedure at their hospitals. *Standards*

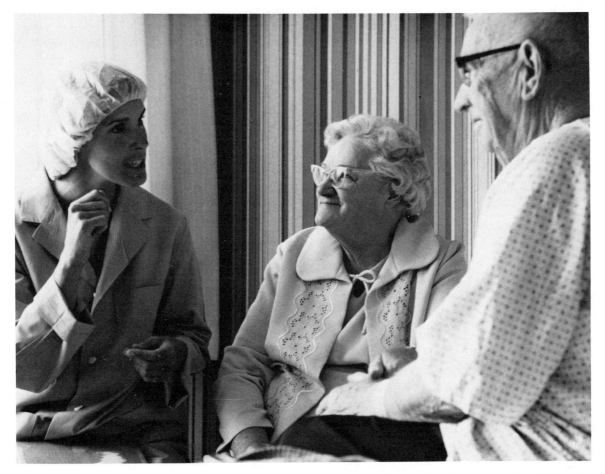

Figure 2.2. Perioperative nurses assess a surgical patient's health status and identify special needs pertinent to the patient's safety and comfort.

of Nursing Practice also became a basis for the concept of a perioperative role for nurses. Project 25, a special committee of operating room nurses, was formed at the 1977 Congress to examine the functions and roles of operating room nurses in the 1970s and to provide a definition and outline of this role.

Delegates at the association's silver anniversary Congress in New Orleans read and approved the Project 25 Task Force's final report. The group defined operating room nursing as (13:1165):

Statement of the perioperative role. The perioperative role of the operating room nurse consists of nursing activities performed by the professional operating room nurse during the preoperative, intraoperative, and postoperative phases of the patient's surgical experience. Operating room nurses assume the perioperative role at a beginning level dependent on their expertise and competency to practice. As they gain knowledge and skills, they progress on a continuum to an advanced level of practice.[13]

Each level of the perioperative continuum was defined by the nursing process, operating room standards, and special goals and objectives for OR nurses.

By the late 1970s and early 1980s, operating room nurses were individually attempting to expand the scope of their nursing practice using the perioperative role as their model.

Nurses in some hospitals were establishing preoperative teaching programs and postoperative follow-up plans for their patients. Others were participating in hospital-wide patient education offerings. Still other operating room nurses had developed and documented patient care procedures, protocols, and standards for their operating rooms. At the core of all these activities was an attempt to integrate the association's proposed perioperative role for operating room nursing into daily practice (see Fig. 2.2).

References

1. Luckes, Eva C. E. *Lectures on General Nursing*. London: Kegan Paul and Co., 1887.
2. MacEachern, Malcolm T. *Hospital Organization and Management*. Chicago: Physician's Record Co., 1935.
3. Finney, J. M. T. *A Surgeon's Life: The Autobiography of J. M. T. Finney*. New York: G. P. Putnam's Sons, 1940.
4. Walsh, James J. *History of Nursing*. New York: P. J. Kennedy, 1929.
5. Bell, Joseph. *Notes on Surgery for Nurses*. Edinburgh: Simpkin Marshall, 1888.
6. Metzger, Ruth S. "The beginnings of OR nursing education." *AORN J* 24(July):73–90, 1976.
7. Robinson, Victor. *White Caps: The Story of Nursing*. Philadelphia: J. B. Lippincott, 1946.
8. Johns, E., and Pfefferkorn, B. *The Johns Hopkins School of Nursing*. Baltimore: The Johns Hopkins Press, 1954.
9. Robb, H. *Aseptic Surgical Technique*. Philadelphia: J. B. Lippincott, 1894.
10. Goodnow, M. *Nursing History in Brief*. Philadelphia: W. B. Saunders, 1950.
11. Driscoll, J. "1949–1957: AORN in retrospect." *AORN J* 24(July):140–148, 1976.
12. *Standards of Nursing Practice: OR*. Kansas City: Association of Operating Room Nurses and American Nurses' Association, 1975.
13. Association of Operating Room Nurses. "Operating Room Nursing: Perioperative Role." *AORN J* 27(May):1165, 1978.

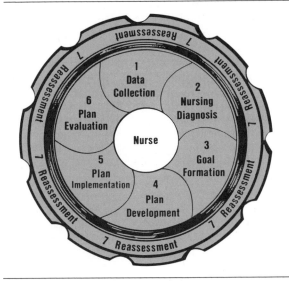

Refinement of nurse's role leads to new dimensions.

Perioperative Nursing Practice: A Dynamic New Focus

"You pursue the only nursing function that still carries a descriptor of geography." When she spoke at the 1977 AORN Congress, nursing leader Ingeborg Mauksch challenged nurses who worked in the operating room to think about their role. She criticized the nurses for thinking of their specialty in terms of a geographical area of the hospital rather than in terms of the patient. "We don't say emergency room nursing any more, we say emergency care or emergency nursing care. When we speak of the intensive care unit nurse we now say intensive, acute, or critical care nursing."

Defining Perioperative Nursing Practice

Mauksch encouraged nurses in the operating room to do more than change the name of their specialty. "As I project to the year 2000, I would like to think of you as perioperative nurse clinicians," she said. It didn't take that long, however, for nurses who worked in the operating room to begin thinking of themselves as perioperative nurses. In 1978, AORN's Project 25 defined the perioperative role, and nurses began to use the term to define a role that encompassed nursing in the preoperative and postoperative periods as well as the intraoperative period. It was not really a new role, but rather a defining and focusing of what many nurses in the operating room were already doing. The term perioperative was suggested by Mauksch because "peri" means around or surrounding, and perioperative would refer to the time and activities in the period surrounding the patient's operation.

The perioperative role gave direction to the many nurses working in the operating room who wanted to extend their practice beyond intraoperative nursing. Traditionally, OR nurses rarely emerged from behind the closed doors of the surgical suite. Other nurses regarded them more as technicians than nurses, and even questioned whether what they did in the operating room was actually nursing. But in recent years, nurses from the surgical suite have expanded their practice to patient assessment before surgery and evaluation of the nursing care given in the operating room after the patient has returned to the unit. In addition to assessing the patient's physical and social needs, nurses from the operating room also instruct patients on complex procedures, such as open heart surgery. For example, a staff nurse and cardiovascular coordinator at a Wisconsin hospital attends the weekly cardiovascular conference with the surgeons, cardiologists, and pump technicians. After a discussion of the individual patients, she then goes to the unit and sees patients who will be coming to the operating room the next day. From these interviews, she can ascertain whether the case can be expected to go well or "may be a tough one." In a major Texas hospital, a nurse from the operating room visits eye surgery patients before surgery. Underlying a patient's cheerful talkativeness, she detects that the woman's grown children are concerned about the operation. While she is circulating during surgery the next day, she goes to the waiting room to keep the children informed. With the support of physicians, other nurses from the operating room have developed extensive patient teaching roles. A nurse in Phoenix who works for a gynecological surgeon interviews and counsels patients in the physician's office before surgery. Although some physicians have resisted the idea of preoperative assessments because they see them as interfering with "their" patient, others welcome this opportunity to have patients better informed. Patients who know what to expect in the operating room are usually more cooperative and less anxious. Recovery also is quicker.

Perioperative nursing is a specialty within medical/surgical nursing. The ANA Statement on the Scope of Medical/Surgical Nursing Practice defines medical/surgical nursing as "nursing care of adults with known or predicted physiological alteration, with trauma, or with disability."(1) Nursing is the care and treatment necessary to provide comfort to the patient, and to assist her in the promotion and maintenance of health, and the prevention, detection, and treatment of illness. Nursing promotes the patient's restoration to the best possible health.

Medical/surgical nursing is based on the four components of the nursing process—assessment, planning, implementation, and evaluation. It encompasses biological, psychological, and social components of the patient's response or adjustment to physiological alterations, trauma, or disability.

The perioperative role is defined as the nursing activities performed by the professional nurse during the preoperative, intraoperative, and postoperative phases of the patient's surgical experience. The three phases of surgery are simply periods of time when prescribed nursing actions take place. The preoperative phase begins with the patient's decision to have surgery and ends when she enters the operating room. The intraoperative phase begins when the patient is transferred to the operating bed and ends when she is admitted to the recovery room. The postoperative phase begins with admission to the recovery area and ends when the patient no longer needs nursing intervention related to her surgery.

Perioperative nursing takes place in different locations. Assessment may begin in the clinic or physician's office and continue after the patient is admitted to the unit and transported to the surgical suite. As the patient enters the operating room, proceeds to the recovery area, back to the unit, and finally to the physician's office, assessment continues.

The location changes, and the nurse making the assessment may also change (see Fig. 3.1).

In performing nursing activities in the perioperative role, the nurse uses knowledge and skills on a continuum. At the basic competency level, the nurse demonstrates application of general principles. For example, the nurse performing a preoperative assessment will do a patient interview, gathering data about previous surgeries. She establishes rapport with the patient, puts her at ease, and determines her usual nursing care needs. These might include relief of anxiety or maintenance of skin integrity. As the nurse progresses on the continuum to excellence she demonstrates a higher level of competency. For example, during the interview the nurse becomes aware that this patient has had previous bleeding problems and recognizes that a potential problem of excessive bleeding exists. The nurse does further investigation of patient, family, and previous records to determine probable cause and takes a course of action demonstrating her ability to apply knowledge and principles to patient care.

Another example of performance at a high level is the case of Mrs. Cross who was having a total hip prosthesis. The perioperative nurse noted she had allergy to glue used in a glove factory. The nurse was quick to realize the implications this might have on the impending procedure. She notified the surgeon and explained the allergy and related it to the methylmethacrylate used on total hip procedures. The surgeon promptly canceled the procedure and began to plan alternative methods of correcting the patient's problem.

The perioperative continuum moves from a basic competency to a level of excellence or mastery as the nurse performs nursing functions during the three phases of surgery (see Fig. 3.2). At the basic level of competency, the nurse applies general principles to specific situations. To perform at the mastery level, the nurse must thoroughly understand all the elements of a specific nursing function. Progression toward mastery is based on continuing acquisition of knowledge and skills.

As nurses from the operating room extend the scope of their practice, they are cooperating and collaborating with other nurses on the unit. No one nurse provides for the patient's care during the three phases of surgery. In interacting with the unit and postanesthesia recovery nurses, the perioperative nurse helps to provide continuity of care for the surgical patient. The perioperative nurse knows the patient and her condition before the patient comes to the operating room; or she communicates facts about the patient's care in the operating room to the unit and the postanesthesia recovery nurses. This communication provides continuity of care for the patient.

The perioperative nurse also interacts with other hospital personnel and services—therapists, social service workers, chaplains, etc. Many of the nurse's responsibilities are shared with other disciplines. For example, during the intraoperative care of the surgical patient, one of the nurse's functions is to maintain safety. This includes performing sponge, needle, and instrument counts, a responsibility shared by the surgeon and nurse. Positioning the patient is a task shared by surgeon, anesthesiologist, and nurse. Ensuring the sterility of instruments and equipment used during the procedure is a responsibility shared by central service personnel and the nurse. Recognizing that many responsibilities are shared with other members of the team is important, yet legal accountability may still rest with the nurse. It is important that a nurse constantly serve in an advocacy role protecting the patient and maintaining safety.

Relationship of Nursing Process to Standards of Perioperative Nursing Practice

In providing care for surgical patients, the nurse uses the nursing process and the *Standards of Perioperative Nursing Practice* (2) to provide a systematic, logical approach to nursing care. Schlotfeldt (3) defines nursing as focusing and assessing people's health status, assets, and deviations from health, and on helping patients regain their health, or the will to maintain their health. The nurse in the operating room uses the nursing process to accomplish this

Perioperative Role Diagram

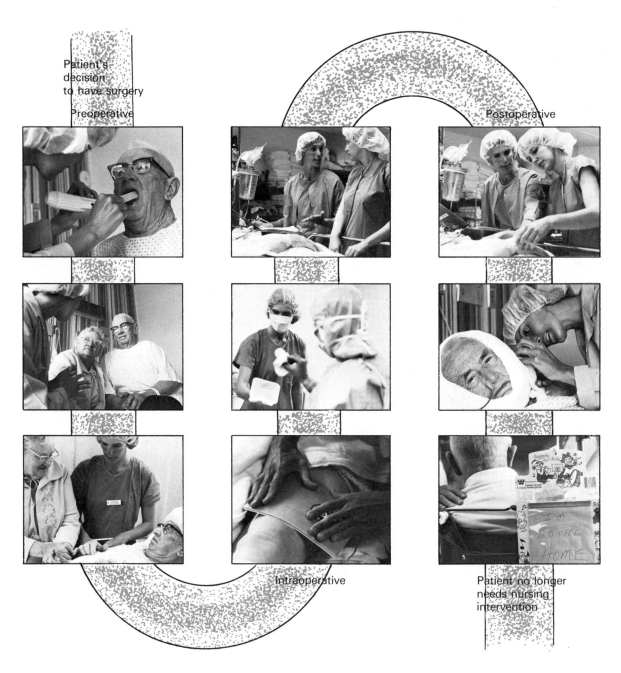

Figure 3.1. Perioperative role diagram showing the scope of the perioperative role, the geographical locations where nursing activities occur, and the three phases of the patient's surgical experience.

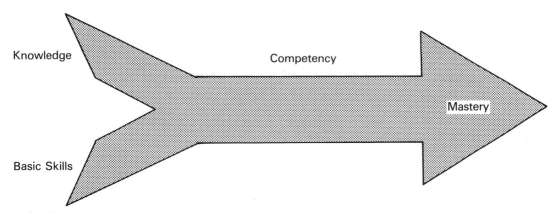

Figure 3.2. *The continuum from basic competency to excellence in performance of nursing functions.*

goal of assisting the sick to regain health or the will to maintain health.

NURSING PROCESS

The nursing process, which evolved during the 1950s, is a problem-solving approach based on the scientific method. The nurse gathers data to identify the problem, then analyzes the problem to determine a solution. An approach is then planned and implemented, with a follow-up evaluation. The nursing process is a planned, deliberate logical progression of activities that result in correction of an identified problem.

The nursing process involves four steps: assessment, planning, implementation, and evaluation. Assessment is a continuous activity the nurse does to identify the patient's existing needs and problems or potential problems. During assessment, for example, the nurse might interview the patient to find out if she has any allergies that could be a potential problem related to medications administered in the operating room or immediate postoperative period. When the nurse has determined a specific problem, she decides on a plan to manage the problem and implements it. If the patient has an allergy to penicillin or other antibiotic, the nurse communicates this to other health care personnel orally and through the nursing care plan and the patient record. The action is then evaluated to measure its effectiveness.

Using the process systematically allows the nurse to make a more thorough assessment and provides a way to plan more effective nursing strategies. The entire process encourages the nurse to focus on the patient, individualizing her care.

Although the four steps of the nursing process are performed in sequence, they are also done concurrently and recurrently. The nurse performs the steps sequentially because she must know what the patient problems are before establishing a plan. But at the same time, the steps may be concurrent. The nurse continually assesses the patient, identifying problems and developing plans to manage them. Several problems may be considered at the same time. A patient admitted for surgery of a fractured hip, for instance, usually has multiple health-related problems that nurses must address. She may be allergic to penicillin. Her immobility presents both potential and actual problems. The care plan includes nursing actions to manage the actual problems and prevent potential ones from occurring. The actions follow the plan concurrently or sequentially, depending on the patient's problems and the priorities established by the nurse.

But the nursing process is also recurrent. Actions taken to manage an identified problem may not have been effective, and a new approach may be selected. To do this, the nurse repeats the steps of the nursing process, starting with assessment of the problem.

STANDARDS OF PERIOPERATIVE NURSING PRACTICE

The *Standards of Perioperative Nursing Practice* are based on the nursing process. In the 1960s, nurses began to look at the need to establish standards that would guide the practice of nursing. Such standards would demonstrate nursing's concern for the quality of care and at the same time provide a method for judging the competency of that care. The first standards, developed by the American Nurses' Association, became the model for standards in specialty nursing. In conjunction with the ANA, the Association of Operating Room Nurses developed *Standards of Practice: OR* (4). When these were revised in 1982, they were published as *Standards of Perioperative Nursing Practice* (1).

A standard is an agreed upon level of practice established by an individual or group. In nursing, the standards are statements of what should be done. Broad in scope, these statements are consistent with the nursing process and expand on its four steps (see Table 3.1). These standards can be used by nurses as models for their practice. They can also be used as a guide for operating room nurses to develop a reliable method of evaluating the quality of nursing provided in any setting.

Perioperative nursing practice takes into account physiological, social, and behavioral problems that affect the patient's response to surgical intervention. The goal of practice is to implement nursing activities that provide continuity of care throughout the preoperative assessment, intraoperative care, and postoperative evaluation and follow-up. The standards direct nursing activities for each step of the process (see Fig. 3.3).

ASSESSMENT STANDARDS

The first step in the nursing process, assessment, includes the standards of collecting data and formulating a nursing diagnosis. The nurse assesses the patient to identify existing or potential problems. There are two steps in the assessment—the first is collecting data, and the second is identifying the patient's problem based on the data obtained or, as stated in the standards, formulating a nursing diagnosis.

In collecting data, the nurse obtains all the information she can pertinent to the patient having surgery. The nurse obtains information through patient interview, physical assessment, review of patient records and reports, and consultation with other members of the health care team. Pertinent information might include the current medical diagnosis, previous hospitalizations, and responses to those hospitalizations, as well as occupational, financial, educational, social, and spiritual data that relate to the patient's work role and habits. Physical and psychosocial status relative to the proposed surgery might also be relevant. These data are collected systematically on a continuous basis and are recorded on the patient record and patient care plan as a means of communicating with others involved in the patient's care.

In collecting and analyzing data, the nurse uses her knowledge and experience. She must be able to apply theory and previous practice experience to the new patient experience. The nurse observes what is happening to the patient and uses her communications skills to obtain information from the patient as well as to relay that information to other members of the health team. Once the information is gath-

Table 3.1. Relationship of Nursing Process to Standards of Nursing Practice.

Elements of Nursing Process	Standards of Nursing Practice
Assessment	Collection of data
	Formulation of nursing diagnosis
Planning	Establishment of goals
	Development of plan
Implementation	Implementation of plan
Evaluation	Evaluation of plan
	Reassessment

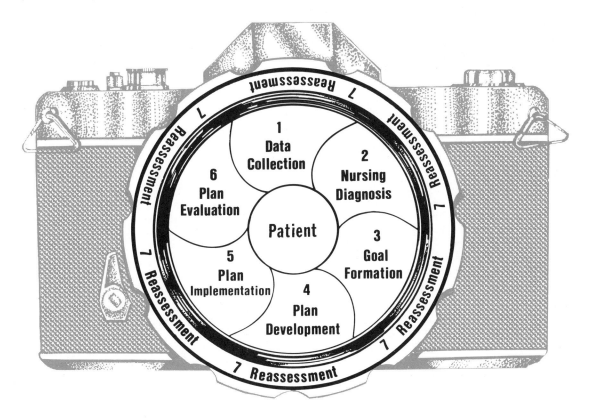

Figure 3.3. The standards direct the activities the nurse performs in a sequential manner.

ered, the nurse sorts, interprets, and analyzes the data and formulates a nursing diagnosis.

A nursing diagnosis, an explicit, concise statement of the patient's health status based on the nursing assessment, is the basis for nursing intervention. Based on established norms and the patient's previous condition, the nurse predicts the patient's problem. If a patient, for example, is thrashing about in bed, disoriented to time and place, and does not respond appropriately to the nurse's questions, the nurse might make the following diagnosis, "Patient confused" or "Patient disoriented." To make a nursing diagnosis, the nurse refers back to the data she has collected and reviews the information to determine if the patient's problems are consistent with the data. The intellectual process of combining, interpreting, and analyzing is essential in every patient situation.

PLANNING STANDARDS

In the second step of the nursing process, planning, the nurse puts into practice two standards —establishing goals and developing a care plan. Planning encompasses setting patient goals, judging priorities, and determining nursing strategies to resolve the patient's identified problem. To plan patient care the nurse needs the skills of effective communication, decision making, nursing judgment, and the ability to apply theoretical knowledge in the clinical setting.

After identifying the patient's problems and formulating a nursing diagnosis, the nurse establishes goals. A goal is the patient outcome or response toward which nursing action is directed. For a patient with a nursing diagnosis of intermittent confusion, one goal might be for the patient to state why she is in the hospital, what day it is, and explain what happened when she fell and fractured her hip.

Goals are stated in terms that can be measured by observing the patient's condition, by the patient's verbalization, demonstration, or psychological responses, or by interpretation of signs and symptoms by the nurse. A patient outcome is measurable in many ways. Patients verbalize and demonstrate behavior patterns or signs and symptoms. They state, explain or describe what they know, what they understand, and how they feel about their illness, treatment, or expectations.

A goal that cannot be measured is inappropriate and not consistent with a realistic approach to providing continuity of care. An example of an unrealistic goal is, "The patient will not experience the phantom limb phenomenon after an amputation."

The patient, as well as her family, significant others, and other members of the health care team, should cooperate in establishing realistic goals for the patient. A patient who is involved and cooperative will participate in achieving the goals. In establishing goals, the nurse must realize that goals must be congruent with the data and attainable. For an amputee patient, it would be unrealistic to expect her to be free of the phantom limb phenomenon. A more realistic goal is, "Patient will have minimal pain at the surgical site." For an elderly patient, the goal, "The patient will ambulate six hours postoperatively," might be unattainable.

As the nurse reviews the nursing diagnosis, she establishes priorities among the goals according to the needs of the patient and the sequence of events that the patient will experience related to surgery. Since patients having surgery generally have multiple problems, the operating room nurse must be realistic in determining which of these problems she can alleviate or for which she can provide supportive care. If material resources or personnel are not available, the nurse needs to consider this in establishing goals.

Goal statements should include a time frame that can be used to ascertain the extent to which the goal has been reached. If the goal is, "Patient will be free of pain at the incision site," a time of 48 to 72 hours might be appropriate. Time is based on two factors: (1) the norm and (2) other data relative to the patient. As an example, the norm will not be applicable to a patient who is a narcotic addict. Research and current nursing knowledge enable the nurse to determine appropriate time periods in which goals should be attained. Time periods for goals are influenced by the patient's condition, so they will need to be determined individually.

In establishing goals, the nurse considers the cost of service, time available, and the expected outcome. The nurse influences the course of action by identifying all possible alternatives that could meet the goal and then selecting those options that will best accomplish the goals for a particular patient.

The next step in the planning phase of the nursing process is to develop the plan—the fourth standard. The care plan is a guide for the nurse to achieve the established goals. In the care plan, the nurse lists nursing activities sequentially, which, if carried out according to plan, should result in attainment of the goals. The care plan should be written so that information is communicated to all members of the health care team. The priorities the nurse has established will be reflected in the sequence of actions. For example, in positioning a patient having pain on the operating table, the nurse determines a sequence of actions that will minimize the pain. For a supine position, nursing actions might be:

1. Place body in resting alignment.
2. Place pillow under head.
3. Apply knee straps in position of comfort.
4. Pad and secure arms and legs.
5. Extend arm on arm rest in a comfortable position.

The plan should be realistic, reflecting available personnel and material resources. The nurse assigned this activity should also have the knowledge and skills to carry it out. The patient is always the focus of the plan. In considering the patient's right to information, the nurse includes in the plan ways to assure that the patient is informed of what is happening.

The patient, family, and other members of the team should know what the plan contains. The nurse needs to discuss the care plan with the patient and family and involve them to the greatest possible extent in its development. The patient and her family need to know what is expected of them and how they can participate in the care. The plan is relayed to other personnel through the written patient care plan and the patient's record.

The care plan specifies what nursing actions are performed, how they are to be done, where they will be performed, and who is to do them. For a patient with a fractured hip, the care plan might reflect:

What? Transferred to operating room with minimal pain maintaining continuous traction.
How? In unit bed, with portable intravenous (IV) pole attached to bed. Note: (1) Secure Foley catheter drainage system. (2) Raise bed to highest position before unplugging from electrical outlet.
When? 30 minutes before surgery is scheduled to begin.
Where? From room to surgical suite holding area.
Who? Two transport personnel (one to push bed, one to pull and guide the bed and stabilize the weights if traction not secured prior to transfer).

As the nurse develops the plan, she uses the assessment data to ensure that the plan is consistent with the information obtained from the patient.

IMPLEMENTATION STANDARDS

The next step in the nursing process is implementation, which encompasses the fifth standard—putting the plan into action. As the nursing actions are performed, the plan becomes a reality. Will the activities planned result in the expected patient outcomes? In this step of the nursing process, the nurse relies on her intellectual, interpersonal, and technical skills to carry out nursing activities. Success of the nursing actions depends upon the nurse's decision-making, observation, and communication skills, and level of competency.

The two elements of implementation are nursing activities and their documentation. Each nursing action performed should be consistent with the written plan of care. For example, the nurse from the operating room has written a plan for transporting a patient with a fractured femur to the surgical suite, keeping the femur in alignment with minimal pain for the patient. If the plan is not communicated to the transport personnel or is not accessible for use, the planned nursing activities may not be followed. In this situation the transport personnel will make decisions about how the patient should be transported without the knowledge and data about the patient which the nurse who developed the plan had and used when determining nursing activities.

Another important factor related to implementing nursing actions according to the plan of care has to do with providing continuity. The preoperative preparation included assessing the patient and determining problems, either actual or potential. The plan was developed to provide consistency throughout the perioperative period. Therefore, it is essential that intraoperative and postoperative nursing actions be based on the identified problems and expected outcomes.

In performing the nursing actions that make up implementation, it is essential that nurses be proficient in technical as well as intellectual skills. In other words, the nurse must know how to do specific tasks that will ultimately result in the desired patient outcome. For example, during the surgical procedure the nurse continuously monitors the patient's position. Damage to the skin, nerves, and muscles may result if the nurse does not carefully monitor the devices and people that can cause harm to the patient during the operation. Demonstrating knowledge that provides safety for the patient is also a factor in carrying out nursing activities. Scientific principles guide the nurse in performing nursing actions.

The second element of implementation is recording the nursing actions performed. This will necessitate that the nurse monitor the patient's response to the nursing actions performed. Monitoring can be accomplished by observing the care as it is given or by obtaining feedback from the patient. The patient can tell the nurse how she is feeling, if the pain has subsided, or if she is warm and comfortable. Members of the family may also give input regarding the effectiveness of care. Documentation provides a method for measuring goal achievement. It serves as proof that the care was given. It also demonstrates the nurse's recognition of accountability. The nurse should be factual in documenting the patient's response and report only observations and signs that accurately reflect the patient's reaction.

EVALUATION STANDARDS

The final step in the nursing process is evaluation, encompassing the sixth standard—evaluation of the plan—and the seventh—reassessment. Evaluation is the appraisal of the quality and results of the care provided to the patient. The written care plan is used to evaluate the extent to which the specified goals were met and the consistency of care. Were the prescribed nursing actions implemented? To determine the extent of goal achievement, the nurse observes the patient's signs and symptoms or has the patient demonstrate goal achievement. For the patient with a fractured hip, the nurse evaluates by observation whether the patient's leg is in physiological alignment when she is admitted to the operating room. The nurse also asks the patient if she has any pain and observes body language to determine if the goal of minimal pain was met. The nurse then records that the patient arrived in surgery with her leg in alignment with continuous traction applied and that she stated she was not having pain at the time.

In evaluating care, the nurse reviews the goals and judges the degree to which they were attained. She must determine whether nursing care made a difference. To do this, the nurse reviews each outcome and evaluates whether the patient expresses, demonstrates, or shows signs and symptoms that indicate the goal was met. The nurse compares current data to the initial information from the assessment.

Each goal statement is measured by criteria. If the goal, for example, is, "Patient will be free from reaction to blood transfusions," the criteria to measure goal achievement are:

1. Patient free of rash on skin.
2. Patient demonstrates no evidence of sudden elevation of temperature.
3. Patient has no evidence of chills.

Because the patient, family, significant others, and health personnel are intrinsically involved in the care, the nurse should consult them regarding their perceptions of the results. How do they feel about their progress toward mutually established goals? What observations do they have? What are their suggestions for future considerations when dealing with patients having similar problems?

When the nurse has made a judgment about the extent of goal achievement, it should be communicated to others involved in the care. Nursing care that results in positive outcomes should be shared with others, as should care that results in deficiencies.

The last standard is reassessment. This is the review and revision of the entire nursing process. Reassessment requires that the operating room nurse gather information continually. New data is used to identify problems, revise or create new goals, and set forth a new or revised plan. The nurse asks if the goals are appropriate for the present situation. If not, new deadlines are set with a restructuring of priorities. The plan is modified, and nursing actions to meet the new goal are selected. The nurse should also examine why the original plan did not result in goal achievement.

A patient having surgery may go into a malignant hyperthermia crisis. When this occurs during the operation, the nurse must reassess the patient's condition. New goals are formulated and nursing actions are consistent with managing the patient's problem and decreasing the temperature to a safe margin.

To demonstrate that the nursing process is an organized progression of activities and at the same time fluid and constantly in motion, examine the following situation: Mr. Miller is admitted for a lumbar laminectomy. The nurse from the operating room conducts a preoperative assessment to plan for individualized care during his surgery. In assessing his psychological status, the nurse perceives that he is frightened about the possibility of being paralyzed from the surgery. The nurse determines a plan to assist Mr. Miller in working through this fear and immediately implements nursing strategies. As she does this, she is also collecting additional data as she continues the physical assessment. In this situation, the nurse is performing more than one activity simultaneously.

Implementation of the Nursing Process

The extent to which the nursing process can be implemented depends on the individual nurse and her level of expertise. How she defines nursing and her philosophy of nursing may influence implementation of the nursing process. Does the nurse see her role as a task-oriented, 7-to-3 job, or a patient-oriented professional role? How she sees her role may be determined to some extent by her educational background. Increasingly, nurses are encouraged to seek the minimum of the baccalaureate degree in nursing.

If the nurse believes her functions include autonomous independent nursing as well as carrying out the physician's orders, the nursing process will include activities that demonstrate that belief. The nurse's personal commitment to her professional role will determine the extent to which she implements the nursing process. As she continues to grow professionally, she will increase her knowledge base and become more proficient in the use of her intellectual skills.

The philosophy of the employing institution may also dictate the competency level and performance of the nurse. If the hospital is dedicated to a high level of patient-oriented care, it will encourage nurses in the operating room to carry out a perioperative role. The standards of performance and philosophy of the surgical suite also set expectations for the level of care.

An operating room suite with established standards of care that expects a high level of care will stimulate nurses to implement the nursing process. Nurses are aware of the institution's expectations and the level at which they must perform to maintain their position in the system.

If nurses are unable to make a preoperative assessment on the nursing unit prior to surgery, the nurse assigned to care in the operating room does not have sufficient information about the patient to plan care during surgery. The plan she devises may not be completely accurate or may have some data missing. For example, Mrs. Carson was having a total abdominal hysterectomy. She did not have a preoperative assessment by a perioperative nurse prior to admission to the surgical suite. When the nurse was admitting the patient she determined that the urologist was planning to insert ureteral catheters. She quickly made adjustments in her plan and set up for a cysto. When it was time to place the patient in lithotomy position the nurse discovered that the patient had a fused right hip. Consequently, she was unable to raise the right leg to place in leg holder. This information was not determined prior to the nurse positioning the patient.

Basic Competencies

What should be expected of the nurse in the operating room after she has been employed from six months to a year? The Statement of Basic Competency (5), developed by the Association of Operating Room Nurses, gives a broad indication of what level of competency can be anticipated at this time (see Figure 3.4). Staff nurses were asked what they were actually doing. In developing the statements, AORN asked OR supervisors at what level nurses who had been employed in the OR for one year were functioning. The 25 basic competency statements serve as a guide for supervisors in evaluating staff nurses and for inservice educators in planning orientation and educational programs for new staff members. These statements cover the basic activities of

I. Physiological and psychosocial statements. The OR nurse who has been employed in the OR for six months to one year:
  A. Assesses the health status of the patient experiencing surgical intervention by collecting pertinent health data through at least three of the following:
    1. Patient interview.
    2. Observation.
    3. Review of records.
    4. Consultation with other members of the health care team.
  B. Assesses the physical status of the patient experiencing surgical intervention by collecting pertinent health data about the patient in at least four of the following areas:
    1. Respiratory, circulatory, and renal status.
    2. Condition of skin and mucous membranes.
    3. Results of diagnostic studies.
    4. Allergies.
    5. Sensory perceptions.
    6. Nutritional status.
    7. Motor ability.
  C. Assesses the psychosocial status of the patient experiencing surgical intervention by being aware of at least three of the following:
    1. The patient's perception of surgery.
    2. The patient's expectations of care during hospitalization.
    3. The patient's fears and anxieties.
    4. The patient's level of understanding.
    5. The patient's philosophical, cultural, and religious beliefs.
  D. Develops a plan of nursing care that reflects use of at least three of the following:
    1. Current knowledge.
    2. Available resources.
    3. Patient rights.
    4. Communication with the individual, family, and health care personnel.
  E. Implements the psychosocial aspects of the nursing care plan for the patient experiencing surgical intervention through all of the following:
    1. Providing support.
    2. Using physical contact in communication when appropriate.
    3. Explaining events and giving information to patient, family, and other health care team members.
II. Skills statements. The OR nurse who has been employed in the OR for six months to one year:
  A. Demonstrates ability in assessing the physical status of patients by checking:
    1. Anticipated incision area.
    2. General condition of skin.
    3. General mobility of body parts.
    4. Vital signs.
    5. Absence or presence of motor or sensory impairments.
    6. Obvious signs of abnormalities, injuries, and previous surgeries.
    7. Presence or absence of prostheses.
    8. Impairments involving cardiovascular and respiratory systems.
  B. Usually demonstrates ability to identify and anticipate patient care needs.
  C. Maintains patient safety by applying principles of body alignment and adapting them to varying situations during positioning.
  D. Knows and applies principles of aseptic practice and recognizes the necessity for following established procedures and adapting them according to varying situations. Adaptation almost always is appropriate for the situation.
  E. Cooperates in team planning and execution of the plan to care for the operative patient effectively.
  F. Usually organizes nursing activities in an efficient manner.
  G. Almost always demonstrates tact and understanding when dealing with patients, team members, members of other disciplines, and the public.
  H. Usually conveys ideas, concepts, and facts related to patient care in a logical and concise manner.
  I. Almost always reports and records information relative to the operative patient.

Figure 3.4. Statement of Basic Competencies. Reprinted with permission of Association of Operating Room Nurses, Denver, Colorado.

III. Professional characteristics statements. The OR nurse who has been employed in the OR for six months to one year:
   A. Demonstrates integrity in aseptic practice and calls attention to and suggests measures to correct breaks in technique by all team members.
   B. Uses judgment in determining nursing actions that are in the best interest of the patient and makes decisions based upon scientific knowledge, nursing experience, and patient information.
   C. Almost always preserves patient privacy through:
      1. Maintenance of confidentiality in communications and documentation.
      2. Physical protection of patients during interviews, examinations, transportation, positioning, and draping.
   D. Usually exhibits professional behavior when interacting with other members of the health care team.
   E. Exhibits flexibility and adaptability to changes in nursing practice.
   F. Accepts constructive criticism and responds appropriately in relation to nursing practice by implementing corrective actions.
IV. Accountability statements. The OR nurse who has been employed in the OR for six months to one year:
   A. Maintains a safe environment by implementing technical and aseptic practices.
   B. Delivers care to surgical patients by:
      1. Checking patient identification.
      2. Proper handling of surgical specimens, completing incident reports, and documenting care.
   C. Respects patients' rights by:
      1. Providing privacy.
      2. Maintaining confidentiality of patient information.
      3. Ensuring the right to ethnic and spiritual beliefs and by recognizing each person's individuality.
   D. Usually collaborates with others to provide nursing care that requires additional skill.
   E. Usually seeks opportunities for continued learning.

Figure 3.4. (continued).

perioperative nursing and are a guide to basic practice in the operating room.

Clinical Ladders

Traditionally, advancement for nurses has meant leaving direct patient care and moving into supervision and management. Nurses who wanted to stay in direct patient care were faced with little reward or recognition for their accumulated years of experience or increased proficiency. The new nurse coming on the unit would be paid almost as much as the nurse with ten years of experience. Also there was no way to recognize different educational levels or specialized knowledge and skills.

As a solution to these problems, clinical ladders have been developed to recognize clinical nursing expertise through promotion and salary increases. Porter Memorial Hospital, Denver, patterned its levels after the model used at the University of California, San Francisco. Four levels of clinical expertise, labeled clinical level I, II, III, and IV, are recognized. Position descriptions for each level include:

1. Qualifications with educational requirements, experience, knowledge, personal attributes, and emotional health
2. Responsibility statements that outline the functions in broad terms
3. Specific functions written in behavioral terms that incorporate the four components of the nursing process, teaching, communication, evaluation, research, and professional growth activities

The clinical nurse I position is for the new employee without experience as a registered nurse. New graduates, nurses completing refresher courses, and nurses without experience in an acute care hospital are hired at this level. The new employee with previous experience enters at the clinical nurse II position. This is also the minimum standard all staff nurses must maintain on a yearly basis to meet employment requirements.

Clinical level III nurses have demonstrated competencies including teaching and management and have applied and been through a promotion review process. Clinical level IV nurses have met higher educational require-

Nursing Process: Assessment
1. Completes OR care plan with preoperative assessment or holding area visit.
2. Assesses patient condition via observation and review of patient record and records on preoperative assessment sheet.
3. Recognizes pathophysiology of assigned patients as evidenced in patient care plan.
4. Recognizes and reports abnormal diagnostic data.
5. Identifies the nursing diagnosis on assigned patients and documents on patient care plan.
6. Validates patient care plan for accuracy and completeness for assigned patients/those delegated.
7. Assesses quality of patient care/unit environment.
8. Assesses entire unit population to determine patient acuity.
9. Assesses complex problem areas as related to scheduled patients, unit environment, staffing, equipment.

Figure 3.5. Clinical level III competencies for assessment by perioperative nurse. Reprinted with permission of Porter Memorial Hospital Nursing Service, Denver.

ments and practice at a level that demands autonomy and leadership functions as well as clinical competency. Figure 3.5 shows how the perioperative nurse functions at the different levels in the first step of the nursing process, assessment.

Operating rooms that have initiated clinical ladders have found that rewarding nurses for competence in clinical practice has encouraged experienced practitioners to stay in direct patient care. This means that experienced practitioners are using their professional capabilities where it counts most—with patients. For the nurse, the incentive for providing direct patient care has increased job satisfaction.

References

1. American Nurses' Association Division on Medical Surgical Practice. *A Statement on the Scope of Medical-Surgical Nursing Practice.* Kansas City: American Nurses' Association, 1980.
2. *Standards of Perioperative Nursing Practice.* Kansas City: American Nurses' Association and Association of Operating Room Nurses, 1982.
3. Schlotfeldt, Rozella, M. "Planning for progress." *Nurs Outlook* 21:766–769, 1973.
4. *Standards of Practice: OR.* Kansas City: Association of Operating Room Nurses and American Nurses' Association, 1975.
5. Ad Hoc Committee on Basic Competencies. "Developing basic competencies for perioperative nursing." *AORN J* 35:871–884, 1982.

II

Assessing the Perioperative Patient

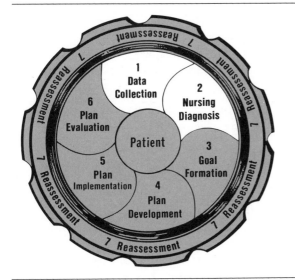

Assessment includes gathering data and formulating a nursing diagnosis.

Performing a Nursing Assessment

Assessment is the most crucial step in the nursing process because the other steps build on it. It has two components: collecting data and formulating a nursing diagnosis. Once the nurse has collected the patient data, he formulates a nursing diagnosis that identifies patient health problems that nurses treat.

To be valid, assessment must be continual. Just as the patient's vital signs change continually, so do other physiological and psychosocial factors. In the assessment process, the nurse must have the ability to use all his senses. He "must be able to *see* changes in the patient's appearance . . . to *smell* to detect odors . . . to *hear* to determine sounds . . . to *feel* to determine skin temperatures and textures as well as body contours" (1).

Just as the detective pursues every clue, no matter how seemingly insignificant, so must the nurse carry out a thorough "investigation," or assessment, of the total patient. Assessment enables the nurse to identify existing as well as potential problems and facilitates the formation of the care plan.

In an effort to save time, the nurse might try to categorize the patient according to his medical diagnosis. It is easy for a nurse to rely on previous experience in dealing with a certain disease and to formulate a care plan based on that experience. But by doing this, he circumvents the assessment process, replacing assessment with assumption. No matter what the medical diagnosis, the patient is foremost an individual who will respond to his illness in his own way. In the long run, the nurse who makes assumptions without first assessing the patient is using his time inefficiently and compromising the quality of care his patient deserves. The nurse's experience has value, but it can also "contaminate" the assessment phase by creating preconceived ideas about the patient. The nurse must continually remind himself that the patient's history is not what he wants to hear, but what he needs to hear.

Before the nurse can do an assessment, he must determine what information is necessary. He needs information regarding the physiological aspects of the patient including skin integrity, sensory perceptions, and the skeletal, cardiopulmonary, and gastrointestinal systems. He needs information about the psychological makeup of his patient, including coping mechanisms, level of anxiety, fear, self-image, mental capability, and the presence of any pathology. Finally, the nurse should assess his patient's sociocultural background, including family, level of education, religious affiliation, position in the family and community, and lifestyle.

The nurse must know where to find this information and devise methods of collecting the data. Sources will be the patient record or chart (including previous medical records), the patient, the family, and significant others (friends, clergy, and neighbors), and the health care team (physicians, nurses, therapists, and dieticians). The nurse's methods of data collection will include interviewing, physical examination or assessment, review of medical records, and observation. Once the nurse has completed a thorough collection of data, he sorts out the pertinent information and proceeds to the next phase of the nursing process, the nursing diagnosis.

Skills Required to Complete an Assessment

To make a good patient assessment, the nurse requires good communication, interviewing, and physical assessment skills.

COMMUNICATION SKILLS

Communication is essential to the development of an effective nurse-patient relationship. "Although the word 'communication' conjures up primarily an image of words, human communication includes much more than words. Gestures, facial expressions, and appearance are all part of communication. The quality and quantity of information the nurse is able to elicit from the patient is directly proportional to [the] ability to maintain open communication" (2). The nurse can readily control her verbal message, but he should be aware that his body language also imparts a message. The key to good communication is fusing the verbal message with the body's message.

When the nurse comes to the patient's room to make an assessment, he is a stranger to the patient. The patient will look at the nurse's nonverbal behavior to help him figure out why the nurse is there, and what he wants from him. If the nurse is controlling the situation, he can direct his nonverbal cues to elicit the desired response from the patient. He sets the mood and provides the opportunity to broaden the depth of the relationship. Imagine the nurse as a transmitter, and the patient as a receiver. The nurse's verbal and nonverbal behavior are the signals he transmits to the patient. For the patient to get the correct message, the nurse's body needs to send the same signal as his words. The nurse who says to the patient, "I'm here to spend time with you," but frequently glances at his watch is sending out a double message. Which signal will the patient respond to? The nonverbal message is often more honest than the verbal or written one (2). Although the nurse might want to spend time with the patient, he may subconsciously be thinking about other work that needs to be done. Through his nonverbal behavior, he has communicated that he does not really have the time to spend with the patient. In this situation, the patient responding to the nonverbal behavior might try to bring a quick end to the communication process by short responses. The astute nurse monitors the message he communicates by analyzing the patient's verbal and nonverbal feedback. Do the patient's words and nonverbal behavior reflect that he received the message that was intended?

The patient may also misinterpret the nurse's words. Some words are ambiguous or vague. Others may be technical terms unfamiliar to the patient. The nurse must be sure his message is clear and understood by the patient. Depending on the patient's level of understanding, explanations may take different degrees of time and patience. The nurse should keep in mind that, even with a complex subject, a simple but adequate explanation will allay patient fears.

INTERVIEWING SKILLS

Once the nurse has a basic understanding of communication, he needs to refine his interviewing skills. Interviewing requires an open attitude as well as basic curiosity—a desire to know more about a person. The interview provides the nurse with the opportunity to establish a relationship with the patient and assess his needs—physiological, psychological, and sociocultural. This provides the framework for the nursing diagnosis. The interview is perhaps one of the most difficult parts of the assessment, but it gets easier with practice.

Nursing students often assume that the interview is simply a series of questions designed to elicit specific information from the patient. In this case, the interviewer can become the focus of attention, with the patient following the cues rather than initiating them. Although it may seem easier to follow a list of questions, the patient could get the idea that the only information the nurse wants is that directly related to the questions being asked. He then might hesitate to give elaborate details, and the nurse would get an inaccurate picture of his patient's health history.

The nurse wants to encourage an open interview where the patient will spontaneously offer information. The nurse can do this by allowing the patient to give as thorough a history as possible with few interruptions. When faced with talking with a stranger, the novice interviewer may want to take control of the interview. It is easier for the nurse to ask direct questions and to keep conversation flowing, quickly filling in any gaps. By doing this, however, the spontaneity is lost, and the nurse may slant the direction of the interview. When taking a nursing history, it is the patient's story the nurse needs, not what the nurse wants or expects to hear (3).

Interviewing skills are learned by trial and error, but certain guidelines help to make the interview more successful. First, an atmosphere conducive to open communication must be maintained. In the hospital, the perioperative nurse needs to let the unit-charge nurse know of his intention to interview a certain patient and how long he plans to spend with him. The charge nurse may be able to prevent some interruptions. The room should be quiet with the door closed. The nurse should not hesitate to ask the patient to turn off the television or radio—not just the sound. If the patient does not have a private room, he should draw the curtain to create privacy and prevent distraction from the other patients or visitors.

The nurse can encourage open communication by developing empathy and the ability to communicate on a one-to-one basis with the patient. Simple nonverbal cues such as sitting close to the patient let him know that the nurse is giving him his full and undivided attention. A patient will quickly respond to a nurse's negative nonverbal signals. For example, if the nurse remains standing, it implies that he is busy and cannot spend much time. Arms crossed on the chest imply an unwillingness to open up. Taking notes or looking at a list is distracting and interferes with the patient's responses.

Above all, the nurse should listen. When we listen, we indicate our recognition of the value of the other person and his thoughts. The nurse also needs to be alert to what is unsaid—what thoughts or feelings are underneath. One way of letting the patient know that he has been heard is to summarize his words or repeat something he has said. For example, the patient might say, "When I had surgery for my hernia in 1975, I had a lot of pain afterward." To encourage the patient to elaborate on the pain, the nurse might say, "You say you had a lot of pain after your surgery . . ."

Patients will not always talk about what the nurse wants to hear. A patient may be angry. It is difficult to listen to a torrent of verbal abuse. The nurse must remind himself that the patient needs to vent his anger, and that he must not take it personally. Often the patient who directs his anger at the nurse is testing him to see just how much he is capable of handling. By listening to both the good and the bad, the nurse shows that he cares about every aspect of his patient and helps to establish a trusting relationship. The experienced listener will be able to read between the lines. By allowing the patient to vent his feelings, the nurse can help the patient focus on underlying problems. Thus the patient is able to recognize that problems exist and participate in solving them. For example, a patient scheduled to undergo exploratory surgery of the bowel for probable carcinoma is angry about the bowel prep he is undergoing, which includes numerous enemas, harsh laxatives, and antibiotics. The anger the patient directs at the nurse is intense and difficult to handle. The nurse should allow the patient time to blow off steam, and then help the patient to distinguish the cause of his anger. In this situation, the patient is able to identify the cause of his anger as fear related to his prognosis.

INTERVIEW TECHNIQUES

Most interviewers use the open-ended interview technique. There are certain techniques the nurse can use to gain greater insight into her patient including silence, facilitation, confrontation, question, direction, support, and reassurance. The first three are the least controlling. Silence and facilitation often go hand in hand (4).

Silence

In normal conversation, especially between strangers, silence often seems awkward and uncomfortable. In an interview situation silence allows the patient time to gather his thoughts and gives the interviewer time to reflect on what the patient has said. There are certain cues the nurse can follow to determine the need to break the silence. If the patient has come to a natural pause or if the nurse needs clarification of a previous statement or if the patient continues to go off on tangents, then the nurse can take advantage of silent moments to bring the patient back to the topic at hand.

Facilitation

When the nurse wants the patient to elaborate on something he has said, he can employ such actions as a nod of the head; verbal statements such as "Mmm-hmm," "I see," or "I understand." He can ask questions such as "Really?" or "Why is that?" A puzzled look or even a change in position communicate to the patient that the nurse is interested and is encouraging him to go on.

Confrontation

What can the nurse do when he reaches an impasse in the interview? The patient does not seem willing to discuss his feelings, yet his verbal and nonverbal communication indicate that his emotions are preventing further communication. The nurse needs to assess the patient's emotional state and confront the patient with his emotion. The nurse can pick up on the patient's anger, depression, or sadness and reflect the emotion back onto the patient. By saying, "You seem angry," or, "You look sad," the nurse will usually promote further conversation. Confrontation can have a detrimental effect, however, if the patient senses hostility, criticism or that he is being forced to continue a discussion of his thoughts upon which he is not yet ready to elaborate. Confrontations should be limited to only one topic during an interview.

Questions

Direct questioning can be useful when the answers are brief but yield good information. Care should be taken when asking questions that require yes or no answers. The patient tends to feel that it is not necessary for him to elaborate, and he will depend upon the interviewer for the content of information required.

Direction

The nurse can make the patient focus on something he has stated. By asking the patient to "tell me more about that," the nurse encourages the patient to elaborate. Asking a direct question, however, limits the amount of information to be gained.

Suggestion

Nurses should avoid making suggestions in the diagnostic interview because it is too easy to guide or redirect the patient's own thoughts and behavior. By suggesting to the patient, the nurse can unknowingly encourage the patient to adopt some of the nurse's thoughts and attitudes. For example, by saying to a patient scheduled to undergo a cystoscopy, "You have probably been experiencing burning upon urination," the nurse could suggest to the patient that this is what he should be experiencing and may cause him to imagine that he has, thus biasing the report.

Support and Reassurance

For an individual to be willing to relate intimate details regarding his personal life, he has to feel that he can trust the person in whom he is confiding. Trust can be brought about through support and reassurance. A patient will naturally respond more readily and willingly to an individual who demonstrates honesty, warmth, and interest and who creates a secure environment. Touching may provide support or restore a patient's confidence and sense of well-being by providing reassurance.

The nurse must be careful to avoid becoming overly sympathetic and reassuring. By promising the patient something that the nurse cannot control or deliver, he can break down the sense of trust and confidence he has worked to develop. Statements such as, "Everything will be all right," or, "There's nothing to worry about," when there very well may be reason for the patient to worry or be fearful, will only lead to breakdown of the relationship when the patient learns that the nurse was wrong.

Collecting Data

SOURCES

Physical Assessment

A physical examination is the classic technique used to obtain data relating to the patient's physical condition. This is done by inspection, palpation, percussion, and auscultation.

- Inspection: The nurse uses his eyes to observe the patient. The nurse becomes skillful at inspection when he knows what to look *at* rather than what to look *for*. For example, the nurse needs to correlate his visual perception with previous knowledge to create an observation. His observation becomes a recordable image.
- Palpation: The nurse uses his hands and fingertips to distinguish temperature variations, between hard and soft, rough and smooth, and stillness and vibration. The fingertips are the most sensitive to touch. The palmar and ulnar regions of the hands are the most sensitive to vibration. In detection of temperature variations, the dorsal and ulnar parts of the hands are the most sensitive. Light palpation is best because sensitivity can be dulled by pressure.
- Percussion: This technique is used to detect tenderness or pain in the underlying surfaces that could indicate pathology such as infection. The nurse lays an outstretched middle finger over the area to be percussed and taps the distal part using the tip of the middle finger of the opposite hand.
- Auscultation: The nurse employs a stethoscope to listen to the quality and quantity of the patient's respiratory, heart, and bowel sounds.

There are two approaches to physical assessment of the patient, the cephalo-caudal (head-to-toe) approach and the major systems approach (cardiovascular, respiratory, digestive). The nurse needs to experiment with both to decide with which one he feels most comfortable.

Medical Data

The history and physical provide information regarding the patient's chief complaint, present illness, medical history, psychosocial background, family history, a review of the systems, physical findings, initial laboratory data, medical diagnoses, diagnostic plans, and therapeutic plan.

The format used in the medical record can be broken down into two major types, the conventional format and the problem-oriented record (POR). The conventional medical record lists information chronologically with little separation of data dealing with one or more illnesses. The progress notes are usually just a documentation of events and observations as they occur. After reading through the progress notes, one is often confused about the progression of the patient's illness or recovery. In the conventional record, emphasis is placed upon a specific diagnosis rather than a synthesis of problems that can relate to more than one diagnosis. Historical findings are separated from the current physical and laboratory findings, and it is sometimes difficult to understand how diagnoses are formulated.

The POR, on the other hand, starts off with a master problem list that includes all the significant difficulties the patient is experiencing. All pertinent data can be assigned to one or more of the problems. The major advantage of the POR is that related data can be listed as a problem until enough information is available to make a specific diagnosis. In other words, it is unnecessary to come up with a list of all the possible diagnoses that could be related to the data. The POR starts off with a data base— patient profile, physical examination, general health history, laboratory data, psychosocial makeup—and proceeds to the problem list which provides immediate information regarding the patient's need for care. The plan, or management of the patient's problems, is included as part of the progress notes. By using the SOAP (subjective, objective, assessment, plan) format when charting, the POR enables any member of the health care team—physician, nurse, health care therapist—to communicate information regarding each specific problem in a concise, organized manner.

The nurse needs to check his institution's protocol regarding who may write on the doctor's order sheet. Usually the sheet is divided lengthwise, with room for orders on one side and progress notes on the other side. The physician as well as health care professionals who have received prior approval by the medical affairs department can write orders on the doctor's order sheet. A registered nurse may write an order he has taken orally from a physician or approved health care professional provided he signs his name and notes the fact that it was an oral order taken from an appropriate individual.

Occasionally a physician will request the expertise of a specialist by writing an order for a consultation. The consulting physician will then fill out a special form rather than record his findings on the progress notes. The rationale behind this is ready access to his report rather than having to shuffle through pages of progress notes. The nurse will see consultation reports made by cardiologists, dermatologists, radiation oncologists, surgeons, internists, and psychiatrists.

Diagnostic Reports

The standard patient will require a complete blood count, urinalysis, chest x-ray, and electrocardiogram. Numerous diagnostic studies may be ordered by the physician to enable him to make a differential diagnosis. Each hospital usually has a manual describing every type of diagnostic procedure done within the institution, and it is the responsibility of the nurse to be familiar with these procedures and the protocol surrounding them (see Fig. 4.1). Some examples of the types of diagnostic reports the nurse will find are given in Table 4.1. Some common laboratory tests are:

- Serology: Studies of the blood to determine malfunctions in heart disease, thyroid, and the presence of syphilis.
- Toxicology: Studies of the blood or urine to screen for presence of drugs, especially barbiturates and anticonvulsant medications.
- Microbiology: Cultures of wound, sputum, urine, vaginal and urethral areas, nasopharynx, throat, eye, ear, stool, etc.

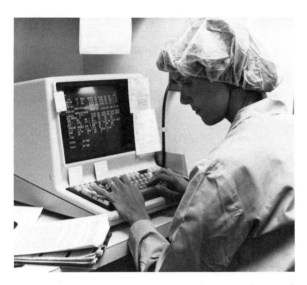

Figure 4.1. Computers assist personnel by storage and retrieval of laboratory analysis and other diagnostic data. Computerized systems for nursing and medical history and clinical problem information have been developed, but are still prohibitive in cost for most hospitals.

- CXR (chest x-ray): Used extensively as a screening test and diagnostic measure, the CXR helps to rule out carcinoma, tuberculosis, and heart disease. It indicates disorders of the soft tissue and bones of the chest wall, tracheobronchial abnormalities, pleural thickening, and fluid in the pleural spaces, as well as any abnormal diaphragmatic contours.
- ECG (electrocardiogram): A graphic record of the electrical activity of the heart muscle, the ECG is usually interpreted for diagnostic purposes by a cardiologist or internist. Ischemia, injury, or infarction of the myocardium as well as other conditions that may or may not be pathological will alter the size, shape, or configuration of the components ot the cardiac complex. A normal ECG does not rule out pathology of the heart because it does not show the actual physical state of the heart or its ability as a pump.
- Diagnostic procedures for the gastrointestinal (GI) system: An upper GI (barium meal) radiograph is taken of the esophagus, stomach, and small intestine after ingestion of a ra-

diopaque substance. The purpose is to detect structural and functional abnormalities in the esophagus and to outline the walls of the stomach to show the presence of ulcer craters and filling defects that could be caused by tumor. The rate of passage of the barium through the small intestine is noted as well as any existing structural defects. Endoscopy of the upper gastrointestinal system involves the esophagus, stomach, duodenum. These areas can be directly seen through a lighted scope. An internist or surgeon may perform the procedure. Endoscopy of the lower gastrointestinal system visualizes the rectum, sigmoid colon, and sometimes the left transverse and right colon. These procedures are referred to as proctoscopy and sigmoidoscopy and are also performed by a surgeon or internist inserting a lighted scope into the rectum.

The nurse will encounter numerous other diagnostic tests and procedures. She will see CT (computerized tomography) scans, which provide the radiologist with a three-dimensional view as opposed to the two-dimensional view of the conventional x-ray. Whereas CT scans were previously used mainly to diagnose neurological disorders, they are now being used more and more frequently for a variety of other purposes, including detection of tumors anywhere in the body, vascular abnormalities such as aneurysm of the aorta, and spinal abnormalities. The nurse will encounter a variety of radiographs when it is necessary to determine the presence of fractures or pathological conditions of the bone (e.g., osteoporosis). Bone scans, brain scans, electroencephalograms (EEGs), electromyograms (EMGs), and ultrasonography are examples of the many types of diagnostic procedures that the nurse will need to understand. He must be familiar with the standard diagnostic procedures. For tests done infrequently, the nurse should research them when they are ordered.

Nursing Data
The data base is the tool the nurse uses after the initial nursing history assessment to record the routine information regarding the pa-

Table 4.1. Diagnostic Laboratory Values.

	Low Range	High Range	Examples of Possible Diagnostic Findings
CBC (complete blood count)			
WBC (white blood count)	2,000	20,000	low: marrow suppression
Hgb (hemoglobin)	7		low: critical anemia
Hct (hematocrit)	20		low: blood loss
Platelets (/cu mm)	50,000		low: potential bleeder
Polys (%)	20	90	low: neutropenia
Bands		20	high: sepsis
Monos		15	
Eos		20	allergy or parasites
Lymphs		70	mono
Reticulocytes (%)	0.05	10	high: rapid RBC turnover
UA (urinalysis)			
Protein		4+	renal disease
Glucose		3+	diabetes
WBC			
Male		10/hpf	genitourinary disease
Female		30/hpf	
RBC			
Male		10/hpf	renal disease
Female		10/hpf	
SMAC (sequential multiple analyzer computer)			
Glucose (mg/dl)	65	115	diabetes
BUN (mg/dl)	6	23	possible renal failure
Creatinine (mg/dl)	0.4	1.4	
Sodium (mEq/liter)	135	147	hypernatremia—cardiac arrhythmia (potential)
Potassium (mEq/liter)	3.5	5.0	hyper/hypokalemia—cardiac arrhythmia (potential)
Chloride (mEq/liter)	95	108	
CO_2 (mEq/liter)	24	32	
Uric Acid (mg/dl)	2.5	8.0	
Calcium (mg/dl)	8.6	10.6	tetany (low)
Phosphorus (mg/dl)	2.5	4.5	
Total Protein (gm/dl)	6.4	8.3	
Albumin (gm/dl)	3.6	5.1	decreased wound healing ability (low)
A/G Ratio	1.0	2.0	
Globulin (gm/dl)	2.1	3.8	
Cholesterol (mg/dl)	150	250	
Triglycerides (mg/dl)	30	170	
Total bilirubin (mg/dl)	0.10	1.3	
Indirect bilirubin (mg/dl)	.0	0.4	jaundice
Alkaline phosphatase			
0–15 years (mU/ml)	50	300	
Adult (mU/ml)	30	115	potential malignancy (high)
CPK (mU/ml)	0	225	myocardial infarction
LDH (mU/ml)	100	225	severe tissue injury
SGOT (mU/ml)	6	41	severe acute liver disease
Coagulation studies			
PTT (partial thromboplastin time) (not diagnostic for platelet disorders)		more than 60 seconds	bleeding disorder due to deficiency of coagulation factor
PROTIME (used to determine dosages of anti-coagulant drugs)		more than 20 seconds	bleeding disorder
FSP (fibrin split product) (indicates fibrinolysis triggered by clotting)		more than 10 mg	DIC (disseminated intravascular coagulopathy)

Note: These values are at above sea level altitude.

tient. He records pertinent facts about the patient's admission to the hospital. For example, he records whether or not the patient came to the hospital by ambulance, and who, if anyone, accompanied the patient. Allergies to food or medicine and a description of the reaction need to be recorded (see Fig. 4.2). He uses the data base to check off whether the patient was oriented to his room and unit, and whether the patient received an information folder. If not, he records the reasons. The nurse uses the form to record in the patient's own words the reason for his admission. The data baseline includes observation and examination. For example, physical assessment includes temperature, respirations, height, weight, pulse, and blood pressure. NPO status is also recorded along with the last approximate time food or drink was ingested. Activity or factors that might influence the care the patient requires are also noted during the nurse's observation. The patient's physical stature and general appearance as well as the emotional status and behavior are assessed and recorded. The nurse needs to record the patient's daily living habits including sleeping patterns, bowel and bladder elimination patterns, and use of alcohol and tobacco. The nurse takes a medical history relating the events surrounding the present illness. A record is made of the type and frequency of medication taken at the present time. Disposition of the medication is also taken care of at this time. The physical and emotional aspects of the history are recorded on a checklist. Anemia, arthritis, cancer, and hypertension are included on this list. Previous hospitalizations

Figure 4.2. Allergies are flagged by notation on the record cover. Personnel's recall of allergic condition is triggered everytime the record is opened.

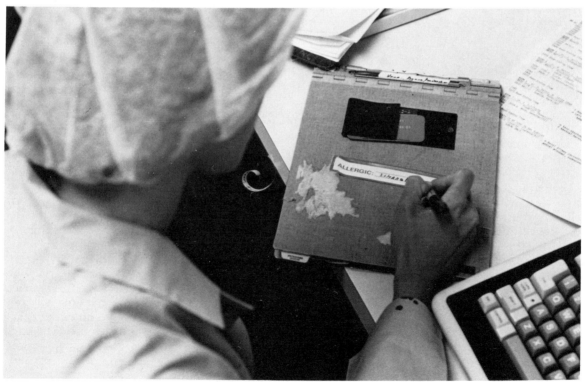

and surgeries are recorded. Previous blood transfusions and reactions are noted. When applicable, pregnancy and date of last pap smear are checked. The nurse needs to check the personal belongings the patient brings to the hospital including contact lens, glasses, hearing aid, dentures, rings, wig, wrist watch, and medical equipment. An accurate list and description of the personal items should be kept in the event of loss or theft.

Once the nurse has completed data collection and filled out the data base form, he is now able to formulate the problem list. The nurse needs to sort through the medical data to get a list of medically oriented problems. He sorts the data collected to devise a list of nursing problems. The problem list then serves as a quick reference point listing the present medical and nursing complications. The problem list provides a numerical index that helps both the physician and nurse with charting. When using the POR it is not necessary to state the problem repeatedly when charting. Each problem is assigned a permanent number, and the problem is referred to by its number when chart notation is necessary. A sample problem list follows:

1. Diabetes mellitus
2. Hypertension
3. Alcohol abuse
4. Alteration in skin integrity (decubitus)
5. Increased risk for infection
6. Alteration in nutritional status
7. Inadequate information related to diabetic diet

The traditional record contains nursing notes that deal with all aspects of patient care including routine daily care and treatments and the psychosocial care. The POR, however, efficiently sorts the data for the nurse by providing "flow sheets." These sheets are broken down, usually graphically, to either check off or record information regarding such things as elimination, activity, treatments, vital signs, diet, hygiene, and comfort. These sheets are color coded to provide quick access to this information. By charting this information separately, the progress notes are left open for

the documentation of the patient's problems and complaints. In the POR the nurse uses the SOAP format of charting.

- S: Subjective information obtained from patient, family, or significant others
- O: Objective information based on the health team's observation of the patient, diagnostic and laboratory tests, and the physical exam
- A: Assessment and examination of the patient's problems
- P: Plan steps the nurse will take to resolve the problem

Patient Care Plan
The patient care plan is in a Kardex that contains an index card for every patient on the unit. Each card lists pertinent data regarding the activity limitations, NPO status, treatments, etc. If the Kardex is used properly, it should contain an individualized patient care plan, including assessment data, nursing diagnoses, goals, plans, implementations, and evaluation. The patient care plan is written in pencil and/or ink. It can be continually updated. The trend is to have a patient care plan which becomes a part of the permanent record when the patient is discharged. The purpose of the care plan is to provide communication to all members of the health care team.

Patient Data
The nurse interviews the patient to get a detailed history of his past and present physical problems (see Fig. 4.3). He talks to the patient about his psychosocial background, as well as any cultural or ethnic differences that may exist. Examples of physical data he collects would include breakdown in skin integrity (decubitus ulcer), dehydration, limited range of motion, sensory distortion (visual and hearing loss), and alteration in vital signs (hypertension). The nurse uses the patient interview to establish rapport and develop a sense of trust in the patient so that the patient will feel comfortable discussing his psychological background. Some examples of the types of feelings he may encounter include anxiety, depression, sadness, fear, as well as any severe psycho-

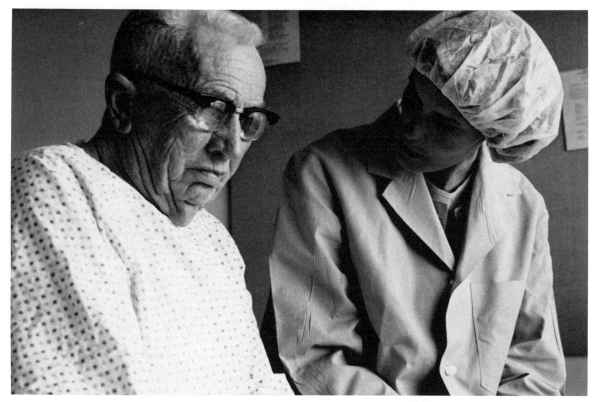

Figure 4.3. Feeling tones and cues are given through body language as well as verbally. Empathy on the part of the nurse gives a patient the freedom to express his feelings.

logical problems which may exist. The patient should also be able to provide the nurse with clues as to the types of coping mechanisms —denial, aggression, and bargaining—he employs and whether or not they are appropriate, therapeutic, or maladaptive. The patient can provide the nurse with information related to his sociocultural makeup including level of education, marital status, family position, financial status, and ethnic background. For example, "Patient describes self as a Hispanic-American, high school graduate, divorced, father of two, collecting welfare." Often the nurse will find out the religious preferences of the patient, be it Catholic, Protestant, Jewish, or agnostic and any effect his spiritual beliefs may have upon the care he receives. Through the interview process, the nurse can discern inadequacies in the patient's level of understand-

ing. The nurse can identify what needs to be taught to the patient to help him learn to manage his illness or disability. Some examples of the types of teaching and learning needs the nurse might encounter would include information regarding colostomy, diabetic dietary changes, insulin management, and cardiovascular exercises.

Data Obtained from Others

Physicians provide information relating to medical diagnosis and progress. They interpret the results of various diagnostic procedures and laboratory values. They plan the medical regimen to meet medically oriented goals designed to eliminate or ease the patient's illness or disability.

Other nurses provide continuity of care by communicating information to the oncoming

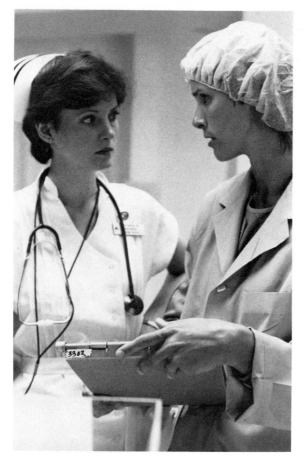

Figure 4.4. Professional consultation with nursing colleagues is an important part of assessment and planning for the perioperative patient's care during the surgical procedure. All nurses share a common concern and interest in the patient's well-being.

shift nurses with the same patient assignments (see Fig. 4.4). Nurses rely upon one another for information when the patient is transferred to another unit or health care facility. The operating room nurse uses data obtained from the unit nurse to plan for the patient having surgery.

Respiratory therapists relay information regarding the respiratory status, as well as the respiratory care and treatment the patient is receiving. They serve as resource personnel in that they are capable of interpreting and explaining to the nurse such things as pulmonary tests, arterial blood gases, and ear oximetry. The information can be communicated orally or through written notes in the chart. Some institutions permit therapists to write on the progress notes, while others supply them with a specific color-coded form.

Dieticians provide information to the nurse regarding the type of diet and caloric intake his patient requires. He can give the nurse some indication as to the teaching/learning needs of his patient with reference to a specific diet. The dietician's information is communicated both verbally and by chart documentation. Here again, the dietitian may have his own form or may write on the doctor's progress notes.

Social workers serve as a resource in providing the nurse with a more in-depth picture of the patient's home life and the way in which his illness may alter his present lifestyle. He can also give input to the nurse about some of the teaching and learning needs of the patient, as well as ways to approach preparation of the patient for his discharge from the hospital. The social worker confers with the nurse for specific information, and documents his visit on the chart on either a special form or in the doctor's progress notes.

Significant others, including family members, friends, and neighbors can provide information similar to what the nurse learns from the patient directly, although bias and misinterpretation may mar the accuracy of the information. The nurse uses significant others when the patient is incapable of communication because of coma, paralysis affecting speech, alteration in level of orientation, chronic organic brain syndrome, or other problems, or if he needs verification of something the patient has stated. The patient may not want to give the nurse necessary information or may withhold significant facts because of embarrassment regarding alcoholism or mental illness. The nurse can turn to others for a more truthful picture of the patient. Significant others can, however, interfere with data collection if their presence during the patient interview causes the patient to withhold vital information.

Clergy can serve as resource personnel to the nurse regarding aspects of different religious beliefs that the nurse might not be knowledgeable about and how these beliefs may affect the care he provides. The hospital chaplain or visiting clergy can often communicate to the nurse how the patient might be using his religious beliefs to help him cope with his illness and hospitalization. These are usually communicated confidentially to the nurse rather than documented on the chart.

The admission information sheet in medical records is a typed written sheet filled out by an admission clerk at the time the patient enters the hospital. The information is obtained from the patient, or if the patient is unable to respond, the information can be taken from a responsible party. Information on the sheet includes patient's legal name, address, phone number, social security number, birth date, sex, marital status, religious preference, place of employment, type of insurance and policy number, name, address, and phone number of next of kin, and person to be notified in case of an emergency. Included also is the patient's current medical diagnosis.

Nursing Diagnosis

The second component of assessment is formulating nursing diagnoses, which identify actual or potential health problems that professional nurses, because of their education and experience, are capable and licensed to treat (5). Although diagnosis is a relatively new concept in nursing and one that many nurses may not feel comfortable with, it is essential for appropriate goal setting and care planning. A nursing diagnosis is simply a concise statement of a patient problem that lends itself to nursing intervention. Nurses have traditionally observed patient symptoms and taken action rather than systematically assessing a patient for the purpose of making a nursing diagnosis. In a nursing diagnosis, the health problem, the etiology, and the symptoms are grouped together to form a statement. For example, a nursing diagnosis for a patient scheduled for a bilateral mastectomy might be,

"Anticipatory disturbance in self-concept (body image) related to bilateral mastectomy. The signs and symptoms she exhibits are fidgeting, elevated blood pressure and pulse, anticipated actual change in body appearance, statements about fear of rejection by her husband, and feelings of helplessness."

In the assessment phase, the nurse has already completed the first step in arriving at a diagnosis—data collection. Now, based on knowledge of social norms, the nurse recognizes critical signs and symptoms and compares them with normal and dysfunctional patterns. Then, she must interpret that data, draw inferences, and group or cluster signs and symptoms related to health problems that nurses treat. This information must also be validated. The nurse then labels the pattern, stating the problem and its etiology.

The process of nursing diagnosis is similar to that of medical diagnosis, but the types of health problems diagnosed and treated by nurses are different. The physician focuses primarily on the diagnosis and treatment of pathophysiological disorders. Nurses direct their diagnostic efforts toward discovery and treatment of health problems that arise from dysfunctional patterns such as deviations in coping strategies, health maintenance, and self-concept. For the patient who is having the bilateral mastectomy, for instance, the medical diagnosis might be, "Carcinoma of both breasts." A nursing diagnosis might be, "Altered physical mobility (level 2) with impaired range of motion related to musculoskeletal alterations."

In Chapter 7, nursing diagnosis is discussed in depth. Although demanding, it is one of the most rewarding activities performed by professional nurses. The patient benefits from the nursing treatment, and the nurse experiences satisfaction in using his intellectual skills and professional abilities.

Assessment provides the perioperative nurse with information about the surgical patient that has direct implications for his safety and well-being throughout the surgical experience. Assessment includes the nursing activities of data collection and diagnosis. Nurses assess the patient's functional health patterns to identify actual or potential health problems and plan care. Communication, interviewing, and intellectual skills are needed for assessment. Sources of data are records and reports, the patient, significant others, and other health team members. The perioperative nurse uses these sources of data rather than duplicating assessments of other health care personnel.

Through nursing diagnosis, the nurse states patient health problems, including the etiology and signs and symptoms, that nurses treat.

A patient situation is used in chapters 5, 6, 7, 8, 15, 16, and 26 to illustrate to the nurse how theory might be applied to practice. An intraoperative care plan, used in conjunction with the patient situation, provides additional emphasis when needed.

Patient Situation

A 79-year-old male admitted for possible surgery, Mr. Ralph Fischer has a diagnosis of recurrent squamous cell carcinoma of the left lateral tongue and floor of the mouth with possible mandibular involvement. Physically he appears well and is well nourished. He weighs 182 pounds and is 5 feet 7½ inches in height. Upon admission, his vital signs are: blood pressure, 120/70; pulse, 82; respiration, 20; and temperature, 99°F orally.

An energetic and active man, Mr. Fischer works part-time in a collection agency. Despite one cataract extraction, he drives short distances. He is supposed to have a cataract extraction on the other eye. He and his wife, who is also 79, live in an upper-class neighborhood of a large southern city. Their chief support is Social Security supplemented by Mr. Fischer's part-time work. Their ground-level home is surrounded by a large garden that they both enjoy, although they are not physically able to attend to all the yard work. The neighborhood is friendly, and neighbors assist them by checking on them daily, running errands, and taking them on outings. An avid baseball fan, Mr. Fischer attends as many games of the city's major league team as possible.

Mrs. Fischer does not drive and must rely on neighbors to transport her to and from the hospital so she can be with her husband. She has several other health problems, including an enlarged heart and COPD (chronic obstructive pulmonary disease). Recently, she was hospitalized for incipient cardiac failure, lung abscess, and gastrointestinal bleeding. The couple have a large family, five sons and two daughters. Both daughters are nurses and live in the immediate area. The sons reside in other cities. Mr. Fischer has one brother and two sisters, all living. A sister was recently diagnosed as having breast carcinoma, but the other siblings are in good

health. Mr. Fischer's mother died of carcinoma of the liver; his father, of "old age." None of the Fischers' children has been diagnosed with cancer.

Although Mr. Fischer has not smoked since 1964, he smoked heavily for 19 years—unfiltered cigarettes, cigars, and a pipe. During World War II, Mr. Fischer worked in an explosives plant that made bombs. His work involved mixing acids and other chemicals. After the war, he managed a business consisting of a grain elevator, lumberyard, and fertilizer operation. During 1962–63, Mr. Fischer was employed in a position that required daily contact with acids. Six years ago, the company discovered that a number of its previous and current employees had been diagnosed with cancer. The company contacted Mr. Fischer regarding any history of cancer, which he did not have, and scheduled him for a complete physical examination at its expense.

Before this examination took place, however, Mr. Fischer was diagnosed with carcinoma of the transverse colon. The examination was rescheduled, and the company continues to monitor Mr. Fischer.

Mr. Fischer's medical history includes a cholecystectomy in 1955 and a subtotal gastrectomy in 1964. In 1975, a subtotal colectomy was performed for carcinoma of the transverse colon. Recovery from these procedures progressed normally with no sequelae. Mr. Fischer has moderate varicosities of both lower extremities. There is moderate septal deviation; otherwise all systems are essentially negative at physical examination except the tongue, alveolar ridge, and floor of the mouth, and a small palpable lesion in the left neck.

The original diagnosis of an epidermoid carcinoma of the tongue and buccal mucous membrane was made in April 1980. A laser vaporization was performed. A month later, a recurrent lesion was vaporized by laser. In January 1981, a squamous cell carcinoma of the left alveolar ridge was excised. Since then, lesions of both left tongue, alveolar ridge, and the floor of the mouth have reappeared. Mr. Fischer is scheduled on September 11, 1981, for a possible left hemiglossectomy, left mandibulectomy, and neck dissection. His surgeon has discussed with him the need for a postoperative tracheostomy and nasal tube feedings while his jaw is wired. He is apparently unaware that the extent of the lesions may indicate a total glossectomy and radical neck dissection.

References

1. Dossey, B. "Perfecting your skills for systematic patient assessments." *Nurs 79* 9(February):42–45, 1979.
2. Douglas, L. M. *The Effective Nurse.* St. Louis: C. V. Mosby, 1980.
3. Hannigan, L. "Nursing assessment of the integument system." *Occup Health Nurs* 26(January):19–22, 1978.
4. Enelow, A. J., and Swisher, S. N. *Interviewing and Patient Care*, 2nd ed. New York: Oxford University Press, 1979.
5. Gordon, M. "Nursing diagnosis and the diagnostic process." *Am J Nurs* 76:1298–1300, 1976.

Suggested Readings

Alexander, C., Schrader, E., and Kneedler, J. "Preoperative visits: The OR nurse unmasks." *AORN J* 19(February):401–412, 1974.

Association of Operating Room Nurses. "Operating room nursing: perioperative role." *AORN J* 27(May):1156–1175, 1978.

Barnett, L. A. "Preparing your patient for the operating room." *AORN J* 18(September):534–539, 1973.

Bird, B. *Talking with Patients*, 2nd ed. Philadelphia: J. B. Lippincott, 1973.

Davis, J. L. Preoperative program prepares children for surgery. *AORN J* 26(August):249–256, 1977.

Fehlau, M. T. "Implementation of standards of practice." *AORN J* 22(November):712–718, 1975.

Gordon, J. C., Jr. *Semantics and Communication*, 2nd ed. New York: Macmillan, 1975.

Hartson, D., and Hartson, K. M. "The five-minute interview." *AORN J* 31(March):605–608, 1980.

Hercules, P. "OR experience teaches continuity of care." *AORN J* 32(November):799–806, 1980.

Jordan, C. H. "If we teach holistic care, can we exclude perioperative nursing?" *AORN J* 32(November):797–798, 1980.

Kneedler, J. A., Reed, E. A., Manuel, B. J., and Fehlau, M. T. "From standards into practice." *AORN J* 28(October):603–642, 1978.

Laird, M. "Techniques for teaching pre and postoperative patients." *Am J Nurs* 75(August):1338–1340, 1975.

Larke, G. A. "Perioperative charting: OR nursing on display." *AORN J* 31(February):194–198, 1980.

Levine, M. E. "Adaptation and assessment a rationale for nursing intervention." *Am J Nurs* 66(November):2450–2453, 1966.

Luckman, J. and Sorensen, D. G. *Medical-Surgical Nursing*, 2nd ed. Philadelphia: W. B. Saunders, 1980.

Price, M. R. "Making a concept come alive." *Am J Nurs* 80(April):668–671, 1980.

Schmitt, F. E., and Wooldridge, P. J. "Psychological preparation of surgical patients." *Nurs Res* 22(March–April):249–256, 1973.

Winslow, E. H., and Fuhs, M. F. "Preoperative assessment for postoperative evaluation." *Am J Nurs* 73(August):1372–1374, 1973.

Wittstock, N. J. "Preoperative evaluation and physical assessment of the patient." *J Am Assoc Nurs Anes* 49(April):197–206, 1981.

Yura, H., and Walsh, M. B. *The Nursing Process*, 3rd ed. New York: Appleton-Century-Crofts, 1978.

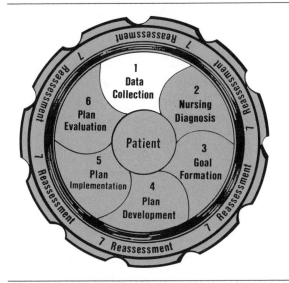

Assessment includes determining the patient's emotional state.

Collecting Psychological Data

All hospitalized patients experience some degree of anxiety. Surgery compounds this anxiety, depending upon the patient's current illness, past experiences, apprehensions, expectations, and coping mechanisms. Each situation is unique and complex. In order to plan and implement comprehensive care for surgical patients, operating room nurses must evaluate a patient's psychological as well as physiological status. Such an assessment allows nurses to individualize care during the intraoperative period and to provide emotional support throughout the perioperative experience.

Consider a 50-year-old man hospitalized for exploratory surgery. A few months ago, he was independent and taking care of himself. Now, he faces possible cancer, a lingering illness, and perhaps, death. He may not be able to continue working and is worried about how he can survive financially in the future. Most of all, he is concerned about being a burden to his family. He finds himself struggling with mixed feelings of anger and despondency. He is ambivalent about having surgery, because his worst fears may be confirmed. How could an operating room nurse assist this patient to cope? Can a crisis be prevented?

Certain situational and maturational events in the life cycle of every person can be described as hazardous. Examples are bereavement, physical illness, alteration of usual living style, adolescence, loss of job, old age, and surgery. Each of these situations can generate emotional strain or anxiety, precipitate stress, and activate a series of adaptive mechanisms that lead to resolution or impairment.

Occasionally, such hazardous events become crises for individuals who are vulnerable due to a distorted perception of the situation, lack of a support system, or inadequate coping mechanisms (1). Obstacles to important life goals appear insurmountable. A period of disorganization occurs during which customary methods of problem solving fail (2). Frequent abortive attempts are made to manage stress and seek a resolution. Thus, a crisis can be an emotional response to a hazard that results in a state of disequilibrium characterized by overwhelming feelings of helplessness and hopelessness. Symptoms of severe anxiety or panic occur. Individuals have difficulty coping because they believe they no longer have control over their own lives. Ability to carry out activities of daily living often decreases. At this point, crisis intervention may be necessary if the process is to be reversed and the patient is to regain her precrisis level of functioning.

Because surgery can be viewed as a psychological crisis for patients, it is imperative for an operating room nurse to understand crisis intervention theories and methodologies. She must also be able to assess mental health status effectively. This knowledge and these skills allow her as a perioperative nurse to assist surgical patients to manage constructively preoperative, intraoperative, and postoperative anxiety. Her intervention can also promote wellness, prevent pathology, and enable adaptive resolution of crises.

Mental Status Assessment

Comprehensive nursing care implies enhancing, maintaining, or restoring a patient's emotional equilibrium. The major focus of a mental status assessment is the determination of an individual's strengths, capabilities, and resources for environmental, social, and intrapsychic adjustment (3). Such an assessment requires nurses to identify cognitive processes, emotions, and behaviors that interfere with a patient's ability to achieve an optimal level of function.

When doing a mental status assessment, the nurse observes aspects of a patient's psychological functioning. For example, she examines:

1. General perceptions about surgery
2. Affective responses or feelings
3. Self-esteem and self-concept
4. Coping and defense mechanisms
5. Support from significant others
6. Attention and concentration
7. Thought processes
8. Sensorium and reasoning
9. Speech characteristics
10. Attitude and motivation

Table 5.1 depicts a concise mental health assessment checklist. After the nurse analyzes the data, she makes inferences about the patient's psychological state. This allows her to plan, implement, and evaluate nursing care for patients during their entire surgical experience.

GENERAL PERCEPTIONS ABOUT SURGERY

The nurse should explore the patient's perception of her surgery. Why is surgery necessary? What is her understanding of her health/illness status? Is she aware of any limitations? What does having surgery mean to her? Do her perceptions appear rational or irrational? Does she see the event realistically, or does she distort its meaning? Will surgery and hospitalization significantly disrupt her current lifestyle? If so, how? What outcomes does she anticipate? Will her future lifestyle be affected positively or negatively as a result of surgery?

AFFECTIVE RESPONSES OR FEELINGS

The nurse should focus on the patient's feelings or affective responses. How does she feel about having surgery? Is her affect (emotional state) appropriate to the situation? Are any of her fears irrational? Is there any discrepancy between how the nurse perceives the person's

Table 5.1. Mental Health Assessment Checklist.

Mental Functions	Appearance	Behavior	Conversation

1. Attitude
  a. Cooperativeness
  b. Interpersonal relationships
	Patient is aloof, unclean, disheveled, indifferent.	Patient is negativistic, uncooperative, hostile, belligerent, passive, drooping, withdrawn, impulsive; has slow gait.	Patient avoids topics; is pessimistic.

2. Affect/mood
  a. Appropriate
  b. Harmony
  c. Swings
	Patient has masklike face, is apathetic, flat, rigid, labile, euphoric, depressed, suspicious, hostile; displays inappropriate affect; shows physical signs of anxiety (flushing, sweating, tremors respirations).	Patient is overactive, underactive, cries or laughs easily; wrings hands; paces floor; strikes head with hands; holds fixed posture for prolonged periods; has silly smile.	Patient displays disharmony with thought processes; talks of guilt, sin, or unworthiness.

3. Speech characteristics
  a. Description
  b. Speed
  c. Quantity
	Patient is soft-spoken, loud, boisterous; has monotonous, slow, or rapid speech.	Patient grimaces, stammers, stutters; displays uncoordinated or exaggerated movement, mutism, echolalia.	Patient displays exaggeration, confabulation, blocking of thought, circumstantiality, tangentiality, autistic speech, incoherence, flight of ideas; is overtalkative; uses neologisms.

4. Thought processes
  a. Logical
  b. Coherent
  c. Perceptual
	Patient is inattentive, easily distracted, preoccupied.	Patient avoids anxiety, displays phobic behavior, compulsiveness, echopraxia.	Patient displays phobias, obsessions, paranoid ideas, illogical flow; has feelings of strangeness, depersonalization, hallucinations, delusions (somatic, grandeur, persecution, alien control).

5. Sensorium and reasoning
  a. Levels of consciousness
  b. Orientation
  c. Memory (recent, remote)
  d. Calculation
  e. Abstract thinking
  f. Judgment/insight
  g. Intelligence
	Patient displays decreased or absent physiologic reflexes, disinterest, peculiarity of dress, bewilderment.	Patient displays stupor, lethargy, coma, confusion, agitation, delirium panic, twilight state, behavior problems, conduct disorder.	Patient displays aphasia, memory defect, disorientation, poor judgment, lack of insight, inability of abstract thinking and calculations.

6. Potential for danger
  a. Self-concept
  b. Harm to self/others
	Patient is docile, sad hostile, angry, apathetic.	Patient has made suicide attempts; is malingering, withdrawn, assaultive, combative, violent; lacks temper control; displays antisocial or criminal behavior (arrests), irritability, explosiveness, excitability, maladaptive coping.	Patient has ideas of self-accusation and condemnation, self-deprecation, suicidal ideations.

7. Patient's psychological assets	Physical assets.	Behavioral assets.	Conversational assets.

This table presents a range of signs and symptoms that may suggest dysfunction. They are not in themselves necessarily reflective of mental illness, nor are they all necessarily confined to a specific area. Some may overlap.

affect and how the patient describes her mood? Does surgery threaten her self-image? Are psychological and physiological symptoms indicative of anxiety?

What is the patient's level of awareness in relation to the degree of anxiety she is experiencing? For example, can she focus on what is happening to her or is her ability limited or greatly impaired? Is she angry? Are there manifestations of aggressive behavior? Is there potential danger of physical aggression by the patient toward others? How powerless does the individual feel? Are there characteristics of depression? Is the patient suicidal? Does she believe life is worth living? Has she ever thought about harming herself? Is she preoccupied with death?

Because these are complex issues, four areas are addressed in greater depth: (1) anxiety, (2) powerlessness, (3) aggression, and (4) depression. Emphasis is placed on factors the nurse should assess, particularly affective responses.

Anxiety
Anxiety is a state of apprehension, tension, concern, or uneasiness in response to a real or imagined danger that is often nonspecific (3, 4). A vague sense of dread, helplessness, isolation, and insecurity is evoked when an individual confronts a situation that threatens her self-image.

Anxiety is a warning to alert us to a dangerous situation. Although all of us feel anxious in the course of our daily lives, the combined effects of illness and confinement usually intensify the emotion. The unknowns associated with surgery further arouse nervousness triggered by the perceived threat we see to our biological and psychological integrity. The stages of anxiety response are (5):

1. Threat to self-image
2. Increased mental and perceptual alertness to threat
3. Physiological reactions largely mediated through the autonomic nervous system
4. Feelings of tension and apprehension
5. Behavior that is successful or unsuccessful in coping with the threat

During a psychological assessment, the nurse first observes physiological reactions to anxiety: pale appearance; cold, clammy skin; muscular tension, especially in the neck; rapid pulse; palpitations; increased blood pressure; frequent wetting of the lips with the tongue due to decreased saliva and drying of mucous membranes; trembling; diarrhea; and increased urination. Noted next are behavioral manifestations of anxiety: restlessness; wringing of hands; difficulty maintaining eye contact; ambiguous complaints; general irritation; sullenness; withdrawal; crying; quarreling; defensiveness; and the inability to concentrate, understand explanations, or retain information.

The nurse evaluates the intensity, appropriateness, and duration of the anxiety attack, if possible. Is the degree of anxiety mild, moderate, or severe? Is there evidence of panic? During mild anxiety, the patient's alertness is heightened because she recognizes her tension as a warning signal. Learning can occur at this level.

Selective inattention and a diminished ability to perceive events accurately characterize moderate anxiety. Learning must be directed. During severe anxiety, the ability to perceive and communicate details is limited. Some distortion of events occurs. Learning usually is blocked. Some patients become panicky; learning is unable to take place due to major impairment of cognitive functions (5).

The nurse should ask herself if the anxiety appears to be provoked by a realistic or imaginary threat or danger. In general, anxiety is regarded as appropriate or normal if it is precipitated by real concerns; it may be considered neurotic if it arises from unrealistic, imagined events. The nurse should estimate the length of time the patient has demonstrated acute symptoms of anxiety.

While assisting the patient to recognize her anxiety and gain insight into its causes, the nurse can continue her psychological monitoring. As additional data are collected regarding the patient's apprehensions, the nurse should try to help the patient identify specific fears. Then the plan of care can be more focused on critiquing the seriousness and realism of the threat, teaching the patient new ways of overcoming the threat, and effectively managing behavioral manifestations of anxiety. The nurse should be sure to assess external environmental factors contributing to the patient's anxiety level as well as internal sources. As she gives clear, concise explanations about current and future events, the nurse seeks clarification from the patient as to any concerns she may have about these situations. The nurse should repeat information as often as necessary, so the patient is able to retain the data. She should remember the correlation between anxiety and learning and be careful not to overload the patient with irrelevant information. The nurse can use touch to calm a patient and encourage coping mechanisms such as talking, crying, or walking.

Powerlessness
When a patient experiences a loss of control over her own behavior and environment or a lack of knowledge regarding her own illness or life predicament, feelings of powerlessness often result (6). She does not feel capable of mastering or coping with unknown, unexpected events.

The nurse assesses with the patient what factors have caused her to feel powerless or helpless. Does the diagnosis of acute or chronic illness generate apprehensions of increased dependency, possible disability, and less control over physical and mental bodily functions? Does hospitalization mean the patient forfeits decision making about her care? Can she retain power through seeking information, clarifying expectations, and questioning aspects of her treatment regimen? Importantly, does she have the right to disagree with health care professionals and to refuse a suggested course of treatment if it conflicts with her values or beliefs?

The administration of anesthesia heightens a patient's concerns about being out of control because she must totally trust members of the surgical team to care for her during altered states of consciousness. The simple fear of saying something inappropriate during induction often illustrates the powerlessness a patient feels over her physiological and psychological functioning. Furthermore, many surgical patients are modest about nudity. They frequently feel as though they have no control over whether their privacy will be respected during the intraoperative phase.

Some patients worry about whether they can protest if surgical outcomes are not satisfactory. What recourse, besides legal action, does a patient have for a grievance regarding her care or treatment? Can a patient be assertive in conveying her comments to appropriate personnel through proper channels? The nurse could refer the patient to the hospital's patient representative, or suggest that the patient write the hospital administrator.

Finally, the nurse needs to determine what behaviors would enhance the patient's sense of power and control. For example, the nurse can reinforce the patient's sense of power over her environment by describing the surgical suite, so she knows what to expect in terms of temperature, general appearance, equipment, and noise. If a patient wants to keep her dentures or a particular piece of clothing until she reaches the operating room, the nurse could make an exception to the usual rule of leaving personal effects in the surgical unit. Frequently, surgical patients want to know how they can communicate with members of the surgical team in the holding area should there be a need, especially since preoperative medication may alter their problem-solving abilities. Finally, how can surgical patients be encouraged to participate actively within realistic limits, in their care during the intraoperative and postoperative phases rather than being passive recipients?

Aggression
One common means of handling a perceived danger and sense of powerlessness is to get angry and become aggressive. Aggressive behavior is a forceful, attacking action that involves injuring another individual directly or indirectly. Such behavior can be verbal, physical, or symbolic and can hurt others by assaulting their self-esteem or damaging their body or property. Aggression is a method for

managing feelings of anxiety, anger, and powerlessness.

Surgical patients may display aggressive behavior by using abusive language; being argumentative; refusing to participate in their care; engaging in fault finding or hypercritical behavior; being extremely demanding; rejecting staff overtures; threatening personnel; being sarcastic; joking at the expense of others; remaining silent when staff try to communicate; removing treatment equipment, such as pulling out a nasogastric tube or Foley catheter; or being physically violent. For the most part, hospitalized patients tend to use passive-aggressive methods of expressing anger rather than active, direct forms. This may make assessment of aggressive behavior more difficult since the variations are more subtle and harder to recognize.

Once the nurse has evaluated the aggressive behavior the patient is using, ongoing assessment may be necessary to determine why aggression is used as a primary coping mechanism. For example, is the behavior a response to increased dependency, loss of control, fear, or deprivation? Can the patient differentiate between aggressive and assertive behavior? Does she understand that aggressive behavior is getting what one wants at the expense of others? If power or control is important to the patient, how can the nurse help the patient exercise greater flexibility in decision making about her care?

Can patients be encouraged to express their anger constructively by fighting fairly? To help them to do this, the nurse must monitor whether they perceive they can discuss angry feelings with staff members and significant others without experiencing retaliation or counter-aggression. Do staff members confront and set limits on destructive aggressive behavior, yet allow patients to verbalize ambivalent, angry feelings?

If a patient is scheduled for a radical neck procedure due to cancer, she may be extremely anxious about the impact of the surgical outcome on her body image. She may also feel angry because she believes it is unfair for her to suffer so extensively. She may resent members of the surgical team for their inability to cure her of cancer. Fears about the ultimate prognosis may magnify feelings of powerlessness, so she becomes demanding of both staff and family to exercise control over the immediate situation. Her caustic remarks communicate her cynicism about the present quality of her life. Gradually, she becomes critical of the team members who are caring for her. She is convinced she will just be another hopeless case for the operating room staff. In fact, she remarks about being another cancer statistic.

At this point, the operating room nurse needs to recognize the different ways the patient is displaying aggressive behavior. Acknowledgment of the underlying anger is essential. Instead of taking the patient's anger personally, the nurse should encourage her to vent it and then encourage constructive conflict resolution. Although limits need to be set on destructive aggressive behavioral patterns, it is critical not to chastise the patient for using aggression as a coping mechanism to adapt to the stressors associated with her illness. Still, the patient needs to be confronted as to her use of aggression and its negative consequences. Once the patient gains insight into her behavior, she should be aided to develop systematic, assertive skills on her own behalf. Although she has the right to express angry feelings, she must channel the feelings into constructive action.

Depression

To some patients and family members, surgery may involve a loss of something of great value. Examples include the loss of a leg due to an amputation, removal of hair because of a craniotomy, change in sexual role identity related to a mastectomy or prostatectomy, or a loss of self-respect because of alterations in the capacity to perform desired family or career roles. Fears about death and dying relate in part to underlying concerns about the inability to control surgical outcomes and the possible loss of life.

Sometimes perceptions of failure and punishment haunt surgical patients, precipitating feelings of remorse and guilt. Because they feel they have failed to live an acceptable lifestyle and properly care for themselves, they believe their illness and treatment, including surgery, are forms of punishment. If the patient views herself as inadequate, incompetent, deficient, bad, or sinful, feelings of despondency and worthlessness can dominate the affective state. Anger may be repressed and introjected, intensifying feelings of sadness, pessimism, helplessness, and hopelessness. These feelings can culminate in depression, a psychophysiological response to a real or perceived failure or significant loss (7).

Psychological assessment includes observing the patient for behavioral manifestations of depression such as:

- Alterations in usual sleep patterns
- Changes in appetite
- Sexual disturbances
- Somatic symptoms
- Inner mood changes
- Inability to concentrate
- Decreased initiative
- Apathy
- Tearfulness
- Self-depreciation
- Negative thinking
- Minimal interest in self, others, or the environment
- Withdrawal
- Suicidal tendencies

The nurse should evaluate major changes or losses the surgical patient has experienced, especially with the past year. If the patient anticipates additional losses due to her scheduled surgery, are there any symptoms of the grief and mourning process? For example, are the patient's responses illustrative of the following steps of the grieving process (8)?

1. Shock and denial
2. Anger
3. Bargaining
4. Depression
5. Acceptance

Engel believes most symptoms of grieving fall into three categories: (1) shock and disbelief, (2) developing awareness of the loss, and (3) restitution (9). Most surgical patients probably do not reach full acceptance or restitution preoperatively, since the process may take up to a year or more.

Assessment of the mourning process is essential, because it is important to differentiate constructive grieving from more severe forms of depression. The nurse can assess the degree of depression by asking some of these questions: How prevalent is distorted or negative thinking? Does the patient perceive life as a series of burdens and obstacles that represent defeat, deprivation, and disparagement? Is surgery just another traumatic event that detracts from her in some manner? What is her self-concept? How negative is her thinking about the future?

The nurse should monitor the patient's expressions for whether she views herself as a failure. Does she discuss feelings of guilt? Does she believe she deserves to be punished for some wrong she has committed? Is she unable to appropriately externalize legitimate feelings of anger? Is she suicidal? What are her perceptions of supportive measures by professional members of the health care team?

SELF-ESTEEM/SELF-CONCEPT

How does the patient evaluate herself? Does she believe herself to be capable, significant, and successful or useless, inept, and unloveable (10)? Does she approve or disapprove of herself? Is she able to identify her assets and limitations? Does she value most aspects of self without harsh censorship or self-hate? How does the patient's self-concept affect her adaptation to surgery? What impact does the perioperative experience have on the patient's body image and self-concept relative to masculinity or feminity?

PHYSICAL APPEARANCE

The nurse should note the patient's physical appearance (11). What is the patient's body build—thin, obese, short, tall, muscular? Does she appear unkempt and dirty or neat and clean? Is she dressed appropriately for the occasion and for her age? If cosmetics are used, are they applied correctly? In terms of body language, what does the patient's posture communicate? Is she relaxed, tense, erect, slouched? Is there a correlation between physical appearance and the patient's self-esteem? Is her behavior influenced by her perceptions of her body-image? What impact will surgery have on physical appearance and, ultimately, body image?

BODY IMAGE

Surgery may raise a patient's concerns regarding body image. Can she adapt to her body, or part of it, in a changed form (6)? If a patient knows she will lose a body part or its usual functioning during surgery, she may worry about coping with the loss associated. She may be frightened that an operation will compound damage, injury, or loss of bodily functions that illness has already precipitated. Some patients fear mutilation, even if surgical outcomes are basically viewed as corrective in nature. Radical procedures trigger anxieties about dismemberment, major alterations in body structure, paralysis, and possible death.

During the interview, the nurse should try to determine what body image alterations the patient perceives will result from surgery (see Fig. 5.1). What do such changes mean? How will they affect the patient's life? Does the patient exhibit feelings that indicate she will

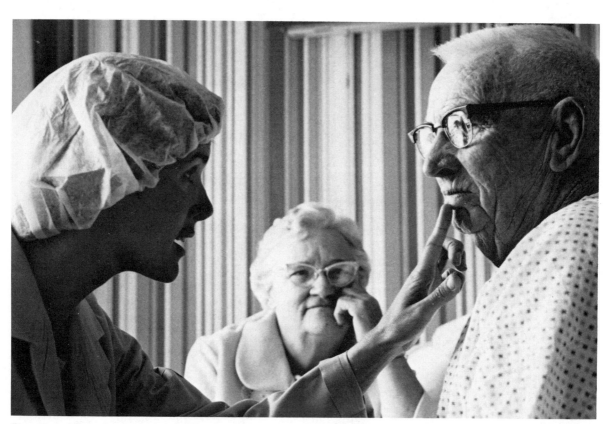

Figure 5.1. The perioperative nurse is determining whether the patient understands that surgery has the potential of disfigurement. This patient is scheduled for a radical neck dissection.

be repulsed or ashamed of physical modifications? Are there any symptoms of depression? Give positive reinforcement about the patient's ability to adapt. Allow expressions of denial, anger, or depression. The nurse should tell the patient which feelings and concerns she regards as normal. If appropriate, the nurse should provide information about groups or prosthetic devices that assist individuals to cope. She should involve other team members, as well as the family, in planning and implementing ways to involve the patient in self-care activities that will facilitate recovery.

SEXUALITY

Sexuality is often ignored or minimized by health care professionals even though it is one of the most crucial dimensions of personality. Sexuality "encompasses those biological, physiological, and psychological characteristics that relate to one's identity as a man or woman" (12:7). It is more than gender, reproduction, or genital sex. Instead, sexuality is a central life force that is a pervasive part of the whole personality and the total of one's feelings and behaviors as male or female (13). Thus, human sexuality should be viewed as a health entity, and human beings should be assisted in the healthy development and expression of sexuality as part of their identity.

Allowing surgical patients openly to vent their concerns surrounding sexuality is imperative. Drugs, procedures, and conditions that can alter either physical or psychological aspects of sexuality should be discussed with patients and significant others. Illnesses that affect a patient's self-concept will also affect sexuality. For example, what does an abdominoperineal resection, cystostomy, colostomy, craniotomy, mastectomy, or hemorrhoidectomy mean to a patient's sexual being?

The nurse should also be aware of the impact of surgical procedures upon sexual performance. She should be knowledgeable about reconstructive measures that could modify or correct physical impairments that adversely affect a patient's sexual self-concept. Guidance and emotional support may be necessary to reassure patients that techniques exist to en-

able individuals to cope with any sexual dysfunction that may result from disease processes or surgical procedures. Importantly, patients must not be treated as asexual beings; their sexuality, including sexual functioning, is affected by illness, hospitalization, treatments, and medication.

COPING AND DEFENSE MECHANISMS

The nurse should ascertain coping devices or defense mechanisms the patient has used in the past to manage anxiety and maintain psychological integrity. How does she usually resolve tension, nervousness, or apprehension? Has she tried any of these methods this time? If not, why? If her usual methods are not working, why does she think they are ineffective at this time? What new, original methods might reduce her anxiety? How can any threat to self-image be overcome? What unconscious defense mechanisms, such as rationalization, projection, displacement, denial, and introjection, are being used to relieve anxiety? Are the coping devices and defense mechanisms appropriate to the situation? Are any addictive coping habits used that might adversely affect the patient's recovery, such as smoking, alcohol, drug abuse, or excessive food intake?

SUPPORT FROM SIGNIFICANT OTHERS

The nurse should ask the patient about support available from significant others. Who is capable of providing emotional support to her, especially preoperatively and postoperatively? Are there family members to whom she feels particularly close (see Fig. 5.2)? Is there someone outside the immediate family who is meaningful to her, such as a friend, teacher, pastor, or colleague? Whom does she trust? How can members of the health care team effectively render emotional support? What support would she like during the intraoperative phase?

ATTENTION AND CONCENTRATION

The nurse should appraise the attention and concentration capabilities of the patient. Often, the attention span is one of the first cognitive

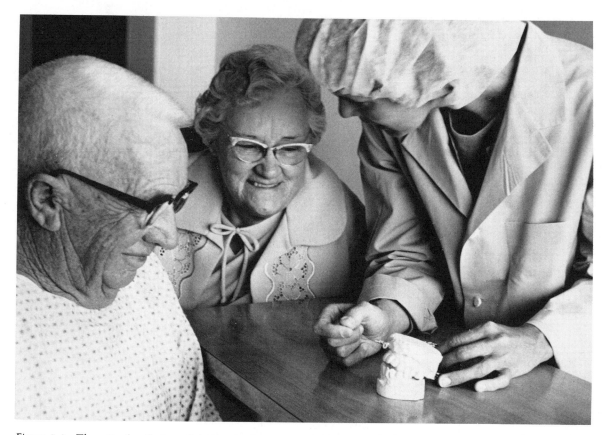

Figure 5.2. *The patient's wife is participating in the preoperative preparation by listening attentively and being interested in what will happen to her husband. Thus, she provides emotional support.*

functions to be disturbed (14). Attentiveness to external conditions can be evaluated to a great degree by the quality of the patient's response to questions, directives, and comments. Also, is she aware of people and objects around her without being inappropriately distracted or confused? Is she able to maintain interest in the interview process and to concentrate so that her replies are thorough? Does the patient have any illusions, misinterpretations of sensory stimuli, or hallucinations?

THOUGHT PROCESSES

Evaluate the patient's ability to be logical, coherent, and relevant. Is there continuity among ideas? Does conversation flow in an orderly sequence, or does the patient ramble and skip from subject to subject? If the nurse interjects a new idea into the interview, does the patient comprehend it and respond appropriately? How negative or pessimistic are the thoughts? Are the thoughts rational or irrational (15,16)? Is there any evidence of the following aberrant patterns (17)?

- Delusions, false fixed beliefs not subject to reason
- Obsessions, recurrent, uncontrollable thoughts
- Errors of reference, misinterpreting events in the world as referring directly to oneself

- Ruminations, repetitive speculative thinking
- Suspicious or paranoid thinking

SENSORIUM AND REASONING

Usually these factors are evaluated within the context of the patient's total health history. The nurse would probably gather most of these data from the patient's record or other team members. During the preoperative interview, however, it is critical that the nurse assess any deviations from the patient's reported normal level of functioning.

LEVEL OF CONSCIOUSNESS

The nurse determines level of consciousness by monitoring the patient's awareness of external and internal stimuli and responsiveness to life's experiences. Is there any lack of clarity or confusion relative to her awareness of self or the environment? Four basic levels of consciousness are (10):

1. Conscious and alert
2. Obtunded (slowed mental processes, lethargy, sleepiness)
3. Semicomatose or stupor (unconscious but can be aroused sufficiently to respond to verbal commands)
4. Comatose or unconscious (cannot be aroused and does not respond to painful stimuli)

A more complex categorization of the levels of consciousness is described in the text, *Health Assessment* (14). Reynolds and Logsdon encourage nurses to evaluate whether the individual is responsive to verbal stimuli, touch, or noxious stimuli (18).

ORIENTATION

The nurse evaluates the patient's orientation by assessing her awareness of person, place, and time. Does she know who she is when asked her name, address, and telephone number? Does she know exactly where she is? Is she aware of her immediate situation? Does she know the hour, day of the week, month, and year? Radical changes in environment—

such as from home to emergency room, to operating room, to recovery room, and to the intensive care unit—can cause disorientation. Sensory deprivation can also precipitate disorientation. Disturbance in place and person usually implies cerebral disorder (11).

MEMORY

The nurse should ask questions that test the patient's recent and remote memory. Usually, such inquiries can be done discreetly in an interview as she explores events of the day or historical data relative to the patient's health. Answers can be validated by checking past records, talking with family members and friends, or questioning other health personnel who have spent time with the patient. According to Grimes and Iannopollo, "Loss of memory is an early sign of pathology of the cerebral cortex in general and of the temporal and occipital lobes in particular. Recent memories are those most affected, since remote memory is seldom disturbed and tends to survive disease" (11:61). Widespread damage of the cerebral cortex or schizophrenia may also impair remote memory (14). The nurse should observe whether there is any tendency to confabulate or make up for memory gaps by substituting fabricated answers. She should inquire directly as to whether the patient has noticed any loss of memory or if she remembers current or past events better.

INTELLIGENCE

The nurse should explore the patient's general fund of information. How well informed is the patient about current world events? Is her level of intelligence average, above average, or below average? How sophisticated or complex is her vocabulary? Intelligence as measured by information and vocabulary is relatively unaffected by any but the most severe psychiatric disorders or organic brain disorders (17).

ABSTRACT THINKING

The nurse should examine the patient's ability to reason abstractly. During the interview, how concrete or abstract are the patient's answers? Could she give the meaning of a familiar proverb or accurately determine the similarity between two items? Concrete explanations may be given by patients with organic brain disorders or schizophrenia (17). Level of education can also affect the depth of a reply, so educational background should be taken into account.

JUDGMENT

The nurse should assess the patient's capacity to compare and contrast facts, ideas, and alternatives to understand their relationships, and to formulate appropriate conclusions (18). How effective are her problem-solving skills? How has she resolved health problems in the past? Does she use information constructively to deal with hospitalization and surgery? Does she use health personnel as resources for improving her decision making?

SPEECH CHARACTERISTICS

The nurse can assess speech patterns by asking herself: What is the pace and volume of the speech activity? For example, does the patient monopolize the conversation, share little information in response to inquiries, or keep up a balanced dialogue? Evasive replies should be noted. What is the quality of the speech activity in terms of loudness, pitch, tone, inflection, and clarity? Are any unusual words or phrases used? Is there evidence of self-coined words or autistic speech? Are any words misused or transposed, thus suggesting aphasia?

ATTITUDE AND MOTIVATION

The nurse should assess whether the patient appears to be cooperative in complying with suggested treatment or prevention regimens in a responsible, informed manner. Is she motivated to maximize her health potential by engaging in self-care practices? Is there any evidence that she is not adhering to parts of her care plan? If necessary, will she modify her lifestyle to adapt to limitations or enhance wellness? The coronary artery bypass patient, for example, will need to follow a specific program designed to facilitate a return to a meaningful level of performance. The colostomy patient may need to modify her diet to adapt constructively.

Assessment of a surgical patient's mental status allows operating room nurses to collect critical data relative to psychological functioning. Such information is essential if the nurse is to aid the patient and family to maintain emotional equilibrium in a hazardous situation or regain it in a crisis state. Some ways of giving emotional support are by correcting unrealistic perceptions, reinforcing effective coping mechanisms, helping with constructive management of anxiety, heightening the sense of power, remedying depressogenic environmental factors, and providing adequate nurturing. Intervention will be enhanced if psychological assessment is based on knowledge of intrapsychic and interpersonal processes because care can then be planned around the unique needs of individual patients. Operating room nurses who practice the perioperative role enrich the psychological care delivered to patients throughout the entire surgical experience. Effective psychological monitoring helps the nurse to capitalize on a patient's strengths to maximize effective adaptation and prevent pathology.

Patient Situation

During the preoperative interview, Mr. Fischer explained that he was having surgery because of recurrent cancer of the left part of his tongue and possibly surrounding tissue and jaw bone. He understood that part of his tongue and mandible would be removed, along with the removal of lymph nodes in his neck. He also realized he would have a tracheostomy. His knowledge of the scheduled surgical procedure appeared excellent. He attributed his comprehension to his physician, two daughters who are nurses, and other supportive members of the health care team. Because of previous surgical experiences, he also knew what generally to expect intraoperatively and postoperatively.

When asked how he felt about his illness, he indicated that he had lived with the diagnosis of cancer for a long time. Mr. Fischer previously had carcinoma of the transverse colon. Although he viewed the disease as life-threatening, he was optimistic that many individuals could be helped medically, including himself. At this point in time, he was slightly frustrated that the "gray, bubbly area" on his tongue kept reoccurring and his jaw was tender, so his dentures hurt. He was also concerned that he could feel a "mass" on his left jaw. He mentioned that he occasionally felt sad to be in poor health, but he had basically lived a very happy, productive 79 years.

As the conversation proceeded, several concerns emerged. First, he would not sign the surgical consent form until he knew the specific results of his whole-body computerized tomography scan. He had struggled with the decision of whether to have or refuse surgery based upon the complexity of the procedure, anticipated outcomes, his age and the concomitant risks, and the impact upon his long-term prognosis. Recently, he had decided that he wanted the surgery if the CT scan did not show evidence of metastatic cancer. If the results of the scan confirmed cancer in other parts of his body, he would not have surgical intervention. As he explained how he arrived at the above decision, it was apparent that his judgment was based upon personal insight and logical, coherent thought processes. Given his past and present health status, his rationale appeared realistic and valid. Mr. Fischer indicated that he expected to be informed by his physician of the results of the scan later during the evening. Arrangements were made by the operating room nurse to ensure that communication regarding the final outcome was clearly conveyed to appropriate nursing personnel. If the decision was to proceed with surgery, intraoperative nursing care could then continue to be planned, implemented, and evaluated.

Next, Mr. Fischer was aware that his daughters had opposing viewpoints about whether he should have surgery. His eldest discouraged him because of her fears that "terrible disfigurement and disability" could result. His youngest encouraged him as long as he understood the outcomes, negative and positive, plus the risks. Although both daughters wanted their father to have all the facts, so he could make his own decision, it was apparent that their interpretation of data provided by various resources led them to two different conclusions. Mr. Fischer indicated that he knew they had had a serious argument over the issue. Although they were

controlled in his presence, he was cognizant of their tension and anger.

The situation made him feel slightly guilty. He said, "They wouldn't be fighting if it weren't for my condition." Gradually, he could recognize that the above thought was probably irrational; still he found he worried about his daughters and felt somewhat depressed because he couldn't assure them that everything would be all right. As a father, he felt he should have been able to protect and nurture more fully, thus facilitating conflict resolution. Still, they, as he, needed to grapple with the facts and manage their concerns.

Support was given to Mr. Fischer by acknowledging that he was a very loving father but that he could not realistically prevent the anxiety and conflict his daughters were experiencing. In fact, his openness with his daughters was a rarer asset than his desire to protect them from truth so they would not suffer. He was assured that other team members would be encouraged to provide emotional support to his entire family, thus allowing him to share the responsibility rather than carry the burden of thinking he had to effectively manage both their and his anxiety.

Next, he talked about some of the "unknowns" associated with his surgery. For example, what would he look like following the partial removal of his tongue and jaw? Would his facial structure be significantly altered? Would the removal of the mandible leave a sunken spot along the jaw line? How much speech would he lose due to impairment of his tongue? How would the surgery affect his eating habits? Would he ever be able to wear dentures again?

Although he could describe where the incision was to be made, there still was concern about the amount of scarring that would occur. Would he be able to withstand the pain? Once he had a tracheostomy, how would he communicate? Was there a danger of choking? How difficult would breathing be? What if he vomited? Did suctioning hurt? How would he look with his jaw wired together?

Would his family be able to accept physical changes in his personal appearance? Would his wife want to kiss him? Although he knew the surgery would impact his self-concept, his age would help to minimize negative ramifications. He was more concerned with the quality of his life than with physical appearance. Also, he believed his wife would not treat him any differently in terms of his masculinity. She would continue to love him, and they would continue their physical intimacy; however, the latter would realistically be affected until he satisfac-

MENTAL HEALTH ASSESSMENT

Identifying Data

Date of Admission _____

Date of Interview _____

NAME *Ralph Fischer*

SEX ___*M*___ AGE ___*79*___ BIRTHDATE ___*7/17/02*___

MARITAL STATUS ___*M*___ RELIGION *Protestant*

OCCUPATION *P.T. worker at collection agency*

DIAGNOSIS *Recurrent squamous cell carcinoma of the left lateral tongue and alveolar ridge*

SOCIAL SECURITY NUMBER *351-13-9167*

RACE/CULTURE *Caucasian*

EDUCATIONAL BACKGROUND *High school - grade 10*

FINANCIAL STATUS *$25,000+ / yr. / S.S. after 65*

ALLERGIES *Ethanol; penicillin*

CHIEF COMPLAINT (IN QUOTES) *"Mass on left side of jaw, plus tenderness"*

1. **Physical Appearance** (a brief description including height, weight, bodily functions, energy level, sleep patterns, and dress)
   5'7"   182 lbs   well-groomed, elderly gentleman; pale, cold, clammy skin; c/o stiff neck due to tension and fatigue due to stress associated with illness; averaging 5 hrs. of sleep at night; wearing pajamas and robe from home.

2. **Motor Ability** (posture, gait, gestures)
   Posture erect and straight; proud bearing; some agitation of hands; general restlessness; slow gait; mild mannered.

3. **Sensory Ability** (see, hear, touch, taste, smell)
   Limited vision in both eyes due to cataracts and macular degeneration. Other senses intact. Responsive to touch.

4. **Level of Consciousness**
   Responsive to:

   Verbal stimuli ___*X*___ Noxious stimuli _____

   Touch _____ Unresponsive _____

5. **Orientation**   Person ___*X*___ Place ___*X*___ Time ___*X*___

6. **Memory**   Recent ___*X*___ Past ___*X*___

7. **Intelligence** (cite supporting data)
   Good - well read; 10th grade high school education only but regards self as committed to taking advantage of ongoing adult continuing-education opportunities.

8. **Fund of Information**
   General _____
   About illness (state specifics) Very well informed about his cancer, scheduled surgery, possible postoperative complications, anticipated surgical outcomes, and possible negative consequences as well as positive. Previous surgical experiences provided him with a good knowledge base of what to expect intraoperatively. Seeks additional data when questions arise.

9. **Judgment/Insight** (cite supporting data)
   Good judgment relative to changes in lifestyle that might result as consequence of surgery. Won't have surgery if positive indicators of metastatic cancer are found on CT scan. Realizes death might be an outcome due to age and condition. Has insight as to historical events that might have contributed to current health status. Also, aware of specific concerns that precipitate current emotional and behavioral patterns.

10. **Thought Process**
    Logical ___*X*___ Coherent ___*X*___ Relevant ___*X*___

    Unusual patterns (cite supporting data) No gross distortion noted. Is not evasive or guarded. Occasional evidence of irrational thinking, especially in relation to need to protect wife and daughters and exaggerated concerns about loss of control or being left alone, including being abandoned in a nursing home.

11. **Speech Pattern** (speed, comprehensiveness, spontaneity)
    Rapid pace but quality of speech activity good in terms of clarity, pitch, loudness, and tone. No unusual words or phrases. No evidence of made-up language. Words were not misused or transposed.

Figure 5.3. Mental health assessment. Reprinted with permission from the August issue of Nursing 79. *Copyright © 1979, Intermed Communications Inc. All rights reserved. (continued)*

12. **Ideation** (cite supporting data)   Self-destructive/suicidal _____
No self-destructive or suicidal thoughts were noted.   Suspicious/paranoid _____
Realistic regarding desire to enhance quality of remaining life, yet accepts death as a possible outcome. Recognizes impact of surgery on self-concept/body image but believes his age mitigates some of negative impact of disfigurement. No suspicious/paranoid thinking.

13. **Affect** (cite supporting data)
Feelings of sadness, frustration, powerlessness, guilt, helplessness manifested through anxious, depressive-dependent and withdrawn behavioral patterns - feelings of anger denied - affect appears realistic, for most part, given circumstances.

14. **Family and Significant Others**
   A. Position in family _Oldest son of 4 children, 2 sisters and 1 brother are living_

   B. Others in family _5 sons and 2 daughters, plus wife are living_

   C. Living arrangements _home in upper middle class neighborhood in large, metropolitan city._

   D. Role/roles in family _husband, father, breadwinner_

   E. Significant others _Neighbors, work colleagues_

   F. Other Support systems _none mentioned_

   G. Interactional ability _good, very authentic, strong sense of honesty, aware that anxious and depressive behaviors are affecting his spontaneity in terms of volume of conversation, responsive to others but initiating fewer interactions._

15. **Addictive/Coping Habits and Amounts** (positive and negative)
   A. Smoking _prior to 1955_   Amount _2 packs x 19 yrs, plus cigars and pipe_

   B. Alcohol __0__ Amount __0__ Frequency __0__

   C. Medications (list all: over the counter, legal, illegal)

   D. Food intake _Normal_   Amount _Appropriate quantities_   When _Regular meals some snacks_

   E. Other _____

16. **Sexual Functioning**
Does not perceive that his masculinity will be negatively impacted due to his close relationship with wife and family. Realizes that serious disfigurement or disability could make him feel less of a man if he allowed such thoughts to dominate his thinking processes. Believes his wife will be affectionate and nurturing in many ways, including sexual intimacy. Verbalized that sexual intercourse had decreased during past 8 years due to many factors and that surgery would not adversely affect present patterns of sexual intimacy.

17. **Need Level**
Physiological, safety, love and belonging, and esteem

18. **Developmental Level**
Mature, elderly man with minimal regression

19. **Coping Devices and Defense Mechanisms** (assess for effectiveness, usefulness, and appropriateness)
Ventilation of feelings. Use of touch. Appropriate increase in dependent behavior. Stoicism. Quiet time to allow introspection about illness. Protective behavior toward wife and daughters. Use of repression and introjection in terms of defense mechanisms.

20. **Assets, Resources, Interests**
Supportive wife and family. Realistic view of cancer and his specific diagnosis. Open discussion of concerns. Willingness to be an active participant in his care. Excellent rapport with physician and nursing staff. Desire to live a full, productive life, including returning to work on a part-time basis. Acceptance of limitations.

21. **Impression/Nursing Diagnoses**
Impression: 79 year old white male responding with depressive behavior to pending changes in lifestyle and altered body image due to anticipated surgical intervention for recurrent cancer.

Other behavioral patterns (anxious, dependent and withdrawn) appear related to possible losses associated with illness, hospitalization, surgery, and unknown outcomes.

NGS DX: Psychological disequilibrium (depressive behavior) related to anticipated changes in body image and self-concept, ↑ powerlessness and dependency, ↑ anxiety associated with the absence of known surgical outcomes, pending lifestyle changes, and possibility of death.

Figure 5.3. (continued)

torily recovered from the postoperative period. He anticipated that most family members would ultimately be able to accept any permanent disfigurement. Initially, they might feel sorry for him, but they would not coddle him.

Another major concern related to Mr. Fischer's perception that he would need to be more dependent upon others. He understood that his postoperative recovery period would be quite long. He worried about the loss of autonomy and control. He anticipated that he would feel powerless, especially during the period when his jaws were wired and he had a tracheostomy. He would be dependent upon others to critically monitor him. They would even need to feed him and suction him if he were to survive.

Because of his wife's precarious health, he did not want to become a burden to her. He believed that his complex care might contribute to physical exhaustion on her part, despite assistance from health care professionals. Because she did not drive, he also wondered about transportation for her between their home and the hospital. This concern appeared to mask an underlying fear of being left alone. Again, he saw this fear as irrational in part because family members would most likely stagger the time spent with him in order to be supportive.

He definitely did not want to be placed in a nursing home for recovery. Such action symbolized total loss of control. Confrontation occurred as to how realistic his belief was. Discussion ensued as to dependency needs during illness and how appropriately to meet those needs. Methods for facilitating involvement in decision making were stressed. Mr. Fischer was encouraged to be an active participant in his care as much as possible.

He did have some financial concerns, since he realized that Medicare would probably not cover all his debts. Some of the extensive dental reconstruction would be in addition to normal allowable hospitalization expenses. Surgery would also prevent him from working for a period of time. This would reduce his income at a critical time. He realized that his large family would assist him economically if necessary, but he took pride in being financially independent.

Finally, Mr. Fischer recognized that his age and condition required him to "face the possibility of his death." He planned to discuss with his family that evening his feelings about dying, as well as personal preferences regarding the management of his death. Although he was aware that he was probably not the best candidate for such extensive surgery (left hemiglossectomy, left hemimandibulectomy, left radical neck dissection with tracheostomy), he be-lieved he should "take a chance if anything could be done to improve his condition." Also, it was imperative to recover, if he could, so he would be able to care for his wife, who was in poor health. Still, what if things went wrong and he was disabled or died? Would surgery have been worth the risks? Periodically, he worried about his wife's ability to withstand the shock of his being severely disabled or dying. He knew she had a strong character, but would the grief be temporarily overwhelming? Would such a crisis precipitate a decline in her health status?

Throughout the interview, Mr. Fischer's anxiety level ranged from mild to moderate. For the most part, he was able to talk about his apprehensions. Occasionally, he minimized the seriousness of his condition. Data was sometimes condensed in a simplistic manner that reflected selective inattention. This was most evident when he talked about death. It was more difficult to listen to the interviewer and to explore alternatives. Things were viewed in a more "black-and-white" perspective. His anxiety diminished his ability to perceive all events accurately.

Mr. Fischer verbalized that he saw himself coping by becoming more introverted, quiet, withdrawn, and silent. He and his family were able to express caring and tenderness through touch. He was extremely grateful that they were so close. Still, he worried that he would experience some depression postoperatively. In reality, he appeared to be struggling with depressive behavior preoperatively as well. The interviewer acknowledged that he was facing a number of losses, even though some were anticipated to be temporary, and that feelings of sadness and powerlessness were normal given the circumstances. He was encouraged to vent such feelings as well as any anger or guilt he might experience. The interviewer reminded him of the hopeful aspects of his surgery and assured him that he would be well taken care of during the intraoperative and postoperative phases. He would not be with strangers in the operating room, since he would know his surgeon, anesthesiologist, and operating room nurses.

Upon conclusion of the interview, the nurse completed a mental health assessment form (see Fig. 5.3). In many institutions, this data is combined on a form along with physiological information in order to expedite documentation. Fig. 5.3 concisely illustrates many of the components that need to be examined within the context of performing a mental status assessment.

References

1. Aguilera, D., and Messick, J. *Crisis Intervention: Theory and Methodology*. St. Louis: C. V. Mosby, 1982.
2. Caplan, G. *An Approach to Community Mental Health*. New York: Grune and Stratton, 1961.
3. May, R. *The Meaning of Anxiety*. New York: Ronald Press, 1950.
4. Bowlby, J. *Separation, Anxiety, and Anger*. New York: Basic Books, 1973.
5. "Anxiety: Recognition and intervention. Programmed Instruction." *Am J Nurs* 65:134, 1965.
6. Neal, M., Cohen, P., Cooper, P., and Reighley, J. *Nursing Care Planning Guides for Psychiatric and Mental Health Care*. Pacific Palisades, Calif.: Nurseco, 1981.
7. Arieti, S., and Bemporad, J. *Severe and Mild Depression*. New York: Basic Books, 1978.
8. Kubler-Ross, E. *On Death and Dying*. New York: Macmillan, 1969.
9. Engel, G. "Grief and grieving." *Am J Nurs* 65:93, 1965.
10. Elkins, Doc, ed. *Self Concept Sourcebook: Ideas and Activities for Building Self-Esteem*. Rochester, N.Y.: Growth Associates, 1979.
11. Grimes, J., and Iannopollo, E. *Health Assessment in Nursing Practice*. Monterey, Calif.: Wadsworth Health Sciences Division, 1982.
12. Calderone, M. "SIECUS as a voluntary health organization." *Calif School Health* (January):7, 1967.
13. Sex Information and Education Council of the United States. *Sexuality and Man*. New York: Charles Scribner's Sons, 1970.
14. Malasanos, L., Barkauskas, V., Moss, M., and Stoltenberg-Allen, K. *Health Assessment*. St. Louis: C. V. Mosby, 1981.
15. Ellis, A., and Harper, R. *A New Guide to Rational Living*. North Hollywood, Calif.: Wilshire Book Co., 1975.
16. Mckay, M., Davis, M., and Fanning, P. *Thoughts and Feelings: The Art of Cognitive Stress Intervention*. Richmond, Calif.: New Harbinger Publications, 1981.
17. Bates, B. *A Guide to Physical Examination*. Philadelphia: J. B. Lippincott Company, 1979.
18. Reynolds, J., and Logsdon, J. "Assessing your patient's mental status." *Nurs 79* 9:26, 1979.

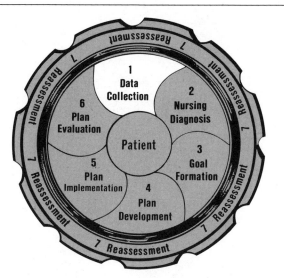

The circular diagram labels, reading around:

1 Data Collection
2 Nursing Diagnosis
3 Goal Formation
4 Plan Development
5 Plan Implementation
6 Plan Evaluation
Patient
Reassessment

Assessment includes information about the patient's physical condition.

Collecting Physiological Data

The perioperative nurse plays a major role in providing safe care for the patient having surgery. To accomplish this goal requires using the nursing process as it pertains specifically to surgical patients. Chapter 4 presents an overview of assessment, outlining the two components, collecting information and formulating a nursing diagnosis. Chapter 5 deals specifically with the psychological data and the perioperative nurse's role. This chapter focuses on the physical data that pertains to the time period surrounding the patient's surgery.

Data collection begins in the operating room before the nurse goes to the unit or holding area to see the patient. It is done in a sequential manner as the nurse moves from the operating room to the patient care unit, emergency room, and outpatient or holding area. Activities performed by the nurse as he obtains data include sorting and interpreting data already obtained by other members of the health care team, obtaining new data from the patient, and performing a physical examination. All this is done to establish a presurgical baseline for setting realistic goals relative to the impending surgery.

Collecting Data

SOURCES

Operating Room Schedule
The operating room schedule provides information regarding the patient's age, sex, planned

operative procedure, surgeon, and anesthesiologist. The operating room nurse begins analysis of this information before he even sees his patient. For example, a tonsillectomy will alert the operating room nurse to check the patient's bleeding time as well as the hemoglobin and hematocrit levels because he knows that this procedure may result in large amounts of blood loss. He also knows that he will need to check the patient's range of motion because the neck will be hyperextended in positioning.

PATIENT RECORD

Next, the operating room nurse reviews the patient's chart at the unit nurse's station. The first thing the operating room nurse looks for is the informed consent for surgery (see Fig. 6.1). He checks to see that the procedure the patient has listed on the consent agrees with the operating room schedule. Another important point when checking the permit is that the correct side, if applicable, is listed. Consent forms are a legal agreement between the patient and the hospital. The nurse should be familiar with the consents used by his hospital. He needs to be aware of protocol, including any state regulations to which he must adhere. For instance, hospitals routinely require the patient or his legal representative to sign an admission agreement. The agreement specifies the type of routine nursing care the patient can expect to receive and the collection of specimens that may be necessary for laboratory and x-ray studies. In turn, the patient agrees to accept responsibility for payment. The agreement provides for the release of certain information to insurance companies, workmen's compensation, and other similar agencies.

The nurse needs to know which diagnostic procedures require an operative consent. Generally any procedure that uses an instrument or introduces a substance into one of the patient's body spaces or cavities will require a consent. This includes bone marrow punctures, cardiac catheterizations, myelograms, and insertion of subclavian catheters.

Informed Consents for Surgery or Diagnostic Procedures
Legally, the person placing his signature on

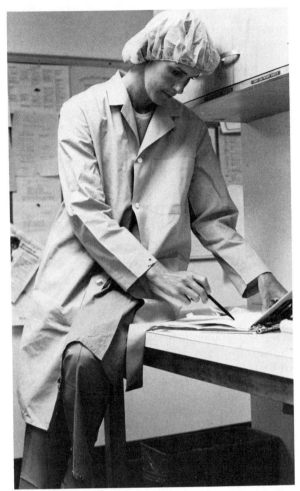

Figure 6.1. *Careful review of the operative consent is necessary to protect the patient's right to informed consent. Consent forms also prevent operative errors and protect personnel and hospitals from lawsuits.*

this type of consent must understand the need for the procedure, what is involved, the risks, expected results, and alternative treatments, as well as the disposition of specimens, if any. Although the physician performing the procedure is responsible for required explanations, the nurse may need to assess the patient's level of understanding and readiness to sign the consent form. In the preoperative interview, the nurse might ask the patient, "What do you understand about your operation?" If the patient does not have an adequate understanding of the procedure, the nurse may request the physician to talk again with the patient. An individual must sign the consent himself if: (1) he is of legal age (varies with states); (2) he is under age but has a valid marriage certificate; (3) he has been designated an emancipated minor (certain states); and (4) he is not presently under legal guardianship. The consent form must be signed by a parent or legal guardian if the patient is a minor or legally considered to be incompetent and is not included in any of the above categories. The nurse must examine the document for the correct date, time, and signatures, which must be in ink (black ink may be necessary for microfilm copying). Consent forms may have a time limit such as 30 days.

Emergency Consent

In a life-or-death situation in which surgical intervention is required and the patient is unable to sign a consent, the surgeon may legally proceed. Every effort must be made, however, to obtain permission from a responsible family member by telegram, telephone, or in certain states by a court order.

In the case of a telephone consent, two witnesses must hear the oral consent of the family member or responsible party and sign the consent form with the name of the responsible party, noting that it is an oral consent by telephone. The surgeon may record the necessity for surgical intervention without obtaining a proper consent in the doctor's progress notes. This may release the hospital, operating room nurses, and other personnel from liability.

Sterility Consents

The nurse should be aware of procedures that require an additional consent form, for example, vasectomy, tubal ligation by laparotomy or laparoscopy, and hysterectomy. The nurse needs to know who is responsible for signing, that is, husband and wife or only the individual having the procedure. The nurse should also be aware of any age cutoff for sterility consent. For a woman over 60 years of age such consent is not required.

Photograph Consent

If the surgeon plans to photograph part or all of the surgical procedure, prior permission from the patient is usually required. A special consent form may be available, or the surgeon may add it to the informed operative consent.

When dealing with consents, the nurse must understand the legal ramifications of his involvement. He must know and follow hospital policies and procedures. By doing so, he will be able to protect himself in the event of a lawsuit (1).

Next the perioperative nurse reviews the history and physical completed by the primary physician. He notes the patient's chief complaint and the reason he is now having surgery. A brief history of the present illness gives the nurse some indication of the value the patient places on health prevention and wellness. If the existing illness has been long term, say 10 years prior to seeking medical advice, the nurse should seek out information to provide reasons for not seeking medical attention earlier. The history of the present illness also provides, from the patient's and physician's perspective, the signs and symptoms that form the basis for the medical diagnosis. Other information important to the operating room nurse is the medical history that outlines the types of surgery the patient has had previously and the complications that may indicate potential problems for present illness and impending surgery. Medications the patient has been taking are of vital importance. Certain medications are contraindicated for patients having anesthesia. Some medications such as coumadin and heparin, which are blood thinners, should be stopped prior to surgery. The potential increased bleeding may cause a complication, which could be irreversible. A review of body systems allows the nurse to collect information that could affect transportation of the patient to surgery, positioning, and other nursing activities performed in the operating room. The physician's physical examination provides information about the physical structure of the patient and a description of the area or body part where existing pathology is located. As the perioperative nurse reviews the history and physical, he makes notes that he uses as he continues to validate all the data obtained from the various sources. It may also be necessary to clarify or provide a more indepth understanding of data that indicate potential complications or problems if corrective action is not implemented. The nurse may seek further clarification from the physician or other members of the health care team.

A review of other documents in the patient record such as consultation notes provides meaningful data related to the impending surgery. The physician's admission note and initial orders give some indication of the medical treatment regime and give the nurse additional data to use in collecting the physiological information.

Diagnostic reports include the admission chest x-ray. If the patient's chest film shows abnormalities, it can have far-reaching implications. Patients with tuberculosis and other infectious disease present a major hazard to other patients and staff in the operating room. Laboratory reports are reviewed by the perioperative nurse to determine such things as electrolyte balance. Chapter 10 discusses the preoperative normal values of electrolytes and how an imbalance has the potential for intraoperative and postoperative complications. Bleeding times are important to assess, as well as the urinalysis and complete blood count. Information about existing infections and abnormalities should be detected, recorded, and communicated to the physician.

A nursing history and baseline assessment will give the perioperative nurse an overview of the patient at the time of admission. This data might include a general review of systems, chief complaint, physical status, habits, daily routines, sleep patterns, nutrition, physical limitations, and prosthetic devises. The nurse makes note of factors affecting the surgery and validates them at a later time with the unit nurse, patient, or family. A complete review of the patient record gives the nurse necessary background information to formulate a nursing diagnosis.

PATIENT INTERVIEW

The next step is the patient interview, which often includes family members or friends. Rel-

atives and friends can be helpful during the interview by providing additional information. There are times, however, when their presence can be distracting or cause the patient to withhold information. The operating room nurse must use judgment when deciding whether they should remain in the room.

In the patient interview, the operating room nurse is specifically looking for objective and subjective data that will help him to plan the intraoperative nursing care. He validates information collected from the patient response. He looks for information regarding height and weight, vital signs, history, and presence of chronic illness. He checks for any alterations in skin integrity (see Fig. 6.2), restrictions in range of motion, or other physical handicaps. He observes if there are any sensory distortions, especially visual or hearing impairment. He asks about medication, soap, or tape allergies, and any specific problems related to previous surgery or anesthesia. He also asks about prosthetic devices and observes for the presence of tubes, drains, parenteral fluid lines, and monitoring lines such as arterial, Swan-Ganz, pulmonary artery, or central venous pressure lines. He determines if there is any alteration in fluid and electrolyte levels and asks if the patient is taking any medications. During the interview, the nurse assesses the patient's level of orientation and notes his cultural and language background.

Through questioning, the nurse will determine the patient's learning needs and what coping mechanisms he uses (see Chapter 5). Chapter 9 discusses the learning needs of the surgical patient and the nurse's role in providing an explanation of what will occur throughout his surgical experience.

FAMILY AND SIGNIFICANT OTHERS

Family members or individuals who are close to the patient often have pertinent information that completes the perioperative nurse's data collection. The nurse can determine the family's beliefs about health, the importance of health to the family, the health practices they employ in the home, who influences what occurs, and the importance placed on wellness and prevention of illness. Through information

The nurse on the surgical unit contributes significantly to the collection of data and the validation of data already collected. These nurses have obtained the initial patient information, and the perioperative nurse uses their knowledge to complete patient data.

Collecting data enables the perioperative nurse to make a nursing diagnosis, set goals, and plan intraoperative care for the patient. The nurse in the operating room works closely with the anesthesiologist in the intraoperative setting. The anesthesiologist frequently depends upon the nurse's expertise and ability to respond quickly when assisting him in a crisis. The more information the nurse can collect about his patient, the more prepared he will be to handle the patient's intraoperative needs, including any crisis situations. This is illustrated in Table 6.1 which depicts the data obtained, validating information, and the activities performed by the perioperative nurse that directly affect the care patients receive intraoperatively.

Just as the patient's blood pressure, pulse, and respirations are the vital signs of life, so must the nurse equate collection of data as one of the vital elements of the nursing process. It is inconceivable that a patient's vital signs would be taken only once during the length of hospital stay. So too with obtaining data. It must be ongoing to validate patient care. The nurse is involved in continual collection of data. Because of his professional experience, he has the analytical capability of sorting the data, categorizing it, and recognizing what is pertinent. He helps to promote continuity of care by documentation of his findings.

Patient Situation

The operating room schedule is posted, and the nurse preparing to do perioperative assessments begins to collect necessary information. One of the patients scheduled for tomorrow is Mr. Fischer. The nurse notes his room number and that he is 79 years old. The schedule states that the operative procedure will be a left hemiglossectomy, left hemi-

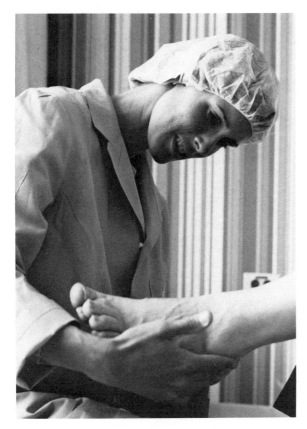

Figure 6.2. Data collection in regard to the integrity of the patient's skin is vital to its protection during the operative procedure. Actual or potential problems are identified so appropriate treatment can be implemented.

obtained from the family, the nurse can predict what might occur postoperatively during recovery. The nurse is concerned about the patient's nutritional habits because they affect wound healing and maintenence of skin integrity. A male patient says he eats well-balanced meals, but his wife says that her husband doesn't eat well, and his diet is not balanced—"He doesn't eat green vegetables, just meat and potatoes."

Thus, in this situation, the nurse will take into account the subjective statements of both the patient and his wife but relay on objective data that he collects. These data include laboratory tests, physical assessment, and the observation of what the patient eats at meal times.

Table 6.1. *Physiological Data, Validating Information, and Nursing Response.*

Data	Validating Information	Nursing Response
Allergies	Medications (antibiotics, narcotics, etc.).	Confirm allergy or sensitivity with patient and communicate to other members of health care team (surgeon, anesthesiologist, scrub nurse, relief personnel, etc.).
	Soap (povidone-iodine, hexachlorophene, baby shampoo).	Check with patient as to what type of reaction occurs and with what agents. Have alternate prepping solutions available. Note reaction, if any, to prep solution and handle necessary documentation and communication to appropriate personnel (i.e., RR, floor).
	Tape (adhesive, plastic, paper, elastoplast, ribbon).	Check with patient as to what type of reaction occurs and communicate to surgeon and anesthesiologist, and RR.
Previous problems with surgery or anesthesia	Patient or family member has a history of excessive blood loss during surgery.	Check current hemoglobin and hematocrit levels. Check for coagulation studies (i.e., ptt); communicate history of blood loss to surgeon and anesthesiologist and check to see if coagulation studies will be required. Monitor blood loss carefully.
	Patient or immediate family member has a history of hyperthermia under anesthesia.	Communicate to anesthesiologist. Have supplies available for possible malignant hyperthermia reaction, including new anesthesia machine tubes, mask, and bag. Have IV Dantrium available. Observe hospital protocol to be followed in the event of such a reaction.
	Patient or immediate family member with history of pseudocholinesterase (low level of enzyme necessary for reversal of anesthetic paralyzing agents—Anectine).	Communicate to anesthesiologist potential need for nerve stimulator. Communicate to RR and/or ICU possibility of postop mechanical ventilation.
	History of postop nausea and vomiting.	Communicate to anesthesiologist and RR potential need for antiemetic drugs. Communicate to surgeon that IV therapy may need to be maintained until patient is able to tolerate oral intake of fluids.
Skin integrity	Rash.	Presence preoperatively will rule out a reaction to anesthetic agents, as well as other medications given in the intraoperative period.
	Decubitus ulcer.	Will require positioning devices to keep pressure off, such as a foam ring, air or flotation mattress.
	Poor turgor.	Potential dehydration and electrolyte imbalance will require careful monitoring of intake and output, and ECG monitoring (potential cardiac arrhythmias).
	Bruising.	Potential bleeding problems will require careful monitoring of blood loss and increased need for replacement. Avoid placement of electrocautery grounding pad over ecchymotic areas to prevent further injury. Use care in moving bruised areas due to possibility of associated tenderness or pain.
	Excoriation 2° to colostomy, ileo-loop conduit, etc.	Increased risk for reaction to prepping solution. Increased risk for infection.
Limited range of motion and physical handicaps	Rheumatoid arthritis.	Potential need for positioning devices to maintain body alignment (i.e., wrist and finger rolls, sandbags, foot board)

Table 6.1. (*Continued*)

Data	Validating Information	Nursing Response
		Potential difficulty with IV and Foley insertion. Potential difficulty with stirrup positioning. Quads.
	Paralysis (2° to stroke trauma, disease—M.S., myasthenia gravis, polio, etc.).	Presence should be noted preoperatively to rule out neuromuscular damage to positioning and length of procedure postoperatively. Need for extra assistance in moving patient. Avoid placement of electrocautery grounding pad over desensitized areas. Increased safety needs of the patient.
	Decreased range of motion of cervical spine.	Potential difficulty with endotracheal intubation. Potential problems with positioning. Increased safety needs.
	Total joint replacement (i.e., total hip, knee, wrist, metacarpal, etc.).	Move joint slowly and carefully. Increased safety needs.
Prosthetic devices	Glass eye, artificial limb, orthopedic hardware (i.e., traction device, internal fixation devices, total joint replacement prostheses).	Potential need for removal. Awareness of internal prosthetic devices with regard to positioning. Plan for extra time when transporting patients with external fixation devices.
Medications	Heparin or coumadin.	Check for blood coagulation studies (ptt, prox). Check for H & H. Assess skin for bruising. Potential need for blood replacement. Monitor blood loss carefully.
	Dilantin.	Be aware that other drugs may potentiate serum drug levels (alcohol, anticoag). Presence of liver and/or kidney disease can also potentiate the serum drug level.
Tubes, drains, IVs monitoring lines	NG tube.	Potential abnormality of electrolyte levels which could in turn produce cardiac arrhythmias. Increased risk of dehydration.
	Arterial line.	Risk of air embolus. Have essential equipment ready for monitoring intraoperatively.
Height and weight	Obesity.	Need for additional positioning equipment to maintain proper body alignment. Be aware of increased risk for infection, cardiovascular problems, respiratory disturbance, etc.
	Excessive height.	Need for table extension to maintain proper body alignment.
Vital signs	Tachypnea.	Assess normalcy for pt. Check pulmonary tests and/or ABG's for abnormal gas concentrations (if not ordered, check with anesthesiologist).
History and presence of chronic illness	Hypertension.	Be aware of medical regimen of patient (meds., exercise, etc.). Potential need for vasopressor drugs (availability of equipment—IVAC, etc.). Check electrolyte levels, esp. K and Na. Potential need for electrolyte replacement.
	Asthma.	Be aware of date and severity of last attack. Be aware of medical regimen (meds., exercise tolerance, etc.). Potential need for bronchodilator drugs.

Table 6.1. (Continued)

Data	Validating Information	Nursing Response
		Check pulmonary tests and/or ABG's for abnormal gas concentrations. Potential needs for oxygen therapy during transport to OR.
	Congestive heart failure.	Check CXR for pleural effusion, degree of cardiac enlargement, etc., and plan care accordingly. Potential for confusion due to cerebral hypoxia. Be aware that restraint may agitate patient and increase cardiac workload. Need for bladder catheterization due to potential need for diuresis. Potential need for cardiac drugs, equipment, etc. Monitor ECG. Potential need for transport to OR on oxygen and life support system (LifePak).
	Diabetes mellitus.	Assess for peripheral vascular disease and peripheral neuropathy. Check pedal pulses; check for ulcerations and presence of infection in feet and legs. Note impaired sensation of feet, fingers, and toes; avoid placement of bovie over desensitive area). Be alert for changes in visual acuity (alteration in glucose levels will produce blurring). Assess presence of lesions of mouth which could interfere with intubation. Check medical regimen (type of meds., dosage, and frequency). Potential for evaluation of blood sugar levels intraop, with subsequent intervention if abnormality presents.
	Myocardial infarction.	Assess patient's current cardiac status by checking ECG, lab, medical clearance for surgery, etc. Increased risk for thromboembolus and potential need for antiembolus stockings. Be aware that cold temperatures can cause vasoconstriction. Need for careful monitoring of ECG if recent: patient may need to be transported on oxygen and life support system. Check ABG's for abnormal acid/base concentrations. Potential need for cardiac emergency drugs and equipment. Be aware that noxious stimuli (loud noises, cold environment, sudden movement or touch, etc.) as well as increased anxiety levels may produce angina and lead to MI (2,3)

mandibulectomy, and left radical neck dissection with tracheostomy. General anesthesia will be administered by Dr. Barry. The surgeon is Dr. Bates, and Dr. Schell will be assisting.

After writing this information on the operating room patient care plan under data collection, the nurse goes to the surgical unit where Mr. Fischer has been admitted. Here the nurse reviews his record and examines Mr. Fischer's surgical consent form. The informed consent states that Mr. Fischer has received an explanation of the proposed operation and has been given the opportunity to question anything he did not understand. Mr. Fischer has signed the form, which has been witnessed by a nurse. The form is dated and includes the time of completion.

The patient's history and physical state the chief complaint as being recurrent carcinoma of the left lateral tongue and alveolar ridge. The patient has a history of carcinoma. Three years previously, he had a subtotal colectomy for adenocarcinoma of the colon. He sought medical treatment approximately one year ago with a small ulcerative lesion on the left tongue. At that time, he underwent laser vaporization of the lesion, which was identified as an epidermoid carcinoma. One month later, he had further laser vaporization of the lesion. Approximately seven months later, he had an area of abnormal mucosa over the left inferior alveolar ridge excised. Recent pain and tenderness in the same area brought Mr. Fischer back to his physician. A biopsy revealed squamous cell carcinoma.

The nurse reviews allergies in the history. Mr. Fischer states a present allergy to ethanol and a possible pencillin allergy. He had not had penicillin in years. The nurse notes the allergy in the data collection section on the operating room patient care plan. The patient's father died at age 82 of natural causes, and his mother died of carcinoma of the liver. There is no history of tuberculosis, diabetes, heart disease, hypertension, or blood dyscrasia in the family. Reviewing the systems, the nurse finds no further pertinent information with the exception of the present node in his jaw. The patient has trace edema in both legs, which the nurse notes on the data collection form.

Diagnostic data include a chest x-ray with no significant abnormalities and a panorex of the mandible. There was no evidence of bone destruction to suggest invasion of the mandible by the existing tissue neoplasm. Admission laboratory data show the patient's chemistry to be within normal limits. Urinanalysis was within normal limits, complete blood count was normal, as was the coagulogram. Blood has been ordered, and the type and crossmatch was compatable for type O positive.

The nursing history provides some additional facts about Mr. Fischer. Mr. Fischer's temperature is 99.1°F; pulse, 84; respirations, 20. His blood pressure is 120/70. He is 5 feet 7½ inches tall and weighs 182 pounds. He wears glasses and dentures. Other data include his sleep patterns, diet and elimination habits, and daily personal hygiene. The nurse adds the vital signs and the information about glasses and dentures to the data. Other data included in the nursing history do not seem pertinent to the surgery.

The unit nurse offers additional data regarding the relationship of Mr. and Mrs. Fischer. They seem to be a close couple who depend a great deal on each other for their individual as well as mutual need. The unit nurse also says that some of the family members were not in favor of the impending procedure. They believe it to be too radical and question the outcome, whereas Mr. Fischer seems to believe that if anything can be done he should take the chance, and he is convinced his surgeon and other physicians are directing him in the right way. The nurse on the surgical unit stated that Mr. Fischer is a man who had a lot of determination and will, which may influence the outcome of his surgery.

With this information, the nurse from the operating room approaches Mr. Fischer's room. When he walks in he finds Mrs. Fischer sitting beside the bed, the couple holding hands and talking. As he enters, they greet him cordially and he makes his initial observation. He notes that Mr. Fischer is a well-developed, well-nourished, white man, who is not in acute distress. He looks a little younger than his age. His hair is white, he wears glasses, and he has a pleasant manner. Mrs. Fischer is shorter than he is and appears thin and somewhat frail. The nurse asks Mr. Fischer to explain in his own words the reason for his hospitalization and his understanding of the surgical procedure. Mr. Fischer responds, "I'm here to find out what's wrong with me. I have a bad place in my jaw, and the doctor has attempted to get rid of it three times. This time he tells me I will have to have more extensive surgery. I might lose half of my tongue, part of my jaw and my neck. I'm not sure of the extent of all of it, but I know my doctor will do what he can for me. He told me I would have a tracheostomy for a few days." The nurse immediately determines that Mr. Fischer will have a communication problem postoperatively due to the surgical resection, jaw wiring, and tracheostomy.

The nurse continues to gather physical data through observation, interview, and physical examination. He assesses that Mr. Fischer has minimal edema in both lower extremities. This indicates the need for prevention of neuromuscular damage and elastic stockings during the procedure. He also determines that the length of the procedure and the required position may require positioning devices and a padding of various areas intraoperatively. An assessment of the skin shows that he has relatively good turgor, no areas of rash, or excoriations, and that the skin is not impaired in any area. He has no evidence of physical limitations, and his range of motion seems normal. He denies any stiffness in his neck or extremities. Mr. Fischer demonstrates moderate anxiety (discussed in Chapter 5).

The nurse completes obtaining data from Mr. Fischer and tells him he will see him in the operating room. After leaving the room, the nurse completes documenting the data collected and continues to develop the patient care plan.

References

1. Wood, L., and Rambo, B. J. *Nursing Skills for Allied Health Services,* 2nd ed. Philadelphia: W. B. Saunders, 1977.
2. Luckmann, J., and Sorenson, K. C. *Medical-Surgical Nursing,* 2nd ed. Philadelphia: W. B. Saunders, 1980.
3. Neal, M. C., Cohen, P. F., and Cooper, P. G. *Nursing Care Planning Guides 1–25,* 2nd ed. Pacific Palisades, Calif.: Nurseco, 1980.

Suggested Readings

Alexander, C., Schrader, E., and Kneedler, J. "Preoperative visits: The OR nurse unmasks." *AORN J* 19(February):401–412, 1974.

Association of Operating Room Nurses, "Operating room nursing: perioperative role." *AORN J* 27 (May):1156–1175, 1978.

Barnett, L. A. "Preparing your patient for the operating room." *AORN J* 18(September):534–539, 1973.

Davis, J. L. "Preoperative program prepares children for surgery." *AORN J* 26(August):249–256, 1977.

Fehlau, M. T. "Implementation of standards of practice." *AORN J* 22(November):712–718, 1975.

Hercules, P. "OR experience teaches continuity of care." *AORN J* 32(November):799–806, 1980.

Jordan, C. H. "If we teach holistic care, can we exclude perioperative nursing?" *AORN J* 32 (November):797–798, 1980.

Kneedler, J. A., Reed, E. A., Manuel, B. J., and Fehlau, M. T. "From standards into practice." *AORN J* 28(October):603–642, 1978.

Laird, M. "Techniques for teaching pre and post-operative patients." *Am J Nurs* 75(August):1338–1340, 1975.

Larke, G. A. "Perioperative charting: OR nursing on display." *AORN J* 31(February):194–198, 1980.

Levine, M. E. "Adaptation and assessment: a rationale for nursing intervention." *Am J Nurs* 66(November):2450–2453, 1966.

Schmitt, F. E., and Wooldridge, P. J. Psychological preparation of surgical patients. *Nurs Res* 22 (March-April):249–256, 1973.

Wittstock, N. J. Preoperative evaluation and physical assessment of the patient. *J Am Assoc Nurse Anes* 49(April):197–206, 1981.

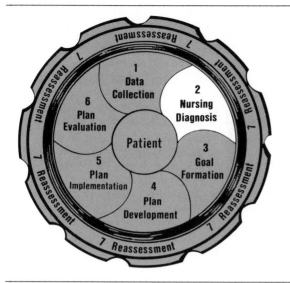

Nursing diagnoses are derived from health status data.

A Nursing Diagnosis

In the nursing process, the outcome of assessment is one or more nursing diagnoses. While assessing a patient's health status to discern actual or potential health problems, the nurse engages in a diagnostic process similar to the one physicians use to diagnose disease or pathology. The diagnostic process involves a systematic search for information that will lead to discovery of a problem or problems. The search in both professions initially takes a broad approach followed by reduction of possible sources for a problem until one becomes reasonably certain the difficulty has been located. Figure 7.1 outlines the sequence of diagnostic steps in nursing.

Although both nurses and physicians use the same diagnostic process for the purpose of treating problems, the focus for each is different. Physicians use a body systems approach; nurses use a functional-dysfunctional health patterns approach. Physicians focus on discovering and treating pathophysiological and pathopsychological problems. Realizing that health management and health conditions influence the quality of human life, nurses have turned their attention to the actions and reactions that take place among individuals families, and their environments. (Environment refers to the internal physical and psychological conditions of human beings as well

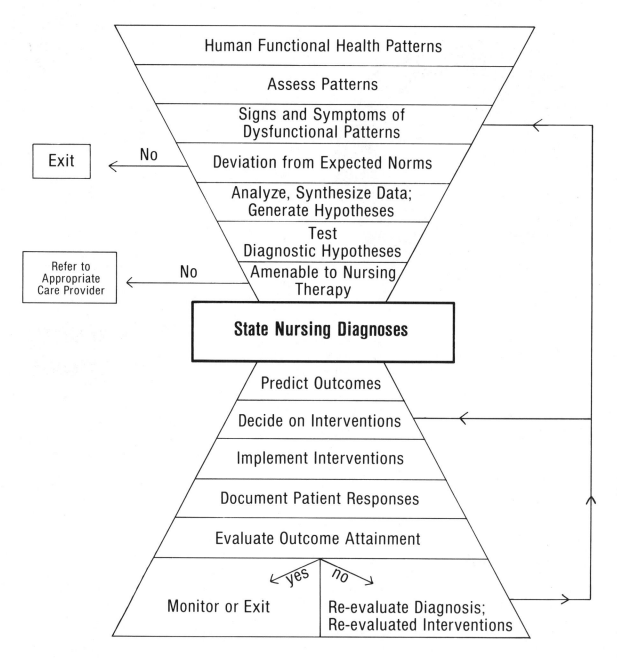

Figure 7.1. Diagnostic steps in nursing process. Adapted from Nursing Diagnosis: Process and Application by Marjorie Gordon. Copyright © 1982 by McGraw-Hill Book Company. Adapted with permission of McGraw-Hill Book Company.

as the external conditions of the surroundings in which human beings live, work, and play.) Unmet health needs create problems, many of which nurses can treat. Identification of these problems is the thrust of the diagnostic process in nursing, and the end products are nursing diagnoses.

Nursing diagnoses are statements about actual or potential health problems that professional nurses, by virtue of their education and experience, are able and licensed to treat. An actual problem is a real difficulty that is preventing an individual or family from responding in a normal, healthy fashion. Potential health problems are those situations in which there are enough symptoms to indicate a high degree of probability that an actual problem could occur in the future.

Only professional nurses can make nursing diagnoses. In most states, professional nurses are accountable by law for directing and supervising the delegated nursing activities of other health care workers. The judgment and decision making involved in determining nursing diagnoses, however, cannot be delegated since the process is primarily mental. Although nonprofessional nursing personnel can make valuable contributions to treatment by carrying out planned interventions and observation of patient reactions, they do so after diagnoses have been made.

Standards of practice and some state nursing practice rules and regulations are encouraging registered (professional) nurses to make nursing diagnoses. These guidelines, and the American Nurses' Association (ANA) *Code for Nurses* (1), are frequently used in courts of law to establish the usual conduct of professional nursing practice.

A nursing diagnosis also represents a class of health problems. It is a label given to a cluster of signs and symptoms. Within such a class, there may be subcategories of related but different health problems. For instance, the diagnostic class potential for injury comprises the subcategories: (1) potential for poisoning, (2) potential for suffocation, and (3) potential for trauma. Classifying and labeling phenomena are a human way of making sense out of the environment to facilitate understanding and communication. Naming health problems treated by nurses serves this purpose. It is a kind of shorthand. A nursing diagnosis, "Impaired physical mobility (level 2) related to postoperative pain," enables a nurse to understand several things about a patient that would otherwise require extensive verbal or written explanation. The nurse will recognize that a patient with this diagnosis needs assistance or supervision from another to physically turn in bed or move about her hospital room (see Table 7.1). Level 2 in the diagnosis signifies that the patient can move although movement causes additional pain. The need for assistance or supervision implies that there is a potential for injury if the patient gets out of bed without another person standing by. The cause of the impaired physical mobility is stated, and in the absence of other contrary diagnoses, either nursing or medical, indicates the patient can be expected to achieve independent movement. The nurse understands that the signs and symptoms of pain with movement are present. Experience with other patients and recall of signs and symptoms of impaired physical mobility and of pain and levels of functional activity enable the nurse to understand what responses can be expected without even seeing the patient.

Structural Elements of Nursing Diagnoses

A nursing diagnosis consists of three structural elements: (1) the problem statement, (2) its etiology, and (3) the defining cluster of signs and symptoms. The problem statement should be clear, precise, and succinct: "Impaired physical mobility (level 2)" and "Impaired verbal communications" are two examples. Certain diagnoses require additional clarifying words so the problem area can be located more precisely. If impaired daily living activities, such as physical mobility and self-care, are the problem, it is necessary to designate the level of impairment using a standard and accepted scheme. Table 7.1 provides such a framework. Other diagnoses, not related to daily living activities, need other clarifying words to indicate the area in which the problem lies. Non-

Table 7.1. Classification of Functional Activity Level.

Score	Activity Level
0	total independence
1	requires use of equipment or assistive device
2	requires assistance or supervision from another person
3	requires assistance or supervision from another person and equipment or device
4	dependent and does not participate in self-care

From Marjorie Gordon. *Nursing Diagnosis: Process and Application*, p. 88. Copyright © 1982 by McGraw-Hill Book Company. Reprinted with permission of McGraw-Hill Book Company.

compliance is one of these. Since noncompliance is a person's informed decision not to adhere to a therapeutic regimen, the diagnosis, "Noncompliance (diabetic diet)," helps nurses understand that the area of difficulty is not in care of the skin or prescribed medication, but in the area of diet.

The second structural component is the etiology or cause of the problem. Etiological indicators consist of patient behaviors, factors in the environment, or an interaction between the two. For instance, with the diagnosis, "Knowledge deficit," possible etiological factors are as follows: (1) lack of exposure, (2) lack of recall, (3) information misinterpretation, (4) cognitive limitation, (5) lack of interest in learning, (6) unfamiliarity with information sources. Without causative reasons, therapy is likely to be hit-and-miss, involving unnecessary time and effort for both patient and nurse. Efficient, effective therapy should focus on the precise need. Table 7.2 gives two other diagnoses with etiological factors and further illustrates the need to narrow the diagnostic focus for adequate planning and interaction.

The final structural part of a nursing diagnosis is the cluster of signs and symptoms characteristic of the category. Just as medical diagnoses have characteristic signs and symptoms, so do nursing diagnoses. The diagnosis, "Alterations in nutrition: more than body requirements," has several signs and symptoms (see Table 7.3). It also has two critical defining characteristics without which the diagnosis cannot be made. If the critical characteristics

are absent, but other noncritical characteristics are present, additional data may indicate that the diagnosis is, "Alterations in nutrition: potential for more than body requirements."

Nurses have just begun naming nursing diagnoses, determining etiological factors, and defining signs and symptoms of diagnostic categories. The examples cited and others have been accepted for validation in clinical practice; however, they have not been published in a taxonomy of diagnoses such as physicians use. Those published in books on nursing diagnoses often need additional work and refinement to be standardized. Consequently, in nursing the field is open for new labels, additional signs and symptoms for ones already identified, and refinement of causative factors. Some already accepted for testing may be discarded or placed in other diagnoses as etiological factors.

Defining Nursing Diagnoses

Could a nurse recognize a nursing diagnosis in a patient's record? Certainly, the presence of the structural components would help identify one. Dispelling a few common misperceptions about nursing diagnoses may also be of benefit. Statements about a patient's therapeutic needs are not diagnoses. "Needs emotional support," and "Turn every two hours" fail to

Table 7.2. Two Nursing Diagnoses with Etiological Factors.

Nursing Diagnosis	Etiological Factors
Impaired physical mobility	therapy/medical regimen pain/discomfort fatigue/decreases strength and endurance trauma lack of physical support neuromuscular impairment psychosocial/depression
Impaired verbal communication	circulatory impairment to brain physical barrier (brain tumor, tracheostomy, intubation) anatomical deficit (cleft palate) psychological barrier (psychosis, lack of stimuli) developmental (age-related)

Table 7.3. Defining Characteristics of the Diagnosis, "Alterations in Nutrition: More than Body Requirements."

Etiology	Defining Characteristics
Excessive intake in relation to metabolic needs	weight 10% over ideal for height and frame weight 20% over ideal for height and frame[a] triceps skinfold greater than 15 mm in men and 25 mm in women[a] sedentary activity level reported or observed dysfunctional eating patterns: pairing food with other activities; concentrating food intake at end of day; eating in response to external cues such as time of day, social situation; eating in response to internal cues other than hunger (anxiety)

[a]Critical defining characteristic.

identify the health problem or its cause, although such statements may indicate ways of treating a problem.

Maslow's hierarchy of human needs (2) and Henderson's basic needs classification (3) furnish nurses with a theoretical framework for their approach to nursing, but they fail to specify patient-oriented health problems. Both frameworks are too general. Every human being, for example, has a need for sleep and rest. Unmet human needs can produce actual or potential health problems, and human needs underlie the functional health patterns approach to assessment, but they in themselves are inadequate to serve as diagnoses.

Just as therapeutic and human needs are not nursing diagnoses, neither are therapeutic nursing or patient goals. Statements such as "to alleviate pain" or "to experience minimal pain" do not tell us anything about the problem causing the pain. Therapeutic goals are derived from nursing diagnoses and, as outcomes, help nurses plan therapeutic measures and evaluate achievement of therapy (see Figure 7.1).

Staff difficulties experienced in treating a patient or managing patient care are not nursing diagnoses. Personnel, for instance, may unethically label a patient as uncooperative, demanding, or stubborn. Such labels, when applied to patients, have no meaning in terms of health problems. In fact, uncooperative, demanding behaviors can be a way of expressing undiagnosed problems and inadequate planning. Such problems are the staff's, not the patient's.

Nursing diagnoses then are not medical diagnoses or tests, treatments, procedures, or equipment. "On respirator," "cholecystectomy," "continuous intravenous therapy" have all been mistakenly referred to as nursing diagnoses. While nurses do make tentative medical diagnoses, these are referred to physicians for affirmative diagnosis and treatment. Certain secondary problems arising from medical diagnoses, complications, tests, and the like, for example, "Fear of death related to surgery," can be treated by nurses. Sometimes symptoms of a medical diagnosis are the same as health problems that nurses treat. For instance, colitis is associated with persistent, copious diarrhea. As a result, the patient with this disease has a high potential for fluid and electrolyte imbalance. Both diarrhea and fluid imbalance are among nursing problem areas. In colitis, however, the symptoms are caused by the pathology. Causative factors are often the source for distinguishing problems treatable by nurses from medical ones.

Just as with medical diagnoses, one or two signs and symptoms do not make a nursing diagnosis—a cluster of related signs and symptoms is needed. Among the cluster must be those that are considered critical, or "defining," signs and symptoms. An actual problem cannot be determined unless the defining characteristics are present. Assumptions based on one or two symptoms are likely to be erroneous and misleading. In the extreme, such assumptions can result in harm to the patient; minimally, they can waste time without patient benefit. A patient might state that she is not concerned with her physical appearance. The nurse cannot automatically think, "Aha, probably a self-image problem," because the statement is only one cue that must be considered in relation to others. (A cue is an indicator that triggers action on the part of the person noting it.) But if the patient is an elected public official, is scheduled for a radical neck dissection, is meticulous in dress, and keeps herself lean and fit, the cluster of cues might perhaps indicate a potential problem in self-image or coping, depending on other cues available.

The diagnostic process is not a series of consecutive, forward steps. It can be separated, however, into four major activities: (1) data collection, (2) interpretation of data, (3) clustering data, and (4) naming the cluster or the problem. These activities may occur simultaneously when the diagnostician is experienced. The nurse may note a cue and almost before the patient is finished speaking or the reading noted process the information mentally. After a blood pressure has been taken, for example, the nurse knows instantaneously whether the systolic and diastolic pressures are within the expected range.

What Data To Collect and How To Collect It

Effective data collection involves knowing what information to collect and how it should be collected. A brief overview of how to collect data is provided in Chapter 4. Chapters 5 and 6 detail what data should be collected for the perioperative patient. This section adds some general information using the diagnostic process as a focus.

Thoughtful nurses may ask such questions about the diagnostic process as: "What areas should I assess?" "How can I structure the data collection process so my search for information will result in identification of problems?" Since a common conceptual framework used in nursing is the human or basic needs one, health care institutions often use an inventory type format based on needs as reflected in health habits. The nurse conducts a physical assessment and then proceeds to interview the patient about health habits related to rest, sleep, food and fluid intake, elimination, and the like. All too often important assessment areas are not considered. Shortcomings might include a patient's home situation and condi-

tions, exercise, recreation, sexual relationships, belief systems, and stress coping strategies. Some nurses have a tendency to pursue data related to possible pathophysiological problems instead of nursing diagnoses. If, for example, the patient says she has one hard stool a week the nurse might immediately think of a medical problem. Questions would be directed toward tentative verification of that rather than a nursing diagnosis. It is possible that the patient's problem might lie in her dietary and/or fluid intake, and nurses could treat it. The structural format used should enable the nurse to organize comprehensive data collection for the purpose of identifying and treating problems. Gordon suggests that the functioning-dysfunctional health patterns structure answers the question of what data to collect (4).

WHAT DATA TO COLLECT

Patients engage daily in activities that promote or damage their health. They have an awareness of those activities and an idea about how good their health is. If problems are to be identified, assessment of a patient's health perceptions and practices is possible and essential. Looking at and talking about a patient's health status by using a structural format— functional health patterns—is an appropriate way to begin the diagnostic process (see Figure 7.2). The nurse constructs patterns from physical examination, observation, and descriptions of current and past practices provided by the patient. A comparison of past and current practices may uncover changes that have occurred. Changes can be indicative of a problem. A patient might say, "I used to go to bed at 11 o'clock every night and sleep soundly until 7 the next morning. Now I find myself having trouble getting to sleep and wake up about 4." Since the statement indicates both past and current patterns as well as a change, the nurse will explore further to gather information about when the change was first noted, any other changes the patient can say happened at the same time, and what if anything she has tried to help regain her previous habit. The information is filed in the nurse's memory, but

Health-perception-health management pattern. Describes clients' perceived pattern of health and well-being and how health is managed.

Nutritional-metabolic pattern. Describes pattern of food and fluid consumption relative to metabolic need and pattern indicators of local nutrient supply.

Elimination pattern. Describes pattern of excretory function (bowel, bladder, and skin).

Activity-exercise pattern. Describes pattern of exercise, leisure, and recreation.

Cognitive-perceptual pattern. Describes sensory-perceptual and cognitive pattern.

Sleep-rest pattern. Describes patterns of sleep, rest, and relaxation.

Self-perception-self-concept pattern. Describes self-concept pattern and perceptions of self (e.g., body comfort, body image, feeling state).

Role-relationship pattern. Describes pattern of role engagements and relationships.

Sexuality-reproductive pattern. Describes clients' patterns of satisfaction and dissatisfaction with sexuality pattern; describes reproductive pattern.

Coping-stress-tolerance pattern. Describes general coping pattern and effectiveness of the pattern in terms of stress tolerance.

Value-belief pattern. Describes patterns of values, beliefs (including spiritual), or gods that guide choices and decisions.

Figure 7.2. Typology of 11 functional health problems. Here, typology refers to a classification system, for areas in which assessment takes place. A pattern refers to sequences of behavior over time (3:82). From Nursing Diagnosis: Process and Application *by Marjorie Gordon. Copyright © 1982 by McGraw-Hill Book Company. Reprinted with permission of McGraw-Hill Book Company.*

will surface again when the patient describes other patterns of behavior because the nurse suspects a sleep-rest dysfunctional pattern.

The overall objective of using the functional health patterns structure is to discover dysfunctional patterns—health problems—within the structural areas. Table 7.4 reviews functional patterns and assessment content areas. Nurses often say they do not have time for a complete assessment on every patient. Screening questions and statements made by the nurse can save time. For instance, the nurse might say, "Let's talk a moment about the things that are important to you in your life. You mentioned that you read the paper and magazines or books every day [patient nods, yes], so keeping up with current events must be important? What are some of the other things?" A patient's response to screening comments and questions often will permit the nurse to determine that no dysfunctional pat-

tern exists. If the patient's response in one functional area conflicts with or reinforces a suspected problem in another, further description and data are pursued. Should a patient respond to the above value-belief screening question by saying, "I read the papers to find out all I can about the crooked politicians and police in this country," then it could be important to find out why this is the focus of the patient's interest. Cues of this nature may be the first indication of another dysfunctional area. Nurses experienced in diagnosing are aware that a problem in one dysfunctional area is commonly the result of a problem in another pattern. For example, Mrs. Carson is a 56-year-old widow. Her husband, who was a truck farmer, has been dead for 12 years. Her only child, a son, now owns the farm and supports her. She lives 25 miles from the farm in a two-room, third-floor walk-up apartment, where she has lived for the past 10 years.

Table 7.4. Assessment by Functional Health Patterns.

Functional Health Pattern	Nursing Assessment Objective	Assessment Content Areas
1. Health perception-health management pattern	obtain perceptions about past and current health status	generalizations about health as child and adult routine physical and dental examinations immunizations as child and adult allergies and reactions employment history description of living quarters and surroundings problems perceived and effectiveness of remedial action
2. Nutritional-metabolic pattern	obtain information about food and fluid intake	daily eating habits including description of usual content of meals weight, height, body structure healing pattern fluid consumption habits growth history problems perceived and effectiveness of remedial action examination of skin, hair, teeth, oral mucosa, temperature, nailbeds
3. Elimination pattern	collect data about regularity and control of excretion	characteristics of bowel, bladder, and skin excretory functions means of disposal for bowel and bladder excreta problems perceived and effectiveness of remedial action gross examination of specimens
4. Activity-exercise pattern	obtain data about energy expenditure activities	description of daily living routine, including self-care activities ability to move body parts type, amount, and frequency of exercise and recreation activity tolerance examination of gait, posture, muscle tone, range of motion, grip, pulse and respiratory rate, and prosthesis or assistive devices problems perceived and remedial action
5. Cognitive-perceptual pattern	obtain information about adequacy of language, memory, problem solving, decision making	observations about use of language, grasp of ideas and abstractions, attention span, learning ability, consciousness, life goals and plans for meeting them hearing, vision, sense of taste, touch and smell, assistive devices used perception, response to pain, and remedial action sensory deprivation or overload compensatory mechanisms
6. Sleep-rest pattern	obtain patient's perception of regularity and control of rest and sleep and satisfaction with amount and pattern	perception of readiness to begin day's activities after sleep usual time of sleep onset and awakening sleep reversal pattern remedial action and its effectiveness for perceived problems sleep pattern within family community sleep-rest disturbances
7. Self-perception-self-concept pattern	obtain patient's feelings and beliefs about self, sense of self-worth	observation of body language (voice, speech, movements, eye contact) cues related to satisfaction with personal physical appearance, competency in social, work, and other life situations; feelings of helplessness, depression, change, loss, and threat

Table 7.4. (Continued)

Functional Health Pattern	Nursing Assessment Objective	Assessment Content Areas
8. Role-relationship pattern	describe the patient's social and family roles	major role currently assumed in family and life (student, worker, housewife, retiree, etc.) satisfaction and dissatisfactions with major role responsibilities and relationships economic status nuclear or extended family, family membership, roles work roles and relationships working environment and hazards to health and safety work stresses, work patterns satisfaction with work role and conditions perceived problems and effectiveness of remedial actions
9. Sexuality-reproductive pattern	obtain patient's perception in relation to satisfaction with sexuality and reproduction	expression of sexual identity sexual relationships with a partner satisfactions, dissatisfaction with expression of sexuality family sexuality patterns and beliefs perception of problems and remedial action stage of current reproductive development age of onset of reproductive milestones (menarche, climacteric, menopause), secondary sex characteristics pregnancies, live births, genetic abnormalities use of contraceptives, effectiveness of types used perception of problems and effectiveness of remedial action
10. Coping-stress tolerance pattern	describe the patient's coping behaviors and level of stress tolerance	recall of life events considered to be stressful how events were managed perception of effectiveness of management strategies perceived current stressors, how they are being handled
11. Value-belief pattern	obtain information about what patient values and effect of belief system on health-related decisions	major philosophical values that guide choices and decisions in life other culture-oriented beliefs

Adapted from Marjorie Gordon. *Nursing Diagnosis: Process and Application*, pp. 81–97. New York: McGraw-Hill, 1982.

Her admission diagnosis is acute, recurrent cholecystitis. She is being considered for a cholecystectomy when the acute episode subsides. She has had the same symptoms periodically over the past two years, but this attack has been prolonged and especially painful. She did not seek medical assistance in the past, but "toughed out" the attacks. A second diagnosis is congestive heart failure. Mrs. Carson denies respiratory symptoms except some dyspnea during her move from home to the hospital.

This is the first illness for which medical consultation has been sought since her only pregnancy. Her son is 27. She claims she has been well most of her life. She has never been hospitalized.

Mrs. Carson's daughter-in-law drives in daily to clean her apartment, run errands, and do her shopping. She also does Mrs. Carson's laundry, dishes, washes her hair weekly and cuts it. Mrs. Carson perspires heavily and has for the last five years. Fluid loss from lower extremities and elsewhere began one week prior to admission with onset of acute upper abdominal distress.

Mrs. Carson eats whenever she feels hungry—probably something "about every two hours." She has no regular mealtimes. She eats raw fresh vegetables and fruit at least twice daily. Milk disagrees with her, and she dislikes all kinds of cereal. She has two soft-boiled eggs upon arising each day and has peanut butter and cheese frequently. She keeps a pot of hot grease on her stove all day and snacks on deep-fat fried bread. She also deep-fat fries meat about twice a week. The fried bread habit is a lifelong one, encouraged by her mother. She has used vegetable oil for the past four years although she prefers lard—"It tastes better, but my daughter-in-law won't buy lard for me. She says it smokes too much, and then she has to clean the kitchen walls more often." Fluid intake averages 16 to 18 eight-ounce glasses daily—about three-fourths water and one-fourth fruit juice. "I need lots to drink because I perspire so much." Tea and coffee are taken in moderation, mostly with friends. Mrs. Carson is grossly overweight, weighing 805 pounds.

Mrs. Carson sleeps sitting up sideways on a single bed with her head against a wall and pillows against her back. She cannot lie flat or on her side because she cannot regain an upright position and she cannot breathe. Her feet are always dependent (i.e., below the level of her heart, thus impeding venous return) because she cannot raise her legs to get them on a stool. She averages about seven hours of sleep nightly in two- to three-hour intervals.

Mrs. Carson says she has many friends and neighbors who visit her frequently. Some are the same age as she is, some are younger. They include both men and women. She "helps them solve their problems," and they discuss many subjects. She plays cards once or twice a week in her apartment with visiting friends. She reads a lot—"everything I can get my hands on."

Mrs. Carson's activity at home consists of moving from her living room-bedroom to and from her kitchen. She reports not standing more than 10 minutes at a time, although she

changes from sitting to standing at least every two hours. Her legs are painful and her knees hurt. The pain in her knees is a new problem since admission to the hospital. (Her legs are not dependent for the first time in eight years.) Range of motion in upper extremities is normal, and movement is not painful. Grasp is good. Gait was not observed.

Mrs. Carson obviously has a number of dysfunctional patterns. Among those patterns reviewed, there are enough data and cues to indicate that the nutritional-metabolic pattern is an area of major dysfunction. The problem in that area has probably caused difficulties in the activity-exercise and rest-sleep patterns. In addition, two cues make one suspect that there might also be a problem in the role-relationship pattern. The cues related to the health perception-health management pattern indicate a probable difficulty in that area as well. Little information is given about the value-belief pattern, but there might be a problem creating the possible one in the health management pattern. Mrs. Carson's history illustrates how a dysfunctional pattern influences other patterns and a problem in one functional pattern might cause a problem in others.

She was hospitalized for six weeks and lost considerable weight—about 200 pounds. Her cardiac condition improved. The surgical risk she presented was too great due to excessive weight, and she was discharged to a rehabilitation center.

HOW TO COLLECT DATA

Information collection during the diagnostic process is not only influenced by a nurse's decision about what data to collect but also by the nature of the information available, the situation in which the data is obtained, and the psychological set or the beliefs and attitudes of the diagnostician. The situation in which data is obtained is addressed in Chapters 5 and 6; the other two factors will be discussed here.

Nurses collect both subjective and objective information about a patient. Subjective data include those things that can be ascertained directly through the senses—color, appearance, temperature, blood pressure, heart rate, and the like. Subjective data consist of things reported by the patient or secondarily by a family member or friend. The patient's perception of her health state is important because it reflects what is real and true to her.

The quality and accuracy of information used in the diagnostic process influences a diagnosis. A nurse must consider how reliable and accurate a particular cue is to prevent diagnostic error. In the case of Mrs. Carson, the reliability of her sleeping pattern is quite possibly good, but there are few data concerning her cognitive-perceptual pattern. Better accuracy and quality cannot be obtained since regular sleep-rest patterns in the hospital often are disrupted. The data concerning Mrs. Carson's nutritional pattern is judged an accurate reflection of the pattern since she is the best source for what she usually eats and drinks. The information concerning her many friends and neighbors, however, was accepted as a perception that needed further data to substantiate it as a good cue to her social relationships. The quality of a cue can be ascertained by other data that verifies it, by checking it with other sources, or by obtaining additional information. The accuracy of cues depends largely upon the source. For example, the hospital admission reading for blood pressure is often taken as the baseline, or standard, against which subsequent measurements are evaluated. If the nurse who takes the reading can hear it, the reading can be judged accurate, but its validity as an indicator of the usual pressure is only moderate because hospital admissions can often elevate blood pressure until the patient has had time to adjust to new circumstances. If the patient reported her blood pressure or took it herself, the accuracy of the reading might be somewhat questionable unless data were available regarding her proficiency and skill. Sometimes cues with less than desirable validity and reliability—for an unconscious patient, for example—have to be acted upon because better data are not available.

A perioperative patient may tell the nurse that her surgeon has explained little about the anticipated procedure. If the nurse has read in the record a full description of what the surgeon told the patient, should she ignore the patient's statement as bad data in favor of the surgeon's report? Certainly not. The cue given by the patient is her perception. Further questioning may provide cues that demonstrate the patient can state everything that will happen to her physiologically but she does not know what to expect before she is given the anesthetic. Her terminology differs from the professional's, but her statement is valid and reliable in the way she is able to express its content. On the other hand, her statement may be one of several indicative of a cognitive-perceptual dysfunction. It can be a reliable as well as a good quality cue for that pattern.

The psychological set of the nurse is another determining factor in how information is collected. Psychological set refers to the tendency to respond to certain cues in a specific way because of attitudes or internal motives. For example, the nurse who responds to a patient's crying by saying, "Don't cry, everything will be all right," is responding, not to the patient's distress cue, but to uncomfortable feelings of her own triggered by the patient's behavior. Focusing on the nurse's feelings and behavior fails to accomplish the aim of the diagnostic process, which should be focused on the patient.

As individuals and as members of society, nurses all hold attitudes about certain circumstances. They frequently encounter patients whose behavior they disapprove of, such as criminals, drug peddlers, child and women abusers, women with several illegitimate children on state aid, patients with untreated venereal disease, and patients who refuse to comply with medical regimens. Individual nurses may have disapproving attitudes toward sexual deviations, tobacco users, obese individuals, and the like.

When the nurse responds to cues given by patients from her own belief system, the diagnostic process becomes blocked, and the patient no longer feels comfortable in the diagnostic situation. The psychological set the nurse must assume is related to her role as a health care professional whose motivation in the diagnostic situation is to work with a patient in discovering problems. That set is not a social one, a self-maintenance one, or a judgmental one, it is a perceptive-interpretive set. Without this set, the end result of the process—the diagnoses—can be faulty.

Interpreting the Data

As the nurse collects clinical health data, the information is subjected to a number of mental processes, which permit the nurse to reduce the possible diagnoses from a great many to a few and finally to one or two. A general term for these thought processes is hypothesizing. Hypothesizing is formulating an explanation for the occurrence of related events, conditions, or behavior. The explanation is a conjecture used to guide the search for additional cues. It is an educated guess, based initially on one or two cues. Hypothesizing involves clinical reasoning and retrieval from memory of theory and experiential data. The process is one that human beings use constantly every day.

Human beings grow up asking the questions, "What is it?" "Why?" and "What is it used for?" We learn from these questions to distinguish between similar objects in our environment, to identify the unknown from the known, and to predict (hypothesize) an event, condition, or object on the basis of cues.

Nurses take this line of reasoning during the diagnostic process. In reviewing functional patterns and observing the patient, a nurse evaluates cues by asking, "What does this mean?" "Why is she saying this?" A conscious decision is made to explore some cues and not others. Or perhaps the nurse will not follow up a cue immediately but return later to it. What is the meaning of a blood pressure of 160/90 in a 20-year-old male athlete? When a patient says, "I'm not concerned with what I look like," what does that mean and what is causing him to say that? A hypothesis is made that the cue is an indicator of a problem. The nurse might even make a tentative hypothesis about the nature of the problem—a tentative explanation. Sometimes there is no need to make a tentative hypothesis because the cues for a problem are obvious, as with Mrs. Carson.

Her weight (805 pounds) and the triceps skinfold measurement (26 mm) meet the two defining characteristics of the problem, "Alterations in nutrition: more than body requirements." The cause of that problem, however, needs to be investigated.

Nurses reason from one or two cues to hypothesize a problem (inductive reasoning) as follows:

1. This patient is scheduled for surgery tomorrow (cue).
2. This patient has the signs and symptoms of anxiety (observation).
3. This patient's anxiety might be related to the proposed surgery (inductive hypothesis).

Nurses also use clinical inferences in inductive reasoning. Inferences can be equated with hypotheses, although there is a slight difference. One infers something that goes beyond the data base. In making an inference, the nurse takes a known principle and applies it to the situation under consideration. Reasoning by inductive inference proceeds as follows:

1. Mrs. Carson belongs to the class, partially physically dependent (inductive inference).
2. Mrs. Carson once belonged to the class, physically independent (inductive inference).
3. Therefore, the change in status from independence to dependence might produce a self-concept disequilibrium (tentative problem hypothesis).

(Dependent and independent in this sense refer to the patient's need or lack of need for support in the activities of daily living, i.e., dressing, toileting, etc.) Inferences 1 and 2 go beyond the actual data to infer circumstances, so that the hypothesis in 3 can be reached. Substantiation of inference 2 is needed, and more information is required to support the hypothesis.

Deductive reasoning is also used to make clinical inferences. In deductive reasoning, a general premise believed to be true in a large number of instances is used to deduce a possible individual problem. For example:

1. Surgical patients experience anxiety (verified by research and experience).
2. This is a surgical patient (cue).
3. Therefore, this patient might be anxious (deductive inference or hypothesis).

A deductive inference is a prediction about the nature of a problem and must be supported by careful collection of additional data to avoid a diagnostic error. The general premise must also fit the circumstances. One could not use the premise, "Surgical patients experience anxiety," as the proposition to support anxiety for a nonsurgical patient. The premises used in deductive reasoning are drawn from the nurse's knowledge of concepts acquired from education and experience.

Data interpretation also involves generating two or more possible explanations for a group of related cues. Because the chances of identifying human problems always are less than a 100 percent, the element of uncertainty stimulates the diagnostician to consider all possible explanations for a problem. Multiple hypotheses enable the nurse to concentrate the search for additional cues. The cue cluster might be: Mrs. Kelso, who is five months pregnant, is admitted for an appendectomy. She is a para ō, gravida III. She says, "I can't believe this is happening—just when I thought everything was going so well!" What are the possible hypotheses to be made in Mrs. K's situation?

- Hypothesis 1: Knowledge deficit (sexual-reproductive).
- Hypothesis 2: Psychological disequilibrium (guilt? depression?).
- Hypothesis 3: Anticipatory grieving related to premature delivery of non-viable infant.

The separation of data collection and interpretation is artificial because the two activities occur simultaneously. The objective of the diagnostic process is to reduce the number of possible problems as rapidly, efficiently, and accurately as possible. For this reason, hypotheses are generated and serve as a focus for the search for additional data. Clinical reasoning also furnishes predictive hypotheses that serve the same function.

Clustering the Data

Clustering information is the third activity of the diagnostic process. Clustering is the realignment of related cues—a mental sorting of data pertaining to hypotheses and inferences. Use of a data-gathering tool based on the functional pattern typology assists in obtaining partially clustered data. As the nurse investigates the meanings of cues, however, the information may fit with another pattern or hypothesis. Mrs. Carson, for instance, offered the information about her daughter-in-law substituting vegetable oil for lard while discussing her nutritional-metabolic pattern. If additional early data seem to support either a family relationship or self-concept dysfunction, the cues are realigned to another hypothesis.

Clustering involves judgmental tasks. One must be aware of inconsistencies among cues—data that refute other cues—and decide which inconsistencies should be held for further study and which discarded. Awareness of these difficulties should open the diagnostician's thinking to include all the possibilities so that diagnostic errors can be prevented.

Once the cues have been clustered, two or three probable diagnoses with probable causes for each cluster are predicted. These are then tested one by one through a search for critical defining characteristics that differentiate one diagnosis from another. The presence of the defining characteristics confirms a diagnosis. If all the critical defining characteristics of a diagnosis are not present, but other characteristics are, the patient is at risk for the actual problem to occur and has a potential problem.

Naming the Diagnosis

The final task in the diagnostic process is to record the diagnosis, its etiologies, and the cues. Only those diagnoses for which critical defining characteristics are present should be recorded as diagnoses. If there is no currently accepted diagnosis available to use, the nurse should record the diagnosis in her own words as briefly and concisely as possible. If adequate supporting data for a diagnosis is not present, signs and symptoms or tentative hypotheses can be recorded.

Efforts To Devise and Classify Nursing Diagnoses

The current work in generating and classifying nursing diagnoses began as an outgrowth of a project initiated at St. Louis University by Kristine Gebbie and Mary Ann Lavin. These two faculty members were attempting to identify the nurse's role in their ambulatory care unit. Difficulties in naming problems treated by nurses made them aware of the need for a taxonomy of nursing diagnoses similar to the medical classification system used by physicians. St. Louis University School of Nursing hosted a conference on the subject in 1973. At that conference, the National Conference Group for Classification of Nursing Diagnoses was formed.

The conference group is made up of nurse practitioners, educators, and researchers. The conference group met every two years between 1973 and 1980 to generate new diagnoses, to refine or discard others, and to identify etiologies and characteristics. Future meetings are projected.

At the first conference, a national task force was appointed to carry out the developmental work between meetings. Marjorie Gordon, a recognized authority on nursing diagnosis, chaired the task force from 1973 to 1980. The national task force is responsible for three major activities: (1) information dissemination and exchange through the Clearinghouse for Nursing Diagnoses; (2) educational activities to encourage implementation of nursing diagnoses; and (3) stimulation and coordination of activities related to development, standardization, and classification of diagnoses. The diagnoses that have been accepted by the conference group are published and available for testing in the clinical setting by practitioners (5). Much work remains yet to be accomplished

if the goal of the conference group and the national task force is to be reached—the publication of an international classification system of nursing diagnoses with a standardized nomenclature.

Perioperative nurses have not yet given much attention to diagnostic labels. But as work on nursing diagnosis progresses, no doubt many will use nursing diagnosis to identify actual and potential health problems of surgical patients. Roy (6) has suggested that nurses in the operating room may become specialists in helping patients cope with fears associated with surgery. It is an intriguing suggestion. As the perioperative role develops and expands, nurses in the operating room may be more involved in treating patient's actual and potential health problems related to surgery.

Patient Situation

The data collected on Mr. Fischer revealed several nursing diagnoses. Because of the extensive nature of his surgery only a few problems are illustrated (see Figs. 7.3 and 7.4). Mr. Fischer was asked in the preoperative interview to explain his understanding of the proposed surgical procedure. The perioperative nurse was attempting to determine his knowledge base. The premise was that coping with the unknown is more likely to produce psychological disequilibrium than coping with the known. The nurse could also be thinking of other predictive hypotheses such as alteration in self-concept, ineffective individual coping strategies, and fear. These would all be appropriate considering the potentially mutilative surgery proposed for Mr. Fischer. All the predictive hypotheses are changed to predictions of potential problems.

When the nurse learns that Mr. Fischer was unaware of the possible total glossectomy and that extensive jaw resection might be necessary, the diagnosis identified is, "Knowledge deficit," related to lack of exposure to information. The second preoperative nursing diagnosis is, "Impaired verbal communication," related to tracheostomy and possible total glossectomy. The nature of the proposed surgery, resultant potentially ineffective airway and

INTRAOPERATIVE PATIENT CARE PLAN
Mr. Ralph Fischer

NURSING DIAGNOSIS	GOAL	PLAN	IMPLEMENTATION	EVALUATION
PREOPERATIVE				
Knowledge, lack of external resources (people or material)				
Communication, impaired verbal due to surgical anatomical resection, jaw wiring, tracheostomy.				
INTRAOPERATIVE				
Potential for neuromuscular damage due to required positioning and length of surgical prodecure.				

Figure 7.3. Intraoperative patient care plan including preoperative and intraoperative nursing diagnoses for Mr. Fischer.

INTRAOPERATIVE PATIENT CARE PLAN

Mr. Ralph Fischer

NURSING DIAGNOSIS	GOAL	PLAN	IMPLEMENTATION	EVALUATION
POSTOPERATIVE Respiratory: Alteration in airway (tracheostomy, hemiglossectomy, mandibular fixation. Increased risk for postop complications due to: 1. History of bronchitis 2. History of smoking 3. Exposure to environmental irritants.				

Figure 7.4. Intraoperative patient care plan including postoperative nursing diagnosis for Mr. Fischer.

ineffective airway clearance (wired jaw) are the cues and inferences from which inductive reasoning generated the diagnoses. With Mr. Fischer, there is no need to search for other cues to test the hypothesis. The probability for the problem to occur is very high.

Because of the extensive nature of the surgery and the extensive reconstructive and plastic work scheduled for the patient's mandible and mouth floor as well as the tongue and mandibular resection, the procedure is likely to take 10–12 hours. Artificial maintenance of neck, head, arm, and other body parts in an abnormal position for a lengthy period causes pressure on nerves that can result in muscular weakness or paralysis. As a consequence, there is a potential in this patient for neuromuscular damage during the operative period. The diagnosis is based on the nurse's knowledge of positioning for the procedure and physiological concepts, an inference about the length of the procedure, and experience. It is a predictive hypothesis and has a high risk factor associated with it.

The perioperative nurse predicts a potential problem for Mr. Fischer during the postoperative phase. Because he will have a temporary, if not permanent, tracheostomy, she formulates the nursing diagnosis as, "Alteration in airway," related to potential ineffective airway clearance. The nurse had a choice based on the cues presented. She could have stated the nursing diagnosis as, "Ineffective airway clearance." Both are correct and valid diagnoses. The second postoperative nursing diagnosis demonstrates the problem of trying to label the cluster of cues. The nurse used the following diagnosis, "Increased risk for postoperative respiratory complications," related to (1) history of bronchitis; (2) history of smoking; (3) exposure to noxious environmental inhalants. This diagnosis is based on cues such as history of smoking, history of exposure to noxious gaseous inhalants, and tracheostomy.

Another diagnosis the nurse might have made based on new information from the National Conference Group on Classification of Nursing Diagnoses is, "Impaired gas exchange related to ventilation imbalance." Another diagnosis the nurse could have used is, "Potential for injury." The etiology consists of interactive conditions between the individual and the environment that impose a risk to the defensive and adaptive resources of a person.

References

1. American Nurses' Association. *The Code for Nurses with Interpretative Statements.* Kansas City: ANA, 1979.
2. Maslow, A. H. *Eupsychian Management: A Journal.* Homewood, IL: Richard D. Irwin Inc. and the Dorsey Press, 1965.
3. Henderson, V. *The Nature of Nursing.* New York: Macmillan, 1966.
4. Gordon, M. *Nursing Diagnosis: Process and Application.* New York: McGraw-Hill Book Company, 1982.
5. Kim, M. J., and Moritz, D. A., eds. *Classification of Nursing Diagnoses: Proceedings of the Third and Fourth National Conferences.* New York: McGraw-Hill Book Company, 1982.
6. Roy, Sister Calista. "The Impact of Nursing Diagnosis." *AORN J* 21:1023, 1975.

Suggested Readings

Gordon, M. "Historical perspective: The National Conference Group for Classification of Nursing Diagnoses (1978–1980)." In Mi Ja Kim and Derry Ann Mortiz, eds. *Classification of Nursing Diagnoses: Proceedings of the Third and Fourth National Conferences.* New York: McGraw-Hill Book Company, 1982.

III

Planning Perioperative Patient Care

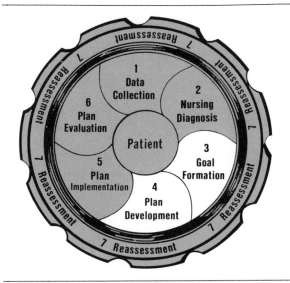

The plan of care includes goals and prescribes nursing actions to achieve the goals.

What is Planning?

Planning is the component of the nursing process that the operating room nurse uses to determine a course of action that will correct the patient's identified problems and prevent potential problems. Two distinct functions in planning are setting goals and prescribing nursing actions. After the priorities of the nursing diagnosis have been determined, the nurse participates in formulating goals to be achieved by the patient. Once goals are developed, nursing activities are planned to meet the patient's individual needs. The nursing interventions selected should produce the desired goals for the patient.

Nursing Competencies Used in Planning

Specific nursing competencies are needed to carry out the planning process. A sound theoretical base is needed because knowledge must be integrated with motor skills in planning and giving nursing care. Organizational skills are essential to coordinate nursing activities in a sequential, consistent, and systematic manner to reach the desired outcome.

Judgment is a cognitive skill essential to the nurse's ability to perceive needs for nursing care and provide that care. Nurses must be able to make sound decisions when developing a plan to correct the patient's problems. The ability to communicate clearly the plan of care in the written nursing care plan and orally to the patient, family, significant others, and members of the health care team is important for all nurses.

ORGANIZATIONAL SKILLS

Organization involves the orderly arrangement of nursing actions. This means nursing actions must be evaluated, ranked, and performed by the appropriate person. Organizational ability is not innate but a skill that can be learned. The first prerequisite is to be knowledgeable. In developing the care plan, the nurse must know what problems surgical patients have and how the surgery will affect those problems. He must have an understanding of surgical procedures and what the patient experiences before, during, and after surgery. He should be familiar with the policies and procedures of the operating room, job expectations of employees, and surgeon's preferences. The knowledgeable nurse will be able to organize the care plan to foster teamwork and cooperation of all involved.

Six questions that will help increase organizational skills are: What? Why? When? How? Where? and Who? The *what* questions provide a list of tasks that must be accomplished. They may be done today, tomorrow, or later during the patient's hospitalization. *Why* questions help determine order. What tests will be ordered first? The *when* questions help the nurse allocate time. Conflicts can be avoided if a time can be specified. In conducting a preoperative assessment, the nurse will have to select a time when the patient is not involved in other preparations for surgery. The *how* questions relate to the institution's policies and procedures. The *where* questions ask the location of the patient when the activity occurs. Finally, *who* questions involve personnel. What are the competencies of members of the team? Who is best qualified to perform the task? Can it be delegated? Choosing the best-qualified individual involves concern not only with the patient's needs but also with the needs of other nursing personnel.

NURSING JUDGMENT

Making judgments is central to nursing practice. The need for judgment sets a profession apart from other occupations. Professionals do not act by rote, nor do they always work under another's direction. They make their own decisions according to their own knowledge and experience. Nurses use judgment to challenge, question, examine, and validate principles and procedures (1).

Making a nursing judgment to decide on a patient's needs and subsequent care follows a prescribed sequence of events. These events begin with the antecedent phase—the time when the perioperative nurse decides to become involved in a specific patient's case. For example:

Antecedent Phase	*Example*
Nurse makes decision to assess a specific patient and form an opinion regarding care needed prior to and during surgery. In this case, the patient is Carol Jones, admitted for a hysterectomy.	Nurse assesses patient's previous surgical experience by conducting an interview.

The second phase in making a judgment is interactive. The nurse begins to focus on the individuality of the patient and to anticipate potential problems based on what is heard and observed.

Interactive Phase	Example
Nurse anticipates potential problems as a result of sensory input (e.g., hearing about a patient's problem).	Patient reports bleeding problem during a previous cesarean section.
Nurse seeks more data from patient and other resources.	Nurse discusses past experience and learns patient received 8 units whole blood intraoperatively and postoperatively. Reviews current hematology report. Discovers hemoglobin of 7.9, hematocrit of 20, and platelet count of 48,000.
Nurse recalls knowledge (concepts) related to hemorrhagic problems.	Nurse reviews current history, finds no mention of previous bleeding problems. Orders previous chart from medical records department and discovers earlier hemorrhagic problem substantiated, plus laboratory records showing clotting times.

	Facts	Knowledge
Nurse integrates knowledge and facts collected.	Carol Jones's bleeding during previous surgical procedure required blood during surgery.	Patient's history of bleeding indicates potential bleeding for this surgery.
	Slow clotting time recorded in previous history.	Slow clotting times indicate bleeding potential.
	Carol Jones's current hemoglobin is 7.9.	Below normal hemoglobin indicates anemia, possibly due to current bleeding.
	Platelet count is 48,000.	Low platelet count indicates potential for bleeding. Normal platelet count is 200,000 to 350,000/cu mm.

Nurse analyzes what the situation might be.	Nurse determines Carol Jones has an above-average potential for bleeding.
Prior to concluding what the situation might be, the nurse reflects on all data presented.	All data support previous conclusion.
Nurse affirms judgment and acts accordingly.	Nurse informs surgeon and other team members of findings.
	Verifies availability of additional units of packed cells.

Acknowledges and communicates order for additional units. Ensures that intravenous fluid is available with blood administration tubing connected.

Increases number of suction bottles on case setup.

Adds additional laparotomy sponges on case setup.

Documents plan to save blood samples should additional type and cross-match be necessary.

Plans for precise measurement of blood loss and irrigation solution.

The final step in the judgment process is the consequent phase. All consequences the final judgment might have are evaluated.

Consequent Phase	*Example*
Nurse assesses the outcome or consequences of the final decision and subsequent actions.	The goal established for Carol Jones was to prevent excessive bleeding and to limit the amount of bleeding. Nursing actions related to this goal were developed.

Preventing excessive bleeding will be a conscious nursing intervention while the plan for care is being implemented. This entire sequence of events becomes part of the experience the nurse will use when faced with similar situations in the future.

COMMUNICATION SKILLS

Communicating is the process by which we understand others and in turn seek to be understood by them. It is a two-way process that involves a series of interactions between two or more people. Touching, observing, reading, sharing, emotional stroking, and listening are all methods of communicating. Communication is an art, skill, and science the nurse, as a therapeutic person, uses.

The nurse needs communication skills to explain information to the patient, provide instructions, or share data with others. His knowledge about how people communicate and how he uses communication skills enable patient goals and nursing activities to be realistic and to be agreed upon by the nurse, the patient, and others involved in care. The interaction between nurse and patient many times determines the success or failure of the plan.

For instance, a patient having a mastectomy is seriously concerned about her body image. She may try to express this concern to a nurse who does not perceive the patient's feelings and attitudes. The nurse ignores the patient's need to discuss her concerns and work through her feelings. This creates a communication barrier. The nurse-patient relationship is jeopardized, as is the possibility to plan constructive help for the patient. The patient is reluctant to express other needs she may have, and meaningful communication ceases.

Effective communication is essential to the nurse-patient relationship. Without it, the plan of care will be unsuccessful. Communication can be verbal, extraverbal, and nonverbal. Verbal communication uses words. The care plan, assessment sheet, other written forms, and the telephone or face-to-face discussion are used to communicate verbally.

Extraverbal communication deals not with what is said but with how it is said. Voice tone, inflection, and speed affect how the receiver translates the message. In written messages, the choice of words and punctuation can be extraverbal messages.

Nonverbal communication involves actions and gestures, or body language. We are constantly saying something with our bodies. We communicate by posture and body movements as well as gestures and touching. Understanding nonverbal communication can enhance a nurse's ability to select nursing activities for the patient's care plan. For example, increased anxiety may be communicated by certain body actions—wringing the hands, pacing, or fidgeting with buttons. When this behavior is observed, the nurse should include in the care plan actions designed to assist the patient with coping.

DECISION-MAKING SKILLS

During assessment, the nurse collects data and makes a nursing diagnosis. The nursing diagnosis identifies the actual or potential problems a patient may encounter during the planned surgery. The nurse studies the identified problems and devises a plan to alleviate or solve the problems and assist the patient to return to his normal activities of daily living.

Ford (2) has developed a model for decision making. The following steps may seem cumbersome but are worth the time involved:

1. Identification, clarification, and ordering of values
2. Formulating behavioral objectives
3. Identifying and stating the problem
4. Generating and screening options
5. Analyzing alternatives for desirability, probability, and personal risk
6. Analyzing the problem situation for desirability, probability, and personal risk
7. Making the decision
8. Evaluating the decision

The values may be those of the nurse, the nursing profession, the hospital, or the patient. A value is an acquired belief or a principle that guides our actions. These values become personal belief systems that are used daily in making decisions. Every nurse and patient has a value system that is gained through experiences and interactions with people throughout life.

Nurses acquire additional values through nursing philosophies and theories they are exposed to during their education. Common values held by most nurses are the worth of life and the preservation of health. All patients do not hold the same values, creating a conflict for nurses. All decisions are based on values held by the individuals involved in the decision-making process. It is helpful to identify carefully values held by those who will be affected by the decision and clarify the impact of those values on the nurse, the institution, the patient, the family, and other members of the health care team. Next, the nurse should rank those values according to his own standards. At some point, a choice may have to be made, and values may help the nurse to choose among alternatives.

The next step is to formulate behavioral objectives. If a nurse's professional value is to provide physical safety to patients going to the operating room, the behavioral objective will be to transport the patient to the operating room without harm. In other words, the objectives are the guidelines for translating values into action. How the patient will get to the operating room without harm will be determined during the decision-making process.

Problem identification is the starting point for the problem-solving process. In identifying the problem, the nurse begins to fulfill the values and objectives. Usually, the problem is stated as a question, "How can I transport the patient to the operating room safely?" This question serves as the basis for possible solutions.

The next step is to generate options. The idea is to brainstorm for as many ideas as possible. At this point, options do not necessarily have to be realistic. Options for transporting a patient safely might be to send three nurses and an orderly—one nurse to monitor and maintain respiration, another to keep traction on a fractured limb, and the third to help the orderly in the transport. Another option is to transport the patient in his own bed, and another is to use a surgical lift. When every option is listed, the desirability of each option is analyzed.

Choosing an option goes back to the nurse's values, determined by what he believes will be best for the patient. Is it possible to use a surgical lift? Perhaps one is not available, or it might not be the best option for this patient. In some cases, more than one option is appropriate. Each option should be fully explored and analyzed. Each alternative selected has the potential of solving the problem. Three criteria can be used to determine which alternative is the most applicable to the situation—desirability, probability, and personal risk. Desirability relates to the nurse's value system and involves ranking the alternatives according to personal preference. Probability deals with the chances the alternative has of succeeding. Personal risk has three elements—physical, emotional, and social.

Physical risk has to do with the threat to body integrity for nurse or patient. The patient being transferred to the operating room has a potential for physical risk if, for example, traction is not maintained and a fractured extremity is not in alignment. Emotional risk can result from exposure to feelings or a loss of self-concept. The patient may experience loss of self-concept due to his illness. Social risk involves a threat to the individual's role in society, the work environment, or the home situation. In decision making, the risks are ranked and the alternative with the lowest risk factor is chosen.

The nurse should choose the option or alternative that will best solve the original problem. Once the decision is made, it should be put into action and then evaluated to determine its effectiveness. If the option selected does not allow the objective to be met, then the nurse must reconsider and go through the decision-making process again.

Decision making is critical in patient care management. Nurses must take responsibility for preparing themselves for the complex problems that demand critical thinking. All nurses are involved in making decisions. The skill with which decisions are made will be one factor in determining the extent to which nurses become autonomous.

Goal Setting

Planning for the care of the perioperative patient, which begins when a nursing diagnosis is made, requires formulating goals and prescribing nursing actions to achieve those goals. Goals are an end toward which action is taken. They also provide a guide for measuring the extent to which intervention was effective and the results accomplished in relation to the patient.

Goals are patient centered. They are established to be able to measure the effectiveness of nursing care. Nurses sometimes confuse patient goals with nursing goals. They may state that a goal is "to prevent," "to maintain," or "to prepare." This indicates what the nurse does to a patient rather than what the patient will do. Therefore, it is not a patient goal, but a nursing goal. Throughout this text, the primary emphasis is on the patient having surgery, therefore, when reference is made to a "goal" it is the patient goal.

Goals state behaviors that can be measured. The patient may indicate progress by verbalizing, demonstrating, or exhibiting signs and symptoms. In verbalizing, the patient will state, explain, or describe what he knows, understands, or feels about illness, treatment, or expectations. Such a goal might be: "The patient will openly discuss feelings about having a radical neck dissection prior to receiving his preoperative medication." The second method for measuring a goal is the patient's demonstration of the behavior expected. An example might be, "The patient will demonstrate coughing and deep breathing exercises prior to receiving the preoperative medication." The third way a patient manifests the desired outcome is by signs and symptoms. One set of observations is compared to another using preestablished norms. Signs and symptoms may be detected from laboratory tests, vital signs, or behavior. A goal to illustrate this type of patient outcome relates to altered venous circulation, "The patient will be free of circulatory system complications 48 hours postoperatively." Goals can be immediate, intermediate, or long term.

Immediate goals are those that may be life-threatening or require immediate nursing intervention. An immediate goal for the patient having surgery is, "The patient will verbalize an understanding of the surgical procedure prior to surgery." An intermediate goal is one that does not require immediate action; nursing care can be delayed for a short period. An example of an intermediate goal is: "The patient will demonstrate maintenance of fluid balance 48 hours postoperatively." A long-term goal will take time to reach. It may be reached at any time between admission and discharge or even be accomplished after discharge. A long-term goal may be staged, with multiple immediate goals that must be met before the ultimate goal is reached. An example of a long-term goal for a patient having a below-the-knee amputation is, "The patient will ambulate with a prosthesis in place prior to discharge."

Goals must be formulated well to assist the nurse in planning nursing actions. The more specific the goal is, the easier it is to measure the extent to which it is met.

There are four parts of a patient goal: subject, terminal behavior, criterion, and condition (3) (see Table 8.1).

1. *Subject:* The patient. The patient is expected to exhibit the behavior.
2. *Terminal behavior:* The action or performance required to meet the acceptable performance standard. What action is required of the patient for him to reach a predetermined health status? For example, "The patient with a below-the-knee amputation will walk using a prosthesis and crutches." The action is the patient walking. In the goal, this is the verb, or the action the subject will perform.
3. *Criterion:* The standard against which the behavior will be measured for acceptable performance. What level of performance are we expecting the patient to achieve? What constitutes "use of a prosthesis"? Will the patient be walking with the use of a prosthesis at discharge, 20 days postoperative, or when? The criterion should always contain a designated time or date for achievement of the behavior.
4. *Condition:* The circumstances or phenomena to which the patient is responding. All goals will not have a condition. The condition for the criterion stated above could be, "Patient walking with a prosthesis and assisted with crutches at discharge." The crutches and prosthesis are the conditions under which the patient will walk.

Table 8.1. *Examples of the Four Parts of a Patient Goal.*

Subject (Who)	Terminal Behavior (Action Verb)	Criterion (When, Where)	Condition (Extent Met)
Patient	will explain what it means to have a colostomy	prior to administration of medication	has knowledge
Patient	will be free of infection	48 hours postoperatively	no infection
Patient	will have minimal pain	24 hours postoperatively	minimal pain
Patient	will ambulate	up and down hall one day postoperatively	with help of walker

Patient goals describe the behavioral outcomes the patient is expected to achieve and provide a means for determining whether that outcome has occurred. They should be stated as concisely as possible and be congruent with assessment data, nursing diagnosis, and current knowledge and practice.

Guidelines in writing goals are as follows:

- *Goals are realistic:* The goal statement is practical and reasonable. It does not exceed what is possible for this particular patient. A goal statement which is realistic might be, "The patient having a lumbar laminectomy will be ambulating 48 hours postoperatively."
- *Goals are useable:* The goal statement will serve the purpose for which it is developed. It is consistent with the patient's problem and based on the nursing diagnosis. If the nursing diagnosis is, "Potential bleeding due to slow clotting time," a goal statement might be, "The patient will not have excessive bleeding due to surgical procedure."
- *Goals are measurable:* The goal statement can be quantified to determine the extent to which the goal is met. In other words, the goal can be measured. For example, did the patient with a fractured femur arrive safely in the operating room with the leg in alignment and free of pain? This is measured by the patient's statement that he has no pain or by the nurse's observation that the patient does not exhibit signs of pain. It is also measured by the nurse's observation that the traction is on and the patient's leg is in alignment.
- *Goals are behavioral:* The patient verbalizes, demonstrates, or shows signs or symptoms that can be used in measuring goal achievement. For example, "The patient states his knowledge and understanding of the surgical procedure and has signed the informed consent form."
- *Goals are achievable:* The goal statement can be carried through and accomplished. The result can be met. For example, "The patient is free of infection 72 hours after an abdominal hysterectomy." Is this a realistic goal? Can it be achieved?

- *Goals have a time element:* The goal states a time for achievement. The time is used to measure the extent the goal has been attained. For example, if the goal is that the patient will walk with crutches, the time element might be 72 to 96 hours postoperatively, depending on the patient.

An operating room nurse must have the ability to predict outcomes of nursing actions. He gains this skill by being exposed to different types of surgical procedures and observing and evaluating how patients progress postoperatively. He needs current knowledge of disease processes, types of surgery, and new technology. He needs to keep up with the current literature and gain experience in completing patient profiles from medical records.

Writing precise goals is a skill worth cultivating. Not only do exact goals enable the nurse to plan systematically for individualized care but they contribute to making nursing more scientific. Based on the scientific method, the nursing process is a way of planning care logically instead of instinctively or haphazardly. The goal is a key point in this process because it distills what the nurse knows about the patient into one concise statement, and it points out what future action the nurse believes will be successful. Each goal becomes a criterion to evaluate the outcome of care.

Measuring Goal Attainment

The *Standards of Perioperative Nursing Practice* (4) demonstrates the use of evaluation criteria. The standard on establishing goals and the criteria included in the standards are a means of measuring the achievement of goals and the effectiveness of nursing care.

The nurse can use the criteria when setting goals during the planning phase. He should ask himself the following questions about a goal he has developed:

1. Is the goal derived from a nursing diagnosis? If the diagnosis is that the patient was having considerable pain, the nurse would

expect the goal to be directly related to pain.

2. Is the goal stated so it has observable outcomes? Will the nurse be able to observe the patient's response to nursing intervention and determine if the goal is met? If the goal is, "The patient will have minimal pain 24 hours postoperatively," the nurse should be alert for signs and symptoms of pain.

3. Is the goal formulated with guidance from the patient, the family, significant others, and other health personnel? Without the cooperation of the patient, family, and others involved in care, there is no assurance that the goals are realistic or obtainable. The amount of the patient's involvement depends on the illness and type of surgery. When planning care, the nurse has a responsibility to involve the patient and family in identifying and defining important information and organizing, analyzing, and interpreting the information (5).

4. Is the goal congruent with the patient's present and potential physical capabilities and behavioral patterns? This question is answered by reviewing the assessment data. Baseline observations made on admission as well as the nursing diagnosis will provide this information. The nurse will also learn about the patient's potential through his own assessment, his family's impressions, and opinions of other health professionals who have worked with him.

5. Is the goal attainable through available human and material resources? Judgment is important in deciding which of the patient problems are pertinent to his surgery. Which problems can the nurse realistically intervene in, and which are appropriate to his specialty? The services provided by the institution will dictate the types of personnel and equipment available. Policies of the operating room also enter in.

6. Can the goal be achieved within an identifiable period of time? To measure goal achievement, the nurse must establish a deadline or a time frame when setting the goal. A goal might be that the patient will be free of wound infection 72 hours post-operatively. The goal has a clear time period. If the patient shows any evidence of wound infection in this time, such as redness, swelling, or drainage at the incision site, the nurse will know that this goal was not met. If the wound is clean and dry with no evidence of redness or swelling at 72 hours postoperatively, the nurse could safely say the goal was achieved.

7. Are the goals assigned appropriate priorities? Once goals have been identified, they are ranked in order of importance. The patient, family, nurse, and other members of the health care team all participate in assigning priorities. The nurse must determine what care is required immediately, what care can wait for a time, and which actions may be long term. Like the nursing diagnosis and patient problems, goals are assigned to be immediate, intermediate, or long term.

Prescribing Nursing Actions

Nursing actions or nursing orders are written for each goal. These are measures that the nurse believes must be taken for the patient to reach his goal. Goals may have one or more nursing actions. Orders must be written in a way that is understandable to those putting them into practice. Since nursing orders must be followed consistently and uniformly, they should be written to minimize any chance of misinterpretation.

Action verbs are one method to describe the nursing actions to be carried out. For example, "Observe and record size and color of ulcerated area on buttock when patient taken to recovery room," or, "Listen to patient express his concerns regarding pending surgical procedure."

It is important to write the orders straight-forwardly. If an order is difficult to understand and cannot be carried out easily, the nurse who is putting the plan into action will choose his own nursing action instead of those prescribed specifically to meet the goal for this patient. Nursing orders about human relationships, such as, "Give emotional support," might be carried out in various ways by different nurses. Therefore, the action for emotional support should be specific, such as, "Listen to Mr. Jones express his anger." The nurse should also be specific about nursing orders relating to observation of signs and symptoms. He might write on the plan, "Check dressing for bleeding, report amount to head nurse, and chart findings." This same approach could be used for pulse, blood pressure, or other signs that need to be closely observed.

Each nursing order consists of five parts—what, how, when, where, and who (see Fig. 8.1). The plan specifies *what* nursing action the nurse should perform to achieve the goal. The activity is usually preceded by an action verb specifying the nature of the action. The operating room care plan will include nursing orders such as:

- "Explain where the patient's family may wait."
- "Identify the patient upon admission to the OR suite."
- "Verify the surgical site with the patient, surgeon, and record."

The order indicates *how* the action is adapted to the individual patient. Any adaptation or change from the usual procedure should be placed in writing. For example, a change is necessary in the plan for a patient having a dilatation and curettage who is to be placed in the lithotomy position. If the patient has a hip prosthesis or fused hip that limits the range of motion, the nursing order should state how the patient is to be positioned. The nursing order should also state, "Additional personnel needed to hold extremity during procedure."

When indicates the timing and frequency of the prescribed order. This simply means the hour, specific time, or the frequency of the order. For example, "Mr. Edwards will receive his preoperative medication one hour before the scheduled time for the procedure," or "The nurse will stand by Mr. Edwards during induction." Knowing when something is to occur allows the nurse to organize his time for the

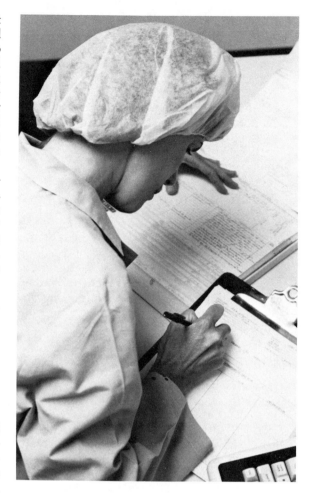

Figure 8.1. The nurse develops the plan specifying the nursing orders during the intraoperative period.

nursing care to be given to a number of patients. An intraoperative example would be counts for instruments, needles, and sponges. In an abdominal case, counts must be done prior to closure of the peritoneum, fascia, and skin. The frequency is three times, and the time is at closure of the specific layers of tissue.

Where concerns the location of the activity. Does it occur on the patient care unit, the holding area, the operating room, recovery area, or critical care unit? This is important because the order might specify that the patient will have a shave preparation prior to surgery, and the person assigned will need to know where this should take place. The order might say, "Shave prep in holding area," or, "Surgeon will shave head in operating room," or, "Shave abdominal area and scrub with antibacterial soap the morning of surgery."

Intravenous fluids are sometimes started for patients in their room or the holding area. The nursing order might read, "Insert 18-gauge intracath and start 5 percent dextrose and H_2O in holding area." Where the activity takes place is important because if an activity is not timed carefully it can affect the time of surgery, hold up the schedule, create a higher potential for infection, or compromise asepsis.

Who carries out the nursing orders relates to the nursing team member who is assigned the responsibility. The plan should indicate whether this is a nurse, licensed practical nurse, technician, or nursing assistant. Prior to assigning personnel to perform nursing activities, the nurse in charge should have a basic understanding of the abilities and educational preparation of the nursing staff. For elective surgery patients, the custom is to have a transport orderly bring them from their room. In every situation, however, the nurse should assess the need for additional personnel, such as for a patient with a fractured femur whose leg must remain in traction during transportation. Here the order might state, "Transport to OR in bed with two orderlies. One orderly maintains leg in alignment with traction." In another situation, a patient in the operating room is showing all the signs of malignant hyperthermia. The nurse in charge carefully selects additional personnel based on their previous experience with carrying out nursing activities necessary for the patient with this condition.

Planning the right nursing activity for each patient having surgery is a major part of professional nursing responsibility. Done thoroughly and carefully, it will involve logic, experience, and scientific knowledge. Most important, it will require devotion to the principle that each patient is an individual who deserves care that is planned for his case alone.

Patient Situation

Goals must be realistic, usable, measurable, behavioral, achievable, and include a time element. To further illustrate how these elements are incorporated into goals let us refer to Mr. Fischer. Mr. Fischer was scheduled for a possible left hemiglossectomy, left mandibulectomy, and neck dissection. Postoperatively he will have a tracheostomy, nasogastric tube, and wired jaw.

Preoperatively the perioperative nurse made an assessment and determined that Mr. Fischer's surgery would create a communication problem. The anatomical resection, jaw wiring, and tracheostomy would impair his ability to talk. Therefore, one goal for Mr. Fischer was that he would be able to communicate postoperatively with his physicians, nurses, and family members. Another preoperative goal that relates to communication is that Mr. Fischer will be able to verbalize understanding of his perioperative care prior to administration of the preoperative medication.

Mr. Fischer did not know what would happen to him throughout the perioperative period, and explanations were necessary to assist him in coping with his fear of the unknown. Both goal statements based on his communication problem meet the criteria described for writing goal statements.

Intraoperatively, Mr. Fischer has the potential for neuromuscular damage because he is elderly, the procedure will be lengthy, and he has some evidence of edema in his extremities. The patient goal is that Mr. Fischer will be free from neuromuscular complications 24 hours postoperatively. These are complications due to positioning and length of the procedure. This goal also meets the criteria for writing goal statements.

During the postoperative period other problems present themselves. One problem Mr. Fischer encounters is a respiratory problem due to alteration of his airway by the presence of a tracheostomy and the mandibular fixation. The goal is simply that Mr. Fischer will have a patent airway until his tracheostomy is closed. A potential respiratory problem is his increased risk for postoperative complications because of his history of bronchitis, smoking, and exposure to environmental irritants. The patient goal is that he will be free of respiratory complications 48 hours postoperatively. Specific complications include atelectasis and aspiration. The intraoperative care plans given in Figs. 8.2 and 8.3 show the goals for Mr. Fischer.

INTRAOPERATIVE PATIENT CARE PLAN

Mr. Ralph Fischer

NURSING DIAGNOSIS	GOAL	PLAN	IMPLEMENTATION	EVALUATION
PREOPERATIVE				
Knowledge, lack of external resources (people or material)	Patient will verbalize understanding of his perioperative care prior to administration of preoperative medications.			
Communication, impaired verbal due to surgical anatomical resection, jaw wiring, tracheostomy.	Patient will be able to communicate postoperatively.			
INTRAOPERATIVE				
Potential for neuromuscular damage due to required positioning and length of surgical prodecure.	Patient will be free from neuromuscular complications 24 hours postoperatively.			

Figure 8.2. Intraoperative patient care plan showing preoperative and intraoperative nursing diagnoses and goals for Mr. Fischer.

INTRAOPERATIVE PATIENT CARE PLAN

Mr. Ralph Fischer

NURSING DIAGNOSIS	GOAL	PLAN	IMPLEMENTATION	EVALUATION
POSTOPERATIVE Respiratory: Alteration in airway (tracheostomy, hemiglossectomy, mandibular fixation.	Patient will have patent alternative airway until tracheostomy is closed.			
Increased risk for postop complications due to: 1. History of bronchitis 2. History of smoking 3. Exposure to environmental irritants.	Patient will be free of respiratory complications 48 hours postop. 1. Infection 2. Atelectasis 3. Aspiration			

Figure 8.3. Intraoperative patient care plan showing postoperative nursing diagnosis and goals for Mr. Fischer.

References

1. Doona, M. E. "The judgment process in nursing." *Image* 8(June):27–29, 1976.
2. Ford, J. G., Trygstad-Durland, L. N., and Nelmsa, B. C. *Applied Decision Making for Nurses.* St. Louis: C. V. Mosby, 1979.
3. Alexander, C., Dodge, G., and Sabbe, J. *Guidelines for AORN Chapter-Sponsored C. E. Activities.* Denver: Association of Operating Room Nurses, 1980.
4. *Standards of Perioperative Nursing Practice.* Kansas City: American Nurses' Association and Association of Operating Room Nurses, 1982.
5. Marriner, A. *The Nursing Process: A Scientific Approach to Nursing Care.* St. Louis: C. V. Mosby, 1975.

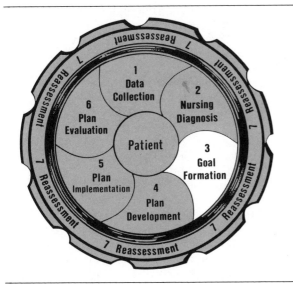

GOAL: Knowledge of the physiological and psychological responses to surgery.

The Patient's Understanding of Surgery

The first goal of perioperative nursing is that the patient will understand the surgery she is about to undergo. The goal is based on the patient's legal right to know. In the last decade it has become increasingly important that the patient has and demonstrates knowledge of the usual responses to surgery. Health consumers today demand this right and refuse to be considered incapable of understanding the details of their illness.

An informed consent for surgical intervention is one that the patient gives knowing and understanding the relevant facts. These include the risks involved, the probability of success of the surgery, and the alternatives. The patient relies on the physician to determine what information is relevant. If the patient has questions or is not completely comfortable about the need for surgery, the nurse is obligated to notify the physician so that further clarification can be initiated.

The commitment of the operating room nurse to the goal of patient understanding is reflected in the *Standards of Perioperative Nursing Practice* (1). The first nursing action described in the standards is: "Assurance of information and supportive preoperative teaching specifically related to the surgical intervention and the operating room nursing care."

The criteria for the goal of patient understanding are that the patient, family, and significant others can:

1. Cite the reason(s) for each of the preoperative instructions provided and exercises explained or practiced.
2. State the time surgery is scheduled.
3. State the unit to which the patient will return following surgery (e.g., intensive care, same unit, recovery room).
4. List anticipated monitoring and therapeutic devices or materials likely to be used postoperatively (e.g., intravenous, catheters, blood).
5. State the location of family and significant others during the intraoperative and immediate recovery periods.
6. Describe in general terms the surgical procedures and subsequent treatment plan (medical and nursing).
7. Describe anticipated steps in postoperative activity resumption.
8. Verbalize expectations about pain relief and the measures likely to be taken to alleviate pain.
9. Express feelings (anger, fear, anxiety, etc.) regarding surgical intervention and its expected outcomes.

In 1972, recognizing that the legal responsibility to the patient is shared by the physician and the hospital, the American Hospital Association (AHA) published the *Patient's Bill of Rights* (2). It is an effort to guide hospitals in rendering more effective care. As a hospital employee and patient's advocate, the nurse in the operating room has an obligation to determine that the patient has given informed consent to surgery and is informed about the perioperative period.

The American Nurses' Association (ANA) *Code for Nurses* (3) refers to the nurse safeguarding the patient from "incompetent, unethical or illegal conduct." The code requires that the operating room nurse seek clarification if, in her judgment, the patient has unanswered questions. Determining which circumstances can be handled without assistance from a physician is a nursing judgment. Good communication between the nurse and physician is needed to prevent misunderstandings and to assure that patients receive correct and consistent information. Table 9.1 provides a comparison of statements from the AHA's *Patient's Bill of Rights* and the ANA's *Code for Nurses*.

The perioperative nurse-teacher faces a challenge. To meet the goal of patient understanding, the nurse must be able to rapidly assess the patient's knowledge and receptiveness to learning. Furthermore, a method of teaching appropriate to the situation must be determined and implemented.

The learning needs of the patient can be identified in several ways. The patient may ask questions that indicate her needs. Comments made during the interview may also give clues to her understanding or lack of it. Another way to determine what the patient understands is by asking questions. It is important not to make assumptions about what the patient does or does not know. Careful observation of the patient's behavior may imply a lack of knowledge, but it should be validated by questioning.

In reviewing the criteria, we discuss ways the nurse can assist the patient to achieve this goal. Explanations of hospital and preoperative routines may be carried out in many ways. Many hospitals prepare videotapes available on a special channel for patient viewing. Printed material of hospital and operating room routines are also used widely. These teaching aids must be supplemented by individualized instruction so the patient will understand the implications of the surgery. Providing information is not the same as teaching. Telling a mother not to give her child anything to eat or drink after midnight or printing it on a list of instructions will not assure that the mother has been taught, only that information has been given. Many parents do not consider a glass of water in the category of eating or drinking. Teaching the mother includes an explanation of the need for an empty stomach and the danger of vomiting. The explanation should be tailored to the assessed ability of the mother to understand. Care must be taken, however, not to alarm parents when discussing potential dangers to their children.

Wherever possible, demonstration should be used as an adjunct to teaching. If the nurse

Table 9.1. Comparison of AHA's Patient Bill of Rights *with ANA's* Code for Nurses.

Statements from *A Patient Bill of Rights*	Statements from *Code for Nurses*
Right to respectful, considerate care.	The nurse respects human dignity and the uniqueness of the individual. Statement reflects patient's right to nondiscriminatory and nonjudgmental health care.
Right to be fully informed about health problems or to have another informed on patient's behalf. Right to know by name the physician responsible for care.	
Right of giving informed consent to all therapeutic measures. Informed consent includes explanation of risks, alternative courses of therapy and length of incapacitation involved.	The nurse respects a patient's right to control what is done with his person. The nurse recognizes the patient's right to information needed to make informed decisions as well as right to refuse treatment.
Right to refuse treatment and be informed of the consequences of refusal.	The nurse protects the public from misinformation by ethical behavior.
Right to privacy.	The nurse safeguards the right to privacy and protects information confidentiality. Judicious disclosure of information to health care team members and others is permitted. Access to records of care is protected and allowed only with patient's written authorization.
Right to expect that all information about himself and his health status and problems is kept confidential.	
Right to reasonable request for services, including evaluation and/or referral.	The nurse is responsible to the public to personally implement and maintain optimal standards of care.
Right to be informed about student participation in his/her care as well as relationships between institutions and other personnel involved with his/her care.	The nurse participates in activities that contribute to development of profession's body of knowledge within the limits imposed by human rights in research. Nurse investigators assure human research subjects' well-being, privacy, and other rights. Nurses recognize patient's right to participate in research by informed consent; to refuse consent and to withdraw from research projects.
Right to be informed about and refuse to participate in research conducted with human subjects.	
Right to reasonable continuity of care, including discharge planning and information concerning care requirements after discharge.	
Right to review and obtain answers to questions about his/her hospital bill regardless of payment source.	The nurse participates in the profession's efforts to implement and improve standards of care. The nurse is responsible to the public to personally implement and maintain optimal care.
Right to be informed of hospital expectations concerning his/her behavior as a patient.	The nurse respects human dignity and the uniqueness of the individual.

from the operating room explains deep breathing, coughing, and passive exercises, for example, demonstration and return demonstration are most effective. Explaining respiratory and circulatory complications should be matter of fact, but the nurse should be continually alert to signs of anxiety when discussing complications. A patient who is not coping well with the stress of hospitalization and impending surgery may overreact and enter a crisis phase when such information is discussed. The nurse should be positive, supportive, and reassuring, presenting a decisive, confident image.

Close communication with the patient's physician is also an important aspect of effective preoperative teaching. Unusual responses of

patients should be reported to the physician immediately so that preoperative anxieties can be handled. It is extremely important for the nurse to realize that a patient sometimes demonstrates a stressful reaction when discussing upcoming surgery. Nurses should not feel guilty if all does not run smoothly. It is not abnormal for a preoperative patient to demonstrate some anxiety and is probably therapeutic, for it can then be discussed and handled.

Informing the patient of the scheduled time of surgery can be tricky at best in some institutions. While there are many operating rooms in many institutions where the time of surgery can be predicted with some degree of accuracy, there are as many institutions where it cannot.

Many variables, including the condition of the patient, make it advisable to discuss an approximate time, explaining that there may be delays, which should not be cause for alarm. Whenever there is the possibility of an alternate plan, it should be explained to the patient. In the unfamiliar hospital world, patients tend to consider information as absolute. The nurse should be certain that absolute status is not given to something that may be subject to change.

The same holds true when discussing the anticipated unit to which the patient will return, the devices which will be used postoperatively for monitoring, and the drains and other therapeutic devices used. Collaboration with other team members is necessary so that accurate preoperative information can be given. Preoperative instruction is useless, and even harmful, if the total plan for the patient is not fully understood. Resource people, who can fill in the nurse prior to the interview and who should be consulted if there are questions, are the unit nurses, the surgeon or resident, the operating room supervisor or person who handles scheduling, and others such as admitting personnel involved in activities that affect the patient.

A waiting area is usually provided for family or significant others during surgery. When giving this information, the nurse should be informed of the surgeon's routines. Some surgeons, for example, instruct families or friends to wait in the patient's room. Between surgical procedures, the surgeon phones the room to talk to the family and give the immediate postoperative information. Other surgeons meet families in the waiting area.

A challenging and demanding aspect of preoperative teaching is the delicate discussion of the surgery itself. The nurse must be sure of her guidelines before this discussion begins. Collaboration with the physician is important. Patients sometimes ask very explicit questions of nurses in an effort to test their surgeon, nurse, or both. If the nurse is to discuss surgical details, she must reinforce the surgeon's prior explanation of the surgery. In some instances, the surgeon may not wish the surgery discussed by anyone else. In other cases, the surgeon and nurse mutually agree on what may be discussed. When on doubtful ground, a good rule to remember is to discuss only activities that the nurse is responsible for and that occur while the patient is awake. Whenever there is a discrepancy between the patient's understanding of the upcoming surgery and its outcome and the actual situation, however, it is imperative that the nurse communicate with other members of the health care team, particularly the surgeon.

Operating room nurses are comfortable with preoperative and intraoperative periods, but sometimes have difficulty with the postoperative period. The demands of the patient preoperatively, both physically and psychologically, are usually well known to the nurse in the operating room. Postoperatively, however, unless there is a problem attributable to the operating room, the OR nurse is not as involved. Therefore, less emphasis is placed on the postoperative phase. Discussion of postoperative activity resumption, pain relief, and concerns about altered body image, changes in lifestyle, or other expected outcomes of surgery are often left to the unit nurse.

The nurse from the operating room, however, should discuss postoperative activity and answer questions the patient may have. The operating room nurse is looked upon not only as knowledgeable but also as sharing in the most critical period of a patient's hospitalization. This is a responsibility that should not be overlooked. For example, a patient may ask if an operating room nurse will accompany her back to the intensive care unit to assist with her care. Desire for continuity is indicated in this question. The operating room nurse must be prepared to support, reassure, empathize with, and inform these patients. Questions which have been forgotten may often be elicited during the preoperative interview.

To determine if the patient understands the usual postoperative course, begin with broad questions. If the patient does not volunteer information, or appears confused, more specific questions can be asked. For example:

Nurse: "Do you have any questions about what happens after surgery?"

Patient: "No, I don't think so." (May indicate the patient does not know what to ask.)

Nurse: "Do you understand that you will have a tube in your throat after surgery to help your breathing, and that it will be a bit uncomfortable?"

Patient: "The doctor said a machine would help me breathe for a while. How long will I have it?"

Nurse: "That will depend on how long it takes for your lungs to resume their normal function. Remember, you won't be able to talk while the tube is in place."

This approach will identify areas that may need reinforcement. Patients may not remember specifics that have already been explained. They only hear what they can cope with, and repetition will help them accept more information as they adapt to the hospital environment. This type of questioning can also be used to determine how much the patient has internalized about therapeutic devices that will be used postoperatively.

The word "discomfort" rather than "pain" should be used, so that the patient's concern will be minimized. The patient can be encouraged to discuss concerns and fears about pain, as well as how she generally tolerates pain or discomfort. For example, explaining why she may have some muscle discomfort will help allay concerns that this is not normal. She may not understand that there is a reason for the discomfort and may think it indicates a complication. The nurse should discuss ways to relieve discomfort by changing positions, for example, and the availability of medication for extreme pain. The patient's expectations about pain and relief of it can be identified by a question such as, "Do you have any concerns about discomfort postoperatively?"

Questions about resuming activities after surgery are more frequently spontaneous, with less need for probing, because patients are eager to talk about the more positive aspects of their recuperation. If the outcome of the surgery is in doubt, however, short-term goals may be all the patient can cope with. The opportunity to express feelings about the surgery and expected outcome can be provided using broad terms, allowing the patient to set the limits on what is discussed.

It is probably unrealistic to expect all the patient's questions to be answered, particularly those related to the outcome of an uncertain diagnosis. As much as possible, though, the entire staff can assist the patient in managing fears and anxiety by providing as much information as the patient needs or requests.

Factors That Influence Goal Attainment

Because the preoperative interview is a complex activity, all phases of the nursing process may occur during this period. Many factors that affect communication between the nurse and the patient occur simultaneously. External conditions such as location and timing of the interview, the involvement of family members or significant others, and the rapport the nurse is able to establish with the patient are important components in attaining this goal. Equally important are internal factors such as the readiness of the patient to deal with the surgical intervention, the prior experience of the patient with hospitalization, and the level of anxiety. When we examine the teaching-learning process, we note the similarity to the nursing process. The first phase is assessment of the learning needs and the learner's ability. Principles of learning are used during the planning and implementation phase. Evaluation of goal attainment occurs throughout the perioperative period.

The assessment phase of the preoperative interview is much more subtle than simply observing for physical disorders such as petechiae, bruises, bumps, or limited range of motion. The operating room nurse must make a nursing diagnosis of the emotional and psychosocial status of the preoperative patient. The teaching plan is initiated with the review of the patient's chart and continues during the interview with the patient and family. A review of some principles of learning illustrates ways the nurse can assist the patient to achieve her learning goals.

Principles of Learning

PERCEPTION AND ATTITUDE

The patient enters the hospital with a preconceived idea of what will happen. This may be based on real experiences or be derived from conversations with others who have had surgery. The nurse assesses what knowledge the patient already possesses and corrects or supplements it with factual information. Questions such as, "What is your understanding of surgery?" or, "Do you have any particular concerns about your surgery?" will often open up areas for clarification.

Just providing information to patient and family such as telling where the operating room is and where the family can wait during surgery, or where they can get coffee, will indicate that the operating room staff are concerned about the comfort of relatives or friends. A rapport between the operating room nurse and the patient will do much to change negative attitudes about the surgical experience and will have a positive effect on learning. How the nurse establishes rapport will depend on the personality of the patient and the circumstances surrounding the interview.

EMOTIONS

Neutral or slightly positive or negative emotions are generally conducive to learning. Extreme emotion, however, will block learning. Patients who exhibit high anxiety as the result of shock or fear will not remember information given to them. Often, after the physician has told the patient about her need for surgery, the patient will hear nothing else until later, when she accepts the situation. Once she has been admitted to the hospital, slight anxiety motivates her to learn what is likely to happen. For this reason, the evening prior to surgery is usually a good time for preoperative teaching. In some situations, the stress level remains high, and the preoperative teaching may need to be deferred, except for minimal information giving. The patient will need time to accept surgery that is potentially disfiguring or that may result in a serious diagnosis. The nurse must also be aware of her own values and not project discomfort to the patient. How teaching is managed will determine how effectively the patient handles the surgical experience.

Patients respond to preoperative stress in the same manner as they cope with other crises or stresses in their lives. If they are unable to cope with stress in a positive way, they may use defense mechanisms temporarily or even as a permanent adaptive behavior. For example, it is common to see denial manifested by an inappropriate cheerfulness in a patient who has a serious diagnosis. She may indicate she has no questions, joke with the nurse, and try to control the conversation. The nurse should not confront the denial; she should offer information in a casual manner, allowing trust to be established with the patient setting the limitations. For example, a man who is director of a very large department is admitted for a ptosis procedure under local anesthetic with sedation and an anesthesiologist in attendance. This man is full of jokes preoperatively and the evening prior to surgery shows little interest in what will happen. He shrugs off teaching attempts with, "Oh, I know you all will take good care of me." The next morning, however, after he is sedated, he is quiet and shows signs of marked anxiety. The nurse says it must certainly feel different to have someone else in charge of everything when he is so used to making the decisions. He immediately expresses his discomfort at feeling helpless and seems to relax as the nurse instructs him on how to assist in his care for the next few hours. As his anxiety level increased, his defense level shifted from denial to repression, and the nurse was able to assist him to manage. The more information a nurse has available about the patient, the more she is able to assist in anxiety management. Perhaps the most important factor, however, is the empathy of the nurse.

Patients are sometimes depressed, and anger and guilt are manifested as the patient emerges from depression. Understanding and management of this emotion are necessary before any learning will occur. The operating room nurse who is confronted by a barrage of complaints about the hospital or staff or is told, "You're the fourth person in an hour to come in here bothering me," might handle this hostility by saying, "I'm sorry so many of us have interrupted you while you're getting settled. Each of us is involved in your care during surgery tomorrow, and we all want to do our best for you. Perhaps I could come back later if you need a little rest."

If the hostility does not have a focus but is simply rude, aggressive behavior, the nurse might ask, "You appear to be angry with me. I'm not sure why." If the patient continues to be hostile, it is best to offer to terminate the interview. Often, however, an open reference

to the anger may assist the patient to recognize her projection and deal with the reality of the surgery more effectively. In this instance, the patient's learning needs can often be met (see Table 9.2).

PHYSICAL AND MENTAL READINESS

A patient who is ill and mentally exhausted from coping with the problems associated with her hospitalization may not remember or fully understand instructions. The nurse should note this limited readiness for learning and docu-

Table 9.2. *Facilitating Learning.*

Response to Anticipation of Surgery	Defense Mechanism	Other Contributing Factors	Nursing Intervention to Facilitate Learning
Anxiety May act jovial and in control. Minimizes or denies symptoms. Misleads the nurse. Uses words such as "just a little," "no problem," "no questions." Appears uncomfortable during conversation.	denial	Patient may not be able to cope with helplessness.	Do not confront the denial. Establish trust. Volunteer some information of a nonthreatening nature and in a matter-of-fact manner. Casually solicit questions. Do not be controlling. Encourage patient through facilitators such as attentive silence, interested posture, etc.
Anger Indicates distrust at questioning. Accusing, suspicious. May complain about physician or other nurses.	projection	Previous authority figure problems, i.e., angry competitive relationship with parent.	Do not be misled into believing that anger against health team is warranted. Ask about anger.
Frustration Expresses feeling of being thwarted. Anger directed at someone or something.		May have had bad experience with other hospital personnel, i.e., long wait in admitting department, lab, or x-ray.	Be tactful and firm. Do not side with patient against others on health team. Listen. Let patient vent feelings.
Depression and self-rejection Appears withdrawn, apathetic, silent	repression	Physical exhaustion due to illness or strain of admitting procedures. Resignation to feelings of helplessness, despair.	Ask tactful, kind questions about depression. Provide empathetic silence. Quietly give major information. Offer availability when the patient feels stronger or feels like talking.
Compulsive behavior Overtalkative, egocentric, hypochondriacal. Tells symptoms in detail. Asks questions, then apologizes for asking.	regression	May have unusually dependent personality. May be embarrassed, nervous. May be attempting to be a "good" patient. Clinging, lonely, fear that interviewer will leave. Elderly patients sometimes ramble.	Reassure and support. Be certain patient understands. Ask patient to repeat instructions. Redirect, as necessary to accomplish teaching goal.

ment the need for repeated teaching as the patient's health status improves. Use of the senses to help the patient know what to expect in surgery will help her remember. Since hearing remains acute after premedication, even when other senses are dulled, the nurse should warn the patient to expect noises or talking to seem louder. Demonstration, pictures, and descriptions of sights and sounds, for example, will assist in preparing the patient for what she can expect in the operating room. Describing the hard mattress or the cold room and the availability of warm blankets is useful. If videotapes, pictures, models, or verbal descriptions of what the patient will encounter are used, they should show how the patient will perceive the experience (see Fig. 9.1). For example, pictures of the operating room should be taken from the stretcher or bed so that the surroundings are shown as the patient will see them.

EFFECTIVE LEARNING REQUIRES PARTICIPATION

Discussion to determine what information the patient already has and to add or clarify instructions is important. Open-ended questions encourage dialogue and help the nurse assess what the patient anticipates.

Broad questions should be used initially, and specific questions can be asked to obtain information the patient does not volunteer. Let us suppose a patient has been admitted for a thyroidectomy. From reading her chart the nurse knows the patient had a cholecystectomy at another hospital two years ago. After introducing herself, the nurse might ask, "Have you had surgery before?" The patient might answer, "Yes, I had my gall bladder out several years ago, but I don't remember much about it. Except, I was really sore for a long time afterward." The nurse could describe some of the hospital routines, referring to the past experience, such as, "Do you remember not having anything to eat or drink after midnight?" By encouraging participation in this way, the interview is a dialogue comfortable for the patient, and not stiff and lecturelike. The patient is contributing to the learning process, not just being bombarded with a lot of information or instructions. What the patient tells the nurse sets the tone for the preoperative teaching. From this information, the nurse can assess what the patient wants to know, what has already been discussed with the physician, and what the patient needs to know.

Figure 9.1. A model is used to show where the surgery will be and how dentures will be replaced.

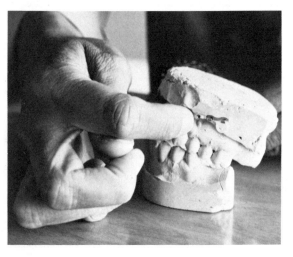

REPETITION AND REINFORCEMENT

Repetition and reinforcement are necessary to increase the amount of information the patient retains. Patients who are having surgery under local anesthetic will particularly benefit from a preoperative evaluation of the procedures. When the instructions are repeated in the operating room, the patient will not be dealing with unfamiliar information and will find it easier to comply.

Information discussed with the surgeon needs to be repeated and reinforced. The patient is often so upset at the prospect of having surgery, she hears little else until her anxiety level decreases. At that time, questions about the perioperative period arise. Frequently, information or instructions must be repeated several times before a full understanding of events surrounding the operation is reached.

The nurse can assist the patient to remember by asking the patient to clarify what her understanding is.

It is important to realize that when a patient says she was not informed about something, most probably the patient has forgotten information. Nurses tend to assume the patient has not been informed, rather than assess the reactions of the patient to the hospital experience.

Significant Others

Another factor influencing goal attainment is the patient's support system. The importance of family and friends to the well-being of the patient must also be determined. The nurse must identify the person or persons who support the patient and consider how to assist them through the surgical experience.

A significant other is that person who provides the major emotional support for the patient (see Fig. 9.2). This person may be a spouse or relative, but not necessarily. The patient may be alone. The nurse must then find out if there is anyone who should be kept informed, or if the staff will be the patient's only support. Professional support may be important for this patient, but the nurse must be careful not to impose, allowing her the right to privacy and dependence on her own inner strength if that is her desire.

Information obtained during the interview is confidential and should be released only to those immediately involved in the care, unless

Figure 9.2. The patient's wife provides emotional support.

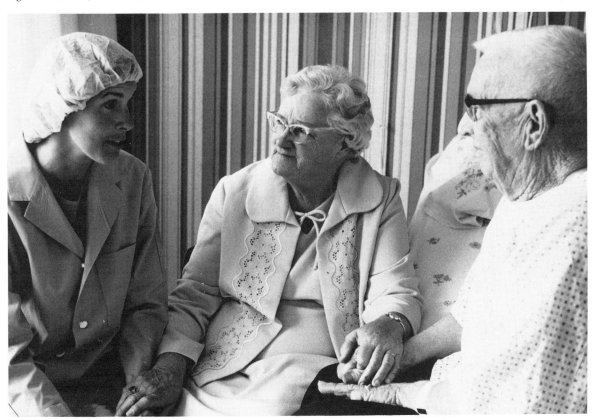

the patient gives permission otherwise. Particular care should be taken with patients in ambulatory surgery. Messages should not be given to family members or others at the patient's phone number unless the patient permits it. The patient may choose not to tell others about the surgery. For example, patients who have cosmetic or sterilization procedures, sometimes do not tell family or friends.

Preoperative teaching is shared by the surgeon, anesthesiologist, and nurses involved in the surgical experience. How effectively the patient goals are met depends on the professional accountability of these individuals. It is important that they not only communicate with each other, but share a respect for each other and for the role each plays in the overall care of the patient. Nurses, in particular, must support each other, if the continuity of care is to be maintained throughout the preoperative, intraoperative, and postoperative phases of care. Communication, both orally and through documentation, will do much to provide this support.

Preoperative teaching is an active process that includes (1) assessment of learning needs and readiness of the patient to learn, (2) teaching, using learning principles, and (3) evaluating the effectiveness of the dialogue by observing the patient's responses.

References

1. *Standards of Perioperative Nursing Practice.* Kansas City: American Nurses' Association and Association of Operating Room Nurses, 1982.
2. *Patient's Bill of Rights.* Chicago: American Hospital Association, 1972.
3. American Nurses' Association. *The Code for Nurses with Interpretative Statements.* Kansas City: ANA, 1979.

Suggested Readings

Annas, G. J. *The Rights of Hospital Patients.* New York: Avon, 1975.

Enelow, A. J., and Swisher, S. N. *Interviewing and Patient Care.* New York: Oxford University Press, 1972.

Francis, G. M., and Mungas, B. *Promoting Psychological Comfort,* 2nd ed. Dubuque, Iowa: William C. Brown Co., 1975.

Gruendemann, B. J., Casterton, S., Hesterly, S., Minckley, B., and Shetler, M. *The Surgical Patient: Behavioral Concepts for the Operating Room Nurse,* 2nd ed. St. Louis: C. V. Mosby, 1979.

Pohl, M. L. *The Teaching Function of the Nursing Practitioner,* 3rd ed. Dubuque, Iowa: William C. Brown Co., 1978.

Redman, B. K. *The Process of Patient Teaching in Nursing,* 4th ed. St. Louis: C. V. Mosby, 1980.

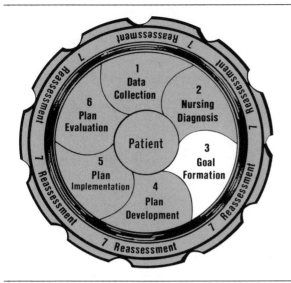

GOAL: Evidence of fluid and electrolyte balance.

Maintenance of Fluid and Electrolyte Balance

Each patient experiencing surgery has the potential for physiological imbalance in body fluids or electrolytes. The patient goal is maintenance of fluid and electrolyte balance during the perioperative period. Attainment of the goal is determined by the following criteria:

1. Ventricular rate is no less than 60 and no more than 110 contractions per minute as compared with the preoperative rate.
2. Diastolic blood pressure is within 20 mm Hg of preoperative pressure.
3. Systolic blood pressure is within 30 mm Hg of preoperative pressure.
4. Respiratory values are within 10 percent of the preoperative values.
5. Central venous pressure (CVP) reading is 6–12 mm H_2O and stable.
6. Cardiac rhythm is a normal sinus rhythm or consistent with preoperative rhythm.
7. Serum electrolytes are within normal limits or consistent with preoperative values.
8. Blood chemistry and arterial blood gas levels are within normal limits or consistent with preoperative values.
9. Physical signs and symptoms do not include those associated with impending fluid and electrolyte imbalance (vomiting, diarrhea, mental disorientation, etc.).
10. Fluid intake is at least 2,000 ml/4 hours unless contraindicated.

11. Urinary output is at least 30 ml/hour per 24 hours.

These criteria are examples of what could be used for patients having surgery. It must be recognized that individual patient responses may differ. Because of this, each person must have a baseline assessment prior to surgery which may be used as a guide in determining goal attainment. This list of criteria is not exhaustive, and other variables may be used for measurement purposes.

Fluid and electrolyte balance is vital to the health of every individual. The healthy individual maintains this balance (homeostasis) through his intake and output. Any disruption of this balance will cause illness or even death. The surgical patient is extremely vulnerable to fluid and electrolyte imbalance due to inadequate intake during the preoperative period or excessive loss of fluids during the intraoperative period. If the patient is unable to consume or retain normal amounts of fluid postoperatively, this problem is compounded. In addition, the patient must replace excess loss during surgery. A person may survive without food for several weeks but may succumb to lack of water in a few days or even a few hours. If fluid is lost through vomiting, diarrhea, or profuse drainage, the patient's problem may worsen from an electrolyte imbalance.

Certain factors influence the attainment of these goals. These factors include, but may not be limited to, the following: (1) fluid and electrolyte balances, (2) water balance, (3) sodium balance, (4) potassium balance, (5) calcium balance, (6) magnesium balance, (7) acid-base balance, (8) nursing care of the patient preoperatively, intraoperatively, and postoperatively.

Fluid and Electrolyte Balance

Body fluid, consisting largely of water, makes up 50–70 percent of adult body weight and 70–80 percent of infant weight. It contains dissolved minerals, proteins, and other nutrients and gases necessary for normal cell func-tion. Water is essential for cell activity. Fluids transport blood cells, oxygen, electrolytes, nutrients, and water to all tissues and cells. They help maintain stable body temperature. Water also carries waste products to excretion organs.

Body water is distributed between three functional compartments: the intracellular, extracellular (plasma), and interstitial. Some experts refer to just two compartments, combining the interstitial and extracellular, since both include all water outside the cells. Homeostasis is maintained by water moving back and forth freely from one compartment to another by osmosis. This occurs because a membrane between two compartments is permeable to water but not to nondiffusible substances or dissolved solutes, such as glucose or urea. The semipermeable membrane allows water to move toward the side of greater concentration from that of lesser concentration. This process does not totally balance the concentration within each compartment, however, because the pressure of the concentrates within a compartment resists water molecules by applying pressure on the opposite side of the semipermeable membrane.

This opposing pressure is called osmotic pressure. Osmotic pressure, or tonicity, depends on the number of particles, their activity, and the electrical charges within a given unit volume. The concentration of osmotically active particles will change when water is added or lost from the extracellular compartment.

Sodium, the major cation in extracellular fluid, accounts for approximately 90 percent of the osmotically active particles. Its presence has much to do with the tonicity of body fluid compartments. For example, when extracellular sodium is depleted, water will move into intracellular space until the two compartments again attain equal osmolarity. Changes in concentration of electrolytes, that is, osmotic pressure, immediately affect water balance by causing a water shift from one compartment to another.

Electrolytes are salts that dissociate in solution into separately charged particles (ions). These ions have either a positive (cation) or a negative (anion) electrical charge and help to maintain the osmotic pressure in body fluids.

Dissociated electrolytes are expressed in terms of their combining activity (equivalents) as compared with hydrogen. The number of ions in solution, or the concentration per given volume, is expressed as the number of milliequivalents per liter (mEq/liter). Positive and negative ions are balanced in the healthy person to create a state called electroneutrality. In other words, the sum of milliequivalents of cations—sodium, potassium, calcium, and magnesium—is equal to the sum of milliequivalents of anions—chloride, bicarbonate, phosphate, organic acids, and proteins. Nonelectrolyte substances, such as glucose, urea, bile salts, creatinine, and cholesterol, do not dissociate in water. However, they affect acid-base balance and osmotic pressure gradients.

The most common fluid imbalance in the surgical patient is an extracellular fluid deficit. Electrolytes are lost as well as water. The loss of gastrointestinal fluids accounts for most of the extracellular fluid loss and may be due to vomiting, diarrhea, draining fistulas, or nasogastric suctioning. The emergency surgical patient is at a higher risk of fluid and electrolyte imbalance, if the emergency condition has involved vomiting or diarrhea, and a lack of fluid intake over a period of several hours. Complete restoration of balance for these patients prior to surgery may not be possible. If an associated anemia and weakening of the patient's total condition accompanies the fluid and electrolyte depletion, an increased risk may exist.

Fluids may be pooled or isolated from normal compartments because of inflammation or infection, such as in peritonitis, or because of extravasation accompanying intestinal obstruction. This pooling is called third-space fluid or third-space edema. The fluid is still within the body but not available for functional use.

Protein is an organic nitrogenous compound that affects fluid balance. Constituting approximately 15 percent of all cell mass, it is the most abundant substance in cells except for water. Plasma proteins have a concentration about four times greater than fluid in the interstitial compartment. Practically all other substances diffuse readily into the interstitial tissue. Therefore, the inability of protein to diffuse freely into the interstitial space maintains effective osmotic pressure between the cellular and interstitial compartments. This is referred to as the colloid osmotic pressure. Since protein is necessary for most biochemical reactions, it also affects acid-base balance and acts as an important buffer.

The debilitated person who has had a major loss of body protein due to anorexia or starvation has several problems related to fluid and electrolyte balance because of the loss of striated muscle and the effects on the heart and kidneys. (1) Cardiac output declines because of slowed metabolic rate, causing an unstable blood pressure with bouts of hypertension. (2) Reduced blood pressure inhibits the kidney's ability to excrete acid. (3) The kidneys may not respond to antidiuretic hormone, and hypovolemia ensues. When there is severe protein deficit, red blood cells and hemoglobin, necessary for oxygen transport, are not adequately produced. When serum albumin levels fall from lack of adequate protein intake, fluid collects in the interstitial compartment because water is not drawn back due to lowered blood osmotic pressure. This is edema. Edema increases total body water, but the patient may remain hypovolemic because of the decreased circulating extracellular fluid. Additional hazards for the surgical patient from protein deficit are delayed wound healing and increased susceptibility to infection (1).

A positive nitrogen balance (anabolism) is needed for normal growth and during periods of special demand, such as pregnancy, tissue replacement following traumatic injury, or healing of surgical trauma. A negative nitrogen balance develops when output exceeds input (catabolism). This may occur when there is a sharp increase in use of protein, such as following major surgery, replacing blood and tissue fluid loss, or from inadequate intake or oxidation of proteins when carbohydrates are not being adequately metabolized.

Water Balance

The average adult man has approximately 40–45 liters of water. The body receives water through oral intake of fluids, water content in food, and the production of water from chemical oxidation of food as it is metabolized. Approximately 8 liters of fluid are secreted daily for digestion by gastrointestinal organs. This fluid is rich in electrolytes, and most of it is reabsorbed by the intestines. The body loses water by kidney excretion, perspiration, fecal discharge, and insensible loss through the lungs and skin (see Table 10.1). Hot weather and exercise increase the amount of water loss, and compensatory water intake is necessary to maintain health.

The kidneys are responsible for water control. They conserve or excrete water in response to deficiency and overload. Water balance control is governed by several major factors involving hormonal and neural regulation.

1. Vasopressin, an antidiuretic hormone, is secreted by the pituitary gland in response to changes in serum osmolarity. Osmolar changes stimulate thirst and also the reabsorption of water by tubular cells of the kidneys. The reabsorbed water is returned to body fluid.
2. Thirst is an important defense against water deficit. Although rare, disturbance of this mechanism may be associated with disturbed levels of consciousness, head injury, or some neurosurgical procedures.
3. Aldosterone is a sodium-conserving antidiuretic hormone produced by the adrenal cortex of the kidney. It is released or inhibited according to serum concentrations of sodium. Sodium, water conservation, and excretion are so closely related that one

can hardly be considered without the other two.

4. Decreased blood volume stimulates secretion of renin with increased formation of angiotensin II. This causes release of aldosterone, which acts on the tubular cells of the kidney to increase water and sodium absorption. Angiotensin II also acts as a vasopressor that diminishes renal blood flow by constricting the arterioles.
5. Decreased cardiac output and blood pressure associated with decreased fluid volume cause a decrease in glomerular filtration rate with resultant decreased water loss.
6. Stretch volume receptors located in the right and left atria respond to excessive blood volume by transmitting nerve signals to the brain. In response, sympathetic nerve signals to the kidneys are inhibited, and the rate of urinary output is increased (2). Under normal conditions, about 125 ml of water is extracted from the kidney each minute. About 124 ml is reabsorbed by tubule cells, leaving 1 ml to be excreted as urine.

WATER EXCESS (OVERHYDRATION)

Water excess, or overhydration, occurs when there is an excess of extracellular fluid, or hypervolemia. This can be the result of excess water intake without sufficient salt, such as may occur after profuse perspiration; prolonged use of intravenous fluids, such as dextrose and water; and pathological conditions, such as congestive heart failure, renal disorders, or adrenocortical insufficiency. Other causes are lymphatic obstruction, as from carcinoma; venous obstruction due to thrombosis or pressure of tumors; hypoproteinemia from cirrhosis of the liver, malnutrition, or severe malabsorption; toxemia of pregnancy; and corticosteroid overdosage or Cushing syndrome.

Signs and Symptoms
Clinical manifestations correspond to the degree of overhydration. These range from headache, mental confusion, delirium, and coma, to death. Other manifestations include muscle

Table 10.1. *Sources of Body Water Gain and Loss per 24 Hours (ml).*

Gain		Loss	
Fluid intake	1,500	Urine	1,500
Water in food	800	Feces	200
Metabolic water from oxidation of food	200	Perspiration and insensible loss	450
		Lungs	350
Total	2,500	Total	2,500

weakness, lack of coordination, puffy eyelids, weight gain, rales in lungs, shortness of breath, blurred vision, tachycardia with full bounding pulse, and moist, warm, flushed skin. There may be anorexia, nausea, and vomiting. Polyuria occurs if kidneys are healthy. Specific gravity falls below 1.010. There may be distended neck veins even when the patient is in semi-Fowler's position. Fluid excess and deficit have significant manifestations on various body systems (see Table 10.2). Both cause acute changes in osmolar concentration (see Table 10.3).

Nursing Intervention

The nurse must watch for the clinical signs of water excess. Nursing care is directed toward relieving symptoms. Discontinuing or slowing the rate of parenteral fluids or restricting oral intake may relieve mild overhydration. The nurse should carefully monitor vital signs since they provide information about the patient's circulatory status. Symptoms of respiratory distress should be reported as soon as detected. Placing the patient in semi-Fowler's position will relieve dyspnea. Diuretics are given as ordered. Accurate recording of intake and output is essential. Daily weights are obtained at the same time each morning and before breakfast if the patient is on oral intake. Special skin care is needed to prevent breakdown due to the poor circulation that accompanies edema. Mental status should be carefully observed as the patient may become disoriented and confused because of the increased intracranial pressure. The disoriented patient should be protected from injury. (When the overload is caused by a specific condition or disease, nursing intervention must be instituted for the problems manifested.)

Table 10.2. Extracellular Fluid Volume.

Signs	Deficit		Excess	
	Moderate	Severe	Moderate	Severe
Central nervous system signs	sleepiness apathy slow responses anorexia cessation of usual activity	decreased tendon reflexes anesthesia of distal extremities stupor coma	none	none
Gastrointestinal signs	progressive decrease in food consumption	nausea, vomiting refusal to eat silent ileus and distention	at surgery: edema of stomach, colon, lesser and greater omenta, and small bowel mesentary elevated venous pressure distension of peripheral veins increased cardiac output loud heart sounds	
Cardiovascular signs	orthostatic hypotension tachycardia collapsed veins collapsing pulse	cutaneous lividity hypotension distant heart sounds cold extremities absent peripheral pulses	functional murmurs bounding pulse high pulse pressure increased pulmonary 2nd sound galloping rhythm	pulmonary edema
tissue signs	soft, small tongue with longitudinal wrinkling decreased skin turgor	atonic muscles sunken eyes	subcutaneous pitting, edema Basilar rales	anasarca moist rales vomiting diarrhea
Metabolic signs	mild decrease of temperature 97–99°F	marked decrease of temperature 95–98°F	none	none

From Sabiston, D. C., ed. *Davis-Christopher Textbook of Surgery: The Biological Basis of Modern Surgical Practice*, 12th ed. Philadelphia: W. B. Saunders, 1981, p. 95. Reprinted with permission of publisher and author.

Table 10.3. Acute Changes in Osmolar Concentration.

Signs	Hyponatremia (Water Intoxication)		Hypernatremia (Water Deficit)	
	Moderate	Severe	Moderate	Severe
Central nervous system signs	muscle twitching hyperactive tendon reflexes increased intracranial pressure (compensated phase)	convulsions loss of reflexes increased intracranial pressure (compensated phase)	restlessness weakness	delirium maniacal behavior
Cardiovascular signs	changes in blood pressure and pulse secondary to increased intracranial pressure		tachycardia hypotension (if severe)	
Tissue signs	salivation, lacrimation watery diarrhea "finger printing" of skin (sign of intracellular volume excess)		decreased saliva and tears dry and sticky mucous membrane red, swollen tongue skin flushed	
Renal signs	oliguria progressing to anuria		oliguria	
Metabolic signs	none		fever	

From Sabiston, D. C., ed. *Davis-Christopher Textbook of Surgery: The Biological Basis of Modern Surgical Practice*, 12th ed. Philadelphia: W. B. Saunders, 1981, p. 95. Reprinted with permission of publisher and author.

WATER DEFICIT (DEHYDRATION)

Water deficit, or dehydration, occurs when there is depletion of extracellular fluids, or hypovolemia. The loss may be due to: vomiting, diarrhea, profuse perspiration, diuresis, hemorrhage, severe burns, draining fistulas, defective thirst mechanism, diabetes insipidus, deprived water and sodium intake, a continued rapid respiratory rate that increases evaporation, and impaired kidney conservation. Also, for each degree celsius of fever, there is a loss of 200 ml of water per day (1).

Infants are extremely vulnerable to fluid loss because of their higher proportion of body fluids. The infant has a daily turnover of over one-half of his extracellular volume as compared to about one-fifth for the adult. Moreover, his immature kidneys are poor conservers of water and he has greater need per kilogram because of increased heat production and rapid growth.

Signs and Symptoms

Manifestations of dehydration include thirst, dry skin and mucous membranes, longitudinal furrows in the tongue, sunken and soft eyeballs, decreased skin turgor (tenting), and a drop in body temperature and blood pressure. Either there is tachycardia or a regular pulse rate, but the pulse palpation can be easily obliterated with pressure. These patients also have oliguria progressing to anuria, constipation, weakness, and lethargy progressing to coma. The pulse may become weak and thready as the patient's condition worsens. Specific gravity levels range above 1.030. Hemoglobin and hematocrit are elevated due to the hemoconcentration. The degree of extracellular fluid loss is classified according to the percentage loss of total body weight: mild, 2–4 percent; moderate, 5–7 percent; severe, 8–12 percent. A 15 percent loss is fatal. (See Tables 10.3 and 10.4 for manifestations of deficit related to specific body systems.)

Table 10.4. *Related Pathophysiology and Causes of Acidosis and Alkalosis.*

Acidosis and Alkalosis	Pathophysiology	Causes
Respiratory acidosis	impaired excretion of CO_2 respiratory depression	drugs, i.e., narcotics, central nervous system depressants anesthetics injury neuromuscular disease pulmonary disorders or disease shock congestive heart failure
Respiratory alkalosis	excess loss of CO_2 acute hypoxia	hyperventilation cerebral hemorrhage high fever bacteremia salicylate intoxication high altitude exercise excessive mechanical ventilation
Metabolic acidosis	excess loss of base bicarbonate retention of fixed acids	severe diarrhea vomiting of lower gastrointestinal contents uremia diabetes lactic acid accumulation excess oxidation of fats and proteins (starvation) small-bowel fistula intestinal malabsorption Addison disease hypoxia
Metabolic alkalosis	loss of fixed acids potassium shift from extracellular to intracellular gain of base bicarbonate	vomiting of gastric contents gastric suctioning severe potassium depletion excess bicarbonate ingestion (alkaline drugs) diuretics excess aldosterone

Nursing Intervention

The circulating volume of fluid must be restored. The nurse must monitor parenteral fluids so replacement does not cause overload. Careful observation of the patient's signs and symptoms, recording, and reporting are essential. The nurse should record accurate intake and output. Output measurements include urine, emesis, suction, and wound drainage. The tongue should be checked for furrows, and overall status of the skin and mucous membranes should be assessed. Good oral hygiene is required because cracked, dry skin, lips, or mucous membranes predispose the patient to infection.

If the patient can tolerate oral fluids, and surgery is not imminent, there may be an order to force fluids. It is easier for the patient to drink in a Fowler's or semi-Fowler's position. The nurse may order fluids that the patient likes or use a small glass to give the patient a sense of accomplishment and thereby encourage him to try more. The nurse needs to know whether any fluids are contraindicated. Certain foods such as ice cream, sherbet, cantaloupe, and watermelon have high fluid content.

Sodium Balance

Sodium, found to some extent in all body fluids, is concentrated in extracellular fluid where it is the major cation. The normal range of sodium is 136–145 mEq/liter in extracellular fluid and 10 mEq/liter in intracellular fluid. It provides about 90 percent of total base in body fluids and 45 percent of base in extracellular fluid. Sodium maintains osmotic pressure of extracellular fluid and moves fluid from one compartment to another by its pump activity and its control over cell permeability. Homeostasis is maintained largely because water follows sodium. Sodium also helps control hydrogen ion balance through buffer action in the blood. About 3–4.5 gm of sodium are required daily. One teaspoon of table salt (5 gm) provides about 2 gm of sodium.

The adult normally has an intake of sodium ranging from 100 to 150 mEq, or about 6–18 gm per day. This is more than an adequate supply for transmission of electrochemical impulses, active and passive transport of other ions (change in cell permeability), buffering, and replacement of that lost through the kidneys, skin, and gastrointestinal tract. The most common source of sodium is table salt. Other food sources are milk, milk products, meat, eggs, fish, celery, asparagus, spinach, and carrots. Kidneys are the primary vehicle for conserving or excreting sodium. With adequate intake, sodium balance is maintained unless abnormal conditions exist.

SODIUM EXCESS (HYPERNATREMIA)

Sodium excess, or hypernatremia, exists when sodium serum levels exceed 145 mEq/liter. Kidney disorders are a major cause of sodium excess. Other causes include steroid therapy, impaired cardiac function, diabetes insipidus, hepatic disease, Cushing disease, and osmotic diureses that may be associated with excess tube feedings of protein. Excess water loss from diarrhea, excess intake of drugs or foods high in sodium, and severe burns causing excess loss of fluid are other contributing factors.

Signs and Symptoms
Clinical manifestations of hypernatremia are nausea and vomiting, flushed, dry skin, thirst, dry, sticky mucous membranes, muscle twitching and weakness, tremors, headache, confusion, convulsions, shock, and death if not corrected. In addition, the patient will have dry skin with poor turgor. If kidneys are functioning properly to conserve sodium and water, urine becomes concentrated with specific gravity above 1.030.

Nursing Intervention
The nurse should monitor the serum levels of sodium and notify the physician of abnormalities and changes. Urine specific gravity should be assessed and recorded. Accurate measurement of intake and output is essential. The patient should be weighed daily at the same time, on the same scales, and with the same weight of clothing. Fluids are given as ordered. Saline laxatives and other drugs with high sodium content are withheld. Substitute salt may be given. It is important to monitor the

patient's vital signs and note any changes. The nurse should institute seizure precautions if the patient exhibits marked hypernatremia.

SODIUM DEFICIT (HYPONATREMIA)

Sodium deficit, by hyponatremia, exists when serum sodium is below 130 mEq/liter. There are many predisposing factors involved with sodium loss:

1. Disease process:
   Diabetic ketoacidosis
   Renal tube acidosis
   Addison disease
   Nephritis
2. Problems related to disease or infectious problems:
   Vomiting
   Diarrhea
   Fistulas
   Profuse perspiration
   Intestinal obstruction with extravasation
3. Iatrogenic causes:
   Nasogastric suctioning
   Series of tap water enemas
   Diuretic therapy
   Creation of ileostomies
   Excessive use of parenteral 5 percent glucose and water without corresponding normal saline

Signs and Symptoms
Gastrointestinal manifestations include nausea, vomiting, diarrhea, and abdominal cramps. The muscular system exhibits weakness and twitching. Also there is poor skin turgor, weight loss, and a specific gravity of urine less than 1.010. The most serious manifestations are those of the central nervous system. Without intervention, these progress from headache to syncope, confusion, convulsions, coma, circulatory failure, shock, and death.

Nursing Intervention
The nurse must act immediately to save the life of the patient with severe deficit. Rapid infusion of isotonic solution may be ordered to correct serious serum level deficit. If it is necessary to continue rapid infiltration for a few

hours, the physician usually inserts a subclavian catheter so central venous pressure can be monitored. The nurse must monitor the infusion to prevent circulatory overload if rapid infusion is necessary over a period of a few hours [see "Water Excess (Overhydration)," above]. Other electrolytes are included with sodium replacement so that overall balance is assured. There should be accurate measuring and recording of intake and output. The nurse institutes seizure precautions. Oral replacement may be in the form of soups, bouillon, sodium chloride tablets, and table salt if the deficit is not too severe.

Nasogastric irrigations should be done with normal saline solution rather than water so excess sodium chloride is not suctioned or washed out. When the order states, "Give enemas until clear return," the physician should be consulted after giving three tap-water enemas. Additional tap-water enemas may lead to sodium deficit. Patients should be taught that they need to replace salt after drinking large quantities of water when there has been profuse perspiration after strenuous exercise or work.

Potassium Balance

Potassium is the major cation in intracellular fluid, with a concentration of about 150 mEq/liter. Intracellular levels of electrolytes are difficult to measure. Since potassium is also found in extracellular fluid in a range of 3.5–5.3 mEq/liter, it is common to measure serum levels when determinations are needed. Potassium helps maintain intracellular osmotic pressure and hydrogen ion balance and thus influences acid-base balance. It regulates neuromuscular excitability, affects cardiac muscular activity, and is necessary for the transmission of nerve impulses that cause contraction of all muscle fibers. Potassium is necessary for the storage of nitrogen as muscle protein. It is lost when muscle tissue is broken down.

The kidneys are ineffective conservers of potassium. Balance is maintained by renal excretion of excess potassium. Ordinarily, 80–90 percent is excreted in the urine, and 10–20 percent is excreted in feces. Sodium may be conserved at the expense of potassium in the exchange across the cell membrane. Since potassium is not conserved, daily intake is essential. It is present in most foods. An average normal daily diet provides 50–150 mEq, or 2–6 gm potassium, which easily supplies the 40 mEq needed. It is absorbed by the small intestine. Foods high in potassium are fresh or dried apricots, avocados, dates, bananas, raisins, watermelon, milk, prune juice, tomato juice, artichokes, bamboo shoots, lima beans, broccoli, raw carrots, cauliflower, celery, lettuce, potatoes, spinach, tomatoes, meat, and fish. Certain commercially prepared carbonated beverages also provide substantial amounts of potassium.

POTASSIUM EXCESS (HYPERKALEMIA)

Potassium excess, or hyperkalemia, exists when serum levels of potassium exceed 5.3 mEq/liter. It may be caused by cell injury or destruction. Crushing injuries and necrosis from trauma, extensive burns, myocardial infarction, kidney disease, or severe infection destroy cells and release intracellular potassium into the extracellular fluid. Intracellular potassium also increases with severe acidosis, due to a shift from within the cells. Hyperkalemia can result from impaired kidney function. It may also be related to renal failure, acidosis, or iatrogenic factors, such as administration of excess potassium or potassium-conserving diuretics. Hyperkalemia is not as common as hypokalemia since normally functioning kidneys excrete the excess.

Signs and Symptoms

Signs and symptoms are related mostly to the gastrointestinal, neuromuscular, and cardiac systems. The severity depends on the extent of excess potassium. Manifestations are nausea, diarrhea, muscular irritability, paresthesia, and diminished reflexes. The serious effect on cardiac function is the most deleterious, causing peaking or tent-shaped T wave, depressed ST segments, widened PR and QRS, dilated and flaccid heart muscle, slow cardiac arrhythmias, ventricular fibrillation, and if not corrected, death.

Nursing Intervention

Hyperkalemia, while uncommon, requires prompt correction because of its life-threatening potential. The nurse's primary role is to administer medications as ordered. Treatment consists of (1) withholding all potassium medications, (2) giving sodium bicarbonate if metabolic acidosis is present, (3) giving parenteral 2.5 percent sodium chloride slowly, (4) giving parenteral calcium gluconate 1 gm slowly over a 15-minute period to counteract the cardiac effect of potassium and the effect on muscular irritability, (5) giving 3–4 gm glucose with each unit of insulin given parenterally to help transfer potassium from extracellular to intracellular fluid, and (6) instituting peritoneal dialysis or hemodialysis if necessary (3). The nurse should never give sodium bicarbonate in the same intravenous line with calcium gluconate because of the precipitate that is formed due to insolubility.

The nurse describes, records, and reports electrocardiogram patterns to the physician. Another key nursing function is to monitor and record all urinary output since good renal function is necessary for potassium excretion. The nurse should note and record the rate, rhythm, and characteristics of the pulse. Neurological status should be assessed. Other nursing measures depend upon the patient's clinical manifestations.

POTASSIUM DEFICIT (HYPOKALEMIA)

Potassium deficit, or hypokalemia, exists when serum potassium levels fall below 3.5 mEq/liter. It is rarely caused by inadequate dietary intake, but may result from alcoholism, poor appetite, or dieting.

Some of the primary causes of potassium deficit are:

1. Gastrointestinal loss because of:
   Vomiting
   Diarrhea
   Nasogastric or intestinal suctioning
   Intestinal fistulas
   Ileostomies
   Enema or laxative abuse
2. Renal loss because of:
   Diuretics
   Acidosis
   Alkalosis
3. Metabolic disorders because of:
   Steroid therapy
   Cushing syndrome
   Adrenal adenomas

Other causes include increased demand from burns, poor absorption because of steatorrhea or regional enteritis, and excessive alkali intake, which causes extracellular potassium to move into the cells.

Signs and Symptoms

Hypokalemia, which may range from mild to severe depending on the serum level, occurs more frequently than hyperkalemia. Signs and symptoms include anorexia, nausea, weight loss, weak, flabby muscles, leg cramps, postural hypotension, manifestations of alkalosis, decreased intestinal motility leading to paralytic ileus, diminished reflexes, congestive heart failure, lowered T wave and prolonged QT interval, supraventricular and ventricular tachyarrhythmias including PVCs, (premature ventricular contractions) and eventually cardiac arrest without corrective measures.

Nursing Intervention

Restoration of potassium balance is the major goal. The amount of potassium replacement depends on the degree of deficit and the patient's clinical condition, and is given according to physician's order. Oral replacement is the best method if the patient can tolerate and retain oral medication. This method is safer because there is less chance of a sudden change from hypokalemia to hyperkalemia. Oral potassium may be given in the form of enteric-coated tablets, liquid, or powder. In powder or liquid form, potassium should be diluted in water or orange or grape juice. This minimizes the unpleasant taste and helps protect the gastric mucosa.

Intravenous replacement requires careful monitoring because of the danger of transition to hyperkalemia and the potential for cardiac arrest. The nurse must know how to evaluate electrocardiogram patterns. The patient's pulse should be taken every 15–30 minutes if the patient is not monitored by electrocardiogram, and the quality, rhythm, and rate should be noted.

Replacement of deficit is more complicated than the common practice of adding 20 mEq to a liter of normal saline to maintain electrolyte balance. To correct severe deficit, no more than 20–30 mEq diluted in 50–100 ml of infusate should be given per hour and no more than 40 mEq diluted in two hours. The nurse should reduce the rate of flow even more as serum levels approach normal.

Potassium should not be given to the postoperative patient until renal function is verified, and there is at least 30 ml/hour of urine output. Low serum potassium potentiates the action of digitalis. Therefore, patients receiving this drug must be observed carefully for signs of digitalis toxicity. The nurse also must be alert for a sudden drop in serum potassium when the patient is receiving drug therapy for correction of acidosis.

Level of consciousness should be assessed, and neurological checks should be done. The nurse should monitor bowel sounds and all intake and output should be accurately measured and recorded. Cardiac rhythm is noted and any change recorded.

Calcium Balance

Calcium is found in both extracellular and intracellular fluid. The normal range for serum (extracellular) levels is 4.5–5.5 mEq/liter. Calcium is present in bones and teeth to a much greater degree than in body fluids. When serum levels drop, calcium is mobilized from the bones to keep serum levels constant. Calcium is necessary for coagulation of blood and gives firmness to bones and teeth. It influences cell permeability and has a role in the transmission of nerve impulses. It becomes more soluble in an acid medium and thus helps maintain acid-base balance. As serum becomes more alkaline, calcium is deposited in the bones, and serum levels are lowered. Vitamin D is necessary for calcium to be absorbed from the small intestine. Increased alkalinity of intestinal fluid decreases absorption. Parathyroid hormone, secreted by the parathyroid gland, is the prime regulator of calcium concentration in body fluids.

Normal daily requirements for calcium are 800 mEq. Food sources are milk, cheese, egg yolk, kale, and cauliflower. Other sources include cabbage, legumes, celery, almonds, dates, oranges, lemons, and apples. Approximately three-fourths of the daily requirements are supplied by milk and milk products. Calcium intake should be increased during pregnancy, lactation, and growth periods.

CALCIUM EXCESS (HYPERCALCEMIA)

Calcium excess, or hypercalcemia, exists when serum levels exceed 5.8 mEq/liter. The most notable cause is hyperparathyroidism. Other causes include bone tumors, renal disorders, hyperthyroidism, excessive milk intake, alkali syndrome, and excessive vitamin D intake. Increased production of vitamin D also may cause excess because vitamin D is used in calcium absorption. A patient's prolonged immobilization causes calcium to move from the bone into serum. Not only do serum levels become high, but there is susceptibility to kidney stones and osteoporosis with depletion of bone stores.

Signs and Symptoms
Clinical manifestations include anorexia, nausea, and vomiting. There may be diarrhea or constipation from loss of intestinal tract tone. There is additional hypotonicity of muscles. The patient is prone to develop kidney or bladder stones, flank pain, and eventually renal failure. Sulkowitch's urine test shows increased precipitation if hypercalcemia is present. Central nervous system signs range from lethargy, headache, mental dullness, and confusion, to coma. Hypercalcemia crisis is manifested by severe nausea and vomiting accompanied by dehydration, coma, and renal failure. Death ensues without immediate corrective intervention.

Nursing Intervention

Prevention of hypercalcemia crisis is the primary nursing goal if intervention has been unsatisfactory. The nurse should be alert for any indications of impending crisis. Keeping the physician apprised of the patient's condition is the nurse's responsibility. Intravenous fluids are given as ordered. Normal saline provides sodium and water. This not only corrects dehydration, but the sodium also promotes renal secretion of calcium. Phosphate drugs lower serum calcium by increasing bone deposit. Other drugs used may include calcitonin, methramycin, and glucocorticoids. These drugs may cause renal toxicity. Thus, the nurse should watch for decreased urinary output. Accurate recording of intake and output is vital.

Cranberry juice may be given to maintain acid urine, which increases the solubility of calcium and also promotes bone deposit. The nurse should strain and observe all urine for stones. The nurse should also encourage the patient to ambulate unless contraindicated because it fosters calcium bone deposit. Active and passive range-of-motion exercises may be instituted.

CALCIUM DEFICIT (HYPOCALCEMIA)

Calcium deficit, or hypocalcemia, exists when calcium serum levels are below 4.5 mEq/liter. Diseases or conditions that cause this deficit include hypoparathyroidism, malabsorption syndrome, magnesium excess, renal insufficiency, and vitamin D deficiency. If the patient receives numerous blood transfusions, the citric acid in the citrated blood binds the calcium in extracellular fluid so it is not available for body use. Excess loss may be due to diarrhea, draining wounds, and acute pancreatitis with increased flow of pancreatic digestive juices. Loss may be precipitated by injury to the parathyroid glands during thyroid surgery.

Signs and Symptoms

Clinical symptoms depend on the severity of the deficit and are mainly neuromuscular, such as fatigue, muscular weakness, muscle twitching, paresthesia, abdominal and muscle cramps, carpopedal spasms, tetany, diplopia, and prolonged QT and ST intervals on the electrocardiogram (ECG). Interference in breathing may come from spasms of the larynx and respiratory muscles. Hemorrhage may occur because calcium is one of the necessary elements for the conversion of prothrombin to thrombin.

Nursing Intervention

The nurse must be alert for any clinical manifestation indicating hypocalcemia. Drug therapy relates to the degree of deficit and is given as ordered by the physician. Oral replacement may be sufficient for treatment of mild deficit. Vitamin D is administered in both mild and severe degrees of deficit with the dosage prescribed accordingly. Calcium gluconate 10 percent is given by slow intravenous for severe hypocalcemia.

Extreme care should be given to avoid infiltration of parenteral fluids containing calcium because tissue sloughing may result. Calcium should never be added to solutions containing phosphate or carbonate because harmful precipitates will form. Following thyroid surgery calcium gluconate 10 percent should be kept at the patient's bedside for emergency use.

When hypocalcemia is likely, the nurse should check for Trousseau's sign and a positive Chvostek's sign. A positive Trousseau's sign is a typical contraction of the fingers and hand when a blood pressure cuff is inflated for 1 to 5 minutes. A positive Chvostek's sign occurs when a tap in front of the ear on the 7th cranial nerve causes spasms of the cheek and corner of the mouth. The patient should be in a quiet atmosphere and allowed to rest.

Magnesium Balance

Magnesium, a cation, is found mostly in bone and muscle. It also exists in minute quantities in body fluids, mainly in intracellular fluid. Like potassium, it is easier to monitor serum levels (extracellular fluid), which range from 1.5 to 2.5 mEq/liter. Balance is maintained through magnesium absorption in the small intestine and through kidney conservation.

Calcium and fat inhibit absorption. Thus, a certain amount is excreted daily in the feces. Malabsorption problems may affect magnesium balance. Because it is a positive ion or cation, it influences fluid and electrolyte balance.

A variety of foods contain magnesium, and the recommended daily allowance of 200–350 mg is easily supplied. Food sources include green vegetables, meat, seafood, milk, grains, fruits, and nuts.

MAGNESIUM EXCESS (HYPERMAGNESEMIA)

Magnesium excess, or hypermagnesemia, exists when serum levels rise above 3. Hypermagnesemia is rare but occurs in patients with renal failure or untreated diabetic acidosis. The excess may be iatrogenic from medications containing magnesium such as antacids and laxatives or self-induced by patients abusing these drugs.

Signs and Symptoms
Clinical signs include nausea, vomiting, diminished or absent reflexes, flaccid paralysis, hypotension, bradycardia, and cardiac arrhythmias. A serum level above 6 mEq/liter results in death. The patient's respiratory muscles may be paralyzed, and cardiac arrest may occur.

Nursing Intervention
When laboratory values reveal magnesium excess, the nurse should withhold the oral and parenteral administration and notify the physician. Patients with renal insufficiency should be taught the hazards of taking medications containing magnesium. The physican may order calcium since it counteracts the magnesium. The nurse monitors vital signs and makes neurological assessments. Comfort measures related to the nausea and vomiting should be instituted. The nurse should make the patient comfortable while he is nauseous or vomiting.

MAGNESIUM DEFICIT (HYPOMAGNESEMIA)

Magnesium deficit, or hypomagnesemia, exists when serum levels fall below 1.5 mEq/liter. Factors causing this include prolonged vomiting or diarrhea, renal insufficiency, malnutri-tion, alcoholism, and hypercalcemia. Iatrogenic causes are prolonged administration of parenteral fluids without magnesium additive, nasogastric suctioning, bowel resection, and diuretic therapy.

Signs and Symptoms
The major manifestations of hypomagnesemia occur in the central nervous system and neuromuscular system. They include tremors, weakness, hyperactive reflexes, dizziness, mental confusion, and convulsions. Cardiac arrhythmias and hypertension may develop if the deficit is severe and prolonged.

Nursing Intervention
The nurse administers the drug therapy ordered by the physician. Oral replacement may be sufficient. Intravenous magnesium is given to the patient slowly to prevent flushing and depression of his central nervous system. The nurse makes frequent neurological checks and periodically monitors the patient's level of consciousness. Vital signs are carefully assessed. Seizure precautions are instituted for severe deficit.

Acid-Base Balance

The hydrogen ion concentration of body fluids is expressed by the symbol pH. Acid solution has a pH below 7.0, whereas base or alkaline solution has a pH above 7.0. Body fluids are maintained in the narrow range of pH 7.35 to 7.45. This slightly basic value must be carefully controlled to maintain health. A pH of less than 6.8 or more than 7.8 is incompatible with life.

Most diets have an acid ash, which could be life-threatening without body homeostasis. The pH of body fluids is regulated by the electrolytes, the buffer systems, and the excretory function of the lungs and kidneys.

The positively charged electrolytes, or cations—sodium, potassium, calcium, and magnesium—have base reactions. The negatively charged electrolytes or anions are chloride, sulfate, phosphate, and bicarbonate. Acids have hydrogen ions that can be released to combine with other substances. Bases have no hydrogen ions but can accept them. Under normal conditions the cations and anions are maintained in balance.

Buffer systems help maintain acid-base balance. A buffer system is made up of a weak acid and a salt of that acid. This combination converts a strong acid or base to a weak acid or base.

The major buffer systems are the carbonic acid-bicarbonate system, the protein system, and the phosphate system. Carbonic acid and bicarbonate are the most important buffer pair in the extracellular fluid because of their concentration there. Both renal and respiratory systems help to maintain the balance of this buffer pair. The kidneys are involved mainly in regulating base bicarbonate, and the lungs release carbonic acid as carbon dioxide. Carbonic acid concentration is expressed as partial pressure of carbon dioxide (PCO_2). Its normal range in the arterial blood is 35–45 mm Hg. The bicarbonate concentration in arterial blood has a normal range of 22–26 mEq/liter.

As long as a 20:1 ration is maintained between bicarbonate (HCO_3), the major blood base, and carbonic acid (H_2CO_3), the major blood acid, there is a normal blood pH of 7.4. This is true regardless of the absolute values of the substances because it takes 20 parts of base to neutralize 1 part of acid.

The Henderson-Hasselbalch equation is used to describe the relationship between pH and buffer compound concentration of carbonic acid-bicarbonate. From this equation, the pH can be determined by the ratio of the salt and acid:

$$pH = pK_a + \log \frac{HCO_3}{H_2CO_3} = \frac{20}{1}$$

For computation, the arterial blood gas value of carbon dioxide is substituted for the carbonic acid since the latter value is difficult to determine.

Problems ensue when there is a base excess or deficit of ±2 mEq/liter more or less than normal. A negative value below 2 mEq/liter indicates a nonrespiratory or metabolic disturbance and is the result of nonvolatile acid accumulations or base excess. A positive value above 2 mEq/liter indicates a nonvolatile acid deficit, or alkalosis. There can be metabolic acidosis, indicated by a decreased PO_2, and respiratory acidosis, indicated by increased CO_2.

The most abundant buffer, the protein buffer system is active in both extracellular and intracellular fluid. It is particularly active in intracellular fluid since the carbonic acid-bicarbonate is the primary extracellular fluid buffer. This buffer system can perform as either acid or base because protein in the form of amino acids has both free acidic (−COOH) and basic (−NH₃OH) radicals that can combine with either acids or bases. Furthermore, as negative ions, proteins attract positively charged ions and repel negatively charged ions. This increases the total colloid osmotic pressure and helps to maintain neutrality. This is called the Donnan effect.

The phosphate buffer system also operates intracellularly to maintain steady body fluid pH. It acts almost identically to the extracellular carbonic acid-bicarbonate buffer system. The intracellular buffer system is further augmented by the pairing up of hemoglobin and oxyhemoglobin with potassium salts.

The lungs perform an important role in maintaining acid-base balance by excreting acid (carbon dioxide) and regulating PCO_2. The rate of pulmonary ventilation is increased as the amount of carbon dioxide increases. This is because hydrogen ions have a direct action on the respiratory center in the medulla oblongata. Conversely, when hydrogen ion concentration falls, the respiratory center becomes depressed until the concentration of hydrogen rises to normal levels.

The kidneys maintain the pH of body fluids by excreting sulfate and phosphate that have paired with hydrogen ion and ammonium ion. They also reabsorb bicarbonate and secrete hydrogen into the urine. Even though phosphate is a weak buffer in blood, by uniting with hydrogen in renal tubular fluid, it becomes a more potent buffer. Ammonia reacts with hydrogen ions in the tubular fluid to form ammonium ions, which are then excreted with chloride.

Any time carbon dioxide concentration is increased in extracellular fluid, the rate of hydrogen ion secretion is increased through the renal tubules. Electrical balance between anions and cations is maintained because for every hydrogen ion that is secreted a sodium ion is reabsorbed. Concomitant with increased hydrogen in the extracellular fluid, bicarbonate ions are reabsorbed by a special process in which they react with hydrogen ions in the renal tubules. Were it not for this special process, the tubules would be impermeable to the large electrically charged bicarbonate ion. The kidneys are effective acid-base regulators because they can remove up to about 500 millimoles of acid or alkali each day. Any excess of this can lead to severe acidosis or alkalosis (2).

Blood gas values are used to assess the adequacy of oxygenation, ventilation, and the acid-base status. Normal levels for arterial blood gases at sea level are: PCO_2, 35–40 mm Hg; PO_2, 80–100 mm Hg; O_2 saturation, 95 percent or more; and HCO_3, 22–26 mEq/liter.

is a major nursing goal. Postoperative patients with chronic obstructive pulmonary disease (COPD) need special care. The condition may be exaggerated because of hypoventilation due to pain and abdominal distention due to retained gas or paralytic ileus. All these may affect normal breathing. Tracheobronchial suctioning may be necessary to remove accumulated secretions and facilitate breathing. Unless contraindicated because of the type of surgery, the nurse should insist that the patient turn, cough, and deep breathe. Splinting over the incisional area will make coughing less painful, and the patient can be more rigorous and effective in his efforts. The nurse must avoid oversedating the patient. Oxygen is administered when appropriate but is used cautiously and in restricted concentration for the patient with COPD. Oxygen should never be withheld from the hypoxic patient since it is not the oxygen flow that depresses respirations in the COPD patient but his PaO_2 (see Table 10.4).

RESPIRATORY ACIDOSIS

Respiratory acidosis occurs when CO_2 is retained and the pH is less than 7.35. The arterial PCO_2 is elevated more than 5 mm Hg initially, while plasma bicarbonate is normal. As a compensation, bicarbonate concentration rises when there are chronic obstructive pulmonary conditions that cause retention of CO_2. Respirations are depressed. (See Table 10.4 for related pathophysiology and causes of respiratory acidosis.)

Signs and Symptoms
Arterial blood PCO_2 is 50–100 mm Hg in respiratory acidosis. When levels reach 70 mm Hg or more, there is headache, mental confusion, weakness, and inhibited response to pain. Total mEq/liter of CO_2 (HCO_3) is greater than 27 and urine pH is less than 6 (3).

Nursing Intervention
Nursing care is directed toward improving ventilation and correcting the underlying disorder. The prevention of respiratory acidosis

RESPIRATORY ALKALOSIS

Respiratory alkalosis occurs when there is excessive loss of carbon dioxide. It may be caused by hyperventilation due to pain or anxiety. Patients who require ventilatory assistance during the postoperative period frequently have respiratory alkalosis. Severe respiratory alkalosis leads to serum potassium depletion as these ions enter the cells in exchange for hydrogen. (See Table 10.4 for related pathophysiology and causes of respiratory alkalosis.)

Signs and Symptoms
The patient with respiratory alkalosis shows symptoms of potassium deficit such as paresthesia, numbness, and tachyarrhythmias. Hypocapnia causes cerebral vasospasm, and patients with severe respiratory alkalosis suffer confusion or loss of consiousness and convulsions. Arterial blood values of PCO_2 range between 20–30; HCO_3 (total mEq/liter) ranges between 15–20; and pH greater than 7.45. Urine pH is less than 6.

Nursing Intervention

The nurse must concentrate on correcting the cause rather than the symptoms of the condition. If the cause is hyperventilation, the nurse should calm the patient and give sedatives as ordered. Rebreathing into a paper bag may aid in restoring carbon dioxide. Vital signs are monitored carefully. Seizure precautions may be taken. The nurse must monitor the patient's level of consciousness and protect him from injury.

METABOLIC ACIDOSIS

Metabolic acidosis results when acids are retained or increased or base bicarbonate is lost. Serum pH level falls below 7.35. In the surgical patient, metabolic acidosis may be due to acute circulatory failure with resultant hypoxemia and accumulation of lactic acid. Or it may occur because the kidneys fail to excrete excess acid. An extreme lowering of serum pH may occur with acute hemorrhagic shock.

Whatever the cause, acidosis occurs when the carbonic acid-bicarbonate ratio does not remain 20:1. (See Table 10.4 for related pathophysiology and specific causes.)

Signs and Symptoms

The rate and depth of the patient's respirations increase hyperventilation because of excess hydrogen ion concentration. Other symptoms may include headache, confusion, fatigue, anorexia, fruity breath, Kussmaul's respiration, vascular shock, and coma. Death may ensue without prompt intervention. Laboratory findings include arterial blood levels of HCO_3 ranging between 2 and 18, pH less than 7.35, and PCO_2 of 15–30 mm Hg. Urine pH is greater than 6 (3).

Nursing Intervention

The nurse gives oral or parenteral sodium bicarbonate as ordered to correct base deficit. In an emergency, nurses may give sodium bicarbonate without an order, but this is done only by nurses specially prepared to assess the critical status of the patient according to hospital protocol. Immediate detection and

treatment often avert life-threatening situations.

Insulin is given for diabetic ketoacidosis. Glucose and saline are given for ketoacidosis related to alcoholism. The nurse must know the implications of abnormal clinical laboratory findings and recognize patient symptoms that indicate metabolic acidosis.

Giving parenteral fluid therapy to correct the acidosis is a nursing function. Sodium lactate may be given to increase the base in body fluids. The nurse must monitor intravenous fluids and continually watch the rate of flow, regulating it according to the physician's order. He must be alert for symptoms of fluid overload or overcorrection of the acidosis. Monitoring the laboratory values aids in detecting overcorrection. Accurate measurement of intake and output is essential.

Mild acidosis may be managed by oral intake. Foods and fluids with alkaline ash are given. However, certain of these foods are high in sodium or potassium and may be contraindicated if the patient has renal failure, diabetes, congestive heart failure, or hyperkalemia.

METABOLIC ALKALOSIS

Metabolic alkalosis is the result of excess loss of acids or the gain of base bicarbonate. It occurs when pH serum level rises above 7.45.

Hypokalemia is present to some degree in most patients with metabolic alkalosis. The patient loses both potassium and chloride when he continually vomits. Nasogastric suctioning may be an iatrogenic cause of metabolic alkalosis. (See Table 10.4 for related pathophysiology and causes of metabolic alkalosis.)

Signs and Symptoms

Patients with metabolic alkalosis show signs and symptoms of hypokalemia, including paresthesia, numbness, and tachyarrhythmias. Other manifestations include slow, shallow respirations, tremors, tetany, and seizures. The patient may be apathetic or confused. Clinical laboratory arterial blood values are pH, 7.45, and HCO_3, 27 (3). Urine pH is around 7.0.

Nursing Intervention

The nurse administers fluids as ordered either orally or parenterally. Potassium, sodium chloride, ammonium chloride, or hydrochloric acid may be given to correct the alkalosis. The physician orders the drugs to be given according to serum levels. Care must be taken to avoid overcorrection. The nurse must know the symptoms of hyperkalemia, which may be the first sign of overcorrection [see "Potassium Excess (Hyperkalemia)"]. Any vomiting or diarrhea should be reported since this may negate the effect of oral replacement therapy and continue to alter parenteral needs. Accurate reporting and recording of all intake and output are important. Seizure precautions may be necessary.

Criteria for ascertaining whether the patient has acidosis or alkalosis are shown in Table 10.5.

Table 10.5. Comparison between Acidosis and Alkalosis.

Acidosis	Alkalosis
Respiratory	
pH: 7.35	pH: 7.45
Bicarbonate: 29 mEq/liter	Bicarbonate: 22 mEq/liter
Compensatory mechanism	Compensatory mechanism
Renal: retain bicarbonate while excreting hydrogen ions	Renal: excrete bicarbonate ions and retain hydrogen ions
Metabolic	
pH: 7.35	pH: 7.45
Bicarbonate: 22 mEq/liter	Bicarbonate: 29 mEq/liter
Compensatory mechanism	Compensatory mechanism
Respiratory: blow off CO_2	Respiratory: depressed, hold back CO_2
Renal: conserve base bicarbonate through preferential excretion of hydrogen ions	Renal: excretion of bicarbonate ions and retention of hydrogen ions

Nurse's Role in Maintaining Fluid and Electrolyte Balance During the Perioperative Period

Surgery has an unavoidable effect on fluid, electrolyte, and acid-base balance. Normal respiration, digestion, circulation, and excretion are all disturbed. This will, in turn, upset delicate fluid and chemical balances. The situation will be even more complicated if the patient has an existing condition or disease that affects his normal intake and output.

Even though surgery disturbs the body's normal equilibrium, the nurse can help to keep problems to a minimum by careful planning. He cannot expect to assess the patient and plan care in this complicated area without a thorough understanding of the intricate relationships of fluid and chemicals in the body. The nurse can develop a plan that anticipates the subtle effects surgery may have. A plan for fluid and electrolyte and acid-base balance should consider the gastrointestinal, cardiovascular, respiratory, and renal systems. Nutritional status is an important preoperative and postoperative consideration. Knowing blood values will assist in hemostasis and hemorrhage control if it happens.

PREOPERATIVE ASSESSMENT

The gastrointestinal system and the kidneys have important functions in maintaining fluid and electrolyte balance. Impairment of either makes the patient more vulnerable to complications from surgery. These systems need to be assessed and baseline values recorded. The nurse checks the patient's chart for laboratory values and past problems with these organ systems.

In assessing renal function, the nurse determines if the patient is voiding adequately. The nurse should note the color of the urine and whether it is clear or cloudy. Any abnormal appearance should be reported and charted. A urinalysis is ordered routinely to determine gross kidney function.

The cardiovascular system should also be evaluated. Cardiac insufficiency may lead to circulatory stasis and pooling of blood and body fluids, all of which affect fluid balance. Pooling of body fluids can make the patient hypovolemic. This puts an added strain on the cardiac system as the heart works harder to meet body needs. Inadequate oxygenation of body tissue due to poor cardiac function may lead to disturbances in acid-base balance.

Whether or not there is electrocardiographic monitoring of cardiac status, the nurse can assess the quality of pulse and check for pulse deficits in the extremities.

Preoperative nursing measures that enhance circulatory sufficiency and respiratory gaseous exchange during the postoperative period include teaching the patient how to turn, cough, and deep breathe. Teaching the patient how to splint when coughing will facilitate his ability to cough after surgery. Shallow breathing may lead to respiratory acidosis as well as promote circulatory stasis. Teaching the patient how to do bicycle exercises, unless contraindicated, will help circulation and deter pooling of body fluids.

The nurse should determine if the patient is eating and drinking sufficient amounts during the preoperative period to assure adequate nutrition and fluid balance. Providing a clean, odor-free, pleasant environment will enhance the patient's appetite. If the patient is allowed out of bed, the unit nurses should encourage ambulation to help increase the patient's appetite and improve circulation, bringing nutrients to all body parts.

Blood values are obtained preoperatively as an adjunct to determining the patient's readiness for surgery. It is important to know the patient's bleeding and coagulation time since hemorrhage is a serious complication. Normal bleeding time is 30 seconds to 6 minutes. Normal coagulation or clotting time is 5–10 minutes. Hemoglobin and hematocrit levels are decreased when the patient is anemic; however, they are increased when the patient is dehydrated due to the concentration of cells proportionate to the fluid volume. Normal values of hemoglobin are 12–15 gm/100 ml for women and 14–17 gm/100 ml for men. Normal hematocrit levels are 37–47/100 ml for women and 40–50/100 ml for men.

The physician may order a type and crossmatch of the patient's blood. The need for blood transfusions may be predicted according to the type of surgery. Often the blood is available in case an emergency arises during the surgery or more blood is lost than anticipated.

Assessing the patient's emotional status is important for physiological as well as psychological reasons. Anxiety may cause the patient to hyperventilate, which can lead to respiratory acidosis.

PREPARATION FOR SURGERY

Gastrointestinal Preparation

The way a patient is prepared for surgery will have a bearing on how well he is able to maintain his fluid and electrolyte and acid-base balance during the procedure. Although these measures may not be part of the OR nurse's responsibility, he should know what has been done for the patient by physicians and unit nurses.

Even if the patient is admitted with adequate hydration and electrolyte balance, this may be altered by preparation for surgery. The patient's stomach should be empty at the time of surgery to prevent the aspiration of vomitus. To ensure an empty stomach, no solid food is given after a regular or a light meal the evening before the surgery. This is followed by clear liquids only until midnight or until six to eight hours before surgery if it is scheduled late in the day. The nurse should encourage the patient to drink fluids until the time they must be withheld because they promote hydration and help the patient's body maintain homeostasis during the remainder of the perioperative period. Children have a much higher metabolic rate and proportionately less glycogen reserve than adults. Thus starvation is more critical for them because of their vulnerability to acidosis. Formula is usually given to infants and clear liquids to children over two years old up to four hours before a general anesthetic. In addition, infants have proportionately more body surface than adults and thus have about twice as much insensible loss per kilogram body weight. This places them at greater risk for the development of dehydration.

The physician may order parenteral fluids for the morning of the surgery if he anticipates a prolonged operation time, if the patient is to receive a blood transfusion or plasma, or if the operation will be late in the day. Intravenous fluids may be started after the patient reaches the operating room.

The nurse may be asked to insert a nasogastric tube so gastric fluids can be suctioned. The trend is to insert the nasogastric tube in the operating room after the patient has been anesthetized. The type of surgery dictates whether insertion of a nasogastric tube is necessary.

Bowel Preparation

The nurse may receive an order that states, "Give tap-water enemas until clear return." This may create an electrolyte imbalance. Many physicians are now ordering, "Fleets enema(s) until clear." This does not pose the potential problem for electrolyte imbalance that tap water enemas do. Some physicians are eliminating the preoperative order for enemas entirely when the surgery does not involve the gastrointestinal system. Others may order cathartics instead if they feel bowel preparation is necessary.

Bladder Preparation

There are two important reasons for asking the patient to empty his bladder completely before surgery: to maintain continence during low abdominal surgery; and to make other abdominal organs more accessible.

The nurse should always ask the patient to empty his bladder before any preoperative medication is given, since he may experience vertigo and syncope from the medication. After the patient has emptied his bladder and been medicated, the nurse should put the siderails of the bed in the upright position to protect him from injury.

Insertion of a Foley catheter may be part of the preoperative orders for patients undergoing abdominal surgery. Current practice is to insert the indwelling catheter after anesthetic induction. This assures an empty bladder throughout the surgical procedure and makes it possible to determine output during the intraoperative and immediate postoperative period. Output of more than 30 ml/hour is essential, especially if the patient is receiving continuous parenteral fluids. It is one indication of adequate perfusion.

Preanesthetic Medication

Preanesthetic drugs reduce the patient's anxiety, the amount of general anesthesia required, and respiratory tract secretions. These drugs have a direct and indirect effect on fluid and electrolyte and acid-base balance because they affect respiratory and cardiac function and circulatory status.

Barbiturates such as pentobarbital (Nembutal) and secobarbital (Seconal) are commonly ordered for the evening before surgery. These drugs have a calming affect and usually allay apprehension and the tendency to hyperventilate, which could precipitate respiratory alkalosis. Opiates such as morphine and meperidine hydrochloride (Demerol) reduce the amount of general anesthetic required. The nurse should be alert for side effects such as nausea, vomiting, hypotension, and respiratory depression leading to respiratory acidosis.

Anticholinergics such as glycopyrrolate (Robinul) and belladonna/alkaloids such as atropine and scopolamine relax smooth muscle, inhibit secretions of duct glands, and prevent laryngospasm. Usual doses temporarily slow the cardiac rate, whereas moderate to large doses increase the heart rate and cause urinary urgency with difficulty in emptying the bladder.

Other drugs used as preanesthetic agents to promote quiescence are droperidol (Inapsine), fentanyl (Sublimaze), and a combination of droperidol and fentanyl (Innovar). These drugs also may cause respiratory and circulatory depression, and they potentiate the action of central nervous system depressants such as sedatives, hypnotics, tranquilizers, and alcohol. Therefore, drugs in these categories should not be used with sedatives. If they are used, the dosage of each should be markedly reduced. Fentanyl may cause laryngospasm or bronchospasm (4).

Patients may be receiving drug therapy for various conditions or diseases. Some of these drugs interact with anesthetic agents or muscle relaxants to cause problems of hypotension, respiratory depression, or circulatory collapse. Drugs of particular concern are antihypertensives, adrenergics, antibiotics, adrenal steroids, and tranquilizers (phenothiazines). Antidepressants may react with anesthetic agents to cause hypertension (4).

INTRAOPERATIVE CARE

The intraoperative period is the focus of the perioperative nurse's care planning. Ideally, the care plan should be written and include the preoperative assessment, potential patient problems that could arise during surgery (nursing diagnoses), and nursing actions. By the time the patient is ready to go to the recovery room, the nurse should be able to evaluate how successful the nursing actions have been to that point. Later, depending on his schedule, the nurse may be able to do a further evaluation in the recovery room or on the unit. Each care plan should be individual. That is, it should address the specific problems a patient may have. This section will discuss how the surgical procedure itself affects fluid and electrolyte and acid-base balance.

Anesthesia

Anesthesia has an effect on a variety of body systems, which in turn can alter fluid and electrolyte balance. (See Chapter 12 for a complete discussion of anesthesia and the nurse's role.) Intravenous anesthetics such as sodium pentothal and sodium methohexital cause respiratory depression. Certain other problems are associated with inhalation anesthetics that vary in severity. High concentrations of nitrous gas causes hypoxia. Cyclopropane may cause postoperative nausea and vomiting and cardiac arrhythmias. It also increases the urine-to-serum osmolarity ratio, reducing urine volume. Halothane (Fluothane) is not as apt to cause postoperative nausea and vomiting but may depress respiration, leading to respiratory acidosis and a depressed cardiovascular system, which reduces cardiac output and hypotension. Halothane has a vasodilator effect. Large dosages of methoxyflurane may cause renal tubular damage. Enflurane may depress respiratory and cardiovascular function (5).

Life-threatening complications may arise from inhalation anesthesia. Peak periods for these to develop are during the induction of anesthesia or the recovery period. Most complications affect fluid and electrolyte and acid-base balance. Cardiac arrhythmia and cardiac arrest may occur because of retention of carbon dioxide and developing acidosis and anoxia. This is because the myocardium is sensitive to its chemical environment. If cardiac arrest occurs, both the scrub nurse and circulating nurse must note the time of cardiac arrest, make available a defibrillator and cardiac pacemaker, provide special drugs, assist with intravenous lines, and prepare instruments for opening the chest if necessary.

Bronchospasm and laryngospasm may be caused by the irritating or allergenic effects of anesthetics on laryngeal and bronchial mucosa. These spasms are more apt to occur in patients with chronic obstructive pulmonary disease and in heavy smokers. Unchecked spasms cause anoxia, which leads to cardiac arrest.

Vomiting and aspiration may occur because protective reflexes are suppressed by anesthetics. Acute anoxia may develop, and death may ensue. Postoperative pulmonary edema and chemical pneumonitis may also develop following aspiration of vomitus. This is why it is important that no fluids or food are taken during the immediate six-hour preoperative period.

There may be mechanical obstruction as well as physiological obstruction (laryngospasm and bronchospasm).

Mechanical respiratory obstruction may be caused by a relaxed tongue, excessive mucus, foreign bodies (teeth), or edema from a tumor or inflammation. Overdose of drugs that depress respirations may cause respiratory failure. Shock and severe hypotension may be caused by hemorrhage, the combination of premedications and anesthetics, dehydration, surgical trauma, anoxia, or neurogenic shock due to vasodilation in response to pain when there is inadequate anesthesia. The most common cause, however, is hemorrhage. Convulsions may occur secondary to cerebral anoxia. Renal ischemia may develop because of operative hypotension. This may result in acute tubular necrosis that may not be evident until postoperative renal failure is detected (6:92–94).

Regional anesthetics affect renal output. Spinal anesthesia reduces the volume of urine production, probably due to increased antidiuretic hormone (ADH). Conversely, epidural anesthesia increases urinary volume, probably due to a suppression of ADH (7).

The nurse must be ready to assist the anesthesiologist in emergencies that arise during the induction, anesthetized period, and emergence from anesthesia in the recovery room.

Management of Fluids

Patients lose blood and body fluids during any surgical procedure. The extent varies with the type of operation. Not only is there frank loss from tissue injury due to dissection, there is functional loss of extracellular fluid because of sequestration or third-space edema. Intravenous normal saline is used as replacement and helps reduce postoperative salt intolerance. Replacement is at the rate of 0.5–1 liter per hour to a maximum of 2–3 liters during a four-hour major abdominal procedure (8). Blood loss is usually not replaced unless it exceeds 500 ml.

Protein loss is often due to hemorrhage but occurs to some extent with plasma loss not associated with hemorrhage. Plasma expanders are not given unless the loss is severe, as in hemorrhage. Loss is also related to the extensiveness of surgery and whether there is considerable resection of tissue as in a pneumonectomy, radical mastectomy, or abdominal peritoneal resection.

Suctioning is necessary during surgery to maintain a clear field but is responsible for additional fluid loss. Suctioning is accomplished by a catheter or tip connected to suction. The amount of suction varies with the vacuum system and degree of pull. Blood and fluid lost through suctioning are collected in graduated containers in bottles in tandem. The nurse is responsible for ensuring adequate suctioning and correcting improper suction pressure. Other fluids may be lost through drains inserted during the closing procedure.

Efforts are made to minimize the loss of blood and tissue fluid by the use of hemostats, pressure, foam or gel, hypothermia, vasoconstricting drugs, and ligation and electrosurgery. Pneumatic tourniquets may be used to control bleeding when surgery is on an extremity.

Estimation of blood loss is important in determining the amount and type of replacement fluids necessary. The surgeon estimates the amount of loss from the accumulated amount in suctioning containers and in sponges. Further discussion of blood loss is found in Chapter 19. Patients undergoing open heart surgery with cardiopulmonary bypass may be on a table that monitors their weight. This is a guide for fluid replacement.

Hemodynamic Monitoring

Adequate cardiac function is necessary to maintain blood pressure and delivery of fluid to body parts. For most general surgeries, frequent blood pressure monitoring with an inflated arm cuff and sphygmomanometer provides an adequate index of the patient's circulatory status and fluid volume. Automatic blood pressure monitoring equipment is used in some operating room suites.

Invasive evaluation may be necessary. One procedure involves inserting a catheter into the arterial system that monitors intraarterial pressure by direct and continuous measurement. Reduced cardiac output may occur when there is hypovolemia. Intraarterial pressure monitoring permits accurate assessment of systolic, diastolic, and mean arterial pressures. Changes, no matter how minute, are recorded. The insertion site of an intraarterial line must be inspected frequently for skin color, pulse quality, and warmth of extremity.

Central venous pressure (CVP) monitoring assesses fluid replacement and determines volume status. CVP indicates pressure in the right atrium, which in turn reflects right ventricular diastolic pressure. A catheter for measuring CVP may be inserted when a change in circulatory status is anticipated, as in major thoracic or abdominal surgery. A normal CVP ranges from 5 to 10 cm of water or 6 to 12 mm Hg when there is adequate perfusion. Pressure rises if the patient is becoming overhydrated, and symptoms of circulatory overload may occur.

The Swan-Ganz catheter measures the pulmonary arterial wedge pressure (PAWP). Readings are more dependable than CVP measurements, but both types of monitoring are important in determining the effectiveness of fluid replacement.

Hemodynamic monitoring has the following advantages over noninvasive blood pressure monitoring:

1. It enables the surgical team to recognize impending shock due to volume deficit or cardiac failure.
2. It permits accurate readings even when the patient is in shock.
3. It reveals minute changes not registered by noninvasive measurement.
4. It reveals circulatory overload.
5. It indicates the patient's response to drugs.

The disadvantages are as follows:

1. There is risk of complications such as bleeding, infection, blood vessel damage, or embolism.
2. Special skills are needed for the insertion, management, and assessment.
3. The patient may worry about the procedure and the monitoring during the postoperative period.

Pulse

Assessing the patient's pulse during induction and the intraoperative period provides the nurse with information about the patient's cardiovascular status and circulating fluid volume. Several sites for palpating the pulse are the radial artery at the wrist, the carotid artery on the side of the neck, the brachial artery along the inner side aspect of the biceps insertion (inner elbow), the femoral artery where it passes over the pelvic bone, the popliteal artery behind the knee, and the dorsalis pedis over the instep of the foot.

When assessing the quality of the pulse, the frequency or number of beats per minute should be noted as well as regular or irregular pulsation. The nurse should note the force of the beat and determine whether each beat is of equal strength. A dicrotic pulse is one in which two beats are felt, but the second one is weaker than the first. The amount of resistance felt by the artery against the finger indicates the blood pressure and fluid volume.

Temperature

Body temperature affects circulation and thereby the circulating fluid volume. In the conscious patient, lowered temperature causes vasoconstriction and the pooling of blood in vital organs. Conversely, increased temperature causes vasodilation with more blood being brought to peripheral areas for cooling of the skin and extremities.

Skin preparation and preoperative drugs contribute to preoperative temperature drop. Furthermore, general anesthesia typically causes a drop of 0.5°C to 1.5°C in body temperature by depressing the heat-regulating mechanisms. These factors lead to postoperative shivering and increase added stress to the cardiopulmonary system. Oxygen consumption may increase up to 400 percent from shivering (9). The nurse should keep the patient warm during the immediate intraoperative and postoperative period and assure adequate ventilation and oxygen intake when the patient enters the recovery room.

When heat-regulating mechanisms have been depressed, as from anesthetic drugs, instead of the usual vasoconstriction to conserve heat, there is vasodilation because shivering and muscle activity are suppressed (9). The patient is more vulnerable to cooling effects. Other factors influencing the patient's body temperature are the infusion of parenteral fluids, which cool circulating body fluids, and the exposure of vital organs in an air-conditioned operating room.

It is better for the patient to have a lowered temperature during certain surgical procedures, such as cardiovascular or cranial surgery, because hypothermia not only decreases metabolism and thus the need for oxygen but has a vasoconstricting effect. All of this affects acid-base balance. The patient must be observed closely for respiratory depression or impending cardiac arrest during hypothermia. Lotion or oil should be used to protect the skin when surface cooling methods are used. The body temperature may be reduced to 82.4–86°F (28–30°C) for anesthesia hypothermia. Blankets are used to slowly rewarm the patient during the postoperative period. The surgeon may order sedatives and muscle relaxants to control shivering.

Positioning during surgery affects fluid balance. Immobility causes body fluids to pool. The lithotomy position may decrease circulatory flow to the lower extremities because of their elevated position. Placing any body part, particularly the extremities, in a dependent (lowered) position to make an operative site more accessible inhibits circulatory flow and causes stasis in that area. Padding helps minimize the effects of pressure that impair circulation. (See Chapter 22 for detailed discussion on positioning the patient for surgery.)

IMMEDIATE POSTOPERATIVE PERIOD

Close monitoring during recovery from anesthesia is as important as it was during surgery. In this period, respiratory function, cardiovascular or circulatory status, and urinary output all indicate how well the body is doing in maintaining or restoring its fluid and electrolyte equilibrium. While the patient is in the recovery area, perioperative nurses may wish to complete their evaluation of nursing measures taken while the patient was in surgery.

The first priority is determining the patient's respiratory status and assuring maintenance of an adequate airway. The patient's color provides a cursory method of assessing ventilation and oxygenation. The rate and depth of respirations should be noted. Stertorous breathing and a weak, thready pulse may indicate hypoxia.

Hypoventilation may be caused by anesthetics, muscle relaxants, or narcotic analgesics. Maximum breathing capacity may be reduced by high abdominal or thoracic incisions. This causes a certain degree of hypoxia and hypercapnia. The patient should be encouraged to turn, cough, and deep breathe as soon as he regains consciousness. He may be reluctant if he is experiencing considerable postoperative pain. The nurse can facilitate expansion of the lungs by turning the patient from side to side. Encouraging the patient to deep breathe improves his respiratory status and reduces the chance of developing atelectasis. It also helps the lungs to expel anesthetic agents. Narcotics should be withheld if the patient is hypoxic since they are respiratory depressants. Other corrective measures will need to be taken to alleviate the hypoxia before pain medication is given. On the other hand, giving pain medication before the patient is conscious of extreme pain may prevent shallow breathing and the development of severe hypoxia.

An oral airway or an endotracheal tube is usually kept in place until the patient has awakened from the anesthesia. This prevents the patient's tongue from falling back and occluding the airway. The nurse may have to suction frequently to remove secretions and assure a patent airway. Positioning the patient on his side will facilitate drainage and deter aspiration. The head should be hyperextended to facilitate adequate ventilation. Tachypnea and dyspnea may indicate cardiovascular complications. Cardiac arrhythmias and arrest may follow if corrective measures are not undertaken.

Narcotic antagonists such as nalorphine hydrochloride (Naline), levallorphan tartrate (Lorfan), and naloxone hydrochloride (Narcan) may be ordered to reverse the effects of narcotics on the respiratory center. These drugs may be administered subcutaneously, intramuscularly, or intravenously. Dosage varies with the age and size of the patient and the degree of respiratory depression. Although effective narcotic antagonists, these drugs do not relieve the depression caused by anesthetics or barbiturates (4).

The nurse must be alert for symptoms of laryngeal spasm that may occur as a complication from the anesthetic. This is manifested by crowing respirations, stridor, and cyanosis. Oxygen should be given and the anesthesiologist notified immediately. An endotracheal tube, if not already in place, is inserted to assure a patent airway. Emergency resuscitation equipment must be available at all times.

Monitoring the cardiovascular status of the patient in the immediate postoperative period requires the nurse to carry out certain nursing activities. The patient's vital signs, pulse, respiration, temperature, and blood pressure should be taken every 15 minutes until they are stable. Fluid and electrolyte infusions are imperative to maintain heart action, satisfactory pulse rate, and circulatory status.

While emerging from anesthesia, cardiac arrhythmias may develop from hypovolemia, hypoxia, or stress. Symptoms of shock may occur. (See Fig. 10.1 for specific endocrine, cardiovascular, and hematopoietic system responses to hypovolemic hemorrhagic shock.) The nurse constantly observes and documents clinical signs of cardiovascular problems. The patient might demonstrate shortness of breath, rapid breathing, hyperventilation, cold, clammy skin, and decreased blood pressure.

Renal function is directly related to the balance of fluids and electrolytes. The patient should have a urine output of at least 30 ml/hour prior to being released from the recovery room. If the urine output is not adequate, the patient is catheterized and an indwelling catheter inserted.

If the kidneys are not producing urine, it may be indicative of hypovolemia, electrolyte imbalance, or impending shock. The nursing responsibility is to maintain the fluid and electrolyte input per order of the physician. In so doing he assesses the patient's response and reports physiological data to the physician. The nurse also measures the output to deter-

Figure 10.1. Hypovolemic hemorrhagic shock. From AACN'S Clinical Reference for Critical Care Nursing, by Kinney, M. R., et al. Copyright © 1981 McGraw-Hill Book Company. Reprinted with permission of McGraw-Hill Book Company.

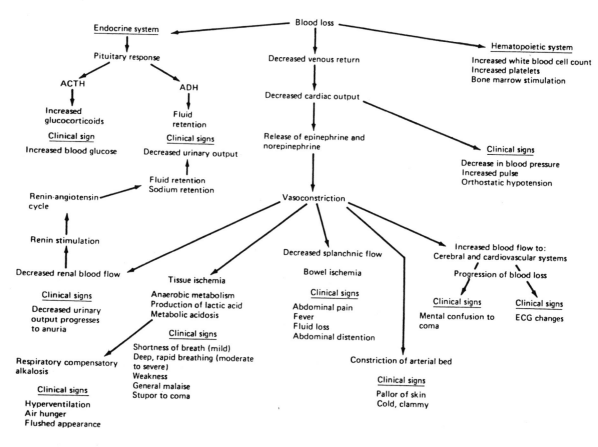

mine the number of milliliters per hour and communicates this to the physician. Intraoperative blood loss can create fluid and electrolyte imbalance. The recovery room nurse must have accurate knowledge of loss of urine, gastric contents, and blood during surgery. He needs to know about any intraoperative crystalloid, colloid, or blood component replacement. An account is kept of fluid and electrolyte intake and output intraoperatively on the anesthetic record. On admission to the recovery area recording continues on the postanesthetic record.

Parenteral Blood Fluids
All blood to be used for transfusion must be cross-matched with a sample of the patient's blood. New recipient serum should be used for cross-matching each day if the patient is receiving repeated transfusions over a period of time. That is because even with the cross-matching and use of compatible blood, antibodies may develop. Excessive blood loss must be replaced to maintain the blood's capacity to carry oxygen.

Each hospital has an established protocol for verifying that the blood to be transfused is identified and double-checked with the patient's name, assigned hospital number, the number on the unit of blood, and the date of collection and cross-matching. This procedure must be followed carefully. Usually, the nurse and personnel in the blood bank are responsible for this final check.

Whole blood and red blood cells should not be used after 21 days except for frozen blood, which may be kept for years but it is usually stored for three to four weeks. Frozen blood is ideal for use during cardiopulmonary bypass and for transplant recipients because platelets and white cells are absent. Its disadvantages are that the red blood cells remain stable for a relatively short time after thawing and coagulation factors are absent. Frozen blood should be used within 24 hours after thawing and cannot be refrozen.

The blood may be heparinized to avoid the problems of blood clotting. In addition, citrate is added to stored whole blood to prevent its coagulation. This combines with calcium ions in the blood and can cause hypocalcemia. [See above, "Calcium Deficit (Hypocalcemia)" for manifestations of hypocalcemia and nursing interventions.] If the blood is administered slowly, the patient's liver can remove citrate.

Transmission of venereal disease and hepatitis through blood transfusions is possible even with careful screening of donors. Another possible problem is hyperkalemia from the loss of potassium from within the red blood cells into the serum. This in turn may precipitate cardiac arrhythmias or arrest. Because of this, blood transfusions are given more cautiously than in previous years.

Autotransfusion is a new technique. The patient's own blood may be salvaged during the operative procedure and reinfused into a vein after it is filtered and heparinized. In autologous transfusion, the patient donates his blood before elective surgery.

Discharge from the Recovery Room
The patient usually awakens from general anesthesia within 2 hours. This time varies with the extent and length of surgery and the anesthetized period.

For fluid and electrolyte balance, the patient is ready for discharge from the recovery room when these criteria are met:

1. Stable vital signs:
   Pulse rate is within 20 beats of preoperative reading.
   Blood pressure is within 20–50 points of preoperative reading with minimal deviation with each monitoring.
   Temperature range is 97–100°F (36–38°C).
   Respirations are within normal limits.
2. Adequate replacement of lost blood or tissue fluid.
3. Absence of excessive draining from any site.
4. A urinary output of at least 30 ml/hour (although this may not be determined until later if the patient does not have an indwelling catheter).
5. A satisfactory level of consciousness.
6. Absence of excessive vomiting.
7. Ability to cough, deep breathe, and move extremities on command. This will improve ventilation and circulation to all body parts.

COMPLICATIONS OF THE POSTOPERATIVE PERIOD

The surgical patient is susceptible to complications arising from either the surgery itself or from associated problems that develop because of inadequate circulation, respiratory insufficiency, or renal impairment. Inappropriate amounts of fluid intake and nutrients compound the hazard. Nurses are in an eminent position to observe, report, and intervene to avert many potential problems that affect fluid and electrolyte balance. These complications are summarized below.

1. Shock due to hemorrhage, cardiac insufficiency, or inadequate replacement of fluids (hypovolemia).
2. Respiratory depression due to prolonged effects of anesthesia, sedation, pain, or tracheal or bronchial obstruction. This leads to respiratory acidosis and eventually metabolic acidosis if the kidneys can no longer retain sufficient bicarbonate to neutralize excess serum acid.
3. Respiratory alkalosis due to anxiety and hyperventilation, or excessive mechanical ventilation.
4. Cardiac arrhythmias due to hypoxia, hypovolemia, and electrolyte imbalance, e.g., decreased potassium, calcium, or magnesium.
5. Phlebothrombosis and thrombophlebitis due to venous stasis, and tissue trauma. Deep thrombophlebitis usually does not occur until after the third or fourth postoperative day. It can be detected by daily ultrasonic examination with the Doppler device. Another method of detection is by checking for Homans' sign. A positive sign is indicated if pain is elicited in the calf of the leg when the patient is asked to dorsiflex his foot when his leg is in extension. However, by the time a positive Homans' sign is evident, the thrombophlebitis usually is quite severe. Phlebothrombosis may lead to pulmonary embolism.
6. Circulatory overload due to rapid infusion of intravenous fluids, retention of fluids because of the increased ADH and sodium in stress response, or continued use of normal saline as parenteral fluid.
7. Renal insufficiency or shutdown due to severe hypotension or hypovolemia.
8. Paralytic ileus due to hypokalemia or manipulation of bowel during surgery.
9. Tetany due to hypocalcemia.
10. Metabolic acidosis due to hemorrhagic shock, acute circulatory failure, or renal failure.
11. Metabolic alkalosis due to persistent vomiting or prolonged nasogastric suctioning.
12. Constipation due to dehydration, narcotic analgesics, and immobilization.
13. Fever due to atelectasis, pneumonia, wound infection, sepsis, or dehydration.
14. Stress ulcers due to the alarm reaction and the psychological and physiological response to the surgery.

The nurse has an important role in performing functions that assist the patient in maintaining fluid and electrolyte balance. It is imperative that manifestations of imbalance are recognized and corrective measures instituted promptly. Many factors affect fluid and electrolyte balance during the perioperative period. The nurse must understand what these factors are and intervene accordingly to meet the patient's needs. Often complications may be averted by appropriate nursing care. Prompt intervention and accurate reporting and recording are essential to the patient's well-being and overall fluid and electrolyte balance.

References

1. Isselbacher, K. J., Adams, R. D., and Braunwald, E., eds. *Harrison's Principles of Internal Medicine*, 9th ed. New York: McGraw-Hill, 1980.
2. Guyton, A. C. *Textbook of Medical Physiology*, 6th ed. Philadelphia: W. B. Saunders, 1981.
3. Harvey, A. M., Johns, R. J., and McKusick, V. A., eds. *The Principles and Practice of Medicine*, 20th ed. New York: Appleton-Century-Crofts, 1980.
4. Bergerson, B. S. *Pharmacology in Nursing*, 14th ed. St. Louis: C. V. Mosby, 1979.
5. Watson, J. E. *Medical-Surgical Nursing and Related Pathophysiology*, 2nd ed. Philadelphia: W. B. Saunders, 1979.

6. LeMaitre, G. D., and Finnegan, J. A. *The Patient in Surgery: A Guide for Nurses*, 4th ed. Philadelphia: W. B. Saunders, 1980.

7. Metheny, N. A., and Sniverly, W. D. "Perioperative fluids and electrolytes." *Am J Nurs* 78(May): 840–845, 1978.

8. Sabiston, D. C. *Davis-Christopher Textbook of Surgery*, 12th ed. Philadelphia: W. B. Saunders, 1981.

9. Ozuna, J. M. "A study of surgical patients' temperatures." *AORN J* 28(August):245, 1978.

Suggested Readings

Felver, L. "Understanding the electrolyte maze." *Am J Nurs* 80(September):1591–1595, 1980.

Hamilton, H., et al., eds. *Monitoring Fluid and Electrolytes Precisely*. Horsham, Penn.: Intermed Communications, 1978.

Kennedy, G. "Total parenteral nutrition: down to the basics." *Can Nurs* 77(March):32–33, 1981.

Lander, J. D. "Nursing care of children with fluid and electrolyte disorders." *Issues Compr Pediatr Nurs* 4(April):41–51, 1980.

Mar, D. D. "Intravenous admixtures." *Am J Nurs* 81(March):574, 575, 1981.

Metheny, N. A., and Sniverly, W. D. *Nurses' Handbook of Fluid Balance*, 3rd ed. Philadelphia: J. B. Lippincott, 1979.

Pratt, M. L. "Blood banks link to OR." *AORN J* 25(May):1058–1068, 1977.

White, S. J. "I. V. fluids and electrolytes: How to head off the risks." *RN* 42(November):60–63, 1979.

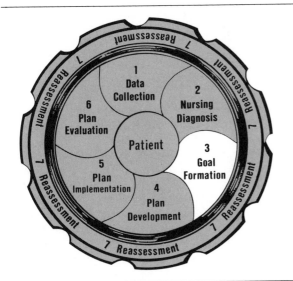

GOAL: Absence of adverse effects related to hazards.

The Patient is Free from Harm

Patients undergoing surgery are exposed to a variety of hazards that have a potential for causing harm or injury. The nurse caring for the perioperative patient is obligated to protect her from harm due to a lack of safety measures. Safety measures must be employed when the patient is exposed to or in contact with anesthesia, electricity, chemicals, radiation, and internal and external disasters.

The patient's goal is that she will be free of harm that may be caused by potential hazards in the operating room. The following criteria are used to measure attainment of the goal:

1. Patient will be free of adverse effects associated with the administration of anesthesia agents. She will:
   a. Emerge from the anesthesia agent as prescribed
   b. Be free of complications due to muscle relaxants, sedatives, and analgesics used
   c. Show no evidence of respiratory complications due to anesthesia
   d. Have an open and functioning intravenous access to the bloodstream
   e. Be free of trauma from intubation or extubation of airway
   f. Be free of postanesthesia signs or symptoms that indicate equipment malfunction

2. Patient will not show evidence of adverse reactions resulting from the use of electrical equipment. She will:
   a. Be free of burns
   b. Be free of neuromuscular damage
   c. Be free of central nervous system complications
   d. Show no evidence of electrical shock
3. Patient will be free of adverse effects due to exposure to chemical hazards. She will:
   a. Be free of skin irritation or burns
   b. Be free of respiratory complications
   c. Be free of neurological symptoms
4. Patient will show no evidence of excessive exposure to radiation. She will:
   a. Have no evidence of loss of hair
   b. Have no reduction in white blood cells
   c. Have no evidence of destruction of healthy cells
   d. Show minimal skin irritation with no ulceration
   e. Be free from nausea and vomiting
5. Patient will be free of harm resulting from an internal or external disaster: She will:
   a. Not be left unmonitored during warning period for pending external disasters
   b. Not demonstrate psychological or physical trauma due to internal disasters
   c. Not be unaccompanied during evacuations

Hazards Associated with Anesthesia

Threats to the surgical patient's safety consist of (1) anesthetic agents and drugs, (2) equipment used to deliver the agents, and (3) the actual process of delivering the agents to the patient. A general understanding of the hazards associated with these threats is needed by nurses even though the anesthetist ultimately is charged with responsibility for the safe delivery of anesthesia. Nursing activities are partially determined by the induction, maintenance, and emergent phases of anesthesia. The chemical, physical, and pharmacological properties of agents and drugs, the working safety of equipment used to deliver agents, and the response of patients in the anesthetic state are among the factors used to plan nursing intervention that will protect the patient from harm while under anesthesia. Certain nursing actions and precautions also protect the surgical team from harm as well.

HISTORY

Lack of effective pain control was, for many years, a major deterrent to surgery, except in dire circumstances, as a treatment modality for human illness. The physiological and psychological shock of exquisite pain associated with surgery was almost as great a threat to life as was the condition requiring operation. Early attempts to render the patient insensitive to pain were recognized as unsatisfactory, as well as unsafe, measures.

In the thirteenth century, the alchemist Raymundus Lullius discovered a fluid called "sweet vitriol." This compound, ether, went unrecognized for centuries as a potential reliever of pain, and few discoveries of clinical usefulness were made until the late eighteenth and nineteenth centuries. During this period, research revealed the basic properties of gases. Oxygen, nitrous oxide, ethylene, and chloroform were isolated. Their anesthetizing properties, however, were not immediately appreciated. More attention was given to their social than their medical use. By the middle of the nineteenth century, "gas frolics" with nitrous oxide and ether were widespread. Students of chemistry and young medical practitioners would use these gases for entertainment at parties, which eventually led to their application for elimination of pain during surgery.

The first clinical demonstration of general anesthesia took place on October 16, 1846, in the "ether" amphitheater of Massachusetts General Hospital. Here a medical student, William T. G. Morton, administered ether to render a patient unconscious during the surgical removal of a lesion under the man's jaw. At the end of the procedure, which the patient tolerated without pain, the surgeon turned to the audience and stated, "Gentlemen, this is no humbug." Oliver Wendell Holmes later coined the words "anesthetic" and "anesthesia."

N_2O, chloroform, and other chemical ether compounds were reassessed for medical value.

These agents were added to the anesthesia armamentarium and a new field of medical practice, anesthesia, was created. The inhalation method predominated, leading to the manufacture of gas contained in cylinders and the development of gas-dispensing machines with flow meters that allowed the anesthetist to accurately control gas and vapor concentrations. The development of the syringe made possible the use of intravenous narcotics and tranquilizers. The first intravenous anesthetic was given with chloral hydrate in 1872.

The discovery of regional anesthesia followed that of inhalation and intravenous anesthesia. Carl Köller in 1884 used the first local agent, cocaine. He instilled cocaine into the eye of a frog and discovered the eye became insensitive to pain. In 1885, Dr. William Halsted introduced the practice of using a solution of cocaine by infiltration to achieve a nerve block. This prompted Leonard Corning in 1886 to produce a peridural nerve blockade. In 1898, August Bier, encouraged by Corning's work, introduced the use of spinal anesthesia. With the development of the three major types of anesthetic techniques: inhalation, intravenous, and regional, it has been the business of contemporary practitioners to refine, delete, and make additions to these categories to provide a safe anesthetic state.

Many theories have been advanced to explain how anesthetics exert their effects. No one theory accounts for all the actions produced by the agents in present use. Researchers continue to look for the ideal anesthetic—new and better agents that will assure an anesthetic state free from harmful effects.

METHODS OF ANESTHESIA

The induction of narcosis, or anesthesia, may be divided into two categories—general and regional. General induction is then divided into inhalational and intravenous, and regional induction into topical and infiltration.

An effective anesthetic will produce a state of sleep, provide analgesia, obtund adverse reflexes, and relax muscles. The agent should be potent, nontoxic, stable when stored, nonflammable, easily eliminated from the body, and reversible in action. One of the most popular means of obtaining this desired anesthetic state is by using inhalational agents.

GENERAL

Inhalation

Inhalational agents are desirable because of their ease of uptake and elimination through the respiratory system. They are delivered to the patient as either gases or vapors of volatile liquids through anesthesia apparatus and a rubber face mask or tracheal tube. One of the advantages of inhalation anesthesia is the high percentage of oxygen that may be delivered concurrently.

Next to oxygen, nitrous oxide (N_2O) is the most commonly used gas in anesthesia practice. N_2O possesses relatively weak anesthetic properties and is used to potentiate the anesthetic state by supplementing drugs such as sedatives and analgesics. It is also used as an adjunct to more potent volatile liquid anesthetics to reduce the percentage concentration necessary to produce an effective anesthetic state.

Halothane (Fluothane), a sweet-smelling volatile liquid anesthetic, is a potent agent used today. It is nonexplosive and nonflammable but decomposes when exposed to light. Due to its chemical properties, it can be destructive to rubber, plastic, and some metal equipment. Halothane is a cardiopulmonary depressant that produces bradycardia, peripheral vasodilation, decreased blood pressure, and reduced tidal volume. The myocardium becomes sensitive to catecholamines, so the concurrent administration of epinephrine should be performed with great caution. Patients often shiver while emerging from halothane anesthesia. This may be due to the vasodilation and decreased body temperature, or may be neurological in origin. Halothane is vaporized for inhalational use in the gas machine from a device known as a copper kettle or other commercially available vaporizers.

Two new volatile agents are gaining popularity. Ethrane (Enflurane) and Forane (Isoflurane) are competing with halothane in clinical practice. Ethrane, like halothane, is a colorless, nonflammable, pleasant-smelling liquid.

Rubber and plastic are soluble in it, so like halothane it may damage equipment made of these substances. Ethrane depresses respiration. Heart rate is minimally altered, but blood pressure is lowered in proportion to anesthetic depth. Ethrane is thought to be free of hepatic or renal toxicity owing to its biotransformation. Less than 3 percent of the administered agent is biotransformed; the remainder is eliminated unchanged via the pulmonary system. Ethrane, like halothane, is dispensed by copper kettle or other vaporizers. There is some myocardial sensitization to catecholamines, but less than with halothane.

Forane, the newest of the volatile agents available, is a stable, nonexplosive, nonflammable clear liquid. It is an isomer of ethrane, but its vapor has a stronger odor. This probably accounts for the respiratory irritation that may accompany its use. Forane is a potent respiratory depressant. The drug does not markedly disturb cardiovascular stability. Blood pressure decreases but returns to normal. The heart rate increases slightly. Forane is metabolized the least of the potent volatile agents and is therefore thought to be nontoxic to the liver and kidney.

Intravenous

Many agents may be given intravenously to cause a safe, reversible state of anesthesia. Barbiturates, phencyclidines, narcotics, and neuroleptic drugs are a few of the commonly used classes of intravenous agents. Short-acting barbiturates have become the predominant drugs used in clinical practice. Unlike an inhalation agent, whose effects can be reversed by turning off the agent and allowing it to be eliminated through the lungs, the intravenous drugs must be metabolized or eliminated by the kidney. Responses to the same dose of the chosen anesthetic drug may vary considerably from patient to patient.

Barbiturates

Thiopental sodium (Pentothal), thiamylal sodium (Surital), and methohexital sodium (Brevital) are the most common short-acting barbiturates used. Dosage is based on body weight and modified to the patient's psychological and pathophysiological status. The short-acting barbiturates have rapid onset and short duration of peak effect. Respiratory and cardiovascular depression occur frequently. Due to these hazards, the anesthetist must have apparatus for artificial ventilation and suction equipment available before infusion of the agent. The drug should be used cautiously in patients with severe cardiac disease, myxedema, multiple sclerosis, and myasthenia gravis. Porphyria is made worse by barbiturates, and they are contraindicated in patients with this condition.

Phencyclidine

A phencyclidine drug causes a state of dissociative anesthesia, i.e., a state of indifference to pain. Ketamine hydrochloride is the phencyclidine used most in clinical practice. Ketamine causes a cataleptic or catatonic state along with analgesia and amnesia. It is used as the induction agent in the patient with shock or hypovolemia because it stimulates both circulation and respiration. There is a transient rise in blood pressure and pulse rate and therefore it must be used cautiously in hypertensive, tachycardiac patients. Salivation often increases.

Postoperative hallucinations have been associated with ketamine use. To minimize this effect droperidol (Inapsine) or diazepam (Valium) may be given.

Narcotics

Morphine, fentanyl (Sublimaze), and meperidine hydrochloride (Demerol) are most often used as adjunct agents. In cardiac surgery, however, they may be used as the sole or primary agents. Their respiratory and cardiovascular depressive effects are well known. (See Chapter 19)

Tranquilizers

Tranquilizers produce sedation and hypnosis. These drug properties have made them important adjuncts to intravenous anesthesia techniques. Diazepam, lorazepam (Ativan), and droperidol are a few of those most commonly employed. These drugs allow the anesthetist to reduce the dosage of anesthetic agents. Most effects of the drugs are dose related and dependent on the patient. Respiratory and cardiovascular depression may occur according to the dosage. A major disadvantage of these drugs is the long duration of action. The advantages are the potent antiemetic effects of droperidol and the amnesia from diazepam and lorazepam.

Neuroleptoanalgesia

Neuroleptoanalgesia developed from the early use of the "lytic cocktail" popular in the 1950s. The cocktail consisted of meperidine, promethazine, and chlorpromazine. The original concept has evolved into the combined use of a potent narcotic and a tranquilizer such as butyrophenone (droperidol). Each drug may be given individually, or in a fixed combination. The combination is an excellent choice for premedication and may serve as an intravenous anesthetic depending on the dose given. The characteristic effect of the drug combination is subcortical suppression, producing marked tranquillity and somnolence. The patient is depressed to a state of indifference to surroundings, but continues to respond to commands. Some amnesia and analgesia, along with antiemesis, are produced.

Neuromuscular Relaxants

Muscle relaxants are adjuncts to anesthetics but are not anesthetic agents in themselves. In addition to the goals of providing unconsciousness and analgesia, there often is a need to provide muscle relaxation for adequate surgical conditions. Muscle relaxation results in reduced tissue trauma created by manipulation during the procedure. There are several techniques to decrease muscle tone.

1. Give high concentrations of an inhalational agent to deepen the anesthesia to a plane where muscle tone is diminished. This is not always desirable, however, because of the adverse effects of deep anesthesia on other organ systems.
2. Block nerve impulses as with regional anesthetic techniques.
3. Suppress transmission of nerve impulse from the motor nerve to the voluntary muscle cell.

Neuromuscular blocking agents are used in the third technique. These drugs interfere with impulse transmission from motor nerves to muscles—specifically at the myoneural junction. The primary indications for use of muscle relaxants are to facilitate endotracheal intubation, to avoid the necessity for deep anesthetic levels, and to provide a relaxed operative field. There are two categories of muscle relaxants clinically used, depolarizing and nondepolarizing agents.

Depolarizing Muscle Relaxants

Within this category are succinylcholine chloride (Anectine, Quelicin) and decamethonium. They exert their activity at the end-plate region of muscle, initiating depolarization of the muscle and muscle contraction. This may be observed as muscle fasciculations noted in patients after injection of the drug. Once the fasciculations have occurred (depolarization), the muscle end plate does not repolarize and relaxation results. Succinylcholine has a rapid onset and lasts no longer than 5 to 10 minutes. Due to its short action, succinylcholine is primarily used as a single-dose injection to facilitate intubation. It may be diluted in an infusion and given in drip form, titrated to patient response. Side effects of the drug are bradycardia, transient rise in intraocular pressure, and increased intragastric pressure. If not hydrolyzed properly, succinylcholine can cause prolonged paralysis. Increased intragastric pressure is always a concern when dealing with a patient who may be in danger of aspiration. Severe bradycardia has been observed with repeated bolus doses. A frequent postoperative complaint is muscle soreness thought to be due to the fasciculations that precede paralysis.

Nondepolarizing Muscle Relaxants

The following drugs are known as nondepolarizing or competitive neuromuscular blocking agents: metocurine iodide (tubocurarine, Metubine), gallamine triethiodide (Flaxedil), and pancuronium bromide (Pavulon). These drugs occupy acetylcholine receptors and block the depolarizing action of acetylcholine at the postjunctional end plate. They have a slower onset than depolarizing agents and a significantly longer duration (45 to 60 minutes). The most common untoward side effect of tubocurarine is hypotension, possibly due to histamine release or to ganglionic blockade. Gallamine and Pavulon increase heart rate and arterial pressure. The safe use of these drugs usually requires securing the airway by endotracheal intubation, along with controlled ventilation.

REGIONAL

Infiltration/Instillation

Spinal, epidural, and other nerve blocks are forms of regional anesthesia, which is an alternative to general anesthesia. It may be advantageous for patients with full stomachs, for brief superficial surgery, or for those patients who are poor risks for general anesthesia. Local anesthetic drugs produce analgesia by interrupting sensory nerve impulses.

Adverse effects of regional anesthetics are either local or systemic. Local reactions include nerve damage, inflammation, and abscess formation. Systemic effects range from allergic responses and muscle paralysis to cardiovascular depression and convulsions.

1. Nerve block entails injecting a local anesthetic in an area blocking the nerve supply to the operative site.
2. Intravenous regional anesthesia is accomplished by injecting local anesthesia in the venous system of an extremity that has been exsanguinated by application of an Esmarch® bandage and occluded from systemic circulation by the application of a tourniquet.
3. Spinal anesthesia is obtained by introducing local anesthetics into the subarachnoid space. Spinal anesthesia is ideal for procedures below the xyphoid process.
4. Epidural anesthesia occurs when a local anesthetic solution is injected in the epidural space outside the dura mater.

Topical

Topical anesthesia is the direct application of anesthetic drugs to skin or mucous surfaces.

Such tissues as the mucous membrane of the nose, throat, mouth, tracheobronchial tree, esophagus, and genitourinary tract and the cornea of the eye can be anesthetized by applying topical agents. The form of the agent used in surgery is most often sprays or drops. Wounds resulting from rectal or minor skin surgery may be covered with anesthetic agents contained in an ointment base. Commonly used agents are procaine, proparacaine (Alaine, Ophthcaine, Ophthetic), benzocaine, and cyclomethycaine (Surfacaine). Cocaine, because of its pharmacologic properties, may still be used on certain types of nasal procedures and most operating rooms keep a small supply of the drug on hand for that purpose.

Water-soluble topical agents are absorbed rapidly by the body, and for this reason, toxic systemic reactions may occur shortly after application. Absorption of agents in the tracheobronchial tree is particularly rapid—almost as rapid as intravenous injection of the agent would be. When these agents are used on the nose, throat, mouth, and tracheobronchial tree, the patient should be discouraged from swallowing the agent in order to decrease the total amount available for absorption, and hence reduce the risk of toxic reaction. In addition, some patients are allergic to the ester form of certain agents. Substitution of an amide form is needed in these circumstances. Agents such as benzocaine that are poorly soluble in water are absorbed too slowly to cause toxic effects.

Administration of topical anesthetics is the responsibility of the surgeon. Anesthesia personnel may not be present to monitor patients during procedures using topical anesthesia. Consequently, the nurse may be responsible for observing the patient's condition as well as for offering both physical and psychological support.

SIGNS AND STAGES OF ANESTHESIA

For anesthesia to be safe, the anesthetist must monitor the patient's physiological status. Depth of anesthesia is one of the factors involved in safety. Since modern anesthesia practice includes a number of agents and drugs, the anesthetist today relies primarily on physiological responses as indicators to gauge the depth of general anesthesia.

Classical indicators of depth were first devised with diethyl ether by Arthur Guedel in 1920 and modified by Noel Gillespie in 1943. These classical indicators are of little practical use today, although anesthetists still refer to the stages of anesthesia. The principle behind classical indicators is still valid. The patient's safety partially depends upon awareness of the level of anesthesia both during surgery and until recovery has been achieved. Thus, postanesthesia care of patients demands that nurses have some comprehension of the "stages" of anesthesia because recovery occurs in a reverse order.

ANESTHESIA MACHINE

The anesthesia machine is a series of conduits that directs a mixture of oxygen and anesthetic gases to the patient to provide an anesthetic state. The safe delivery of agents to the patient requires the anesthetist to understand the machine's construction and capabilities.

A number of anesthetic machines are available on the market for clinical use. They range from very simple models to complex systems with multiple accessories. Each machine, regardless of design, has basic elements common to all. In general, anesthetic machines have the following components:

1. Oxygen source, given alone as supportive therapy, or in the anesthetic mixture
2. Anesthetic gas source
3. A flow device to measure and control the amount of oxygen or gas delivered
4. A mechanism for vaporizing and dispensing liquid agents
5. A breathing system for exchanging gases
6. A means for eliminating carbon dioxide

Gas cylinders, which may contain nitrous oxide, oxygen, air, or helium, are attached to the anesthesia machine. These cylinders are color coded for easy identification as well as safety. An additional safety feature is known as the "pin-index system." The neck of each cylinder has two pin settings that correspond to two holes in the machine cylinder yoke. This prevents inadvertent attachment of a cylinder to the incorrect flow meter. Flow meter devices measure the flow of gases being delivered and are color coded to be compatible with the cylinder codes. If gases are delivered from a wall source, the "diameter index safety system" (DISS) is used. DISS assures connection of the wall source hose to the correct gas line leading to the machine. Gas pressure gauges, which indicate the volume of gas present in the cylinders, also conform to the color code.

Most machines have two types of vaporization equipment: the "out-of-series" vaporizer (copper kettle) and an "in-series" vaporizer (Fluotec, Pentec). When the anesthesia machine is in use, oxygen and anesthetic gases are mixed (this is known as the anesthetic "mixture") and directed to an outlet that connects to the breathing circuit. The breathing system consists of a pair of breathing tubes, a "y" connector, and a mask for ventilation. A reservoir bag is incorporated within the breathing circuit, which allows the anesthetist to assist or control the ventilation of the patient.

A mechanism for eliminating expired carbon dioxide is an essential part of the anesthesia machine. A carbon dioxide absorption system neutralizes expired carbon dioxide. Another method to eliminate carbon dioxide is an escape valve contained in the breathing system. In addition, the later models are equipped with a gas scavenger system to remove anesthetic gases that could otherwise escape into the room. This mechanism was devised to eliminate hazards to personnel associated with concentrations of agents in the operating room.

SAFETY REGULATIONS AND CARE MAINTENANCE

Fires or explosives require three components: source of ignition, oxygen, and a combustible element. With the general use of nonflammable anesthetic agents hazards of explosion have diminished in the operating room. However, many of the current anesthetic agents, although nonflammable, do support combustion. Therefore operating room personnel should be cautious when working around these agents and other flammable materials.

A number of regulatory agencies are involved in developing and enforcing safety standards for anesthetic equipment and anesthetic environments. The U.S. Food and Drug Administration, the Interstate Commerce Commission, the Compressed Gas Association, the National Fire Protection Association, and the Department of Transportation are a few of the agencies concerned with safety in manufacturing, handling, and use of anesthetic agents. Detailed code information may be obtained from the Code for Use of Flammable Anesthetics, published by the National Fire Protection Association and the Compressed Gas Association. Electrical standards are recommended by the National Fire Protection Association, National Electrical Code. City building codes specify the safe installation of hospital electrical and gas piping systems.

To reduce human error, a number of safety features have been devised for anesthesia-related equipment. In addition to the color coding and pin index system associated with the cylinders and machines, there is a fail-safe system that prevents the delivery of hypoxic admixtures. In the event of a loss of the oxygen source, the delivery of other inhalation agents stops. Anesthesia machines and auxiliary equipment have lighting systems or alarm devices that alert anesthetists to minimal safety limits. The anesthesia machine, related breathing circuits, and auxiliary equipment associated with anesthesia are the direct responsibility of the Department of Anesthesia.

All equipment used must operate safely. Equipment should be cleaned daily and checked routinely by trained service personnel for reliability. When possible, anesthetists should use disposable apparatus. Nondisposable equipment may be cleaned with chemical solutions or gas sterilized. The Association of Operating Room Nurses has published *Standards for Cleaning and Processing Anesthesia Equipment* (1) as a guide for nursing and anesthesia personnel engaged in this task. The manufacturer's directions should also be consulted for appropriate cleaning. Most hospitals have an infection control committee that routinely assesses microbial growth and makes recommendations regarding infection prevention.

Each operating room should have a scavenger system. Controversial research suggests that long-term exposure to trace gas elements may contribute to a higher incidence of spontaneous abortions, birth defects, and malignancies among OR personnel. As a safety precaution excess gas flow escaping through the elimination valve on the machine may be diverted out of the room by a sophisticated method of venting the excess elements to a wall source vacuum system.

ANESTHESIA-RELATED EQUIPMENT

Auxiliary equipment used by anesthetists helps provide safe and homeostatic anesthesia. The items basic to most general anesthetic procedures are:

1. Suction apparatus
2. Blood pressure cuff and sphygmomanometer
3. Electrocardiographic monitor
4. Monaural and precordial stethoscopes
5. Mechanical ventilator
6. Nerve stimulator
7. Temperature probe
8. Oxygen analyzer

With difficult surgical procedures or seriously ill patients, additional devices will be required:

1. Thermal blanket
2. Hemodynamic monitors (arterial pressure, central venous pressure, pulmonary wedge pressure)

Most of the equipment monitors the physiological status of the patient. In addition to the monitoring equipment, the anesthetist assesses urinary output, fluid intake, blood loss, and blood gas values. Even the most sophisticated equipment does not replace the importance of constant surveillance by the anesthetist. Extensive discussion of the physiological response of the patient is given in Chapter 19.

PREANESTHESIA ASSESSMENT

Assessing the current and past physical status of the patient preoperatively is necessary for safe anesthesia administration. The anesthetist uses this information to develop and implement the patient's anesthesia care plan. After reviewing the chart and evaluating laboratory data, the anesthetist interviews each patient prior to surgery. Establishing rapport between the anesthetist and patient may reduce the patient's anxiety. The anesthetist's visit prior to the surgery may decrease the inductive dosage needed and diminish the need for premedication.

The anesthetist should discuss the proposed anesthesia plan and the alternatives available to meet the patient's needs. Together they agree on the plan to be followed. For example, spinal anesthesia may be the best and safest choice for a patient. However, the patient may refuse this option despite the anesthetist's convincing arguments for it. A second option would then have to be chosen. The process of induction should be explained, as well as what the patient can expect upon emerging from anesthesia. The presence of an endotracheal tube or airway, oxygen devices, nasogastric tube, intravenous lines, monitoring equipment, muscle soreness, mental cloudiness and pain are all subjects upon which the patient should be informed. A well-informed patient who knows the expected conditions will be more cooperative and feel more secure.

Hazards Associated with Electricity

As a power source for sophisticated equipment, electricity is an important ally of health care providers. Lifesaving devices, such as defibrillators, electrocardiographs, and dialysis machines depend on electricity. The operating room has many important and complex electrical devices. The most common are electrosurgical units, microscopes, monitors, and lights. Many of today's operating room tables are electrical. Endoscopes are electrically powered, as are lasers, x-ray machines, drills, and video equipment.

Although electrical equipment provides important advantages in surgery, it also introduces potential hazards to patients and personnel. Electricity has been called "the single greatest hazard to the life of the surgical patient at the present time" (2:27). A respect for electricity and basic knowledge of the principles of electricity will do a great deal toward avoiding problems. Basic courses on the theory and application of electricity to patient care should be in the nursing curriculum because perioperative nurses need a working knowledge of electricity to protect patients properly.

BASIC THEORY AND PRINCIPLES OF ELECTRICITY

To understand the basics of electricity, it is important to review the following definitions.

- Electricity: A form of energy produced by a flow of electrons. Electron movement is caused by creating a higher positive electric charge at one point than at another point on the same conductor. The amount of current flowing is known as *amperage*, or *amps*. The force of the current is known as *volts*. The force (volts) multiplied by the amount of current (amps) equals *watts*.
- Conductivity: Capacity of a material to transmit electricity.
- Resistance: Impedance in an electrical circuit to flow of current; measured in *ohms*.

The behavior of electricity can be compared to the functions of the sensory nervous system: The brain acts when it has power (calories) and a stimulus (such as hitting the finger with a hammer). An electrosurgical unit, microscope, or drill also react when there are power (electricity) and a stimulus (on-off switch). The power capacity and stimulus produce a reaction.

Think of an electrical device as a brain and the electrical cords as peripheral nerves. Both the cord and the nerves carry messages (currents) to generate an action. The force that drives electrons through a wire conductor is voltage, and the conductors allow the flow to be continuous. The force that drives a sensation along a nerve is a combination of chemical reactions that also allow the flow to be continuous.

In either case, resistance or blockage of the flow results in improper reactions. If impulses are blocked in the nervous system, say by medication, the arm does not pull back and the person does not say "ouch." If electrical current is blocked, the result is also no action; however, if current is blocked inadvertently, say within a person's body, it will seek a path of least resistance until it reaches ground. This may cause burns or even electrocution.

COMMON HAZARDS AND SAFETY PRECAUTIONS RELATED TO ELECTRICITY

The three most common hazards relative to electricity are fire, burns, and electric shock.

Fire

Many texts say that the fire hazard in the operating room has been reduced because explosive anesthetic gases are no longer used. But what new equipment has been introduced? Lasers, ultrasonic devices, and cryosurgery units all have electrical connections, so fire is a possibility. In one case, four alcohol sponges used for skin preparation were placed back into the basin. The basin was set on the lower shelf of the prep table. An OR nurse pushed the table back against the wall as she rushed to prepare for the procedure. Having finished induction, the anesthesiologist stepped back to plug in the radio. Because the radio was turned on, a spark struck out as connection was made and ignited the basin of alcohol sponges. The startled anesthesiologist jumped back, upsetting the table. Flames poured across the floor, striking the feet of the circulating nurse, who suffered minor burns on the ankles.

The threat of fire and the control of such a disaster should be on the mind of every hospital employee. Methods of fire prevention should be well ingrained in personnel working in patient care areas. The same is true for patients. They should plan an escape route when they are admitted to the hospital, as they would when checking into a high-rise hotel. A fire in an operating room can cost lives, or it can be

nothing more than an unpleasant memory if personnel are prepared through adequate planning and rehearsal.

Faulty wiring, extension cords, poorly maintained equipment, and lack of current safety measures are all contributing factors to fire. If a fire starts, the first measure is to remove the patient from the danger zone. Second is to shut off anything that is contributing to the fire—electricity, oxygen, or chemicals. The third measure is to activate the disaster plan by reporting the fire and getting help. Precautions against fire include:

1. Memorize telephone numbers and rules for reporting fires.
2. Know the location of fire fighting equipment and its proper applications, e.g., water hoses and fire extinguishers.
3. Allow only flame-retardant garments or blankets in the operating room.
4. Know the guidelines for the prevention of fire hazards in an oxygen-enriched atmosphere.
5. Eliminate the use of explosive gases and liquids.
6. Check all electrical equipment before each use for integrity of function. Are cords intact? Do plugs fit well? Are fixtures securely mounted?
7. Establish and enforce maintenance routines necessary to keep all electrical equipment in perfect operating order.
8. Remove and send for repair any questionable electrical equipment.
9. Assess and plan for sufficient backup equipment to allow for maintenance downtime.
10. Be aware of substances that can be ignited with sparks, e.g., alcohol and skin degreasing prep solutions.

Electrical Burns

Burns occur directly from contact with hot electrical wires or indirectly from items overheated by electrical wires. High frequency currents that are dissipated through patient grounding systems, such as those used with electrosurgery or defibrillators, may cause burns. The burn may be due to inadequate contact of the electrode with the patient or faulty wiring of the ground wire while the current is passing through.

The three major kinds of burns associated with electricity are contact, flash or arc, and flame. Contact burns are caused by electrical and thermal coagulation as current enters and leaves the skin. The flash or arc burn results from intense heat generated by electrical current passing through the air from one conductor to another. Arc burns usually produce serious injury to the skin but do not affect internal organs. The defibrillator causes these kinds of burns if the paddles are not placed correctly. The flame burn is the result of an explosion or fire.

Burns are generally classified as first, second, and third degree. First-degree burns damage the epidermis and cause a reddening of the skin area. Second-degree burns damage both epidermis and dermis and result in blistering of the skin. The black charring and tissue desiccation seen in third-degree burns is almost always the result of direct contact with electric current. When a burn occurs, three basic principles of treatment should be kept in mind. First, maintain an airway at all times. If the burn is in the head and neck area, there is potential for laryngeal edema and tracheal obstruction. Second, take corrective action to maintain fluid and electrolyte balance. Third, maintain an environment that will prevent infection. With severe burns, there is gross tissue damage and the threat of contamination by bacteria. Usually if there is necrosis of skin and muscle, debridement can help clean the area, making it easier to thwart the potential infection.

Electric Shock

The third common hazard associated with electricity is shock or electrocution. Any direct contact with 110 or 220 voltage wiring has the potential of electrocuting patients and employees. This is common household current, which is also used in hospitals. If the voltage is high enough, it can cause damage to the brain and respiratory center resulting in apnea. In contrast, low-voltage currents frequently affect the heart, causing ventricular fibrillation.

One of the most common complications of electric shock is vascular injury, caused by current following blood vessels. The result may be necrosis, thrombosis, or hemorrhage. Loss of consciousness is another complication due to electrocoagulation of brain tissue. Damage to the respiratory center or paralysis of respiratory muscles leads to cerebral edema, hemorrhage, thrombosis, or apnea. Infections may occur because anaerobic organisms thrive in tissue destroyed by electric current. Cardiac arrhythmias are possible because of the heart's increased susceptibility to extopic activity after electric shock. Eye damage may also be a complication, with blindness occurring due to electrocoagulation of the lens. Precautions against electrical shock include:

1. Establish an uninterrupted power supply to each operating room with a back-up emergency power source.
2. Establish and maintain a functional ground detector system that has both audio and visual alarms in each operating room.
3. Know proper grounding devices and secure utilization to grounding panels.
4. Establish policies and procedures for the testing of electrical patient care equipment when newly installed and at intervals of not more than six months.
5. Do not use equipment that has frayed cords or poor connections.
6. Discontinue the use of any equipment that demonstrates an excessive need for power, e.g., electrosurgical units that do not seem to function unless dials are set at unusually high levels.
7. Use laboratory-approved patient grounding systems compatible with the electrosurgical units in use.
8. Develop a habit of "nontouch" when electrical equipment is being activated, i.e., do not rest against or touch patients, operating room tables, or machinery.
9. Be aware of and stay current with records of equipment maintenance including repairs made.
10. Keep instructional material on the use of equipment available for all personnel.

Basic safety regulations governing hospitals are found in the standards, guidelines, or codes of local, state, and federal agencies as well as voluntary standard-setting groups. The Joint Commission on Accreditation of Hospitals (JCAH), the Occupational Safety and Health Administration (OSHA), and the National Fire Protection Association (NFPA) are some of the strongest, most important voluntary agencies setting guidelines for patient safety. State and city regulations are promulgated by health boards, licensing bureaus, and commissions on health. The U.S. Department of Health and Human Services (DHHS, formerly the Department of Health, Education and Welfare) issues regulations governing all hospitals. Findings of these agencies can influence a hospital's accreditation, certification, or licensure. More important, the hospital's level of compliance can affect the life and safety of patients and employees.

An awareness of the safety standards published by such agencies is the legal, ethical, and moral responsibility of every employee who provides direct patient care in a hospital. Electrical safety features should be planned and designed from the time of construction of every operating room suite and must be followed routinely every day thereafter. Regulations governing construction of hospitals and operating room suites are set by the city, county, and state health departments.

An example of a JCAH regulation is: "There shall be a written policy for the testing of electronic and electrical patient care equipment." The rationale for this regulation is supported by surveys that reveal as much as 40 percent of all electric and electronic patient care equipment requires some kind of mechanical repair or calibration prior to its initial use.

It is impossible to list here all the regulations governing patient safety. The ones governing electricity alone would take many pages. For instance the National Fire Protection Association has over 50 publications dealing with safety in health care, each containing many regulations and standards regarding the hazards associated with electricity. The JCAH publishes multiple manuals regulating health care of facilities and the related hazards. The DHHS offers a significant number of publications, many of which are relevant to hospital facilities. A specific example might be a regulatory body such as JCAH which has a requirement, "Operator's manual shall be made available to all those who use electrical equipment." The purpose of this is to provide instructions for use of equipment and eliminate the hazards associated with misuse. A manual of this type will contain specific information regarding proper operating, safety considerations, and special warnings related to use. What is important is to know (1) these rules exist, (2) who and how to contact the agencies establishing the regulations, and (3) that the safety measures are to be followed in all patient care areas including the operating room. Each hospital must have an established method for receiving the information from regulatory agencies and for communicating the safety measures to all concerned. Usually the administrative manager responsible for planning and development is the resource person who has possession of these regulations. The biomedical department and the safety committee are other important resource contacts.

The safe use of electrical appliances in the operating room environment is a realistic goal for nurses and patients. To attain this goal, personnel should know the purpose of the electrical equipment being used and the precautions for preventing accidents. Typical electrical problems are inadequate insulation of cords and cables, faulty grounding, leakage of current, and static charges.

Insulation protects the user from the electricity traveling through a wire. Insulation material varies but usually consists of rubber or plastic over cotton. Copper wires are usually used as the conductors of the current. In the operating room, lightweight cords, heavy-duty cords, and building cables are used. Use of lightweight cords, which typically have two wires, is generally discouraged because they are not as sturdy as the heavy-duty cord. Heavy-duty is preferred for OR equipment. This three-wire power cord is much heavier and has two layers of insulation, one layer for each wire plus a separate outer layer. This cord can stand up under heavy use, particularly when there are multiple users of each cord. The building cable, which brings electricity to the wall outlet, usually encased in steel or flexible spiral-steel tubing, is a conduit.

All these power cords protect users against contact with "hot" power wires. If the insulation breaks down, electric current flows between the conducting wires, generating heat, which may start a fire. If a fire starts in the power cord attached to equipment, the electric current can be shut off. If the fire goes to the wall outlet, the steel tubing or conduit prevents it from spreading.

Grounding electrical equipment is one of the most important safety measures associated with the use of electricity. The basic grounding system for a building includes two cables, one "hot" and the other "cold." The cold cable carries the electricity from a power company generator. At the generator, the cold side is connected to an earth ground through large copper rods or pipes driven deep into the ground. One of the best ways to eliminate electrical hazards is to make sure all metal surfaces in an electrical system are connected to ground. Three-prong safety plugs should be used with all equipment in the operating room. One of the three prongs provides a reliable connection to ground, and the plug is constructed so it grips the power cord firmly. The three-prong plug can be easily opened for inspection of the connections.

The electrosurgical unit deserves special attention because it is used in almost every operating room. Although usually used without incident, it can be dangerous. In electrosurgery, high-frequency electrical energy cuts tissue and provides hemostasis. The functions of the electrosurgical unit are coagulation, cutting, and fulguration (see Figs. 11.1–11.3). Coagulation eliminates bleeding by thermally sealing the ends of blood vessels as they are dissected. The cutting (separation) of tissue is accomplished by high temperatures exploding the cells contacted by the hot active electrode. Fulguration is the destruction of tissue by electrical sparks.

The electrosurgical generator delivers high-energy electrical waves into the patient's body through a small, active electrode. The wave of

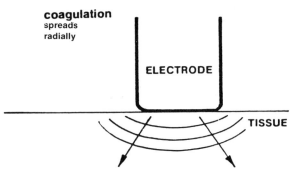

DESICCATION

coagulation
spreads
radially

ELECTRODE

TISSUE

Results: hemostasis
light brown eschar

Figure 11.1. The desiccation function of electrosurgical units. The coagulation spreads radially. Results are hemostasis and light brown eschar. Used with permission of Valleylab, Inc., Boulder.

electricity virtually explodes the tissue cells it contacts, causing cutting and coagulation. The electrical wave continues to travel, leaving the body and returning to the generator. Originally, lead or steel contact plates were used to complete the current flow back to the generator. Today, pregelled disposable adhesive pads are used and take most of the danger out of grounding plates. This modern version of the old plate ensures contact with the patient by adhering to the body skin surface, thus allowing the electrical current continuity of flow, which if interrupted may result in a burn. The gel reduces tissue heating and eliminates air spaces between the patient and the conductive surface.

The size, shape, and placement of the grounding pad is important to the prevention of patient burns (see Fig. 11.4). The shape must provide for uniform contact with the patient's body. This is critical. If there are gaps between the pad and the body, the electricity may arc across the gap, causing a burn. Also, the pad must be of sufficient size to cover enough body surface to avoid high thermal contact points. Selection of the patient contact site is crucial as well. Nothing can be allowed to interfere with the contact surface of the ground. The pad is not placed over bony prominences, excess hair is removed, and fluids are not allowed to run or pool near the pad. The patient's position should be established prior to pad application. Repositioning of a patient during a surgical procedure requires reassessment to be sure there is secure contact between the patient and the grounding pad. Poorly applied grounding pads are not the only burn hazard associated with electrosurgical devices. Burns can also occur as electrical current seeks alternate paths out of the body. Electrocardiogram electrodes are one of the most common alternative paths. Other locations are points of contact between the patient and metal objects such as intravenous poles and stirrups.

Bipolar electrosurgery is best for specific surgical procedures. Bipolar refers to the means by which the current travels back to the generator. The active electrode is usually similar to a forcep in design. Electricity travels along one side of the forceps and returns along the other side when the tips touch or grasp tissue, which completes the flow of current. Because the cutting instrument provides for a complete circuit, a pregelled grounding pad is not needed during the use of a bipolar unit.

Routine inservice education for circulating nurses is the best prevention for hazards

FULGURATION

surface coagulation

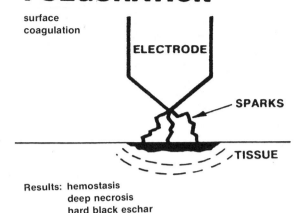

Results: hemostasis
deep necrosis
hard black eschar

Figure 11.3. The fulguration function of electrosurgical units. There is surface coagulation. Hemostasis, deep necrosis, and hard black eschar results. Used with permission of Valleylab, Inc., Boulder.

related to electrosurgical devices. Critical topics for the inservice session would be:

- Alternative paths for electricity
- Positioning the patient prior to grounding plate placement
- Placement of the grounding plate as close to the wound site as possible
- Inspection for insulation against any patient-metal contact points
- Use of rubber, cotton, or foam pads or drapes as insulation between the contact points

No matter how impressive the safety features seem, the nurse should always go through a mental checklist to protect her patient from the potential problems related to electrosurgical units. Electrosurgery is so necessary in performing rapid, precise surgical procedures that its use is worth the risks involved. Risks are minimized when nursing personnel are alert to potential hazards. Ongoing hazard prevention includes:

1. Establish a routine maintenance check program with manufacturers and hospital biomedical engineering personnel.
2. Establish procedures for cleaning per manufacturer's recommendations.

Figure 11.2. The cutting function of electrosurgical units. Hot continuous sparks separate cells, resulting in cut tissue and hemostasis. Used with permission of Valleylab, Inc., Boulder.

CUTTING

hot continuous sparks separate cells

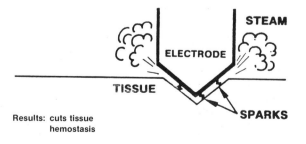

Results: cuts tissue
hemostasis

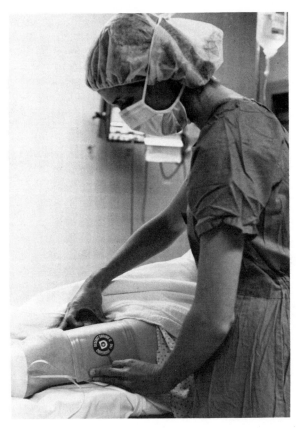

Figure 11.4. The size, shape, and placement of the electrosurgical unit grounding pad is important to the prevention of patient burns.

3. Replace adapters that do not provide tight connections.
4. Avoid use of the unit as a dispensing table. Machine settings can inadvertently be changed if the unit is bumped, and fluid will cause damage if spilled into the unit.
5. Establish a system of shelf rotation for all accessories, such as gelled electrodes and sterile cords.

Immediate preoperative plans for precautions against burns include:

1. Inspect all patient contact areas. Patients must be insulated from contact with metal objects, e.g., stirrups and head or shoulder braces.

2. Plan the placement of all electrodes (ECG leads, grounding pad, EEG leads, and any other conductor of current) after the position of the patient has been determined and established. Repositioning during the intraoperative phase may cause loosening of attached conductive electrodes.
3. Be cautious in the use of skin degreasers because they promote adhesion of electrodes but can cause burns if not totally removed before electrode application.
4. Be sure gels used to enhance conduction are moist and uniform in quantity.
5. Be sure contact areas between the skin and conductive electrodes are clean and dry. This includes removal of hair if necessary to secure tight, close adhesion.
6. Place patient grounding devices and ECG monitoring leads away from bony prominences or scar tissue.
7. Place grounding pads close to wound site.
8. Place monitoring lead electrodes as far from wound site as possible.
9. Do *not* let moisture or liquids come in contact with conductive electrodes.

LASERS

The laser is rapidly gaining acceptance as a surgical tool because of patient advantages such as less bleeding, reduced swelling, and minimized scar tissue formation. The laser's most important function is tissue vaporization. The carbon dioxide laser operates at such high temperatures that the water in cells boils and evaporates so fast that the cell explodes and vaporizes. This action separates tissue with minimal thermal damage to surrounding tissue. Other lasers are of lower energy levels but function much in the same manner.

The laser brings old and new potential hazards to the intraoperative setting. The old hazards are those previously explained related to any piece of electrical equipment in the operating room. The new or additional hazards are those related to the high degree of temperature and thermal action caused by the laser light. The amount of electricity (expressed in wattage) used by the laser will determine, along with other factors, the power density of the laser light beam. The more wattage used the more power converted to light and thus the higher degree of thermal effect emitted by the light. The thermal effect can be at several hundred degrees celsius which will vaporize, cauterize and sterilize tissue. Laser energy is light amplification by stimulated emission of radiation. It is not an ionizing radiation such as with x-ray.

Carbon dioxide, argon, and yttrium aluminium garnet are mediums most commonly used to create laser beams. Each of these mediums has different physical properties. The most important safety aspect for all of them is that the beam and its direction must be controlled to prevent undesired tissue damage. The most critical damage to tissue is burn of the eye or skin.

To prevent injury to personnel working with lasers, place a warning sign on the door leading into the room where a laser is in use. Protective eye wear should be worn by awake patients as well as personnel. The incidence of damage has been minimal in the 17 years that lasers have been on the commercial market. In the eye, the radiation is absorbed in the cornea and causes "welder's flash" or "photokeratitis." Because of this potential hazard, one of the most important safety aspects of the laser in use includes the wearing of safety glasses by personnel to protect their corneas. Patients who are anesthetized have their eyes covered with moist cotton and eye pads. These serve to protect the corneas in the event of a reflected beam. A reflected beam could vaporize the tissue on the surface of the cornea, thus producing destruction of cells and ensuing damage. It is imperative that the cotton stay moist to absorb any reflected beams with the eyepads serving to hold the cotton in place.

Few serious eye injuries due to lasers have been reported; however, there is a potential for radiation damage to the retina and also the lens. The lens is affected like a cataract formation and is called "glassblower's cataract."

Surgical instruments with high-gloss surfaces should be ebonized or covered with wet sponges to prevent inadvertent beam reflection. Another potential hazard is the possibility of a laryngeal fire. The literature recommends several methods for counteracting this hazard. One is to wrap the endotracheal tube with a foil tape designed to reflect the beam rather than absorb it. An alternative to wrapping the endotracheal tube is the Norton metal endotracheal tube which offers flexibility and decreases the possibility of vocal cord damage. This tube has as its chief composition metal. It is airtight, easily sterilized, atraumatic to tissues, indestructible, and absolutely noncombustible with flows of 100 percent oxygen. A third method is the use of silicone, metal reinforced, endotracheal tubes that are wrapped with cloth adhesive tape. The adhesive tape wrapped tube is soaked in distilled water for five minutes prior to insertion.

Personnel working with lasers should have special training classes related to the function of the specific laser to be used. Credentialing committees must determine the criteria for use. The Bureau of Radiation Hazards (BRH), a part of the Food and Drug Administration, sets regulations for use, and all personnel should be familiar with safety precautions. Precautions against laser hazards include:

1. Never activate the laser without full control of beam direction.
2. Wear protective eye glasses specific to the laser medium.
3. Place a warning sign on the door that laser is in use.
4. Implement criteria to prevent indiscriminate application.
5. Cover high-gloss metal instruments with wet sponges in the presence of CO_2 laser beam.
6. Protect endotracheal tubes from contact with laser beams by wrapping with metal or cotton water-soaked tape.
7. Cover with a wet sponge.

Hazards Associated with Chemicals

In the operating room, personnel and patients are exposed to chemical hazards. There are two sources of hazards associated with the chemicals. One is due to the inherent properties of the material, and the other is from the toxic products of combustion or decomposition.

OR personnel should be aware of chemical hazards and safety precautions. Reading labels and following manufacturer's directions for use of products is important. Chemicals that may be used in the operating room include ethylene oxide, methyl methacrylate, phenols, acetone, alcohol, and ether. These chemicals are all flammable as well as water soluble. The extent to which a chemical is water soluble is useful in determining the type of extinguishing agent that will be most effective. Alcohol-resistant foam is usually recommended for water-soluble flammable materials.

Hazards related to these chemicals are placed in three categories: health hazards, flammability hazards, and reactive hazards. Each chemical is properly labeled to comply with the National Fire Protection Association Standards. Health hazards are labeled with blue; flammability hazards with red, and reactive hazards with yellow. Specific information about hazards related to flammable chemicals can be obtained from the National Fire Protection Association.

ETHYLENE OXIDE

Ethylene oxide (EtO) is a colorless gas used to sterilize instruments that cannot be exposed to steam sterilization. EtO is highly explosive and flammable in the presence of air. It is moderately toxic by inhalation and irritates the eyes and respiratory tract. If it contacts the skin for a prolonged period of time, burns may result. EtO has been shown to be a mutagen, which means it can cause changes in the genes of live animal cells. Workers at the American Hospital Supply Corporation exposed to EtO were found to have abnormalities in their chromosomes. The National Institute for Occupational Safety and Health (NIOSH) states that EtO should be considered as a potential occupational hazard and recommends that workers be monitored for both acute and chronic effects. Upper respiratory irritations and skin rashes are among short-term acute effects. The gas may have long-term effects on the reproductive, hemotalogical, and neurological systems.

The current Occupational Safety and Health Administration (OSHA) exposure limit for an eight-hour work day is 50 ppm, on a time-weighted average (TWA). This regulation is currently under examination and may be significantly reduced. EtO in the air can be measured by a portable infrared analyzer or by absorbing EtO into activated charcoal tubes. In working with EtO, the following precautions are recommended:

1. Use of EtO should be limited whenever possible. Materials that can withstand moist or dry heat should not be sterilized with EtO.
2. The biggest source of EtO exposure occurs when items are removed from the sterilizer. This exposure can be significantly reduced by increasing the number of exhaust cycles and providing local exhaust ventilation over the door.
3. Exposure while the sterilizer is being used can be reduced by using local exhaust devices on table top sterilizers and cycle purges on the larger sterilizers.
4. All equipment should be vented directly to the outside. The outside exhaust should not be near the air intake for the department or other parts of the hospital.
5. Without proper aeration, residues remain that can burn workers and patients. Aeration should be done preferably in an aeration cabinet. Materials which do not absorb EtO (metal, glass) do not need to be aerated *unless they were wrapped*. If they were wrapped in muslin, they need at least 30 minutes aeration. Aeration times depend on the composition, form, and weight of the material sterilized. Items made of polyvinylchloride require the longest time. The Association for the Advancement of Medical Instrumentation (AAMI) recommends the following aeration times:

At room temperature	7 days
122°F in aeration cabinet	12 hours
140°F in aeration cabinet	8 hours

For other materials, the manufacturer's recommendations should be followed. When in doubt about aeration time for a particular item, follow the recommendation above.

6. Regular monitoring of the workplace, especially in and around the sterilizer, is important.

METHYL METHACRYLATE

Methyl methacrylate, which is mixed in the operating room, is used as a bone cement in artificial joint replacement surgery. A flammable liquid whose vapor forms explosive mixtures in the air, methyl methacrylate is slightly irritating to the eyes, skin, and respiratory tract. Some patients have experienced hypotension and cardiovascular irregularities. The current OSHA exposure limit is 100 ppm. When methyl methacrylate is mixed, exposure levels immediately after mixing can be higher. Local exhaust hoods should be used, or mixing should be done in a separate ventilated area. When stored, methyl methacrylate should be protected from physical damage. Outside storage is preferred.

Iodine and iodophors are bactericidals used in skin preparation. A major drawback is that they stain the skin, but they are one of the best solutions for skin preparation. They can irritate the skin if the solution is in too high a concentration. These solutions should not be used on instruments because they cause corrosion. Alcohol is also used in skin preparation and because it is flammable, caution needs to be taken to prevent pooling under the patient. It is also used as a disinfectant for instruments and anesthesia equipment.

HOUSEKEEPING CHEMICALS

Several chemicals used in housekeeping are potential hazards, especially if used incorrectly. Phenol (carbolic acid) and phenolic derivates are germicides, and are colorless or come in white crystals. Phenol is flammable and emits vapors that, when warm, can form explosive mixtures with the air. The phenolics are toxic and can cause severe tissue burns. Systemic absorption of hexachlorophene may lead to convulsions or liver damage. Hexachlorophene, a phenolic compound, was once used for routine hand washing, but it is not recommended for this purpose since it is absorbed through the skin, causing systemic toxicity. The phenolics can also be irritating to the respiratory tract. Personnel should be cautious when handling phenolics. If the solution does come in contact with the skin, water should be used to dilute the phenol and a solution of caustic soda applied to neutralize it.

Chlorine compounds are also used for housekeeping purposes in the operating room. These include sodium hypochlorite or chlorinate lime. They are highly corrosive to instruments. When using these chemicals, personnel should protect themselves against physical contact because they are irritating to the skin, eyes, and respiratory tract. These compounds should be stored in a well-ventilated, cool, dry area away from combustible materials. The National Fire Protection Association (NFPA) code for the storage of liquid and solid oxidizing materials provides additional information on these chemicals.

Formaldehyde is another potential hazard in the operating room. It produces a colorless gas with a highly irritating odor. It is used in formalin, an aqueous solution of 40 percent formaldehyde, and as a disinfectant and sporicide for cold sterilization or disinfection. It is a poor choice, however, because of the length of time necessary for sterility and the hazards associated with skin contact. It is highly damaging to tissue and is irritating to the eyes and respiratory tract. Water should be used for spills or to rinse any materials that might come in contact with patients.

Once a common anesthetic agent, ether is now rarely used in the operating room. It has been replaced by nonflammable anesthetic gases, but on occasion it is used to remove substances on the patient's skin that are difficult to remove with other chemicals. Extremely flammable, ether gas is heavier than air and can travel considerable distances to a source of ignition. Ether should never be stored in the operating room and must be isolated from other combustible material.

GASES

The hazards associated with anesthesia gases in the operating room are included in the first section of this chapter. Other gases used in the operating room include nitrogen (N_2), which is used for air-powered instruments, carbon dioxide (CO_2), used for laser equipment, and helium, used in the intraaortic balloon pump. These gases are all nonflammable, noncorrosive, and have low toxicity. Carbon dioxide is a colorless gas, liquified at high pressure, and slightly acidic. Nitrogen is a colorless, odorless gas compressed to a high pressure, as is helium.

Carbon dioxide, helium, and to a lesser degree nitrogen can act as asphixiants by displacing air and causing suffocation. For this reason, the gases should be stored in well-ventilated areas or kept covered in an outdoor area. When used in the operating room, it is important that ventilation be adequate. The proper exchanges of air per established standard provides adequate ventilation.

The staff should know how to handle and use gas cylinders. Cylinders of gas in the operating room should be chained to a solid support. If knocked over and the neck broken, the cylinder becomes an uncontrollable projectile. Cylinder valves should be closed at all times when not in use. When a tank is empty, the valve should be closed prior to moving. If there is a fire, the cylinders should be moved away if possible, otherwise they should be cooled by spraying with water. Cylinder inspection is another safety precaution. Connecting valve outlets are critical to the safe use of gas. The Compressed Gas Association, a manufacturers' association that establishes standards for safe use of gases, has publications that can be used for teaching purposes. Two groups that also establish standards for chemicals in the operating room are the American Gas Association Laboratories (AGAL) and the National Fire Protection Association (NFPA). The AGAL conducts research and laboratory examinations to ascertain if manufacturers are complying with standards related to labeling, handling, and storage of gases. The NFPA is the principal organization establishing fire protection standards. These standards may be used as operating standards or legal requirements. Other groups concerned with safe use of hazardous materials are the Institute of Makers of Explosives and the National Safety Council.

Hazards Associated with Radiation

Diagnostic x-rays, radium implants, and radium-substitute implants are sources of ionizing radiation in the operating room. A less common source are patients who have radioactive substances in their bodies and may require surgery. Personnel and patients in the operating room are exposed to the same radiation hazards as personnel in the radiology department. Although the amount of exposure may not be as high, the same education and safety rules should apply in any area where there is a potential hazard due to ionizing radiation.

Radiation is a hazard because it has the ability to modify molecules within body cells. This may cause cell dysfunction, alteration or halt in cell replication, or cell destruction. Cells may be able to recover from radiation damage if exposure is not too high. Effects of radiation are both somatic and genetic. Somatic effects can be observed in patients who are receiving large doses for treatment. The skin gets very red, they may have a temporary loss of hair, ulcerations may occur, cataracts form on the eyes, and there may be a reduction in white blood cells that predisposes them to infections. Somatic effects vary with the amount of radiation, the age of the person, and what part of the body is exposed. Children are more sensitive than adults, and the unborn fetus is highly sensitive. Radiation effects on offspring are genetic. Radiation is associated with reproductive abnormalities such as birth defects and childhood leukemia. Radiation exposure during pregnancy slows down the normal growth of the uterus, and children of mothers exposed to radiation show reduced growth and an increase in mental retardation and leukemia. Radiation exposure is associated with all kinds of cancer and a general shortening of life expectancy.

X-RAYS

Sources of x-ray radiation exposure in the operating room include the portable x-ray machine used to take films in cholangiography and orthopedic manipulations; diagnostic radiology and radiotherapy, fluoroscopy, which directs large doses of intermittent radiation at the patient, and image amplification with television circuitry. Radiation is present from x-rays only while the x-ray tube is energized.

For personnel exposed to radiation, government regulations limit permissible levels to 5 rems/year (5,000 millirems/year) for workers over the age of 18. A dose that exceeds this level is overexposure and requires investigation by a regulatory agency. The purpose of all protection measures is to reduce the exposure as much as possible and to ensure that the radiation received does not exceed the maximum permissible dose equivalent (MPD). Unnecessary exposure can be avoided in three ways: minimizing the time of exposure, increasing the distance from the source, and placing a shield between the radiation source and the body.

Radiation exposure is monitored by a film badge clipped to the body. The film badge should be worn for one month, then evaluated. The most commonly recommended location for the film badge is at waist or chest level inside the protective apron. This, however, does not measure exposure to arms and legs or head and neck. If the film badge is worn outside the lead apron, it doesn't measure radiation to the body.

For pregnant women, the monitoring device should be worn on the waist. If a lead apron is worn, it should be under the lead apron. The pregnant employee is of great concern anywhere in the hospital where there is radiation exposure. The American Society of Radiologic Technologists has adopted guidelines for radiation safety practices for pregnant radiation workers. The recommendations include: (1) during gestation the MPD equivalent to the fetus from occupational exposure should not exceed 0.5 rem; (2) pregnant employees should disclose their pregnancy as soon as they know they are pregnant and cooperate with safety practices; (3) the employer should make available to the employee the mandates of "The Pregnancy Disability Law," the National Council on Radiation Protection and Measurements (NCRP) guidelines, and the Equal Employment Opportunity Commission (EEOC) "Guidelines on Sex Discrimination and Questions and Answers."

Increasing distance from the source is another way of reducing exposure. At 1 foot, four times the radiation is received than at 2 feet. Therefore, removal from the source as far as possible will decrease the hazard. Shielding also decreases exposure. Aprons, gloves, and walls that contain or are made of lead material reduce the radiation exposure by a factor of 10 to 30 depending on the lead equivalence in the material used.

Every hospital radiology department should have a radiation safety program that involves the x-ray department and other departments where radiological diagnosis and treatment occur. Because the operating room has areas where special procedures are done that require personnel and patients to be exposed to radiation hazards, the safety program should include that area.

Regulations for use of ionizing radiation have been established in most states. The State Department of Health has a Radiation Control Division that establishes standards. Regulations for the Administrative and Enforcement of the Radiation Control for Health and Safety Act are also available. Compliance with the regulations is important and should be included in a safety program. The Bureau of Radiologic Health is another regulatory body that sets standards for radiological safety.

Compliance with safety regulations is difficult to mandate. A philosophy of safety and caution must be developed that permeates the entire staff. Potential hazards are real, but at the same time proper handling and caution will greatly decrease any dangerous hazard.

Safety for patients having x-rays during surgery includes efficiency in preparation of the patient and the operation of equipment. Functions related to radiologic studies include positioning of the patient so the area of study is exposed to the film or fluoroscopy, ensuring that the contrast media selected is effective for the type of study being done, and checking that all equipment is in working order. The patient should be protected by gonadal shielding when appropriate.

Radiologic technologists have a responsibility to protect the patient as much as possible by selecting exposure factors that reduce the incidence of multiple x-rays being taken. The level of exposure is important for viewing purposes, but overexposure simply adds radiation. Focusing the beam of the x-ray to the specific area of study also reduces area exposed to radiation. The technician should always be cognizant of other members of the health care team and allow them to leave the room or wear a lead apron or gloves.

RADIUM AND RADIUM SUBSTITUTES

Radium and radium substitutes are used in treatment of cancer. Usually double-sealed in metal tubes, radium remains radioactive indefinitely and is potentially hazardous for thousands of years. When radium or radium substitutes are present in the operating room, the nurse should attempt to stay several arm lengths away from the source. But it is necessary to be close to the patient, 15 minutes at a half-arm length is no more hazardous than an hour at one arm length. If a radium source is dropped in the operating room, it should be picked up and placed in a lead container with long forceps. The source should not be squeezed too hard. An empty emesis basin can be used as a temporary receptacle, but should be located several feet from personnel. The source should not be touched directly. Lead aprons and gloves should not be used. They are not thick enough to offer protection against radium radiation, and usually only increase handling time, which increases exposure. To ensure that no radium is lost in the operating room, linen and trash should be checked with a radiation detector prior to removal.

Radium substitutes (iridium 192, cesium 137, and cobalt 60) are less hazardous because of the principal type of radiation rays they emit. More radiation is absorbed by the body, but they have less ability to penetrate lead.

Distance from the source reduces the hazard. The substitutes only remain radioactive for a few years. The hazards of implantation have been reduced by afterloading techniques. The radioactive sources are not inserted in the operating room, but after the patient is returned to her room.

Some treatments consist of permanent implants of short-lived radioactive materials. If these patients require surgery before the material has decayed to a low level, there may be a hazard of radiation. Precautions are similar to those for patients with radium implants. In addition, radioactive fluids or tissues removed in surgery should be put in strong bottles and handled carefully to avoid breakage. Linens and other waste should be checked for contamination to reduce exposure through distance and shielding.

As with any potential hazard associated with the operating room, personnel and patients can be protected against the dangerous effects of radiation exposure by safe practices. In the health care field there may be a tendency to negate the effects because of the common usage of ionizing radiation. All personnel should be reviewed on safe radiation practices on an ongoing basis. Regulations should be reviewed and updated practices implemented. Personnel safety measures such as monitoring exposure, wearing protective clothing, and following guidelines for the pregnant employee are essential.

Hazards Associated with Disasters

Every hospital should have plans for external and internal disasters. For accreditation by the JCAH, the plan must be written and rehearsed at least twice a year.

EXTERNAL DISASTERS

An external disaster is one that originates outside of the hospital such as an airplane crash, a train wreck, nuclear accident, or explosion at a chemical plant. Because the hospital has a responsibility to serve the residents in the community, it must be prepared to provide care when an emergency arises. The overall external disaster hospital plan is established according to JCAH recommendations. The operating room, like other units within the hospital, uses the master plan and individualizes it for the operating room. The plan for the operating room includes the same components as the overall hospital plan. The plan must provide a method of notifying operating room personnel when a disaster occurs. When they are notified, they must have an assignment. All personnel may not be assigned to perform surgical procedures. Other areas may need additional assistance, and staff would be assigned to those positions. Medical staff coordination is done through the hospital team. Surgeons are assigned to patients needing surgical intervention. The operating room plan includes the availability of supplies, equipment, and instruments, plus their distribution. Procedures for transferring patients to the operating room or surrounding patient care areas are outlined and specific types of personnel capable of monitoring critical patients are specified. The plan includes a physical layout of space available for patients and the type of patients that could be treated in the allocated space.

The hospital has special medical records to be used for disasters. These are available in the operating room for use when needed. When a disaster occurs, there is a need to maintain security. The plan established provides direction as to who should give information to the press or family members calling the hospital.

INTERNAL DISASTERS

In addition to the external plan, an internal plan should be written and available to personnel. Internal disasters include events that would necessitate moving patients from one unit to another or evacuating them from the hospital. The plan for an internal disaster must include methods of transferring critical patients to other medical facilities in the immediate vicinity.

Fire is an internal disaster. Hospitals provide personnel with specific instructions as to what they should do in case of fire. Besides ongoing education of personnel, regular drills are conducted to evaluate the effectiveness of the plan. Copies of the fire plan are located in an accessible place in the operating room. Personnel are drilled on notification of a fire and how to contain it. They are instructed on use of hospital fire extinguishers, including the types of extinguishers to use on different materials and the removal of patients. Fire drills are conducted quarterly in an effort to keep staff in a state of readiness.

The purpose of rehearsing the disaster plan twice a year is to maintain readiness of administration and other hospital personnel and the medical staff. Simulated disaster drills help all involved to evaluate how they would function in a crisis situation. It is helpful to determine whether equipment used is in proper functioning order and if the physical facility is adequate to treat the victims. The operating room, as well as other units, must evaluate its participation. This includes an assessment of personnel's effectiveness, documentation of problems, and identification of strengths and weaknesses.

There are voluntary agencies that require hospitals to maintain personnel readiness for disasters. The JCAH, NFPA, and the NFPA Life Safety Code are examples. These agencies recommend that employees have formal training on a cyclical basis and that each sign a form indicating that she has been trained and knows her responsibilities related to the plan. The form signed by the employee should be maintained as a part of the employee's personnel file.

Additional Hazards Associated with the Operating Room

Patients have a right to assume that instruments, implants, and equipment are safe and have been tested in accepted ways. Hospital policy should provide for this. Unauthorized adaptation of equipment and supplies is a difficult hazard to prevent yet imperative to deal with if patient safety is to be maintained.

Ahlstrom remarks on the history of surgical instruments, "In the old days the doctor brought his own instruments to the hospital and handed the nurse the instruments needed for the particular operation scheduled." Today, hospitals provide instrumentation (3).

There is a legal risk involved with instrumentation no matter who provides it. Hospitals bear the responsibility for making instruments available in sound working order.

Instruments can be damaged from repeated washing, handling, wrapping, and sterilizing. Thus, all instruments require routine inspections for damage, wear, and loose parts. Every operating room should have a *standing* policy of equipment and instrument inspection. Responsible hospital personnel should (3):

1. Set standards related to handling, processing, and use of instruments.
2. Demand quality when purchasing.
3. Demand and support good service from manufacturers.
4. See that all new and repaired instruments are carefully inspected by qualified persons.
5. Reject inadequate instruments at time of delivery; accept them only when satisfied with precision.
6. Delay marking instruments until they are inspected and accepted.
7. Ascertain what guarantees are promised and insist that they be kept.

The professional nurse employed in a hospital is expected to be alert to what she considers potential causes for harm to patients. When she recognizes danger to patients, she is responsible for putting the appropriate administrative and clinical personnel on notice.

The practice of some surgeons of altering or improvising devices for use in surgery is dangerous. The Bureau of Medical Device and Diagnostic Products establishes compliance standards which manufacturers must meet. Also, manufacturers will not stand behind their products if these products have been changed or applied in an unorthodox manner. The various publications and standards set by the bureau are available from the Food and Drug Administration and should be accessible in every operating room.

Inadequate air exchange in the operating room creates a hazard of potential infection. Controlled, filtered air reduces the possibility of contamination and air pollutants. Every operating room should have a controlled, filtered air supply. The number of air exchanges that take place each hour is regulated by the JCAH.

Improper handling of wastes is one of the major causes of employee lost-time and accidents in the hospital. Hazardous items include needles, knife blades, and other objects that may cause punctures. The disposal of contaminated drapes, suction canister content, and other waste that can cause infection should be of concern to the operating room nurse. Trash compactors, incinerators, and other means of containing and disposing of contaminated materials are required.

References

1. Association of Operating Room Nurses. "Standards for Cleaning and Processing Anesthesia Equipment." *AORN J* 25(7):1268–1274, 1977.
2. Rhodes, M. J., Gruendemann, B. J., and Ballinger, W. F. *Alexander's Care of the Patient in Surgery*, 6th ed. St. Louis: C. V. Mosby, 1978.
3. Ahlstrom, G., and Ahlstrom, H. "Hospital's instrument problems and some suggestions for relief." *AORN J* 15(January):77–87, 1972.

Suggested Readings

Buchsbaum, W. H., and Goldsmith, B. *Electrical Safety in the Hospital.* Oradell, New Jersey: Medical Economics Co., 1975.

Churchill-Davidson, H. C., ed. *A Practice of Anesthesia*, 4th ed. Philadelphia: W. B. Saunders, 1978.

Code for the Storage of Liquid and Solid Oxidizing Materials, (NFPA 43A). Boston: National Fire Protection Association.

Collins, V. J. *Principles of Anesthesiology*, 2nd ed. Philadelphia: Lea and Febiger, 1976.

Day, J. L., and Lightfoot, D. A. "O.R. radiation hazards." *AORN J* 20:249, 1974.

Dorsch, J. A., and Dorsch, S. E. *Understanding Anesthesia Equipment.* Baltimore: Williams and Wilkins, 1975.

Dripps, R. D., Eckenhoff, J. E., and Vandam, L. D. *Introduction to Anesthesia,* 5th ed. Philadelphia: W. B. Saunders, 1979.

Electricity in Patient Care Areas of Hospitals (NFPA 76B). Quincy, Mass.: National Fire Protection Association, 1980.

Fire Hazard Properties of Flammable Liquids, Gases, Volatile Solids (NFPA 325M). Boston: National Fire Protection Association, 1977.

Gary, C. T., Nunn, J. F., and Uttling, J. E. *General Anesthesia,* 4th ed. Boston: Butterworths, 1980.

Gruendemann, B. J., Casterton, S. B., Hesterly, S. C., Minckley, B. B., and Shetler, M. G. *The Surgical Patient,* 2nd ed. St. Louis: C. V. Mosby, 1977.

Handbook of Compressed Gases. New York: Compressed Gas Association. [n.d.]

Harris, F. W. *Desiccation as a Key to Understanding Electrosurgery.* Boulder: Valleylab, 1978.

Hazardous Chemical Data (NFPA 4A). Boston: National Fire Protection Association, 1975.

Hospital Safety Compliance Guide. Chicago: Inter Qual, 1977.

Keys, T. *The History of Surgical Anesthesia.* New York: Dover Publications, 1963.

Lichtiger, M., and Moya, F. *Introduction to the Practice of Anesthesia,* 2nd ed. New York: Harper and Row, 1978.

Life Safety Code (NFPA 101). Boston: National Fire Protection Association, 1973.

Manual of Hazardous Chemical Reaction (NFPA 491M). Boston: National Fire Protection Association, 1975.

Miller, R. D., ed. *Anesthesia,* 2 vols. New York: Churchill-Livingstone, 1981.

"Radiation protection." *Radiologic Technology* 51:525, 1980.

"Radiation protection." *Radiologic Technology,* 52:321, 1980.

Rhodes, M. J., Gruendemann, B. J., and Ballinger, W. F. *Alexander's Care of the Patient in Surgery,* 6th ed. St. Louis: C. V. Mosby, 1978.

Safer Electrosurgery. Dayton, Ohio: NDM Corp., 1981.

Specialty Gases: Safety Precautions and Emergency Procedures. New York: Union Carbide Corporation, 1976.

Tuck, C. A., Jr., ed. *NFPA Inspection Manual,* 4th ed. Boston: National Fire Protection Association, 1976.

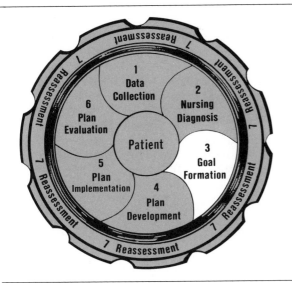

GOAL: Skin does not show adverse effects from surgery.

Maintenance of Skin Integrity

A major focus in the perioperative care plan is the surgical patient's skin. This chapter deals with maintaining the patient's skin integrity, or wholeness. Normal anatomy, preoperative skin preparation, wounds, and the wound repair process are discussed.

Since the goal being considered focuses on skin wholeness, the following criteria are indicators of satisfactory achievement:

1. During the postoperative course, the nurse will observe the patient's surgical incision. The incision will:
   Evidence only minimal signs of inflammation
   Be covered by a dry crust formation
   Not exhibit signs of epithelial growth down skin suture tracts
   Have the edges approximated
   Not be associated with excessive pain (determined by objective nursing judgment and subjective patient response)
2. Postoperatively, the nurse will observe no burns, lacerations, abrasions, contusions, or reddened areas that were not present prior to surgery.
3. Postoperatively, the patient will not exhibit unanticipated sensory impairment.

Certain factors influence how well the criteria are met. The maintenance of skin integrity is influenced by the preoperative condition of the integumentary system, preparation of the skin for the surgical procedure, and the patient's wound-healing capacity.

Anatomy and Physiology

To plan perioperative care effectively, the nurse must have an understanding of the integumentary (skin) system. Human skin is composed of three layers: subcutaneous tissue, the deepest layer; the dermis, or middle layer; and the epidermis, or outer layer. Each layer has specific components and functions, but all work together to form a protective covering for other body systems. The integument makes up about 15 percent of total body weight. It has three functions:

1. Protecting the inner body from injury
2. Preventing fluid from escaping from within and external fluid from entering
3. Enabling the person to communicate with and respond to the environment

SKIN LAYERS

Subcutaneous Tissue
This inner-most layer is the area for fat formation, metabolism, and storage. It is the supporting layer for blood vessels and nerves. Hair follicles and sweat glands originate here. Subcutaneous tissues serve as an insulating layer for the internal body structures.

Dermis
The dermis, sometimes called corium, is composed of connective tissue and cellular and ground substance. This layer supports the epidermis and separates it from the fatty subcutaneous tissue.

Connective tissue contains collagen and elastic fibers that contribute to support and elasticity of the skin. Collagen fibers are responsible for 25 percent of human protein mass. These fibers are composed of thin fibrils held together by cementing ground substance composed of cross-linked, overlapping units of tropocollagen molecules. Elastic fibers, also composed of pro-

tein, are thinner than collagen but entwined among it.

Three types of cells in the dermis are: fibroblasts, which form connective tissue, including collagen; macrophages, which clean up bacteria, debris, and particulate matter; and leukocytes, which increase in number during inflammatory processes.

The ground substance of the dermis is a gelatinous matrix that contains proteins, enzymes, and immune bodies. This cements the collagen and elastic fibers.

Epidermis
This outer covering is composed of five layers (see Fig. 12.1). This tough surface enveloping the body is the human's point of contact with the outer world. Its entire thickness averages 1 mm, or the width of a sharp pencil mark.

The basal layer of the epidermis contains cells called keratinocytes that produce other cells in the epidermis. The prickle cell (malpighian) layer is composed of a network of cytoplasmic threads or intercellular bridges. In exceptional circumstances, these cells may contain glycogen in preparation for rapid proliferation during the wound repair process. Granular layer cells contain protein granules and are flatter than the cells previously mentioned.

The lucid layer is a translucent layer of flat cells that occurs only on the palms of the hands and soles of the feet. The granular and

Figure 12.1. The five layers of the epidermis.

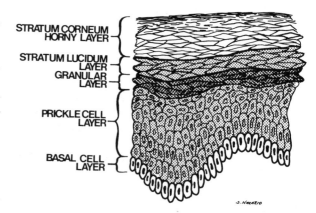

lucid layers act as a barrier to outward water loss and inward transfer of noxious substances. The outer horny layer is composed of dead keratinized cells that are constantly shed. The protein in these cells is capable of absorbing vast amounts of water, as is seen when feet and hands become white and swollen after submersion in water for an extended time.

VASCULAR AND NERVE SUPPLY

A continuous arteriovenous network traverses subcutaneous tissue and extends into the dermis. This network regulates heat and maintains nutrition for skin cells. After an injury, new capillaries quickly form to bring nutrients to the wound repair area.

Nerves that run through the subcutaneous tissue are divided into sensory and motor nerves. Sensory nerves mediate the sensations of touch, temperature, and pain. Motor nerves control sweat glands, arterioles, and smooth muscle.

Itching and goose flesh are two interesting phenomena involving the integumentary nervous supply. Itching is a mild, painful sensation but differs from frank pain by having a lower impulse frequency that travels along the nerve fiber. Goose flesh is due to traction of the muscle (arrector pili) attached to the hair follicle.

APPENDAGES

Skin appendages are of two types, cornified and glandular (see Fig. 12.2). These are further separated into more specific groups. Cornified appendages take the form of hair and nails, both of which are keratinized structures. Hair arises from follicles, which are an invagination of the epidermis. An individual's life-long complement of hair follicles is present at birth. No new follicles will be formed during the life time. Hair growth is cyclic, with the anagen (growing) phase or telogen (resting) state being influenced by hormones. This hormonal influence is the most important internal factor in hair growth. A premature resting stage may be caused by stress such as massive illness or childbirth.

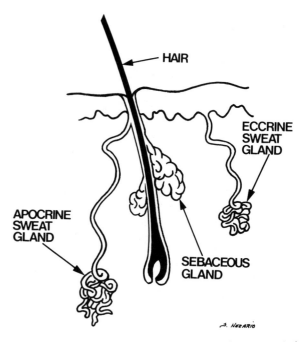

Figure 12.2. *The two types of skin appendages, cornified and glandular.*

With each scalp hair growing approximately 0.35 mm per day, over 100 linear feet of hair is produced daily. Excess male hormone produces baldness; castrated males do not lose their hair.

Nails are also cornified appendages. These are produced by an invagination of the epidermis. Their growth is continuous, although fingernails grow more rapidly than toenails. They protect the tips of fingers and toes, which have a delicate sense of touch.

The other type of skin appendage is glandular. There are two major types of glands—sebaceous and sweat. Sebaceous glands are present everywhere except on the palms of the hands and soles of the feet. They continuously secrete the products of cell breakdown and produce sebum, a thin lipidal film that covers the skin. Sebum is mildly bacteriostatic and fungistatic. It also retards water evaporation.

Sweat glands are divided into two categories —eccrine and apocrine. Eccrine glands, opening directly onto the skin surface, are controlled by the autonomic nervous system and flood the exterior skin with water for cooling purposes. Eccrine glands are a major factor in maintaining a stable temperature inside the body. Their prime stimulus for function is heat.

Apocrine glands are located in the pubic and axillary areas. The sweat produced in these areas is sterile until it is contaminated by bacteria. It then decomposes, producing body odor. These adrenergic glands are activated by emotional stimulation.

FLORA

Healthy skin is host to innumerable bacteria. Normally, these bacteria and the human organisms coexist peacefully. Normal skin bacteria—*Staphylococcus epidermidis*, *Corynebacteria*, and *Candida*—are especially concentrated in hair follicles and moist areas such as the axilla, groin, and perineum. Their populations remain fairly constant on an individual unless disturbed by such factors as climate changes or antibiotics. People with oily, moist skin harbor more bacteria than those with dry skin. Drying is the principal method by which the skin prevents overpopulation of bacteria.

There are two types of bacteria on the skin—transient and resident. Resident bacteria live and multiply on the skin. These bacteria are shed from the body with the movement of old cells and skin secretions from the dermal to the epidermal layer. In this manner they serve as a source of contamination for any break in the skin. Resident bacteria need 6–10 minutes of soap and water scrubbing to decrease their population by 50 percent. Bacterial regrowth begins immediately, and in 24 hours, 25 percent will be replaced. Transient bacteria are loosely attached to the skin surface. They are effectively reduced by a 3–5-minute scrub.

When planning for maintenance of skin integrity, the perioperative nurse continues the assessment that began with the surgical patient's admission. The primary nurse has assessed the overall health status and specific condition of the patient's skin. He has considered factors that differ from normal skin and incorporated these into the plan of care (see Table 12.1). The perioperative nurse's responsibility is to continue that assessment and plan intraoperative interventions based on it.

Preoperative Skin Preparation

Inherent in the goal of maintaining skin integrity is rapid, uncomplicated wound repair. To achieve that goal, a nurse's activities will be based on the "minimal interference concept." Aimed at removing all interference to wound repair, this concept means preventing contamination and minimizing tissue trauma. Damage to tissues is minimized by gentle handling of wound contents during the surgical procedure. Manipulation of tissues is reduced to the minimum necessary to complete the surgical procedure. One of the criteria for maintenance of skin integrity is, "Postoperatively there will be no burns, lacerations, abrasions, contusions, or reddened areas that were not present prior to surgery." Presence of any of these increases the body's healing effort for the surgical wound.

Preventing contamination begins with the patient prior to the surgical procedure. To prevent contamination, the preoperative hospital stay is as short as possible to prevent unnecessary exposure to bacteria in the environment. The preoperative skin preparation is aimed at making the skin as clean and germ-free as possible.

SURGICALLY CLEAN SKIN

Preparation of the surgical patient's skin begins before his admission to the surgical suite. The evening before the operation, the patient will be asked to shower using an antiseptic or hexachlorophene-based soap. Depending on the procedure, the patient may be asked to repeat the shower procedure the morning of the surgery. He will be asked to pay particular attention to scrubbing the operative site. For example, joint replacements require careful skin preparation because of the potential for infection.

Although some institutions may do a preoperative shave the night before surgery, it is preferable to remove hair, if necessary, in the holding area immediately prior to surgery. Preoperative shaving the night before surgery has been associated with increased wound infection. According to Seropian and Reynolds (1), a standard shave done 24 hours prior to

Table 12.1. Factors That Influence Preoperative Skin Preparation.

Areas of Assessment	Influencing Factors	Considerations
Overall health status		
Age	pediatric patient geriatric patient	Most pediatric patients will not be shaved. Skin may be dry and lack resiliency.
Nutritional status	malnourished, obese, hypovolemic	Skin texture and tone may be altered.
Allergy history	possible sensitivity to soaps and antimicrobial solutions	Select a solution that will not produce a skin reaction.
State of consciousness	degree of alertness	Positioning may be difficult and require extra personnel for the semiconscious or unconscious patient.
Medical condition	diabetes (for example)	Diminished circulation to extremities, impaired healing ability. Extra caution exercised during shave.
Previous surgeries	presence of scars, degree of keloid formation	Scars and keloids are fragile tissue and must be avoided when shaving.
Limitation of motion	arthritis, contractures, etc.	Attention given to comfortable positioning.
Condition of skin		
Color	palor, cyanosis, jaundice, pigmentation changes	These features of skin may not have individual considerations but should all be noted by the person doing the skin preparation. Any unusual skin changes such as obvious lesions or evidence of bleeding which become obvious only after the hair has been removed should be reported upon completion of the prep.
Vascularity	evidence of bleeding or bruising	
Obvious lesions	allergy reactions, acne, psoriasis	
Edema	injury or underlying medical procedures	
Moisture	dry or sweaty	
Temperature	warm, hot, cool—bilaterally	
Texture	rough or smooth	
Thickness	paper thin, fragile, or thick	
Mobility	decreased due to edema	
Turgor	decreased due to dehydration	
Examples of surgical disease		
Carotid artery disease	plaque in the artery	Gentle scrub and shave to avoid dislodging the plaque.
Breast biopsy	possible breast carcinoma	Gentle scrub because of possible spread of carcinoma. Axilla and upper arm will be shaved.
Fractures	unstable or open	May be prepped following induction of anesthesia. Attention directed to maintaining alignment of fracture. This will require additional personnel.
Skin lesions	raised areas on skin surface, i.e., melanomas, basal cell carcinomas, or lesions erupting through skin	Location of lesion noted prior to beginning prep so that the razor will not inadvertently traumatize these areas. Hair on these areas should be closely trimmed with scissors.
Preps following cast removal	buildup of desquamation skin and scab-like patches adhering to skin	The skin will be very sensitive, requiring time to gently soak away any adherent patches.

surgery has an infection rate of 20 percent; when the shave is done just prior to surgery, it is 3.1 percent. With a depilatory, the infection rate is 0.6 percent. Cruse (2) showed that when hair is not removed, the infection rate is 0.9 percent; when hair is clipped, it is 1.7 percent; and with the standard shave less than 24 hours before surgery, it is 2.3 percent. Shaving destroys the natural skin defenses and also can create superficial cuts and nicks that encourage bacterial growth. The longer the period between the shave and the surgery, the greater the potential for bacterial growth.

Hair removal should be done only when

necessary. Facial hair from women and children should never be removed. The method that is least damaging to skin is recommended—use of a depilatory if the patient is not allergic to such agents. Hair can also be clipped about 1 cm from the skin with electrical clippers. If hair must be shaved, a wet method should be used, and the razor should be disposable or a terminally sterilized reusable one. Several points should be kept in mind when removing hair:

1. Hair removal should be done as closely as possible to the time of surgery to decrease the possibility of wound infection.
2. The patient's privacy should be respected at all times.
3. Skilled personnel should be responsible for hair removal.

Under optimal circumstances all hair is removed with a depilatory, preps are done immediately prior to surgery in a holding area adjacent to the surgical suite, and patient privacy is provided.

Wound Healing

The wound repair process begins the moment an injury occurs, and may go on for years. This is true regardless of the type of wound. The injuries may be made with a planned incision during a surgical procedure, or the damage may occur due to some type of skin-tearing trauma.

There are two types of wounds — those with no tissue loss and those with tissue loss. Incised or sutured wounds with no tissue loss heal by primary union or first intention. The edges of the wound are approximated rapidly with no complications. Contamination is minimized by good aseptic technique and lack of dead space. Wounds with tissue loss, such as traumatic injuries and burns, heal by secondary intention. The wound may be infected or there may have been excessive loss of tissue, and the skin edges cannot be adequately approximated. There may be infection or necrosis, and the wound is left open to heal from the inside toward the outer surface by granulation.

Some body tissues are capable of regeneration. This occurs in "like" cells, such as in an injury involving exclusively epithelial cells. Most injuries involve more than one layer of tissue. Wounds in these tissues heal by scar formation. This is the most common repair process. It involves fibroplasia, contraction, and scarring.

Wounds heal in three phases. These phases overlap and may extend for many years after the injury or incision. The first phase is a *defensive* phase that lasts one to four days. Also known as the *inflammatory* or *exudative* phase, it begins the moment the surgical incision is made or the moment a traumatic injury occurs. The immediate response is vascular, with vasoconstriction and clot formation to control hemorrhage. Vasoconstriction lasts 5–10 minutes and is followed by dilation of the vennules. Blood fills the area, and clots form a matrix of fibrin that provides a framework for repair. The surface scab that forms maintains hemostasis and provides protection from contamination.

For approximately three days, a substantial amount of fluid containing plasma proteins, water, and electrolytes leaks into the tissues surrounding the injury. As the fluid enters the region, cells become sticky and trap large amounts of interstitial fluid. Therefore, the area becomes edematous and warm to the touch.

Leukocytes are the first cells to arrive at the injured area. They squeeze through a vessel wall by a process called *diapedesis*. Macrophages also move to the site and digest and mobilize debris from the injury.

Several hours after the damage, basal cells are activated and begin migration down below the clot that seals the wound. The cells migrate from both sides of the wound and meet within 24 to 48 hours. When both sides meet, cell mitosis begins. Epithelial cells can also migrate down into suture tracts to form so-called stitch abscesses. These are not really abscesses but rather a localized inflammatory reaction.

Fibroblasts begin to multiply 24–36 hours after the injury. They move randomly into the wound as the inflammatory process subsides.

New capillaries quickly form to provide nutritional substances to newly developing cells.

The second, or *fibroblastic*, phase, also known as the *proliferative* or *reconstructive* phase, begins approximately the 5th postoperative day and continues to day 20. This phase overlaps the earlier inflammatory stage and will likewise overlap into the later maturing phase of wound repair.

Fibroblasts synthesize collagens, glycoproteins, and mucopolysaccharides. Collagen molecules form into fibers that crisscross into large bundles and give strength to the new connective tissue. New capillaries are also formed to provide nutrients to the growing, emerging cells. As more collagen is deposited, capillaries begin to disappear. At the end of this phase, the collagen synthesis and destruction will balance itself. These new connective tissue fibers are associated with the breaking strength of the wound. By the time skin sutures are removed, the wound has approximately 5 percent of its original skin strength. In one month, the wound has regained 35–50 percent of its original strength. It will never achieve more than 70–80 percent of its preinjury skin strength. The wound reaches this maximum strength in approximately three months.

During the third and final *maturation* phase, the size and shape of the scar undergo slow, progressive change. This phase may last a number of months or years. Open wounds decrease in size by contraction, caused by inward movement of fibroblastic cells.

PREOPERATIVE FACTORS
THAT INFLUENCE WOUND HEALING

When the perioperative nurse is doing the assessment, he identifies data pertinent to the patient's total surgical experience. Postoperatively, the incision site and healing process are major concerns. During the preoperative interview, the nurse makes observations and asks questions that relate directly to the patient's ability to respond physiologically to the trauma of the incision.

The nutritional status of the patient is a major factor in wound healing. In response to stress and injury, the basal metabolic rate markedly increases. Protein is essential for collagen formation. In complex wounds, there is increased protein waste. Cortisol levels increase, and blood glucose may rise, leading to increased glucose accumulation in cells. This produces an environment conducive to bacterial growth. Vitamin C assists in collagen synthesis and capillary formation. In the aged patient and the patient who smokes, vitamin C levels are lower. Vitamin A encourages formation of granulation tissue in healing skin incisions. It also seems to have an opposing effect on cortisol during the wound-healing process.

Specific groups of patients have more nutritional problems than the average person. Since the surgical procedure or trauma increases the basal metabolic rate of the body, these patients require careful, preoperative nutritional assessment. Frequently the aged patient is in poor nutritional state and hence exhibits retarded wound healing. Diabetics, obese patients, and those with disease processes requiring irradiation exhibit unique nutritional needs, and therefore increased healing time. Electrolytes, enzymes, antibodies, and vitamins are important in wound healing. Known deficiencies should be identified preoperatively and corrected if possible. Surgery may be delayed while patients receive nutritional support. Enteral nutrition is preferred, but some patients may need total parenteral nutrition to overcome nutritional deficits.

The patient's weight may be a factor. Obese patients are candidates for wound-healing problems. Systemic diseases associated with obesity such as cardiovascular disease, hypertension, respiratory disease, and diabetes increase the risk of wound complications. In obese patients, impaired circulation and respiration result in less blood flow and oxygen at the wound area, both important to wound healing. Potential wound complications are infection, incisional hernias, wound dehiscence, and seroma formation. The risk of infection is increased by the longer operating time and trauma to tissue from retraction. Adipose tissue, which is relatively avascular, has less ability to resist infection. Incisional hernias may be caused by increased strain on the incision. Wound dehiscence, often associated with infection, is a common complication. The surgeon may not be able to close the wound so that it will maintain its integrity. In obese patients, there is a greater potential for dead space, which can lead to formation of seromas.

Some disease processes, such as cancer and diabetes, are a concern to the nurse during the preoperative assessment. In the diabetic patient, wound healing is delayed, and wound infections are more severe and prolonged. Assessment should include the patient's current therapeutic regimen and how well the disease is controlled. Medical history is important, including the age of onset. Obesity is also common among diabetics. The cancer patient may be malnourished and generally debilitated. His wound-healing ability may also be affected by therapeutic regimens. If the cancer patient has received radiation, skin in the irradiated area may be fragile and sensitive. The amount of radiation the patient has received, his response to it, and his overall health should be included in the assessment since they are indicators of postoperative wound healing. Both cancer patients and diabetics may be immunosuppressed, also a factor in wound healing. Other patients who are immunosuppressed include those with congenital, acquired, or age-related deficiencies. Malnourished patients as well as those with uremic disease also have impaired immune response. Immunosuppressive drugs include steroids, anti-inflammatory agents, and cytoxic drugs.

The data on skin integrity obtained by the nurse is communicated by the patient care plan or patient record to other members of the health care team so that any treatment that might counteract potential complications in wound healing can be instituted preoperatively.

INTRAOPERATIVE FACTORS THAT INFLUENCE WOUND HEALING

Wound healing and the potential for infection are affected by intraoperative events. The perioperative nurse is primarily concerned with maintaining environmental asepsis during this period to prevent exogenous contamination of the wound. He assures the sterility of the instruments and supplies, and is responsible for the skin preparation of the patient. To minimize the potential transfer of contamination from OR personnel to the patient, he ensures that all members of the team are properly gowned, gloved, and masked. He observes any breaks in technique and takes corrective action.

The surgeon is responsible for the surgical technique, which influences wound healing. Good surgical technique leads to good wound healing. In some procedures, antibiotics are used prophylactically before surgery and during surgery in wound irrigation. A sharp, clean incision heals better than one with ragged edges. An electrosurgical knife damages the wound edge and increases the risk of infection. Other factors that affect wound healing are the length of time the wound is open, the handling of tissue, pressure from retractors and other instruments, and hemostasis. Dead space or poor drainage, which permit pooling of fluids, creates a potential for contamination.

The type of suture, needle, and stitch used have a bearing on wound healing and susceptibility to infection. Sutures are foreign bodies that the body reacts to. In a study on sutures and wound infection, Sharp and colleagues reported that "synthetic monofilament sutures were far superior to any of the braided sutures, and the synthetic sutures were better than the natural sutures" (3:62). They recommend that natural sutures not be used for wounds with potential for infection. Sixteen types of suture were tested for their resistance to both Gram-positive and Gram-negative infections. The diameter of the suture material should be as small as possible. The least amount of suture with the least tension is the best. Staples, now used extensively in surgery, are essentially nonreactive and minimize infection. The B-shape of the staple does not crush the skin, and nutrients can pass through the staple line to the edge of the incision, reducing necrosis and promoting wound healing. Because the staples are inserted with mechanical devices, tissue handling and operating time are reduced.

The swaged or eyeless needle minimizes tissue damage and is now more commonly used than eyed needles. The suture is swaged to the needle by mechanical pressure and only a single strand of suture is drawn through the tissue, causing less tissue damage and leakage of fluid. The interrupted suture stitch is the most widely used and most efficient. Fewer stitches are used, and the skin edges are inverted or everted, promoting wound healing. The fewer the stitches, the less foreign body in the wound to cause a reaction.

POSTOPERATIVE FACTORS THAT INFLUENCE WOUND HEALING

Healing is strongly influenced by nursing interventions throughout each phase of the wound repair process. During the initial inflammatory phase, observations of the wound, dressing, and surrounding tissue can detect hematoma formation or frank hemorrhage. Drain sites demand the same careful observation as the suture line. Flawless sterile technique must be used to guard against bacterial contamination. Inspection of drainage devices to assure proper function will facilitate correct calculation of the patient's intake and output. The area surrounding pressure dressings must be checked for adequate circulation. Edema of surrounding tissues can lead to increased pain. Elevation of an injured or incised limb above the level of the heart will ease drainage and decrease edema.

Control of circulating fluids is critical for oxygenation of the wounded tissues. Oxygen tension of greater than 15 mm Hg at the wound edges is required for collagen formation. Adequate respiratory movement allows for proper oxygenation of tissues during the healing process. Deep breathing, sighing, yawning, and use of an incentive spirometer increase oxygen exchange as well as stimulate secretory movement from the lungs.

Abdominal stress can seriously affect proper wound healing. Vomiting, the Valsalva maneuver, and deep coughing can produce intra-abdominal pressures up to 150 ml water. Contrast this to 29 ml for getting out of bed and 18 ml while walking. Muscles and the wound are stretched, inhibiting network for-mation and endothelial and fibroblastic migration necessary for wound healing. Deep coughing can be contraindicated since it can raise intrathoracic pressure to 300 mm Hg. Excessive coughing can occasionally cause abdominal wound or muscle disruption.

Although nasogastric (NG) tubes are used to prevent abdominal distention, they can also cause it, since the presence of the NG tube in the throat causes many patients to swallow excessively and take in large amounts of air. Also, channels may form along the tube through which secretions flow and bypass the suction ports. Turning the patient helps collapse these channels and aids maximum, efficient function of the NG tube. A distended bladder also causes muscles to stretch beyond normal capacity and contributes to retarded wound healing.

PAIN CONTROL, REST, AND SLEEP

Pain can affect wound healing. In the postoperative period, pain can lead to vital sign changes. The heart rate increases, and blood pressure exhibits instability. Pain medication can effectively return these hemodynamic changes to their normal limits, thus delivering required oxygen to the wound site for healing.

Pain also produces changes in metabolic activity. As metabolism increases, cortisol is produced and in turn retards wound healing. Patients experiencing pain have a poor appetite and diminished food intake, creating an extra drain on the already compromised nutritional state.

As an adjunct to medication, relaxation can be taught preoperatively to enable the patient to participate in pain control.

Rest and sleep are important factors in wound healing. Since the greatest amount of growth hormone is released during sleep, special times of rest should be included in the care plan. Growth hormone influences protein synthesis, which again influences wound healing by collagen production. Explanations to the patient and visitors about the importance of rest may be necessary to promote maximum wound repair.

WOUND COVERING

Wounds are covered for two reasons: immobility and protection. If no dressing is used, the dermis at the edges of the incision dehydrate and become part of the crust covering that forms a barrier to epithelialization.

Although the wound is sealed with fibrin within several hours after the incision is closed, a wound covering or dressing of three layers is generally used: a contact layer of nonstick material that will not adhere to the wound; a middle layer, usually gauze to absorb drainage; and an outer layer to protect the wound. The absorbent gauze layer will collect fibrin, blood products, and debris. If the contact layer is made of gauze that adheres to the wound, the reparative process can be disrupted when the dressing is removed.

Sometimes the skin incision is covered with a vapor and gas-permeable transparent covering that acts as a second skin. These semipermeable dressings allow oxygen to communicate with the wound and promote faster regeneration of epithelial cells. If an occlusive dressing is used, it maintains a moist environment that hastens epithelialization. The major disadvantage is the culture medium for bacteria that is formed by wound exudate trapped in the dressing.

Nursing responsibilities for wound healing include observation and protection of the dressing from contamination (e.g., urine, feces, bath water) and dressing changes necessary to meet wound needs.

COMPLICATIONS

Even with meticulous nursing and medical care, wounds in the repair process are subject to complications. Keloids, fistulas, adhesions, hematomas, infections, and wound disruptions may complicate healing.

Keloid formation is a hypertrophic scar that results when collagen synthesis exceeds destruction. Fibrous tissue varying in color from white to red extends above the skin surface. This type of scar is treated by injection with corticosteroids or surgical excision. In either case, the keloid tissue tends to recur. It is more common in blacks and dark-skinned Caucasians.

Fistulas may develop during the fibroblastic phase of healing. A tract develops between two epithelium-lined surfaces allowing drainage that is not expected from a particular organ. Patients having surgery of the head and neck, bowel, or genitourinary system are candidates for fistula formation. Some small fistulas may heal spontaneously but most require surgical intervention.

Wound disruption or dehiscence occurs on approximately the fifth day. Fifty percent of patients with dehiscence will exhibit serosanguineous drainage. Total dehiscence leads to evisceration, in which wound contents protrude. If this occurs, the area should be covered with saline dressings and a sterile towel, and the surgeon should be contacted immediately.

Incisional hernias most often occur in patients with abdominal surgery and complicated postoperative courses. Patients exhibit peristalsis under the skin and abdominal protrusion when standing but not while lying down. Incisional hernias can lead to bowel obstruction and must be surgically corrected.

Hematoma formation can occur in the immediate postoperative course, or it may not be evident until days after the surgical procedure. Immediate formation is evidenced by unexpected blood on the dressing and vital sign changes. This may be caused by a vessel not ligated or a slipped ligature. These patients are returned to the operating room for surgical correction of the problem.

If the hematoma does not become evident until the wound is in the fibroblastic stage, a small vessel may be slowly leaking blood into the wound space. Evidence of this type of hematoma is generally dehiscence with old, dark-red blood being discharged. On occasion, the surgeon will tie the vessel and pack the wound, thus allowing for healing by secondary intention.

Adhesion formation is a problem during the final phase of healing. Two surfaces in the operative area will adhere to one another. For example, loops of bowel may bind together causing pain, dysfunction, and gangrene, necessitating surgical intervention.

This chapter explores the goal of maintenance of the patient's skin integrity. Criteria to achieve that goal and factors affecting that achievement are given. Anatomy of the integumentary system is reviewed, and preoperative skin preparation is considered. Nursing observations related to the minimal interference concept, oxygenation, and nutrition of the wound are examined. Physiology of wound healing and nursing interventions influencing the repair process are discussed.

References

1. Seropian, R., and Reynolds, B. M. "Wound infections after preoperative depilatory versus razor preparation." *Am Surg* 121:251, 1971.
2. Cruse, P., and Foord, R. "A five-year study of 23,649 surgical wounds." *Arch Surg* 107(August): 206–210, 1973.
3. Sharp, W. V., Belden, T. A., King, P. H., and Teague, P. C. "Suture resistance to infection." *Surgery* 91(January):61–63, 1982.

Suggested Readings

Association of Operating Room Nurses, "Standards for preoperative skin preparation of patients." In *AORN Standards of Practice*. Denver: AORN, 1978.

Bernard, L. A. "Wound healing." *AORN J* 35(May): 1067, 1982.

Besset, J. A., and Wallace, H. L. "Wound healing: Intraoperative factors." *Nurs Clin North Am* 14(December):701–712, 1979.

Brooks, S. M. *Fundamentals of Operating Room Nursing*, 2nd ed. St. Louis: C. V. Mosby, 1979.

Bruno, P. "The nature of wound healing." *Nurs Clin North Am* 14(December):667–682, 1979.

Cooper, D. M., and Schumann, D. "Post surgical nursing intervention as an adjunct to wound healing." *Nurs Clin North Am* 14(December): 713–726, 1979.

Finn, K. "Wound healing." *Crit Care Update* 7(April): 14–16, 18, 1980.

Frogge, M. H. "Promoting wound healing in the irradiated patient." *AORN J* 35(May):1088–1093, 1982.

Groszek, D. M. "Wound healing in the obese patient." *AORN J* 35(May):1132–1138, 1982.

Hannigan, L. "Nursing assessment of the integumentary system." *Occup Health Nurs* 26:19–22, 1978.

Harris, D. R. "Healing of the surgical wound: II. Factors influencing repair and regeneration." *J Am Acad Dermatol* I(September):208–215, 1979.

Keithley, J. K. "Wound healing in malnourished patients." *AORN J* 35(May):1094–1099, 1982.

Kottra, C. J. "Wound healing in the immunosuppressed host." *AORN J* 35(May):1142–1148, 1982.

Luckmann, J., and Sorensen, K. C. *Medical-Surgical Nursing*, 2nd ed. Philadelphia: W. B. Saunders, 1980.

Montagna, W., and Parakkal, P. F. *The Structure and Function of Skin*, 3rd ed. New York: Academic Press, 1974.

Pillsbury, D. M., and Heaton, C. L. *A Manual of Dermatology*, 2nd ed. Philadelphia: W. B. Saunders, 1980.

Pinkus, H., and Mehregan, A. H. *A Guide to Dermatohistopathology*, 3rd ed. New York: Appleton-Century-Crofts, 1981.

Sauer, G. C. *Manual of Skin Diseases*, 4th ed. Philadelphia: J. B. Lippincott, 1980.

Schumann, D. "Preoperative measures to promote wound healing." *Nurs Clin North Am* 14(December):683–689, 1979.

Schumann, D. "The nature of wound healing." *AORN J* 35(May):1068–1077, 1982.

Winters, B. "Promoting wound healing in the diabetic patient." *AORN J* 35(May):1083–1087, 1982.

Yordan, E. L., Jr., and Bernhard, L. A. "The surgeon's role in wound healing." *AORN J* 35 (May):1078–1082, 1982.

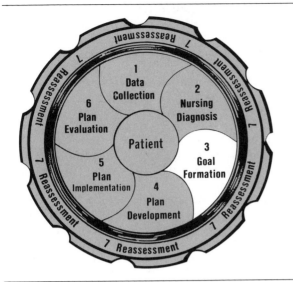

GOAL: *No evidence of infection related to surgery.*

Absence of Infection

Infection is usually defined as the presence or growth of pathogenic microorganisms (pathogens) in body tissues or fluids accompanied by a clinically adverse effect either locally or systemically in the patient. Infection can be distinguished from colonization, which is the persistence of microorganisms on skin or in body fluids or tissues, but without a clinically adverse effect. Therefore, nurses need to know the clinical signs and symptoms of infections and be able to interpret the results of laboratory tests conducted on cultures of body tissues or fluids to detect the presence of infecting microorganisms.

The perioperative nurse is very conscious of the fact that all patients having surgery have the potential of acquiring an infection. The goal established for patients is that they will be free from infection postoperatively.

The clinical signs and symptoms of infection differ according to the site of infection; nevertheless, heat, pain, swelling, and redness occur with most infections. The heat associated with infection may occur either locally at the site of infection or systemically as fever; the pain associated with infection may vary in degree from mild tenderness to severe distress. In addition, the presence of purulent discharge strongly suggests an infection; the purulence may appear as pus in wound drainage, as pyuria (pus in urine), or as purulent sputum.

The isolation of one or more microorganisms from a properly collected and processed culture of body tissues which appear to be clinically infected usually confirms the presence of an infection and the identification of the infecting microorganism(s). Indirect evidence of infection such as serologic or biochemical results from laboratory tests and radiologic evidence such as infiltrates on chest x-rays can be useful in diagnosing an infection but cannot be used alone in the absence of clinical or microbiological data.

Factors influencing goal attainment relate specifically to sources of infecting microorganisms, the process of infection, and activities the nurse engages in to prevent infection. Activities that the nurse performs to produce a controlled aseptic environment protect the patient from infection. The sterilization of instruments and equipment and the packaging of supplies and their storage in a safe, clean environment are essential to reduce the incidence of infection related to the patient's stay in the operating room.

Sources of Infecting Microorganisms

Various microorganisms are capable of causing infections. Those capable of causing infections in healthy persons are commonly referred to as *pathogens*. Less pathogenic microorganisms, often referred to as opportunistic pathogens, are capable of causing disease in persons whose defense mechanisms may be deficient or compromised. Commensals, microorganisms which normally inhabit skin, mucous membranes, and the gastrointestinal tract, are also frequent opportunists in some perioperative patients. Saprophytes, microorganisms abundant in the environment where they are ordinarily of little concern, may cause infections in perioperative patients whose defense mechanisms are deficient or compromised.

Microorganisms capable of causing infections can arise from endogenous or exogenous sources. *Endogenous* sources of infections come from the patient's own microbiological flora (the "normal flora" of the skin, nose, pharynx,

and gastrointestinal tract). For example, peritonitis in a patient after a ruptured appendix spills bowel contents into the peritoneal cavity is due to endogenous microorganisms and is therefore referred to as an endogenous infection. On admission to the hospital, the patient's microbiological flora may become altered, particularly in the pharynx and gastrointestinal tract, by acquiring "hospital strains," especially Gram-negative bacilli. Infections may arise from these newly acquired flora. Such hospital strains are often involved in aspiration pneumonia.

Exogenous sources of infection, on the other hand, are those that arise from outside the patient, such as infected or colonized patients and hospital personnel, or inanimate objects in the hospital. For example, epidemics of *Staphylococcus aureus* and Group A *Streptococcus* wound infections usually arise from exogenous microorganisms acquired through person-to-person contact with infected or colonized members of the surgical team. In contrast, the source of *Pseudomonas cepacia* blood stream infections is usually contaminated intravenous preparations or patient care objects used intravascularly during the perioperative period.

The Chain of Infection

Microorganisms are ubiquitous. Nevertheless, infection will not occur unless the essential components for infection are present and in interaction or a chain of events occurs among the components. Three components are essential for infection: an infectious agent, a susceptible host, and a means of transmission (see Fig. 13.1). These components are analogous to links in a chain. For an infection to occur, the following must be present: (1) an adequate number of pathogenic microorganisms (an infectious agent), (2) an individual who is susceptible to infection (a susceptible host), and (3) a means for the infectious agent to have appropriate contact (a means of transmission) with the susceptible host. When these conditions are met, the chain of infection is completed and infection occurs.

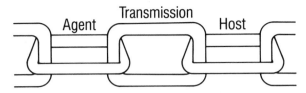

Figure 13.1. Chain of infection.

INFECTIOUS AGENTS

The first link in the chain of infection is the infectious agent. Infectious agents can be bacteria, fungi, parasites, or viruses. Bacteria, however, are the most common microorganisms isolated in culture from infections in hospitals. Bacteria are identified in the laboratory by various characteristics including their staining reactions and their requirement for oxygen for growth. One of the most important and widely used differential staining techniques for bacteria is the Gram stain. This stain rapidly identifies bacteria as Gram-positive or Gram-negative and shows their size and shape when viewed under a microscope.

Bacteria can also be classified according to whether they will grow in the presence or absence of oxygen. Aerobic bacteria grow in the presence of oxygen (i.e., on the skin), whereas anaerobic bacteria grow in the absence of oxygen, a condition that can occur in some deep body organs or tissues. Bacteria commonly isolated in culture from infections in the hospital are grouped according to their oxygen requirements, Gram stain, and shape in Table 13.1.

SUSCEPTIBLE HOST

The second link in the chain of infection is the susceptible host. Host susceptibility is determined by various factors such as age, immune status, and type of underlying disease. For example, the extremes of life—infancy and old age—are associated with decreased resistance to infection. Likewise, patients with chronic diseases such as certain types of cancer and kidney disease, diabetes mellitus, leukemia, or lymphoma may be more susceptible to infection

than other patients. Additionally, factors such as nutritional status and lowered local resistance are important contributors to infection in perioperative patients. For example, an incision in the skin interrupts the anatomical barrier to infectious agents, allowing them to penetrate. Moreover, anesthesia interrupts the cough and sneeze reflex and compromises other normal defenses of the respiratory tract such as the mucous cells and cilia that tend to repel invading infectious agents.

Host susceptibility also depends on the effects of diagnostic and therapeutic procedures such as biopsy or surgery and treatment with antimicrobial or immunosuppressive agents. Furthermore, the use of invasive devices during the perioperative period such as intravascular and urinary catheters increases host susceptibility to infection.

MEANS OF TRANSMISSION

The final link in the chain of infection is the transmission of the infectious agent to the

Table 13.1. Common Bacteria Isolated in Culture from Infections.

Gram-Positive	Gram-Negative
Aerobic	
Coccus	Coccus
Staphylococcus sp.	*Neisseria* sp.
Streptococcus sp.	*Moraxella* sp.
Bacillus	Bacillus
Bacillus sp.	*Acinetobacter* sp.
Corynebacterium sp.	*Enterobacter* sp.
Listeria sp.	*Escherichia coli* sp.
	Haemophilus sp.
	Klebsiella sp.
	Proteus sp.
	Providencia sp.
	Pseudomonas sp.
	Salmonella sp.
	Serratia sp.
	Shigella sp.
	Yersinia sp.
Anaerobic	
Coccus	Coccus
Peptococcus sp.	*Veillonella* sp.
Peptostreptococcus sp.	
Bacillus	Bacillus
Clostridium sp.	*Bacteroides* sp.
Propionibacterium sp.	*Fusobacterium* sp.
Lactobacillus sp.	

susceptible host. Transmission of infectious agents can occur through one or more of four different means of transmission: contact, airborne, common vehicle, or vectorborne.

Contact Transmission

Contact transmission is the most frequent means of transmission of infection in hospitals and can occur by direct, indirect, or droplet contact between the source of the infectious agent and the susceptible host. Direct contact transmission occurs when there is person-to-person contact that results in the transfer of infectious agents between the infected or colonized source and a susceptible host. Such transmission can occur between the nurse and patient and vice versa during routine hands-on activities of perioperative patient care such as preoperative skin preparation and postoperative dressing changes. Direct contact transmission can also occur by self-inoculation when microorganisms from the patient become the source of the infection.

Indirect contact transmission occurs when the contact between the source and susceptible host involves a contaminated intermediate object, such as some piece of patient care or surgical equipment that transfers the infectious agent. Droplet contact transmission involves the brief passage of relatively large infectious particles through the air when the infected source and susceptible host are in close proximity, usually within several feet. Such transmission could occur between an infected circulating nurse and the patient during a surgical procedure in the operating room.

Other Means of Transmission

The remaining three means of transmission of infection—airborne, common-vehicle, and vectorborne—occur less frequently in the hospital than contact transmission. Airborne transmission, in contrast to droplet transmission, is relatively infrequent but involves a true airborne dissemination of infectious agents in droplet nuclei or dust particles that remain suspended in the air for prolonged periods of time and move about as a result of air currents or mechanical movement of air. Common-vehicle transmission occurs when a contami-

nated inanimate vehicle such as liquid antiseptics, disinfectants, or food is the medium for transmission of the infectious agent from the contaminated source to multiple susceptible hosts. Vectorborne transmission occurs when the infectious agent is transmitted through vectors such as mosquitoes or tsetse flies. Vectorborne transmission rarely occurs in U.S. hospitals.

Breaking the Chain of Infection

While completing the chain of infection requires all three essential components to be present under the right conditions, breaking the chain of infection involves altering or removing only one of the three components or links. Thus, the chain of infection can be broken by: (1) destroying the infectious agents; (2) increasing the resistance of the susceptible host; or (3) interrupting transmission of the infectious agent.

DESTROYING THE INFECTIOUS AGENTS

Without the presence of an adequate number of infectious agents, infection cannot occur. Thus, the chain of infection can be broken by destroying or reducing the number of infectious agents. Although various cleaning and disinfection procedures reduce the number of microorganisms on objects, the complete destruction or removal of infectious agents on objects in the hospital environment can be accomplished only through the processes of sterilization and incineration.

Sterilization

Sterilization involves completely removing or destroying all forms of microbial life, as compared to disinfection, which only kills some microorganisms. Though it is impossible and unnecessary to attempt to destroy all microorganisms in the hospital environment, it is important, from an infection control standpoint, that surgical instruments and certain patient care items used during the perioperative period be sterile. For example, any object or instrument that will enter tissue or the vascular system or objects such as tubing and catheters that blood will flow through should be sterile (1).

The most convenient, effective, inexpensive, and widely used method of sterilization in hospitals is steam under pressure. Steam sterilization is unsuitable, however, for processing certain items such as plastic tubing and catheters with low melting points and delicate objects that might be damaged by heat or moisture. In contrast to steam sterilization, ethylene oxide gas sterilization is more complex and expensive and requires special aeration to remove toxic residues of the ethylene oxide gas. Its use, therefore, is usually restricted to delicate objects such as lensed instruments and plastics that might be damaged by heat or moisture (1).

Liquid chemicals such as glutaraldehyde, formaldehyde (8 percent), and alcohol (70 percent) solution, and 6 percent stabilized hydrogen peroxide can also be used for sterilization if the objects are precleaned with a detergent until they are free of organic matter such as blood or mucus. However, the contact time for sterilization with liquid chemicals ranges from 6 to 18 hours. Moreover, because of their chemical makeup, these agents often cause skin reactions and dermatitis unless personnel using them wear gloves during contact and splashes are prevented. Therefore, sterilization using liquid chemicals may be impractical for most reusable patient care items requiring sterilization in hospitals (1).

Recommendations from the Centers for Disease Control (CDC) for hospital sterilization of various objects that will enter tissue or the vascular system are shown in Table 13.2.

Incineration

Infectious agents can also be destroyed by incineration. Some hospital solid wastes such as pathology wastes and isolation wastes from infected patients may be highly contaminated with infectious agents. Infectious agents in such wastes can usually be destroyed more easily and economically through incineration than through steam sterilization. Even with strict air pollution regulations, incineration of small quantities of potentially hazardous wastes is still possible in most communities. Relatively small amounts of heavily contaminated high-

Table 13.2. Methods of Sterilization for Objects That Will Enter Tissue or Vascular System or That Blood Will Flow Through.

Object	Procedure	Exposure Time (hours)
Smooth, hard surface	A	mfr. rec.
	B	mfr. rec.
	C	10
	D	18
	E	6
Rubber tubing and catheters	A	mfr. rec.
	B	mfr. rec.
	E	6
Polyethylene tubing and catheters[a]	A	mfr. rec.
	B	mfr. rec.
	C	10
	D	18
	E	6
Lensed instruments	B	mfr. rec.
	C	10
	E	6
Thermometers (oral and rectal)[b]	B	mfr. rec.
	C	10
	D	18
	E	6
Hinged instruments	A	mfr. rec.
	B	mfr. rec.
	C	10
	E	6

Modified from "Guidelines for Hospital Environmental Control." In: *Guidelines for the Prevention and Control of Nosocomial Infections.* Atlanta: Centers for Disease Control, 1981 (rev. July 1982).
Procedure Key:
  A Heat sterilization including steam or hot air.
  B Ethylene oxide gas (for time, see manufacturer's recommendations, mfr. rec.).
  C Glutaraldehyde (2 percent).
  D Formaldehyde (8 percent)-alcohol (70 percent) solution (corrosion inhibitor needed if formulated in hospital).
  E 6 percent stabilized hydrogen peroxide (will corrode copper, zinc, and brass).
[a]Thermostability should be investigated when indicated.
[b]Do not mix rectal and oral thermometers at any stage of handling or processing.

risk materials must be disposed of in this manner (2).

INCREASING HOST RESISTANCE

Without a susceptible host, infections cannot occur. Nevertheless, host resistance is often the most difficult component to alter when attempting to break the chain of infection, particularly for increasing resistance in patients who undergo a surgical operation. Some factors that predispose a patient to infection, however, may be altered during the perioperative period if the operation can be delayed until attempts have been made to increase host resistance. For example, the risk of infection in uncontrolled diabetic patients can be reduced if such patients can have their blood sugar better controlled during the perioperative period. The risk of infection in severely malnourished patients can be reduced if they receive parenteral nutrition perioperatively. Increasing host resistance to infection can also be accomplished by the judicious use and care of invasive devices such as urinary catheters and pressure-monitoring lines. The benefits of such attempts to increase host resistance must be weighed against the risks associated with the intervention. For example, the infection risk associated with total parenteral nutrition in some hospitals may outweigh any potential benefit of such therapy to increase host resistance.

INTERRUPTING TRANSMISSION

Since it is difficult to increase host resistance and often impossible and unnecessary to destroy all potentially infectious agents in the hospital environment, attempts at breaking the chain of infection should be directed toward interrupting transmission of microorganisms responsible for infection. Because nurses spend more time with perioperative patients than other health care professionals, it is particularly important that they direct nursing activities toward interrupting transmission of infection. Important methods for interrupting transmission of infection in the hospital include frequent and careful handwashing, compliance with isolation techniques, and use of preventive patient care practices during the insertion and management of urinary and intravascular catheters.

Handwashing
Handwashing is generally considered to be the single most important method for interrupting transmission of microorganisms and preventing infections. Numerous agents ranging from soap to antiseptics are usually available for handwashing in most hospitals. Soap and detergent handwashing agents suspend easily removable microorganisms on the skin and allow them to be washed off. Antiseptic handwashing agents control or kill microorganisms that contaminate the skin and other superficial tissues. Although handwashing agents, including antiseptics, do not sterilize the skin, they can reduce the amount of microbial contamination and interrupt or prevent transmission of infection. The degree of reduction of microbial contamination depends on the amount and type of contamination on the hands, the type of handwashing agent used, the length of exposure to the agent, the presence of residual activity of the handwashing agent, and the handwashing technique used (3).

In the absence of a true emergency, CDC recommends that personnel *always* wash their hands (3):

1. Before performing invasive procedures, whether or not sterile gloves are worn
2. Before and after contact with wounds, whether surgical, traumatic, or associated with an invasive device (e.g., an intravenous cannula entrance wound)
3. Before contact with particularly susceptible patients
4. After contact with a source that is likely to be contaminated with virulent microorganisms or hospital pathogens, such as an infected patient or an object or device contaminated with secretions or excretions from patients (e.g., a urinary catheter system)
5. Between contacts with different patients in special care units

When handwashing is indicated during routine patient care, CDC recommends a vigorous washing under a stream of water for at least 10 seconds using bar soap, a nonantimicrobial liquid soap, granule soap, or soap-filled tissues. When handwashing is indicated during care of patients in isolation or in precautions for infections with multiply-resistant bacteria, antiseptic handwashing agents containing chlorhexidine, hexaclorophene, iodophors, or alcohol are recommended by CDC. Antiseptic handwashing agents should also be used before invasive procedures and should be available for use in special care units (3).

Isolation Precautions
The chain of infection can also be broken by using isolation precautions to interrupt transmission. The means of transmission of an infectious agent determines whether a private room is necessary for the patient and whether protective attire (gowns, masks, and gloves) are indicated for hospital personnel and visitors. Cloth or disposable gowns are worn to prevent contamination of clothing when infections can be transmitted by direct or indirect contact. When gowns are indicated to interrupt transmission of infection, they should be used only once and then placed in an appropriate receptacle before the user leaves the isolation area. Masks (high-efficiency) that cover the nose and mouth are worn when infections can be transmitted by droplets, aerosols, or air. When masks are indicated to interrupt transmission of infection, they should be used only once and then placed in an appropriate receptacle before the user leaves the isolation area. Masks should never be lowered around the neck and reused. Gloves are worn when infections can be transmitted by contact with articles contaminated by patient discharges or body fluids. When gloves are indicated to prevent transmission of infection, nonsterile gloves are adequate. If sterile technique is necessary, then sterile gloves should be worn.

The means of transmission of an infectious agent also should determine whether articles and linens used for the patient on isolation precautions need special handling to prevent or interrupt the transmission of infection. Only a small proportion of infections that require isolation precautions need all these provisions (4).

Preventive Patient Care Practices
Diagnostic and therapeutic interventions, such as those that involve the use of urinary and intravascular catheters, increase the risk of transmission of infection in perioperative patients. This risk can be minimized if nurses comply with preventive patient care practices for the insertion and maintenance of urinary and intravascular catheters.

Urinary catheterization should be done only when necessary for medical indications. Alternative methods to indwelling catheters, such as condom catheters or adult-type diapers, should be considered and used when possible. When indwelling urinary catheters are necessary, CDC recommends the following practices to prevent catheter-associated urinary tract infections (5):

1. Wash hands immediately before and after any manipulation of the catheter.
2. Insert the catheter using aseptic technique and sterile equipment.
3. Secure the catheter properly to prevent movement and urethral traction.
4. Maintain closed sterile drainage.
5. Obtain urine samples aseptically from the sampling port or drainage bag.
6. Maintain unobstructed urine flow.

CDC's "Guidelines for the Prevention of Intravascular Infections" (6) contain preventive patient care practices for insertion and maintenance of intravenous therapy and intravascular pressure-monitoring systems. CDC's "Guidelines for Prevention of Nosocomial Pneumonia" (7) contain perioperative measures for preventing postoperative pneumonia and recommendations for suctioning the respiratory tract.

Nosocomial Infections

Infections in perioperative patients can be classified as either hospital (nosocomial) or community-acquired infections. Nosocomial infections are infections that occur during hospitalization that were not present or incubating when the patient was admitted to the hospital. Infections with onset after discharge from the hospital are also considered to be nosocomial if the infecting microorganism is judged to have been acquired during hospitalization. The term nosocomial infection, therefore, includes potentially preventable infections from exogenous sources as well as those from endogenous sources that may be regarded, by some, as inevitable.

Nosocomial infections in surgical patients can either be surgery- or nonsurgery-related. Surgery-related nosocomial infections are those that involve the surgical wound or surrounding deep organs, tissues, or cavities exposed during the operative procedure. Examples of surgery-related nosocomial infections include an incisional wound infection in a patient after laminectomy, a subphrenic abscess in a patient after gastrectomy, or an empyema in a patient after thoracic surgery. Infections that arise in surgical patients but do not involve tissue exposed or manipulated during the operative procedure are not considered surgery-related. For example, a purulent thrombophlebitis, a postoperative pneumonia, or a urinary tract infection in a patient after gastrectomy would not be considered surgery-related.

Surgical patients, more than any other patient group in the hospital, have a high risk of developing both surgery- and nonsurgery-related nosocomial infections. Data from the CDC Study on the Efficacy of Nosocomial Infection Control (SENIC Project) (8) show that almost three-fourths of nosocomial infections occur among patients undergoing surgery. This means that surgical patients are at about three times greater risk of acquiring a nosocomial infection than nonsurgical patients. However, most infections in surgical patients are not related to the surgical wound but to instrumentation of the urinary and respiratory tracts during the perioperative period. Of all nosocomial infections detected among surgical patients in the CDC SENIC Project, 42 percent were urinary tract infections, 40 percent surgical wound infections, 14 percent pneumonia, and 4 percent bacteremia (blood stream infections) (8).

Data from another CDC study, the National Nosocomial Infections Study (NNIS) (9), suggest that the frequency of surgical wound infections may have declined slightly from 1975 to 1979. Since surgical wound infections are second only to urinary tract infections as the most frequent nosocomial infection, they remain an important cause of increased cost, morbidity, and mortality in surgical patients and therefore deserve special emphasis.

SURGICAL WOUND INFECTIONS

A working definition of a surgical wound infection is any wound that drains purulent material. One of the most important factors determining the likelihood of a surgical wound becoming infected is the degree of wound contamination at the time of surgery. More than two decades ago, the National Research Council developed a system for classifying wounds based on the degree of contamination of the wound and surrounding tissues during the operation (10). This system of wound classification, also recommended by the Committee on Control of Surgical Infections of the American College of Surgeons (11), has been widely adopted for research studies to determine wound infection rates in various settings. The classification system divides all surgical wounds into four classes: clean, clean-contaminated, contaminated, and dirty or infected wounds. Since the classification of a surgical wound can vary depending upon the findings and circumstances during operation, usually only a member of the operating team can accurately determine the ultimate classification of the wound. Ideally, the classification should be made and recorded at the completion of the operation.

Class I: Clean Wound
This category of wounds includes nontraumatic surgical wounds in which no inflammation was encountered, no break in surgical technique occurred, and no entry was made into the respiratory, alimentary, or genitourinary tracts. Examples of clean wounds are thyroidectomy, mastectomy, herniorrhaphy, and laminectomy. Clean wounds have a 1–5 percent likelihood of becoming infected (10, 12).

Class II: Clean-Contaminated Wound
This category of wounds includes nontraumatic wounds in which only minor breaks in surgical technique occur or wounds in which no significant spillage occurred if the gastrointestinal, genitourinary, or respiratory tracts were entered. Examples of clean-contaminated wounds are cholecystectomy and resection of

the small or large intestine when no inflammation or infection was present, hysterectomy, oophorectomy, and cesarean-section delivery. Clean-contaminated wounds have an 8–11 percent likelihood of becoming infected (10, 12).

Class III: Contaminated Wound
This category of wound includes any fresh traumatic wound from a relatively clean source or any wound in which there is a major break in surgical technique, gross spillage from the gastrointestinal tract, or entry into the genitourinary or biliary tracts if there is acute nonpurulent inflammation. An example of a contaminated wound is an inflamed but unruptured appendix or gallbladder. Contaminated wounds have a 15–17 percent likelihood of becoming infected (10, 12).

Class IV: Dirty Wound
This category includes wounds in which acute bacterial inflammation or a perforated viscus is encountered and wounds in which clean tissue is transected to gain access to a collection of pus or abscess. Surgical drainage of an intraabdominal abscess is an example of a dirty wound. Dirty wounds have more than a 27 percent likelihood of becoming infected (10, 12).

MICROBIOLOGY OF SURGICAL WOUND INFECTIONS

Recent reports from the CDC National Nosocomial Infections Study (NNIS) (13) indicate that there has been a shift in pathogens responsible for nosocomial surgical wound infections from predominantly Gram-positive to Gram-negative bacteria. For example, the rate of *Staphylococcus aureus* wound infections reported to NNIS has decreased substantially from 1975 to 1979, but the rate of infections caused by *Serratia marcescens* has slightly but steadily increased.

The percentage of pathogens isolated from surgical wound infections as reported to NNIS from 1976 to 1979 are shown in Fig. 13.2. As mentioned previously, as a group, Gram-negative bacteria (*Escherichia coli, Proteus-Providencia* sp., *Pseudomonas aeruginosa, Kebsiella* sp., *Enterobacter* sp., and *Serratia* sp.) make up the

majority of surgical wound pathogens. Other microorganisms such as fungi and viruses are rarely reported as surgical wound pathogens.

Preexisting Infections and Implications for the Operating Room

Patients undergoing surgical procedures who have a preexisting active bacterial infection, even if it is remote from the surgical wound, have a higher risk of acquiring a wound infection than those without such infection. Therefore, most surgeons will attempt to identify, treat, and control infections before the operation, particularly in elective cases.

Occasionally a patient with an active infection will require surgery. If the infection involves the operative site and frank pus is encountered during the operative procedure, the case is often referred to as a "dirty" or infected case. In the past, it was common practice to use extraordinary cleaning procedures in the operating room after such cases and then seal the room with tape for up to 48 hours before permitting another surgical operation to be performed (14). This practice is no longer considered necessary or cost-effective, provided appropriate cleaning procedures are used and the air-handling system is adequate (a minimum of 25 air changes per hour).

Detailed recommendations for routine housekeeping between cases in operating rooms are available (11, 15, 16). Such detailed cleaning procedures are based on the rationale that every operation is potentially, if not actually, infected. The routine cleaning procedures between cases are intended to provide a margin of safety; therefore, additional cleaning procedures for "dirty" or infected cases are not needed nor recommended. Moreover, it is no longer necessary or cost-effective to set aside a separate room for infected or "dirty" cases when appropriate cleaning and air-handling procedures are used.

THE INFECTION CONTROL NURSE

The need for infection control nurses (ICNs) was recognized as a result of outbreaks of

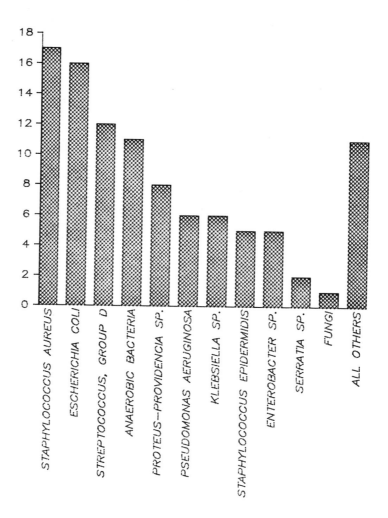

Figure 13.2. Percentage of pathogens isolated from surgical wound infections, NNIS, 1976–1979.

Staphylococcus aureus wound and skin infections in hospital patients and personnel in the mid-1950s in both the United Kingdom and the United States. Infection control as a nursing specialty originated in England in 1959, when a nurse was appointed to act as liaison among all persons concerned with infection control (17). The infection control nurse concept spread to the United States in the early 1960s when Stanford University appointed an ICN as the "central figure of the infection control program." The goal of the program was to "assist

in providing a high level of patient care by reducing the ever present risk of nosocomial infections through consistent surveillance of infections and personnel education (18).

The value of the ICN in infection control activities was summarized in 1970 by Moore, a pathologist who believed that a nurse can more reliably assess the general standard of nursing care and morale of the nursing staff of a hospital ward than a physician (19). During the same year, Garner and coworkers (20) from CDC concluded that the ICN was essential for hospital infection surveillance and control programs. Before 1970, only 6 percent of U.S. hospitals had an ICN, but by the end of 1976, 80 percent had instituted such a position (21).

ICNs in U.S. hospitals perform a wide range of responsibilities and activities. On the average, ICNs spend 46 percent of their time performing surveillance of nosocomial infections, 23 percent researching and developing infection control policies, 13 percent training hospital personnel about infection control, 10 percent consulting with physicians, nurses, and other personnel or hospital departments, and 8 percent investigating outbreaks of infection (22). Through these activities, the ICN works with clinical, administrative, and support service personnel associated with the hospital. These contacts with hospital personnel range from informal interaction with nurses about specific patient care or personnel health practices, and teaching sessions with nurses, physicians, or other members of the hospital staff, to conferences with administrators, department heads, or chiefs of medical services.

The ICN is usually a member of and works with the infection control committee, which is responsible for the infection control policies and procedures in the hospital. The ICN also acts as liaison between the infection control committee and hospital departments such as the operating room when policies and procedures are proposed, reviewed, implemented, and evaluated. Moreover, the ICN keeps the director of the operating room informed about the occurrence and outcome of surgical wound infection problems and trends of such infections. Recent data from the CDC SENIC Project indicate the need for the ICN to spend a substantial amount of time on infection surveillance and control activities for patients undergoing surgical procedures for these reasons (8): (1) 70 percent of all nosocomial infections occur in such patients; (2) 75 percent of pneumonia cases (the nosocomial infection with the highest case-fatality rates) occur in such patients; and (3) surgical wound infections may be the type of infection most amenable to reduction by surveillance and follow-up activities.

RELATIONSHIP BETWEEN THE INFECTION CONTROL NURSE AND THE DIRECTOR OF THE OPERATING ROOM

The formal relationship between the ICN and the director of the operating room will depend, in part, on the organizational structure of the hospital and the administrative placement of the operating room and infection control departments. Regardless of the organizational structure, the ICN and the director of the operating room should be able to share information about prevention of infections in patients and personnel.

In past years ICNs often were recruited from the ranks of OR nurses because OR nurses learn to be very conscious of the necessity for policies and procedures to prevent infections. The current trend, however, is toward recruitment of ICNs who have had ward or intensive care nursing experience and who have also come from a baccalaureate nursing program that included epidemiology, biostatistics, and other related science courses. Unfortunately, such nurses have often had only limited OR experience. Therefore, it is often necessary for the OR director to orient the new ICN to the various activities of the operating room.

Although the new ICN may lack experience in OR nursing, the ICN's background and experience with infectious diseases and in reviewing scientific studies can be valuable to the OR director when new products or equipment are considered. The ICN will not only be concerned about whether the product or equipment will be likely to reduce or prevent infections, but also whether the infection control benefit of the product outweighs its cost. Cost-benefit studies have been done that relate to infection control and the ICN should have copies of such studies available for discussion with the OR director.

The ICN and the OR director have the same goal of prevention of infections in patients and personnel. Each brings different knowledge, experience, and perspective to the goal. This goal can be more readily achieved if they have a positive relationship built on mutual respect.

Staff nurses also have certain responsibilities for prevention and control of infections. Staff nurses providing perioperative patient care in the operating room, special care units, or the surgical ward have a responsibility for conducting their nursing activities so that the risk of infection is minimized. It is particularly important that staff nurses know and comply with preventive patient care practices for the insertion and care of invasive devices, such as urinary and intravascular catheters, for tracheostomy care including suctioning, and for dressing techniques for surgical wounds. Staff nurses should also comply with the infection control policies set forth by the infection control and personnel health departments that pertain to known or suspected illnesses, or exposures, if susceptible, to rubella or varicella-zoster virus infections (23). Moreover, staff nurses have the responsibility for reporting known or suspected infection problems in patients and personnel to their supervisor. These responsibilities also apply to students assigned to perioperative patient care.

The Role of Centers for Disease Control as a Resource

The Centers for Disease Control (CDC) is the principal public health agency of the federal government responsible for preventing and controlling the spread of infectious diseases. For the past 25 years, CDC epidemiologists have been assisting state health departments and hospitals in investigating epidemics occurring in hospitals. A summary of 22 such outbreaks in surgical patients has been reported (24). In addition to epidemic investigations, CDC has published a number of infection control recommendations and guidelines that have been widely accepted by hospitals and incorporated into their routine practices (1–6). For example, 87 percent of U.S. hospitals in 1976 reported using the CDC recommendations for isolation precautions (25). A new CDC guideline for prevention of surgical wound infections was published in 1982 (26). Other

CDC activities related to hospital infection control include providing written or telephone consultation to hospital personnel and conducting or participating in training courses for infection control nurses, OR nurses, and other hospital personnel.

Controlling the Environment

During the preoperative assessment, the nurse identifies host factors that influence the risk of infection such as nutritional status, age, and underlying disease. These factors, however, are not usually amenable to change through nursing action during the immediate perioperative period. The primary focus of the nurse in reaching the goal of freedom from infection for the patient is control of the number and types of microorganisms present during surgery.

Surgery has been described as controlled assault on the human body. Surgical intervention breaks down some of the body's primary defenses against infection. Infection can adversely affect the outcome of surgery and even endanger the life of the patient.

While not all the principles and activities described in this chapter are carried out by nurses, the nurse should understand what is involved in minimizing the microbial population present during surgery. This enables the nurse to coordinate supplies, equipment, and a physical environment that are safe for use in patient care. The nurse must also recognize when conditions or events might make an item or area microbiologically unacceptable for use in the care of the surgical patient.

Control of microorganisms starts with control of the physical environment of the operating room. The factors to be considered and the methods of control also apply to other areas where items are prepared for and undergo sterilization. Most infections associated with surgical intervention are caused by bacteria, although certain fungi and some viruses are also of concern. Environmental measures are, therefore, aimed primarily at control of bacterial contamination. The temperature of the operating room is maintained between 20° and

24°C (68° and 75°F), except in situations where the risk of hypothermia for the patient outweighs the benefits of lower temperatures. Such might be the case when the patient is an infant because infants have immature temperature-regulating mechanisms and physiologic intolerance to cold. Normally, however, the patient can tolerate the 20–24°C range with no difficulty, especially after the surgical drapes are applied. It is thought that most bacteria pathogenic to humans metabolize and reproduce best at temperatures at, or near, normal body temperature, 37°C (98.6°F). By keeping the room temperature below this level, bacterial growth may be inhibited to some small degree.

A stronger argument for keeping the temperature at these levels is the comfort and thermal regulation of the operative team. When dressed in scrub suit or dress, cap, mask, and fluid-impervious gown and gloves, surgical team members have little body area exposed for heat loss through convection or radiation. If a member of the scrub team becomes overheated, the principal cooling method will be evaporation of perspiration. This means possible soaking through of clothing and possible dripping of perspiration onto the surgical field. This moisture carries the bacterial flora and could be a source of infection. Temperatures below 20°C (68°F) may be too cold, even for those dressed in full surgical garb, and involuntary shivering may occur. The attention of the surgical team should be on the patient. Variations from the suggested temperature range can produce discomfort and distraction even without provoking the extremes of diaphoresis or shivering.

The relative humidity in the operating room is maintained at 50 percent ± 10. Bacteria are thought to multiply best in moist environments above 60 percent relative humidity. The 40–60 percent relative humidity range does, however, allow some bacterial growth. The primary reason for the convention of maintaining relative humidity at this level goes back to the time when explosive anesthetics, such as ether, were in wide use. The potential for static electricity buildup and discharge is greatly lessened if the relative humidity is about 50 percent. Provisions for the control of relative humidity remain a part of most voluntary and regulatory standards for the surgical suite even though explosive anesthetic agents are no longer used. Controlled discharge of larger electrostatic charge accumulation sometimes interferes with the operation of electrical monitoring equipment and can cause actual damage to electrical equipment. Also, static shocks that might occur when the operation team member touches the patient could be uncomfortable if the materials in use and the humidity conditions were conducive to static buildup. Therefore, even without explosive anesthetics, there are still reasons to control electrostatic charge buildup through control of humidity.

AIR QUALITY

The air that passes over the surgical wound site and supplies being used contains airborne microorganisms that could settle into the wound, introducing contamination. Air-handling or ventilation systems of operating rooms being built today are designed to minimize the introduction of contaminants from outside the operating room. The optimal ventilation system delivers air to the room at or near ceiling level from the center of the room. Air exhaust vents are in the periphery of the room, just above floor level. The air currents set up move air down through the surgical field, carrying most airborne particles to floor level and away from the surgical field. In new operating rooms, the rate of air exchange should be 25 room volumes per hour. Up to 80 percent of the air may be recirculated, providing the exhausted air is adequately filtered. Recirculation of air conserves energy because minimal heating, cooling, and humidity adjustments are necessary.

The filtration or cleaning of the air is important. In the modern operating room, air-handling systems include a series of filters that remove almost all particulate matter coming from the outside, fresh air, or contained in the recirculated air. The air delivered to the operating room is almost sterile. The particle count and thus the bacterial burden, however, rise sharply as the air travels through the operating room because of microbial shedding from the patient and members of the operative team. This shedding increases with activity and cannot be totally eliminated even with modern and effective surgical attire. The 25 air exchanges per hour is sufficient to dilute the bacterial debris from the surgical team to a level considered safe for most types of surgery.

Some procedures, however, are thought to require a greater margin of safety because of the potentially catastrophic results of postoperative infections. These include total joint replacements and other procedures where large amounts of foreign prosthetic material are left in the patient. Procedures on patients who have severely compromised host defense mechanisms, such as severe bone marrow depression, might also fit into this category.

For these patients, some surgeons use laminar airflow systems to create an ultra clean environment where even shedding from the surgical team is minimized as a source of airborne contamination. Laminar airflow means unidirectional, nonturbulent airflow. The airflow direction can be either horizontal or vertical, depending on whether the plenum containing the high-energy particulate air (HEPA) filters are on the ceiling or on a wall. In a vertical flow unit, the air enters from the ceiling and exits at floor level. In a horizontal flow unit, the air enters from one side of the room and travels in straight currents, across to the opposite wall. What makes this air-handling system different is not the filtration, since most air-handling systems for the operating room have efficient filtration mechanisms, but the speed at which the air travels, which maintains the unidirectional flow. There is a perceptible breeze in rooms using laminar airflow equipment.

Laminar airflow equipment introduces virtually sterile air into the room and blows it across the field at such a rate that particles shed by persons in its path are suspended in the unidirectional currents and not allowed to settle onto the surgical field. It then carries the particulates away from the field to a point where they are captured in a vent or can safely settle out on the floor. In reality, in an occupied operating room, true unidirectional airflow is almost impossible to achieve because the air must pass over and around people and objects that break up the laminar flow pattern.

When using laminar airflow equipment, careful planning of the positioning of personnel and equipment is essential. If possible, nothing should obstruct the flow of air from the filter plenum to the wound site. All objects and people should remain downwind or peripheral to this airflow. This is extremely difficult to do, especially in vertical flow units, because the head and shoulders of the surgical team may be over the wound. In these cases, some surgical teams wear special headgear that totally covers the head and face. This may be a plastic face guard similar to those worn by astronauts and a sterile nonwoven hood. An exhaust system to remove expired air from the plastic face dome is sometimes used, often more for cooling than for respiratory needs.

There is still a great deal of controversy as to laminar airflow's effectiveness in reducing postoperative infections. Many authorities dispute the claim that it reduces infection by pointing out that the surgeon's speed, proper tissue-handling techniques, appropriate wound drainage, elimination of wound dead space, and the use of prophylactic antibiotics are all significant in keeping the infection rate low. Laminar airflow equipment is expensive, and many hospitals are reluctant to install it until its efficacy is clearly demonstrated. If the laminar airflow equipment is misused because of inadequate planning and positioning, the results could be an increase in infection because particles may be driven into the depths of the surgical wound.

Another characteristic of air-handling systems for the surgical suite is the creation of pressure gradients between so-called clean and dirty areas. The actual operating room is considered clean, and the adjacent hallway and substerile or scrub areas are considered less clean. The operating room is kept at a slightly (about 10 percent) higher air pressure than the surrounding space so that if a door is opened, air from the less clean space cannot enter the clean space. In surgical suites with a clean core where only sterile supplies are stored and all personnel wear masks at all times, the clean core has slightly more positive pressure relative to the operating room. Thus, when the door to the clean core is opened, air flows from the "cleaner" core area into the "clean" operating room.

These pressure gradients are effective only when the doors to the operating room are kept closed except when someone is entering or leaving. Leaving the door open or opening two doors at once disrupts the pressurization and causes turbulent airflow that could increase airborne contamination. In addition, the air-handling system must work harder, thus using more energy and increasing costs.

If air-handling systems are allowed to function as they were designed, they deliver high-quality, well-conditioned air. Older operating rooms, built more than 20 years ago, may not have these sophisticated systems in place and extra care with regard to environmental cleaning, OR apparel, and surgical speed may be appropriate.

TRAFFIC

The greatest source of bacterial contamination, however, is the people in the room at the time of surgery, including the patient. This contamination increases with movement and talking.

Every effort should be made to minimize the number of people in the room during a surgical procedure. The higher the risk of infection or the greater the consequences of infection for the patient, the more stringent should be the controls on access to the room. This is particularly difficult in teaching hospitals, where residents and students need legitimate access to operative procedures to complete their training. Highly technical or complex procedures that last a long time or require much technical equipment are also of concern. Examples of these are limb replantations and cardiopulmonary bypass procedures.

In these cases, careful planning by the nursing personnel can minimize excess movement in and out, as well as within, the operating room. Anticipating supply needs, checking out equipment before the patient arrives, and using the intercom or telephone if available can reduce trips in and out of the room. Identifying

each person in the room and ascertaining her purpose in being present are essential. It may be appropriate to challenge some visitors, using tact and the appropriate channels of authority for each institution. The nurse must serve as the patient's advocate in this matter to minimize the risk of infection and to protect the patient's right to privacy.

Traffic flow within the operating room is governed by the principles of asepsis. Traffic flow within the suite in general, outside the actual operating room, is largely dependent on the physical design of the suite. Three components that make up the traffic within any surgical suite are patients, personnel, and supplies and equipment. For each of these, the ideal pattern is unidirectional, with entry in one area, travel through the suite, and exit in another area. But few surgical suites are built to permit this ideal traffic pattern, and compromises are usually necessary. These adjustments can be effective and safe in minimizing contamination if they are well thought out and judiciously adhered to. In fact, constructing an ideal surgical suite can be prohibitively costly because of the wasted space involved in providing separate corridors and access to them.

For personnel traffic flow, the surgical suite is usually divided into three zones. The first of these is the unrestricted or semipublic area where people in street attire may enter and mix with those in scrub attire. Examples are the locker rooms, some offices, and the administrative control desk if it is located at the entrance to the surgical suite. The second zone is the semirestricted area where scrub attire, cap, and shoe covers or clean shoes are required. Examples are the hallways adjacent to the operating rooms, work rooms, and offices located in the interior of the suite. The third zone is the restricted zone where full scrub attire and mask are necessary. Examples are the actual operating rooms, scrub areas, and the clean core area if the suite is designed around that concept. Personnel can move freely between all three zones if they are appropriately attired. After leaving the suite, however, reentry should be permitted only through the locker room areas where some or all items of scrub apparel may need to be changed.

Patients usually enter the suite through the public or unrestricted zone and may wait in a holding area where some preoperative assessment and actual care, such as hair removal, may take place. As patients enter the semirestricted area, their hair is usually covered with a bouffant disposable cap or some other method of containment to minimize particulate shedding during surgery. The time spent by patients in the semirestricted zone is usually only during transport to the operating room. Patients are not asked to don masks when entering the operating room in the restricted zone. Masks would hinder access to the face and airway and might increase the patient's anxiety, outweighing any small benefit in minimizing bacterial contamination. Masks prevent the spread of respiratory droplets, which usually travel less than 10 feet even with forced exhalation. By keeping the sterile setup well away from the head of the OR bed until after the patient is draped, the nurse can minimize the possibility of contamination from the patient's respiratory tract. After surgery, the patient usually goes to a recovery room area by the same path taken to enter the operating room through the semirestricted area. If the surgical suite has a clean core, patients are never allowed into this area.

Supply and equipment traffic is probably the most variable within the surgical suite. Separation of clean and dirty items is paramount. Clean and sterile supplies should be transported to the surgical suite on carts that are covered to prevent contamination of the wrappers by dust and respiratory droplets during transport through hospital corridors and on elevators. Corrugated paper boxes and any outside shipping containers should be removed before the items enter any sterile storage or patient care area because corrugated boxes generate and collect dust, and the shipping containers are contaminated by handling and transport on common carriers.

At the surgical suite entrance, the dust cover should be removed from the carts and discarded or reprocessed, depending on the material used. Supplies may then be moved to storage locations within the suite or, if a case cart system is in use, directly to the operating room. In a case cart system, all sterile supplies and instruments needed for a patient's surgical procedure are collected and transported on a mobile cart. The cart is usually prepared in the central sterile processing department of the institution and sent to the surgical suite. The cart is taken into the operating room and, if of the appropriate design, may be used as the back table during surgery. At the end of the procedure, all dirty or used items are loaded back onto the cart and the cart is returned to the decontamination area of central sterile processing for item disposal or recycling.

Whether or not a case cart system is used, all soiled items leaving the operating room must be contained to prevent cross contamination. These soiled items never enter the clean core if the suite has one. In most instances, soiled items travel approximately the same pathway as clean items, except in reverse. As long as they are contained and are not left next to clean or sterile items for any length of time, this is no problem. Soiled items should not ride on elevators at the same time as patients, food, or clean and sterile supply items, even if enclosed in plastic bags. The turbulent air currents that accompany the rise and descent of the elevators can cause cross contamination to occur. A separate elevator for soiled material is the ideal, but seldom accomplished, situation. If items such as linen and trash are stored in the suite for future pickup and disposal, the storage area should be enclosed and separate from corridors, lounges, or other storage areas.

In addition to traffic patterns, the OR team must be alert to the need for handwashing. All the separation of clean and dirty breaks down if a nurse goes from the lunch table to opening sterile supplies without washing hands.

Equipment that comes from outside the suite must be damp dusted with a clean cloth moistened with a germicide safe for use on the equipment. This should be done before the equipment enters the semirestricted zone of the suite. Items that cannot be adequately cleaned, such as compressed gas cylinders with flaking or chipped paint, should be covered with a drape or a cover specifically designed for that purpose before they are moved to the restricted area of the suite.

The use of tacky mats at suite entrances to remove debris from the soles of shoes and from cart wheels is controversial. While the mats collect noticeable amounts of debris, it is questionable whether this debris, already at floor level, represents any real threat of contamination, if the surgical suite is properly cleaned each day. The mats also require monitoring to make certain they are changed when dirty. The cost-effectiveness of the mats is questionable. Most of the dust and other airborne contaminants in the operating room are generated in the room by the handling of textiles and nonwoven materials and by bacterial dispersion from the people present. Nonetheless, some institutions take this extra step and use tacky mats on the floor adjacent to entryways to the surgical suite.

Processes Used in the Preparation of Supplies

In addition to control of the environment, the nurse must also be knowledgeable about the preparation and handling of supplies and instruments used during surgical procedures. In the past, the tasks involved in this were the sole responsibility of the nurse working in surgery. Now, however, these duties are more often assigned to ancillary personnel trained by the nurse. The preparation of supplies and instruments from the surgical suite is performed by trained personnel in support areas such as materials management and central sterile processing.

This frees the nurse to spend more time with the patient or in planning patient care. Some nurses see this as a positive move because it allows broader implementation of the perioperative role without increasing staff. On the other hand, some nurses see this shift of responsibilities as negative, fearing that quality control for sterilization may be lessened. In general, however, quality control programs in a modern hospital's central processing department meet or exceed those in the surgical suite. The nurse who cares for patients as well as prepares supplies must divide efforts between the two. Central processing's prime objective is the preparation of supplies and equipment safe for use in patient care.

The division of responsibilities does not relieve the nurse of the accountability for determining whether an item is safe for use. That accountability is shared with other health care workers, but not diminished for the nurse. Therefore, the nurse must still have an understanding of sterilization and disinfection processing, as well as storage and handling of sterile supplies. In many institutions, the move to centralize sterile processing is just beginning, so nurses may be involved in actual sterilization and disinfection procedures in the surgical suite.

The following discussion is theoretical in nature. Techniques and instructions for specific products or equipment will not be discussed. If not familiar with an item, the nurse should always consult the operator manual for any equipment and the label instructions on any cleaning agent or solution before use.

The preparation of sterile or disinfected supplies is a series of tasks, not a single event. There are three commonly used processes: (1) decontamination; (2) disinfection; and (3) sterilization.

DECONTAMINATION

Decontamination means literally to remove contamination. In health care it has two meanings: (1) to render an object safe for handling by removing infectious material; and (2) to clean an object as the first step leading to sterilization or disinfection. Decontamination assumes that an object has a high, but unknown bioburden. Bioburden is the amount and resistance level of microbial contamination on an object at a given time. Blood, feces, sputum, and soil all represent substances that could produce a high bioburden on an object. But it is not necessary for gross debris to be visible for the bioburden to be very high. Bacteria are invisible to the naked eye, and millions of them could be present. Decontamination lowers the number of organisms to a level that is assumed to be safe because the body's defense mechanisms can usually cope with small to moderate numbers of bacteria. Except in rare instances where a known, very dangerous pathogen such as the Jackob-Creutzfeldt virus is present, decontamination processes are not designed to produce sterility, even if the same equipment is used that might be used for sterilization processing.

DISINFECTION

Disinfection is classically defined as the killing of all pathogens by a chemical, usually a liquid. Today, however, we recognize the ability of microorganisms to adapt, transform, and mutate quickly so that an organism such as *Serretia marcescens*, which was once a nonpathogenic organism cultured in microbiology laboratories for use in demonstrations of bacterial dispersion, is now a highly feared cause of sepsis in hospitals. Therefore, the definition of a pathogen is too variable to rely on in preparing supplies for use in surgery.

Earl Spaulding and others (27) have developed a method of classifying levels of disinfection that has been widely adopted. According to Spaulding, there are three levels of disinfection: high, intermediate, and low. Disinfection is an inexact process and so the definitions of each level are also imprecise. High-level disinfection means that all vegetative forms of bacteria, all fungi, and all viruses have been killed. Highly resistant bacterial spores, however, may survive. Intermediate-level disinfection kills most vegetative bacteria, including the tubercle bacillus. Most viruses are also killed, although an agent that claims to kill the tubercle bacillus may not necessarily be an intermediate-level virucide unless that claim is specifically made. Viruses differ in their susceptibility to chemical disinfectants. Low-level disinfection kills most common vegetative pathogens such as *Staphylococcus* and *Streptococcus.* Low-level disinfectants may be used as cleaning agents for inanimate objects. When referring to the preparation of supplies and instrumentation for use in surgery, high-level disinfection is usually meant unless otherwise indicated.

STERILIZATION

Sterilization is a process that is supposed to result in the absolute absence of microbial life on an item. Absolutes, however, are difficult to prove. In this instance, to prove that all life is absent for every object sterilized, each item would have to be cultured thoroughly, rendering it unusable, and the test would still be subject to error. Therefore, science deals with the probability of an item being sterile. In general, an item is considered sterile if it has been subjected to a process that gives a 10^{-6} assurance level of sterility. That is, there is a 1 in 1 million (10^{-6}) chance of a single organism surviving.

Because sterilization deals with probability, everything that can affect it is relative. Two hemostats, one grossly soiled with blood, the other washed with soap and water, are placed in two identical steam sterilizers. Each sterilizer is run for the same time at the same temperature and steam quality. The time chosen is according to the manufacturer's instructions for sterilization of unwrapped stainless steel instruments. Both items have been through a "sterilization" process. But are both items sterile, according to the 10^{-6} probability level? No. The clean instrument can be considered sterile. The dirty instrument cannot. Why? Bacteria and other microbes vary, even within the same species, in their resistance to being killed, just as humans vary in their ability to withstand adversity. Studies have shown that, when subjected to heat or a chemical process, not all microorganisms die at once. Ninety percent die in a specific period of time that can be calculated for each species. If you continue exposure for a repetition of that period of time, 90 percent of those surviving the first time will be killed. Successive repetitions of this time will continue to reduce the surviving microbes by 90 percent each time. Thus, if you start with 1 million organisms, the first time period will leave 100,000 still alive. The next exposure period will leave 10,000 alive; the next 1,000; the next, 100; the next, 10; the next, 1. But 90 percent kill of one organism does not mathematically produce zero—or absolute sterility. It produces 0.1 organisms, or 10^{-1}. Obviously, there is no such thing as 0.1 bacterium, but this is where the 10^{-6} assurance level comes in. Just how safe is safe? A 1 in 1 million chance of a survivor or 0.0000001 bacterium is the accepted answer.

If there were 10 million organisms to start with (not a very big clump of bacteria) or if the sterilizing agent had to spend some of the exposure time penetrating organic or inorganic soil to get to the bacteria, as might have been true for the dirty hemostat, there would be less than a 10^{-6} assurance level. Indeed, there might be one or two or more whole survivors if the organisms were highly resistant and well shielded.

In hospitals, with many different types of items being sterilized by several different methods, how are sterilizers set to achieve this magic number of 10^{-6}? The sterilizer manufacturers set them. They base the length of time for each cycle on how long it takes to produce a 10^{-6} assurance level for a highly resistant bacterial spore that has been dried to increase its resistance. Most vegetative bacteria and fungi are killed in seconds in a steam sterilization cycle and within minutes with ethylene oxide. Some viruses take longer, and bacterial spores take the longest of all. Bacterial spores are of primary concern to nurses in the operating room because several organisms causing postoperative infection, including *Clostridium perfringens*, which causes gas gangrene, are spore-formers.

Because of the variability of items being sterilized, there is a certain amount of overkill or safety level built into the sterilization cycle by the manufacturers. But manufacturers state in their instructions that items must be clean prior to sterilization.

Decontamination, disinfection, and sterilization each provide a different level of safety. Choosing the correct processing method for an item that will be used in surgery depends on several factors. Where and how will the item be used? What, if any, are the limitations placed on processing because of the structure or composition of the item? What are the costs involved, both in materials and time, especially if alternatives are available?

There are some general guidelines depending on where and how the product will be used. If an item will contact the vascular system or will penetrate the skin, it should be sterile. If the item will contact mucous membranes or be used in respiratory therapy or anesthesia gas administration, it should be high-level disin-

fected. All items that contact blood, body fluids, tissue, or that may have indirectly been contaminated by these, should be decontaminated prior to further reprocessing or disposal.

Items that will be implanted and left in the patient should be packaged appropriately and sterilized. Optionally, these items should be held in quarantine until the biological sterilization indicator has been incubated for at least 48 hours with no growth evident. As with all generalities, there are exceptions to these guidelines in some circumstances. For instance, there is a long-standing controversy over whether laparoscopes and arthroscopes, two types of telescopic apparatuses used to look into body spaces through small incisions, should be sterilized or disinfected. According to the above guidelines, both should be sterilized since they penetrate the skin and contact normally sterile tissue. Yet even the CDC indicates that, for laparoscopes, while sterilization is recommended, high-level disinfection is considered adequate. Orthopedic surgeons are divided on the issue of arthroscope disinfection, and no standard-setting body such as the CDC has officially spoken to the issue. Until that occurs, each institution must be governed by its own policy based on the opinions of the administration, the surgeons, the infection control officer, and the institution's liability insurance carrier.

In both cases, the key to safety with high-level disinfection is thorough cleaning prior to disinfection. Without this step, organisms other than a few rare bacterial spores may survive a sterilization process if they are shielded from the sterilizing agent.

Some materials and types of devices will not tolerate some sterilization or disinfection methods. Polyethylene plastic will not tolerate the heat needed for steam or dry heat sterilization, yet polypropylene can be steam sterilized. Teflon will not tolerate radiation sterilization. Electrical appliances may not tolerate immersion in chemicals or the high humidity level in steam. Controls of flexible fiberoptic endoscopes cannot be immersed in liquids for disinfection.

If an item is to be processed or reprocessed in the health care institution, the manufacturer of the device should provide specific written instructions for cleaning, sterilization, or disinfection. Sales representatives for that manufacturer can provide such instructions.

The cost of various sterilization and disinfection methods varies greatly. In general, steam sterilization is the least expensive and fastest method. Dry heat sterilization is not expensive, but it takes several hours and is suitable for only a few types of products. Ethylene oxide sterilization is relatively expensive and, although sterilization may take only 2–4 hours, the aeration process that must accompany ethylene oxide sterilization takes an additional 8–12 hours at least. Therefore, if an item can be steam sterilized, this is the method of choice.

Tasks in the Preparation of Supplies

DECONTAMINATION

Adequate cleaning is basic to sterilization and disinfection. This cleaning can be accomplished by machine, by hand, or a combination of the two. For contaminated items that will tolerate immersion in water and exposure to high temperatures (132°C, 270°F), the automatic washer/sterilizer is the method of choice for initial decontamination. This machine combines a short wash cycle that soaks the items in detergent and water, rinses, and then exposes them to steam under pressure at 132°C (270°F) for three minutes.

Some operating rooms have washer/sterilizers opening directly into them, built into the wall, or have access to a washer/sterilizer in a substerile room. This arrangement is good for the immediate decontamination of instruments and utensils. Some institutions, however, have developed the practice of considering the instruments sterile after this process and immediately reuse the instruments in the next surgical procedure in the adjacent room. This is a dangerous practice because the wash cycle in a washer/sterilizer may not remove all debris that could shield microorganisms, and the steam-under-pressure cycle may be too short to produce sterility at the 10^{-6} assurance level. Items processed in a washer/sterilizer should be hand inspected and cleaned further if necessary before being sterilized for the next patient.

Hospitals that have centralized instrument processing may have large tunnel washer/sterilizers that load from the dirty or decontamination area of central processing and automatically empty into the clean area. Not all of these tunnel apparatuses are washer/sterilizers. Some may be washer/sterilizers that substitute a short exposure to water at 71–82°C (160–180°F) for the steam under pressure exposure at 132°C. This equipment is an effective decontamination method for many items used in patient care. Grossly soiled surgical instruments and utensils, however, should be processed through a washer/sterilizer for decontamination.

Some hospitals have neither device available, and some items will not tolerate immersion or high temperatures. Handwashing is an acceptable alternative for decontamination, providing it is done conscientiously by trained workers wearing appropriate attire. As a minimum, anyone doing handwashing of items used in surgery should be wearing rubber gloves (not necessarily surgeons' gloves), eye protection, and a water-proof apron. Some institutions also require a mask, hair covering, and rubber boots. All these items protect the worker from splashes and spills of contaminated waters. To reduce the risk of splashing and the creation of aerosols, the item being cleaned should be held low in the sink or basin being used. If a brush is used, it should be kept under water when in use. Items should be cleaned with a solution of water and an appropriate detergent-germicide. The concentration should be mixed according to the detergent manufacturer's instructions. Careful selection of all cleaning agents is important so that maximum microbicidal effect can be achieved without harm to the item. In general, it is best to avoid extremes in pH of cleaning solutions, especially when cleaning stainless steel or other metal hand-held surgical instruments. A pH of between 5 and 10 is generally satisfactory. Very acidic or alkaline solutions can damage the inert passivation layer that keeps the instruments from corroding through multiple uses and may react with the metal itself to produce damage.

Sometimes, after washer/sterilizer decontamination, inspection reveals that the instruments or other items are still dirty. The box-lock portions of ring-handled instruments are especially prone to this. Further handwashing may be necessary before the item is ready for resterilization and reuse. Neglecting this important inspection step may allow the buildup of debris that may eventually interfere with the function of the instrument or other device.

An alternative to hand inspection and further hand cleaning for surgical instruments is the ultrasonic cleaner. This machine uses high-frequency sound waves to dislodge debris from the surface of objects. When combined with an appropriate detergent, it is an excellent adjunct to the washer/sterilizer and produces clean instrumentation. However, ultrasound has no microbicidal properties and the ultrasonic should be used only after processing instruments through the washer/sterilizer or otherwise decontaminating the instruments. After cleaning in the ultrasonic, instruments should be rinsed to remove the loose debris. Otherwise the material will once again adhere to the instruments. Not all surgical instruments can be placed in the ultrasonic. Some manufacturers of microsurgical instruments advise against it. Likewise instruments with telescopic lenses should not be placed in the ultrasonic.

The care of endoscopes is different from that of other types of surgical instrumentation. This is especially true of flexible fiberoptic endoscopes. As with all other devices, these instruments must be thoroughly cleaned, rinsed, and dried prior to disinfection or sterilization. The endoscope manufacturer should be consulted for recommended care, and the same personnel should perform the task to avoid damage to these expensive instruments. Many of the accessories for the telescopic piece can be washed and steam sterilized. Because some of the accessories, especially those for flexible scopes, have very fine springs, extra care is needed in washing and inspecting prior to disinfection or sterilization.

PACKAGING

The second step in sterilization and disinfection is packaging the material, if necessary. Items that are going to be disinfected by

chemicals do not require packaging. All items undergoing sterilization, however, require some type of packaging, whether the items are actually wrapped or are sterilized in an open pan. The packaging selected must be appropriate to the sterilization method and to the conditions of storage and handling that the item will undergo prior to patient care use.

Packaging used for steam sterilization must allow rapid penetration of steam and rapid air removal. For surgical instruments, packaging begins with selection of an appropriately sized tray with holes in the bottom to allow for steam and air movement. Next, thought should be given to how the items will be arranged in the tray and how they will be kept in order. Heavy items should be on the bottom or separate from more delicate items. There are many devices on the market to hold, string, clip, or arrange surgical instruments in a specific order, even if the tray is tipped. These can save effort and avoid exasperation on the part of the scrub person asked to set up for the next procedure in five minutes or less. Some institutions line the bottom of the instrument tray with a woven fabric towel or other highly absorbent material before beginning to place the instruments. This helps to absorb condensate formed on the instruments during the steam sterilization cycle and speeds drying. Instrument pans or trays should weigh no more than 16 pounds when full. Exceeding this weight concentrates too much metal mass, which can act as a heat sink during the early stages of the sterilization cycle and interfere with the sterilization process.

Pans, basin sets, or other items that can be nested should have a layer of porous material between each closely nested layer to facilitate steam penetration. Endoscopes that can be steam sterilized and some microsurgery instruments come with special packaging containers to prevent dislodging or inadvertent crushing should a heavier object be placed on top of the delicate item.

Textiles and small items require no tray or pan for steam sterilization. Textiles are folded so that they are ready to use, that is, gowns are folded with the inside out so they can be donned without contamination. Bundles containing several different items are arranged in the order of use, and the warp direction of one item is placed perpendicular to the warp of the next item to facilitate steam penetration and air removal.

Textile bundles must measure no more than 12-×-12-×-20 inches and weigh no more than 12 pounds. The maximum density of the pack should be no more than 7.2 pounds per cubic foot. If these measurements are exceeded, steam may have difficulty penetrating the pack, air may be trapped, and sterilization failure can result.

Wrappers used for steam sterilization may be woven or nonwoven disposables. If a woven reusable textile is chosen, it should have a thread count higher than 140 threads per inch. Cotton muslin is not an acceptable textile for use as a wrapper or aseptic barrier. The textile material may be treated with a chemical that renders it highly resistant to liquid penetration, also known as strike-through.

There are many types of nonwoven disposable flat wrappers and peel-open type pouches available today. Whatever the outwrap chosen, it should be permeable to steam and resist tearing and puncture. If seals are involved, they should not reseal once opened so that tampering or damage can be detected. The wrapper must be resistant to penetration by airborne bacteria and dust. It should have minimal or no lint, and ideally, if not totally impervious to liquid penetration, the material should discolor or otherwise indicate that it has been inadvertently wet and therefore contaminated, since liquid penetration carries microorganisms with it. The material should be in ready supply, and the cost should be in line with the item's perceived value to the institution.

Packaging items for ethylene oxide sterilization is not much different than for steam except that trays are seldom used except to contain items like endoscopes or power tool parts. The wrapping material must be ethylene oxide compatible and must allow gas penetration and elution. Nylon and aluminum foil are not acceptable. Selection of packaging material involves the same parameters and desirable characteristics discussed under steam sterilization.

For dry heat sterilization, packaging materials should be selected that will not be damaged by high heat—160°C (320°F)—for long periods of time. This usually means metal or glass only. Textiles should be avoided since they will char and burn.

STERILIZATION PROCESS

The third step in the preparation of supplies is the actual sterilization or disinfection process. There are four methods of sterilization commonly used in hospitals and other health care institutions: steam under pressure, ethylene oxide, dry heat, and liquid chemical. A fifth type of sterilization widely used in industry for medical devices is irradiation. There are two common methods of disinfection used in hospitals: liquid chemical and pasteurization. Each of these will be briefly discussed from the point of view of what the nurse needs to know to carry out the care of the surgical patient.

Steam Sterilization

This involves the use of saturated steam under pressure so that the temperature of the steam in the closed sterilized chamber will rise. It is the synergistic action of the moisture and temperature on the microorganism that produces death through coagulation of protein. Direct contact with the steam is needed to produce assured sterility. Thus, any items with ratchets or with removable parts should be processed in the open or disassembled position. While some vegetative bacteria might be killed just through dry heating at the temperatures involved with steam sterilization, others, and certainly bacterial spores, might survive without the synergy of the water and heat at points where metal is tightly approximated to metal, as in a closed hemostat.

There are two basic types of steam sterilizers, commonly referred to as "autoclaves." The first of these is the gravity displacement sterilizer. This type of unit relies on gravity to remove air, which is heavier than steam, from the sterilizer load to allow steam penetration. Saturated steam does not mix with air and air acts as an insulator to prevent the heating and moisture contact necessary for sterilization. Thus, items placed in a gravity displacement sterilizer must be loaded in such a way as to aid air removal. Textile drape bundles or other bulky porous packages are placed on end or on their side. Basin sets or any other item that could hold water are placed so that any water runs out. Once the cycle begins, the air will "run out" as if it were water. Packs containing metal are not placed above textile packs because condensation at the end of the cycle when the door is opened could drip onto and contaminate the textile packs. The entire chamber cannot be overloaded or air will remain trapped in some packages, resulting in sterilization failure.

Once the chamber is loaded, the door is closed and the chamber becomes a pressure vessel. Steam enters the chamber through the upper rear and hits a baffle that disperses it. As steam enters, it displaces the heavier air, which exits through a drain in the bottom front of the chamber near the door. In this drain, there is a temperature sensor reflected in a temperature gauge at the front of the sterilizer. There is also a gauge that registers the pressure inside the chamber. As steam continues to enter, all of the air is eventually forced out, if the load is properly arranged. The pressure and the temperature gauges continue to rise. The pressure is necessary to raise the temperature of the steam vapor. At sea level, saturated steam under 15 pounds per square inch pressure according to the gauge (psig), which measures the pressure above the ambient atmospheric pressure, will have a temperature of 121°C (250°F).

Commercially available steam sterilizers, by common convention, are set to run at either 121°C or 132°C. At 132°C, the pressure gauge at sea level should read 27 psig. Atmospheric pressure decreases with altitude. To compensate for the lower initial gauge setting, the maximum gauge reading must be increased by 0.5 psig for every 1,000 feet of altitude above sea level. Thus a steam sterilizer running at 132°C in Denver (altitude 5,280 feet) must have a pressure gauge reading of 29.5 psig to reach the desired temperature.

The second type of steam sterilizer speeds up the evacuation of air by drawing a partial vacuum in the chamber at the beginning of the cycle, which removes the air. This type of steam sterilizer, known as a "hivac" (high prevacuum), is slightly more forgiving of errors in loading some items, but the same rules should be used. In both types of sterilizers, the sterilization cycle has the same elements: the come up time, during which air is eliminated and steam penetrates the load; the holding time, which is the period necessary to assure lethality at the 10^{-6} level; and the come down time, which involves the reintroduction of air to the load. If the load contains wrapped articles, a drying time is added onto these before the door can be opened.

Articles can be processed either wrapped or unwrapped in either type of sterilizer at either temperature. Unwrapped articles are most commonly sterilized in the gravity displacement type at 132°C (270°F). This is referred to as a "flash," or emergency, sterilization. It is frequently used for items needed suddenly but not sterile or for instruments that are dropped or otherwise contaminated. Cleaning of these instruments is necessary if sterilization is to occur. In the past, prosthetic devices, such as orthopedic implants, were often "flash" sterilized. Although the practice is still widespread, this is now discouraged because of the short holding time. Cycle duration for steam sterilization varies with temperature and with the type of air evacuation used. The come up time for the hivac or prevacuum sterilizer is almost instantaneous (see Table 13.3).

The advantages of steam sterilization are that it is inexpensive, usually readily available, reliable, free of toxic residue, generally safe to use, and fast. The disadvantage of steam sterilization is that not all items can tolerate the high moisture, pressure, and temperature necessary.

Steam sterilization is monitored by periodically placing a special pack containing textiles and meeting the 12-×-12-×-20-inch limit, in the bottom front of the sterilizer. This pack also will contain dried, live bacterial spores of the *Bacillus stearothermophilus* species, in a known concentration. Commercially available spore strips or vials are usually used. This particular species has demonstrated high resistance to destruction by heat. The pack is run through an appropriate sterilization cycle for the type of

Table 13.3. Time/Temperature Relationships for Steam Sterilization.

Type of Sterilizer	Temperature	Load	Exposure Time (minutes)
Gravity displacement	121°C (250°F)	wrapped, mixed	15 plus drying time
	132°C (270°F)	unwrapped, nonporous only	3
		unwrapped, some porous	10
		wrapped	10 plus drying time
Hivac	132°C (270°F)	unwrapped	4
		wrapped	4 plus drying time

sterilizer and the temperature selected. The spore strip or vial is retrieved under aseptic conditions and incubated along with a non-exposed control strip or vial from the same lot number, according to the biological indicator manufacturer's instructions. It should be noted that *B. stearothermophilus* likes high temperatures and should not be incubated in the customary 37°C (98.6°F) clinical incubator. The sterilization cycle is said to be efficacious if there is no growth of *B. stearothermophilus* in the test culture and in the control. The first, presumptive reading is usually done at 24–48 hours incubation. However, 7–10 days may be necessary to make sure there is no growth since some spores may be alive but slow to recover. Biological monitoring is recommended at least once a week for every steam sterilizer and in each load containing implantable devices.

In addition to biological indicators, there are other process controls often used with steam sterilizers. These include a recording chart that registers maximum temperature and duration for each cycle. That chart is usually on the upper front of the sterilizer and requires frequent changing of the chart paper. Various chemical indicators are also used to monitor temperature, moisture, and time. Not all indicators measure all parameters, and not all indicators are equally accurate. It is important to read the instructions that come with the indicator and be familiar with the color changes or other indications to be expected. With some chemical indicators, it takes a great deal of practice to produce reliable readings.

Hivac sterilizers are checked daily with a Bowie-Dick type test for adequate vacuum for air removal. There are commercially available sheets with various patterns of heat-sensitive ink on them. The sheet is contained in a specially constructed pack of woven fabric towels placed in the center of an otherwise empty sterilizer. The object of the test is to check for uniformity of color change on the test sheet. Lack of uniformity indicates a problem with the vacuum portion of the cycle. The Bowie-Dick type test does not in any way measure sterility and should not be confused with chemical indicators that measure one or more of the conditions necessary for sterilization to occur.

Ethylene Oxide (EO)Sterilization
This involves the use of the highly poisonous gas under controlled circumstances to produce microbial death. EO sterilizers may resemble the pressure vessels used for steam, or they may be as simple as a cannister with an ampule of EO. EO sterilization generally occurs at temperatures ranging from room temperature to about 60°C (140°F). Four interrelated parameters are necessary to produce sterility using EO: gas concentration, temperature, relative humidity of 30–50 percent, and time. Temperature is inversely related to time, so the lower the temperature, the longer the exposure time needed. Gas concentration varies with the type of sterilizer used and also has an impact on the exposure time. Adequate relative humidity in the load is vital since dessicated organisms can

be highly resistant to EO penetration of the cell wall or cellular membrane. Because of the great variety of sizes and types of EO sterilizers available and the lack of standardization, it is not possible to give time guidelines for the sterilization cycle using EO. Manufacturers' instructions should be followed.

Precautions must be taken when using EO because it is a highly toxic gas that can pollute the working environment. EO also leaves residuals in the products sterilized. These can be harmful. The current Occupational Safety and Health Agency (OSHA) limit for exposure to EO is 50 parts per million (ppm) as an average exposure over an eight-hour period. Recent studies have indicated that the limit is too high. Long-term inhalation and skin exposure to 50 ppm have been implicated as being dangerous to human health and reproductive ability. The limit is currently under review but a lower standard has not been set either for industrial workers using EO as a raw material in plastic manufacture or for workers using EO as a sterilant in industry and hospitals.

Worker exposure during EO sterilization can occur at two times. If the gas is not properly vented directly to the outside or to a sanitary sewer through a separator, exposure may occur when EO is eliminated from the sterilizer chamber. If there is not a continuous fresh filtered air purge cycle in the sterilizer unit, exposure may occur when the sterilizer is opened. Many hospitals are now retrofitting EO sterilization equipment with dedicated exhaust ventilation systems to reduce worker exposure to a safer level. To minimize exposure when opening an EO sterilizer, it is important to follow the manufacturer's instructions closely. These units differ greatly in determining when the lowest possible concentration in the chamber is reached and in what direction the gas will exit the chamber, which depends on its temperature relative to the ambient temperature in the room.

The threshold for human detection of the odor of EO is approximately 700 ppm. If a nurse smells a strange odor around the EO sterilizer or aerator, she should leave the area immediately and report the smell to appropriate administrative officials with her suspicions as to its source.

Because EO penetrates all porous materials and time is required for the EO to dissipate, all items sterilized by EO must be aerated before use. The method of choice is to use a filtered, heated forced air aeration cabinet vented directly to the outside atmosphere. The length of aeration time necessary depends on the nature and composition of the material being sterilized and the type of packaging material used. The manufacturer of the device being sterilized as well as the manufacturer of the sterilizer and aerator can be consulted for guidance. In general, polyvinyl chloride is very resistant to the elution of EO and, therefore, is used as the benchmark for aeration times. For polyvinyl chloride:

Type	Temperature	Time
Forced air	60°C (140°F)	8 hours
cabinet	50°C (122°F)	12 hours
Open shelf in	Ambient room	7 days
separate room	temperature	

Other materials may require less or more aeration time.

If an aeration cabinet is used, the aeration chamber should not be opened until aeration for all items is complete. To do otherwise may expose the person opening the cabinet to unsafe concentrations of EO. If some items require brief aeration and some require longer aeration, ideally they should be separated and sterilized in different loads and aerated in different units. Sorting an EO sterilized load after the sterilization cycle can expose the worker to high levels of EO. If more than one aeration cabinet is available, one alternative is to arrange the load by aeration time, putting each aerator load in a separate metal basket or tray that can be quickly picked up and moved to the appropriate aerator without handling each package.

There may be times when a physician insists on retrieval of an instrument or device that is not fully aerated or is in a load that is not fully aerated. This request should not be honored unless everyone involved, with full knowledge and consent, believes that the risk to a patient of not having the device is worth the risk to the worker who must retrieve the device. Hospitals have a responsibility to both patients and personnel to make sure that there is a sufficient supply of such critical devices so that this situation does not arise.

In addition to the EO itself as a toxic residue, two other chemicals can also form during the sterilization process. Both are toxic and neither is diminished by aeration. Ethylene glycol forms when EO contacts water. Ethylchlorhydrin forms when EO contacts water and available chloride ions. The key to preventing the formation of both byproducts is the elimination of free-standing water from the load. Thus all items placed in an EO sterilizer should be dried so that no visible water droplets are present before the item is packaged.

EO is an effective sterilant for medical devices. Items must be clean prior to sterilization because dried crystalline debris can effectively block the penetration of EO and allow even vegetative organisms to survive.

The efficacy of the EO sterilization process is monitored using live spores of the species *Bacillus subtilis* or *B. globigii*, which have demonstrated resistance to EO, although there are contaminants with suspected greater resistance. As with steam sterilization, the biological indicator is run in a regular load and then incubated and compared to a nonexposed control. Because of the high degree of possible variability in conditions within the EO sterilizer, each load of an EO sterilizer should be monitored.

Chemical process indicators for EO are available but they have not yet reached the sophistication of some indicators available for steam. Development is taking place in this area.

Dry Heat Sterilization

This is seldom used now in hospitals except in the laboratory for glassware. Dry heat at temperatures of 160°C (320°F) will produce microbial death by incineration in approximately two hours after the item reaches the required temperature. Dry heat sterilization is the method of choice for powders and oils that cannot be sterilized by steam or retain EO or its byproducts, if these items must be sterilized by the hospitals. Most powders and oils that might be required are commercially available in a sterile state.

Chemical Sterilization

Some chemicals that can produce high-level disinfection are capable of sterilization. They are sporicidal if the exposure time is greatly extended. For instance, 2 percent alkaline glutaraldehyde will produce sterility in 10 hours. Obviously, this requires immersion of the clean, dry device in the chemical for an extended length of time. Few devices will tolerate extended immersion and frequent repetitions. In addition, the object must be thoroughly rinsed to remove any residue of the chemical sterilant, and then moved to the point of use without contaminating it. This is difficult to do. Also, chemical sterilization is expensive. Both steam and EO sterilization should be considered before deciding upon chemical sterilization. Furthermore, there is no means of testing the efficacy of the process without destruction or contamination of the item being sterilized. There are no biological or chemical indicators for liquid chemical sterilization or disinfection.

Radiation Sterilization

This is used widely in the medical device industry but is not currently used in hospitals in this country. Briefly, radiation sterilization involves the use of gamma ray or electron beam radiation exposure of a product, its package, and usually shipping container for a specific amount of time so that a carefully calculated dose of radiation is administered. The necessary dose may be determined by minimal government standards and a careful analysis of the known bioburden of the product at the conclusion of manufacture and packaging. The sterile medical device industry maintains careful control and records of the personnel and environment involved in the manufacture of medical devices. They use protective clothing, special air-handling systems, traffic regulation, and personnel monitoring to control bioburden much more effectively than can be done in the diverse hospital environment. Thus, exact computations of bioburden are possible in industry. The radiation passes right through the entire product, killing organisms through alteration and interference with metabolism and nucleic acid synthesis. Radiation sterilization leaves no radioactive residue. Not all materials can withstand radiation sterilization because the process may alter chemical structure.

So much is known about the response of certain materials to radiation that some of these substances are used as dosimeters to measure the amount of radiation received by the load. Thus, although biological indicators may be run, the product is released for sale based on the dosimetry readings before any biological monitoring could be read.

Radiation sterilization requires special physical facilities and a large degree of technical support. Because of the high cost of initiating a sterilization facility, radiation sterilization is not likely to be used by hospitals.

DISINFECTION PROCESS

Not all items require sterilization prior to use. Some procedures performed in the operating room do not require sterile instruments, but rather, only disinfected instruments. These procedures usually involve entry through a body orifice, such as the mouth or vagina, that cannot be washed and prepared in the same vigorous manner as intact skin. Thus, the operative area remains grossly contaminated with the patient's own organisms. The general principles of asepsis are still applied in these procedures to minimize the introduction of exogenous microorganisms. However, because the body's defense mechanisms are less altered in these procedures than in procedures involving incision through the skin, high-level disinfection is considered adequate preparation for smooth, hard surface devices that can readily be cleaned, such as endoscopes.

Anesthesia and respiratory therapy devices may be a source of cross contamination if the devices are reused for several patients. The microorganisms of concern here are vegetative bacteria, fungi, and some viruses, but not bacterial spores. Therefore, cleaning followed by high-level disinfection between each patient use should be adequate protection.

Chemical Disinfection

This involves immersing the clean, dry item in a solution that will produce microbial death in a reasonable period of time. The U.S. Environmental Protection Agency (EPA) requires manufacturers who make sterilization or disinfection claims for their products to register with the EPA and submit data in support of these claims. If found acceptable, the product will be given a registration number as a sterilant, a disinfectant, or both. This number is to be displayed on the product label. When selecting a chemical disinfectant, look for the EPA registration number and read the label claims carefully to make certain that it is a high-level disinfectant that will kill everything but bacterial spores.

The most commonly used chemical disinfectant is a 2 percent solution of glutaraldehyde; a phenolic combination that has a glutaraldehyde concentration of 0.1 percent when diluted for disinfection is also acceptable. Halogenated compounds such as sodium hypochlorite (household bleach) are also effective if used in the proper concentration as are some iodophors. Quaternary ammonium compounds are not acceptable high-level disinfectants and should not be used.

Even though these solutions may produce disinfection, all chemicals are not safe for all devices. For instance, soaking stainless steel instrumentation in sodium hypochlorite will damage the surface of the instrument. Therefore, manufacturers' recommendations should be followed in selecting chemical disinfectants. Precautions and contraindications on the disinfectant label should be read to determine if the solution is compatible with the type of device to be disinfected.

Chemical disinfection usually takes 10–30 minutes of soaking. Much longer periods are required for sterilization. Some people refer to the short exposure period as "cold sterilization," but this is a misuse of the term sterilization.

As with all other processes, disinfection requires that instruments or other devices must be clean before immersion. Chemicals require direct contact to kill, and dirt and organic debris can effectively shield microorganisms from the effects of the disinfectant. Devices should also be dry when placed in the disinfectant to avoid further dilution of the chemical by the addition of water.

After the appropriate soaking time has elapsed, the device must be adequately rinsed. Sterile distilled water should be used to avoid reintroducing microorganisms such as those found in tap water. Merely dipping the instrument in a basin of water may not be adequate rinsing, especially if the device has a lumen. Disinfectants are potentially toxic chemicals, and any residue left on the instrument may cause injury to the patient's tissues when the device is used. If the device is not going to be used immediately, it should be dried thoroughly prior to storage. Water in lumens or on the surface can be a suitable environment for bacterial growth over several hours.

Reusable devices should be washed and disinfected immediately after each use to minimize the possibility of environmental contamination. If a device will not be immediately reused and will be stored for more than a few hours, it should be disinfected again prior to use, if the procedure calls for high-level disinfection. This is because bacterial spores not killed by the chemical could return to the vegetative state and multiply during this interim. Also, it is difficult to package and store an item aseptically after disinfection with any degree of assurance that no contamination occurred during the drying and wrapping process.

Physical Disinfection
This involves boiling or pasteurization. Boiling is seldom used, because if an item can tolerate that temperature and moisture level, steam sterilization is a better option. Pasteurization is the process of heating the device in water, to temperatures at or above 71°C (160°F) and holding the device there for a period of time, depending on the temperature, but usually 15–30 minutes. The process is modeled after that used to treat milk or other liquid foods. It kills vegetative bacteria, the tubercle bacillus,

some viruses, and some fungi. It is not truly high-level disinfection, but more accurately, intermediate level. The process is suitable for some respiratory therapy devices and anesthesia masks and tubing that do not directly penetrate deep into the airway. Special equipment is used to accomplish pasteurization. Since the process involves nothing but heated water, no rinsing is necessary, but items must be dried before storage in a manner that will not recontaminate them. There are forced air heated cabinets for this purpose.

HANDLING AND STORAGE

Although disinfected items cannot be stored for any length of time and still be considered free of everything but bacterial spores, wrapped materials that have been sterilized are stored for long periods of time and still considered sterile. The safe storage of sterile items depends on four factors: whether or not the item was sterile initially; the type of wrapper or barrier used; the amount and type of handling the product receives after sterilization; and the actual conditions of storage. The first factor is obvious but often forgotten. The second factor, the wrapper, deserves discussion. A package wrapper should be resistant to contamination from any condition it may encounter during the handling and storage process. This may include airborne contamination through passive settling of particles. If the package may encounter rough handling, the wrap or packaging should resist tearing and the entry of airborne organisms through forced compression and release. If the item may encounter moisture, even as little as the perspiration of workers' hands, the wrapper should be resistant to this.

There is no one type of wrapper or packaging that suits all needs and conditions. The more controlled the handling and storage process, the less concern for the wrapper. Most hospitals, however, do not have well controlled processes that strictly monitor the number of times an item is subjected to events that might cause contamination. As a general rule, a sterile package should be handled as few times as absolutely necessary between sterilization and use. Everyone handling or transporting the package must be aware of any condition that might lead to contamination. If such a condition is encountered, the package should be regarded as of doubtful sterility and not used.

Storage of sterile items that will be longer than one or two days should be in closed cabinets to minimize dust accumulation. If open shelf storage is used, the packaging material should be resistant to dust penetration and be capable of having any dust accumulation removed before the package is opened. Otherwise, dust from the surface of the package can contaminate the package contents during opening.

Wire mesh shelves are preferred to solid shelves to minimize dust accumulation. Shelving should be at least 10 inches from the floor to prevent splashing during cleaning. If open shelving is used, the shelves should be at least 2 inches from the wall and 18 inches from the top of items to the ceiling to allow for adequate air circulation. Sterile items should be stored separately from clean items and away from soiled or used items.

There are no standard answers for the shelf life of a particular item. Shelf life is the result of the interrelationship of the four conditions identified earlier. A sterile item can be contaminated at any point after the opening of the sterilization chamber. Only planning and awareness by all personnel involved can guarantee delivery of sterile items at the moment when needed for patient care. Each institution must set its own guidelines for shelf-life duration both for products sterilized within the institution and for those purchased sterile, based on the conditions existing in that facility. A package that is sterilized and wrapped in a sealed impervious wrapper will remain sterile forever if the package is not damaged or opened. Shelf life is event related, not time related.

The preparation of supplies for use in surgery involves careful attention to the following tasks: cleaning, packaging, sterilization or disinfection, and handling and storage. Inadequate care in any process invalidates the whole sequence. The nurse working in the operating room must work with other health care personnel involved in these tasks, sharing responsibility and accountability with them for the ultimate delivery of products that are safe for the patient and will further the goal of freedom from infection.

References

1. Centers for Disease Control. "Cleaning, disinfection and sterilization of hospital equipment." In: *Guidelines for the Prevention and Control of Nosocomial Infections*. Atlanta: Centers for Disease Control, 1980.

2. Centers for Disease Control. "Disposal of solid wastes from hospitals." In: *National Nosocomial Infections Study Report 1974*. Atlanta: Centers for Disease Control, 1977.

3. Centers for Disease Control. "Antiseptics, handwashing, and handwashing facilities." In: *Guidelines for the Prevention and Control of Nosocomial Infections*. Atlanta: Centers for Disease Control, 1980.

4. Centers for Disease Control. "Guideline for isolation precautions in hospitals." In: *Guidelines for Prevention and Control of Nosocomial Infections*. Atlanta: Centers for Disease Control, 1983.

5. Centers for Disease Control. "Guideline for prevention of catheter-associated urinary tract infections." In: *Guidelines for the Prevention and Control of Nosocomial Infections*. Atlanta: Centers for Disease Control, 1980.

6. Centers for Disease Control. "Guidelines for prevention of intravascular infections." In: *Guidelines for Prevention and Control of Nosocomial Infections*. Atlanta: Centers for Disease Control, 1981.

7. Centers for Disease Control. "Guideline for prevention of nosocomial pneumonia." In: *Guidelines for Prevention and Control of Nosocomial Infections*. Atlanta: Centers for Disease Control, 1982.

8. Haley, R. W., Hooton, T. M., Culver, D. H., et al. "Nosocomial infections in U.S. hospitals, 1975–1976. Estimated frequency by selected characteristics of patients." *Am J Med* 70:947–959, 1981.

9. Allen, J. R., Hightower, A. W., Martin, S. M., and Dixon, R. W. "Secular trends in nosocomial infections: 1970–1979." *Am J Med* 70:389–392, 1981.

10. Howard, J. M., Barker, W. F., Culbertson, W. R., et al. "Postoperative wound infections. The influence of ultraviolet irradiation of the operating room and various other factors." *Ann Surg* 160(suppl):1–192, 1964.

11. American College of Surgeons Committee on Control of Surgical Infections. *Manual on Control of Infections in Surgical Patients*. Philadelphia: J. B. Lippincott, 1976.

12. Cruse, P. J. E., and Foord, R. "The epidemiology of wound infection. A ten-year prospective study of 62,939 wounds." *Surg Clin North Am* 60:27–40, 1980.

13. Brachman, P. S., Dan, B. B., Haley, R. W., Hooten, T. M., Garner, J. S., and Allen, J. R. "Nosocomial surgical infections: Incidence and cost." *Surg Clin North Am* 60:15–25, 1980.

14. Laufman, H. "The operating room." In: Bennett, J. V., and Brachman, P. S., eds. *Hospital Infections*, pp. 129–136. Boston: Little, Brown and Co., 1979.

15. Lange, K. "AORN standards for OR sanitation." *AORN J* 21:1223–1231, 1975.

16. Mallison, G. F. "Housekeeping in operating suites." *AORN J* 21:313, 1975.

17. Gardner, A. M. N, Stamp, M., Bowgen, J. A., and Moore, B. "The infection control sister." *Lancet* 2:710–711, 1962.

18. Wenzel, K. "The role of the infection control nurse." *Nurs Clin North Am* 5(1):89–98, 1970.

19. Moore, B. "The infection control sister in British hospitals." *Int Nurs Rev* 17:84–92, 1970.

20. Garner, J. S., Bennett, J. V., Scheckler, W. E., Maki, D. G. and Brachman, P. S. "Surveillance of nosocomial infections." In: *Proceedings of the International Conference on Nosocomial Infections*, Center for Disease Control, August 3–6, 1970, pp. 177–181. Chicago: American Hospital Association, 1971.

21. Emori, T. G., Haley, R. W., and Stanley, R. C. "The infection control nurse in U.S. hospitals, 1976–1977." *Am J Epidemiol* 111:592–607, 1980.

22. Emori, T. G., Haley, R. W., and Garner, J. S. "Techniques and uses of nosocomial infection surveillance in U.S. hospitals, 1976–1977." *Am J Med* 70:933–940, 1981.

23. Kaslow, R. A., and Garner, J. S. "Hospital personnel." In: Bennett, J. V., Brachman, P. S., eds. *Hospital Infections*, pp. 27–52. Boston: Little, Brown and Co., 1979.

24. Garner, J. S., Dixon, R. E., and Aber, R. C. "Epidemic infections in surgical patients." *AORN J* 34:700–724, 1981.

25. Haley, R. W., and Schachtman, F. H. "The emergence of infection surveillance and control programs in U.S. hospitals: an assessment, 1976." *Am J Epidemiol* 111:574–591, 1980.

26. Center for Disease Control. "Guideline for prevention of surgical wound infections." In: *Guidelines for Prevention and Control of Nasocomial Infections*. Atlanta: Centers for Disease Control, 1982.

27. Spaulding, E. H., et al. "Chemical disinfection of medical and surgical materials." In: S. Block, ed. *Disinfection, Sterilization and Preservation*, pp. 654–682. Philadelphia: Lea and Febiger, 1977.

Suggested Readings

American Society of Hospital Central Service Personnel. *Ethylene Oxide in Hospitals: A Manual for Health Care Personnel*. Chicago: American Hospital Association, 1982.

Association of Operating Room Nurses. "Guidelines for cleaning and disinfection of flexible fiberoptic endoscopes (FFE) used in GI endoscopy." *AORN J* 30(November):907–910, 1978.

Association of Operating Room Nurses. "Guidelines for preparation of laparoscopic instrumentation." *AORN J* 32(July):65, 1980.

Association of Operating Room Nurses. "Proposed recommended practices for OR sanitation." *AORN J* 33(June):126, 1981.

Association of Operating Room Nurses. "Recommended practices for inhospital sterilization." *AORN J* 32(August):222, 1980.

Association of Operating Room Nurses. "Recommended practices for traffic patterns in the surgical suite." *AORN J* 35(March):750, 1982.

Association of Operating Room Nurses. *AORN Standards of Practice*. Part III: *Standards of Technical and Aseptic Practice, OR*. Denver: Association of Operating Room Nurses, 1978.

Beck, W. C. "Guest editorial: Asepsis, super asepsis, and ultra asepsis." *Am Surg* 42(April):227, 1976.

Beck, W. C. "The open door in the operating room." *Am J Surg* 125(May):594, 1973.

Bennett, J. V., and Brachman, P. S., eds. *Hospital Infections*. Boston: Little, Brown and Co., 1979.

Burke, J. F. "Host defects caused by surgical operation." In: J. F. Burke and G. Y. Hildick-Smith, eds. *The Infection-Prone Hospital Patient*, pp. 175–182. Boston: Little, Brown and Co., 1978.

Centers for Disease Control. "Cleaning, disinfection and sterilization of hospital equipment." In: *Guidelines for the Prevention and Control of Nosocomial Infections*, p. 7. Atlanta: Centers for Disease Control, 1981.

Corson, S. L., et al. "Sterilization of laparoscopes: Is soaking sufficient?" *J Repro Med* 23(August):51–55, 1979.

Ernst, R. R. "Sterilization by heat." In: Seymour

Block, ed. *Disinfection. Sterilization and Preservation*, pp. 592–602. Philadelphia: Lea and Febiger, 1977.

Glaser, Z. R. *Special Occupational Hazard Review with Recommendations for the Use of Ethylene Oxide as a Sterilant in Medical Facilities.* Rockville, MD: U.S. Department of Health, Education and Welfare, 1977.

Good Hospital Practice: Ethylene Oxide Gas-Ventilation Recommendations and Safe Use. Arlington, Va: AAMI, 1981.

Good Hospital Practice: Steam Sterilization and Sterility Assurance. Arlington, Va: AAMI, 1980.

Hargiss, Co. "The patient's environment: Haven or hazard?" *Nurs Clin North Am* 14(December):671–688, 1980.

Harris, W. H. "The etiology and prevention of deep wound infection following total hip replacement." In: J. F. Burke and G. Y. Hildick-Smith, eds. *The Infection-Prone Hospital Patient*, pp. 183–192. Boston: Little, Brown and Co., 1978.

Infection Control in the Hospital, 4th ed., pp. 103–122. Chicago: AHA, 1979.

Karki, M., and Mayer, C. "Assessing reuse of disposables: An interdisciplinary challenge for the 1980s. *Med Instru* 15(May-June):153–156, 1981.

Laufman, H. "Air handling in operating rooms." In Laufman, H., ed. *Hospital Special Care Facilities*, pp. 157–167. New York: Academic Press, 1981.

Laufman, H. "The control of operating room infections: Discipline, defense mechanisms, drugs, design and devices." *Bull NY Acad Med* 54(May):465–483, 1978.

Litsky, B. Y. "Microbiology and postoperative infections." *AORN J* 19(January):37–52, 1974.

Minimum Requirements of Construction and Equipment for Hospital and Medical Facilities. Washington, D.C.: U.S. Department of Health, Education and Welfare Publication No. (HRA) 79-14500, 1978.

Perkins, J. J. *Principles and Methods of Sterilization in Health Sciences*, 2nd ed. Springfield, Ill.: Charles C Thomas, 1969.

Pflug, I. J., and Holcomb, R. G., "Principles of thermal destruction of microorganisms." In: S. Block, ed. *Disinfection, Sterilization, and Preservation*, pp. 933–994. Philadelphia: Lea and Febiger, 1977.

Phillips, C. R. "Gaseous sterilization." In: S. Block, ed. *Disinfection, Sterilization, and Preservation*, pp. 592–602. Philadelphia: Lea and Febiger, 1977.

Polk, H. C., and Stone, H. H. *Hospital-Acquired Infections in Surgery.* Baltimore: University Park Press, 1977.

Ritter, M. A., et al. "The operating room environment as affected by people and the surgical face mask." *Clin Ortho* 3(September):147–150, 1975.

Ryan, P. "Basics of packaging." *AORN J* 21(May 1975):1091–1112.

Schultz, J. "Traffic and commerce in the surgical suite." In Laufman, H., ed. *Hospital Special Care Facilities*, pp. 233–242. New York: Academic Press, 1981.

Silverman, G. J., and Sinskey, A. J. "Sterilization by ionizing irradiation." In S. Block, ed. *Disinfection, Sterilization and Preservation*, pp. 542–556. Philadelphia; Lea and Febiger, 1977.

Standard for the Use of Inhalation Anesthetics NFPA 56A-78. Boston: National Fire Protection Association, 1980.

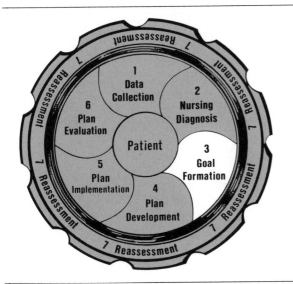

GOAL: *Patient participates in activities designed to restore normal functioning.*

Patient Participation in Rehabilitation

In planning effective perioperative care, the patient's participation in the rehabilitation process must be given major consideration. To participate successfully, the patient and his family or significant others need to:

1. Participate with health care providers in setting realistic rehabilitation goals to follow surgery.
   a. Identify strengths conducive to goal attainment.
   b. Identify hindrances to goal attainment.

2. Participate with the nursing staff in determining methods for overcoming hindrances and using strengths for rehabilitation purposes.

3. State physiological and psychological sequelae of surgery.
   a. Use healthy coping mechanisms to manage psychological consequences.
   b. Relate plan for follow-up care.
   c. Repeat instructions for care after discharge.
   d. Relate feelings associated with the surgical experience.

4. Pace resumption of activities realistically.
   a. Perform stir-up routine (turning, coughing, and deep breathing) without supervision.

223

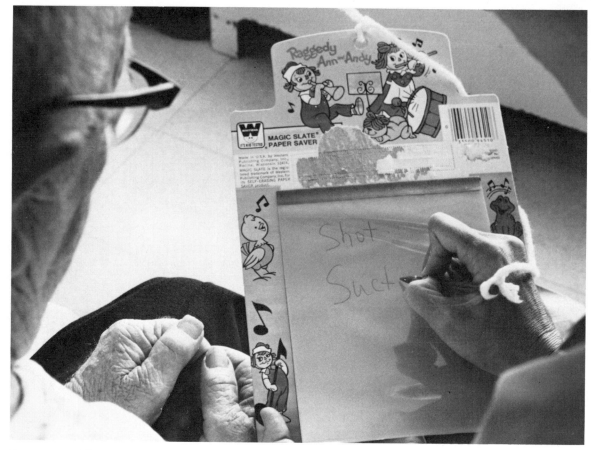

Figure 14.1. *The nurse recognizes the effect that a tracheostomy and wired mandible will have on the patient's ability to communicate postoperatively. A child's magic slate (A) and telephone signals (B) are substituted for oral communication. A patient must be able to initiate or respond to communication if he is to participate in his rehabilitation.*

b. Assume greater responsibility for self-care each postoperative day.

How well these criteria are met is influenced by:

1. Involvement of the patient, family, or significant others in planning and implementing care
2. Whether goals to be met are realistic and achievable
3. How much care-givers impose their culture, such as language and customs, on the patient and how the patient responds
4. Discharge planning and follow-up

In patient-centered rehabilitation, communication between all departments will be focused on the discharge potential or goals of the individual patient. Every person in the hospital who is involved with any aspect of care will need to assist the patient to participate as completely as possible with his care (see Fig. 14.1).

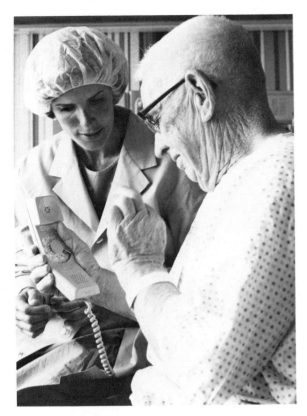

Figure 14.1(B).

A perioperative nurse is involved with the patient's rehabilitation as he goes through the nursing process of assessment, goal setting, implementation, and evaluation. During the relatively short time he spends with the patient, he assists him in the rehabilitation process.

By using the nursing process in the perioperative role, the nurse expands his contribution to the patient's rehabilitation. The patient cannot consciously focus on his goals during the operation, but the perioperative nurse is able to continue work toward those goals during the surgical procedure. This can be successful only if the plan of care has been communicated to various members of the team so that all involved in the care are aware of the goals and can contribute to fulfilling them.

Rehabilitation is a relatively new concept. Formerly, the ill person usually relied entirely on the judgment of those caring for him and had little to say about the process for regaining his former state of well-being.

Nursing has always emphasized caring for and nurturing the ill. Yet, nurses were subservient to physicians. Physicians prescribed the care regimen and neither patients nor nurses were encouraged to think for themselves. The patient did as he was told and did not question decisions made by the physician.

As cultural values and roles have slowly shifted, nursing has moved toward a more collegial relationship with physicians. Patients, too, have begun demanding and taking a more active role in their care. Health practitioners are encouraging patients to take charge of their bodies, to "own" their illnesses, or to accept them, and take the responsibility of collaborating with the health care team in returning to wellness.

The concept of health has also changed. Being ill and being well are no longer seen as two absolute states but rather as opposite ends of a continuum. The patient, family, or significant others have been encouraged to participate in the process the patient follows from illness, through rehabilitation, to wellness. For rehabilitation to be successful, it must be individualized for each person. The contemporary nurse is educated and skilled in individualizing care and assisting patients in their own specific rehabilitation process.

Rehabilitation Defined

Rehabilitation varies considerably in scope. It may involve a change in lifestyle due to a catastrophe, such as an auto accident leading to quadraplegia, or it may simply involve a return to the former lifestyle after a minor procedure, such as a carpae tunnel release. A general definition by the National Council on Rehabilitation states: "Rehabilitation means the restoration of the individual to the fullest physical, mental, social, vocational, and economic capacity to which he is capable" (1:11).

Dr. Sedgwick Mead sees rehabilitation as: "A transient episode during which a human being with a physical or psychological impairment is given the opportunity to realize in himself latent potentialities for improved independency of action and personal care" (1:15). Stryker describes the process in another way, focusing on prevention: "Rehabilitation is a creative process that begins with immediate preventive care in the first stage of an accident or illness. It is continued through the restorative phase of care and involves adaptation of the whole being to a new life" (1:15). Alice B. Morrisey, a pioneer in rehabilitation nursing, covered its scope with a single statement: "Rehabilitation extends from the bed to the job" (2:ix). For the purpose of perioperative patient care, rehabilitation is defined as the process that brings the person from a state of illness to the state of wellness. The person participates in the process by setting realistic goals of wellness and works with assistance to achieve those goals.

Patient Participation in the Rehabilitation Process

How does the surgical patient set goals for achieving a return to wellness? He begins by defining a problem that places him at the beginning of the process—he seeks assistance from a physician, who determines that he needs surgery. The patient makes a decision from the information he has received from his physician and possibly from family and friends. If the patient proceeds with the suggested surgery, he has set a goal for himself and thus begins his rehabilitation. The patient may also choose to reject surgery. In this case he accepts the consequences, whatever they may be.

The rehabilitation process continues when the patient is admitted to the hospital. The primary nurse assesses his overall health status. The patient, family, or significant others and the nurse set specific goals that will assist him in rehabilitation. The nurse explains the routines for the specific surgical procedure and points out how those routines assist the pa-

tient in his anticipated return to wellness (see Fig. 14.2). Involving the family or significant others in the explanations tells the patient that he will not be abandoned. It also may decrease the anxiety of those who can be most supportive of the patient.

During the assessment, the nurse assists the patient to identify strengths conducive to goal attainment, and together they determine factors that may limit success. The nurse guides the patient in setting realistic, achievable goals and not in setting them so high that he will fail in attempting to reach them.

The following example shows how nurses are involved in the nursing process, how they assist the patient in goal setting, and how the patient and his family participate in the rehabilitation process. Mr. Forbes is a 68-year-old man with the diagnosis of osteoarthritis of the right hip. He has been unable to walk without pain for several years, and his physical activity has been markedly diminished. He is entering the hospital for a total hip replacement.

STRENGTHS IDENTIFIED

During the admission assessment, the nurse identifies Mr. Forbes's major strength as his determination to walk without pain after the surgery. Several of his friends have had hip replacement surgery and were able to resume activity previously curtailed by pain. They had actively participated in rehabilitation by doing their exercises faithfully, getting proper rest and sleep, eating recommended foods, gradually increasing activity, and fostering positive thoughts about the surgery and their own participation and involvement in the process. Mr. Forbes says he will not be outdone by his friends and believes he will be able to go through the surgery and convalescence without a great deal of difficulty.

Mr. Forbes identifies another strength—his wife. She is eager for him to be able to continue his previous activities without pain and its hampering effects on their previous lifestyle. She respects his wishes and decision about the surgical procedure and is eager to work with the health care team in Mr. Forbes's rehabilitation.

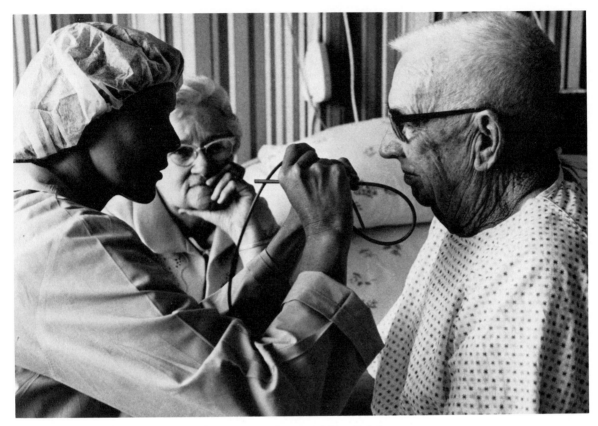

Figure 14.2. The nurse explains surgical routines to a patient and his wife before surgery.

HINDRANCES IDENTIFIED

Mr. Forbes tells the nurse, "My eyes really aren't too good. I absolutely have to wear my glasses to read, eat, walk, or do anything." The nurse identifies this as a hindrance to his goal of learning to ambulate after surgery. The nurse and patient together determine that the glasses will always be available to him. They decide to keep the glasses in a particular drawer in the bedside stand so Mr. Forbes will not have to call for help to find them when he awakens. The nurse makes a special notation in the plan of care about the limited vision and where the glasses are to be kept. She also notes that he must have them available at all times to accomplish his goal of ambulation after surgery.

Another hindrance to goal attainment is a 10-year history of diabetes. Although this is controlled by diet and oral hypoglycemics, Mr. Forbes is aware of complications that can accompany surgical procedures. "The surgeon and I have discussed increased healing time and chance of infection," he says. "I know these are very real problems since I have diabetes. It may be that I have to stay in the hospital longer than the usual patient." Together the nurse and patient decide to check his urine four times a day and have the dietitian assist in menu selections to assure that food choice will aid the healing process while remaining within the diabetic food intake restrictions. The nurse also tells Mr. and Mrs. Forbes about the diabetic classes given by the diabetic nurse specialist. They say they would both like to attend the classes to review the disease and how they can cope with it. Mrs. Forbes says she will attend the classes even if Mr. Forbes will not be able to get to all of them. The nurse tells them she will arrange for the nurse specialist to come talk with them.

The Forbeses and the nurse have discussed his major goal for the surgery—ambulation and activity without pain. He has identified strengths and hindrances to goal achievement and participated with the nurse in determining methods of attaining his goal.

PHYSIOLOGICAL AND PSYCHOLOGICAL SEQUELAE OF SURGERY

Several hours later, while discussing preoperative and postoperative routines for the surgery, the nurse discovers Mr. Forbes does not have a clear understanding of the anatomical changes that will take place during surgery. His surgeon has shown him pictures of the surgery, but he is still a bit puzzled. The nurse shows him an anatomical hip model, a sample hip prosthesis, and responds to his questions. The nurse also tells him he will be shown the postoperative x-rays after the surgery, when he is feeling well enough to be interested.

Since the surgeon is using a posterior approach for the procedure, the nurse demonstrates the abduction device that Mr. Forbes will use to maintain hip abduction during the first few days of the postoperative period. The nurse tells him he will be using a pillow between his legs by the time he leaves the hospital to maintain abduction. He will use the pillow for six to eight weeks after his return home. The nurse also demonstrates the proper method of slide-sitting into the chair. This maintains proper hip extension and prevents prosthesis dislocation. Mr. Forbes tries this method but discovers he has too much pain and limited movement to be successful. He is able to direct the nurse how to do the maneuver, however, showing that he understands the procedure.

The nurse tells Mr. Forbes that he will be asked to do a deep breathing, coughing, and turning routine at two-hour intervals during recovery to prevent postoperative complications. Coughing and deep breathing will help prevent lung problems, while turning will help prevent the pressure sores from developing over bony prominences. The nurse tells him that other nurses will periodically direct him to do the routine, but as he improves, he will be expected to assume the responsibility to do the routine by himself. He demonstrates the routine and has both Mr. and Mrs. Forbes return the demonstration until they do it correctly. In this way, Mrs. Forbes can assist with care after surgery and participate in his rehabilitation.

The nurse discusses the suction drain and shows the Forbeses a sample. He tells them its purpose is to draw out fluid and blood that has collected inside the hip joint. The staff will periodically empty the drain to check the amount of fluid collected in it. The surgeon will order its removal approximately forty-eight hours after the operation. The nurse tells Mr. Forbes he will wake up after the surgery with the abduction device and suction drain in place.

He also tells Mr. Forbes that he will probably have an oxygen tube in his nose, and that the nurses in the recovery room will be taking his blood pressure and pulse frequently. Since Mr. Forbes has never had a general anesthetic, he needs to know that taking vital signs is routine for the immediate postoperative patient in the recovery room. If he lacked this information, he might become anxious, thinking something was going wrong because the nurses were checking his vital signs so frequently. He will also be asked to do the turning, coughing, and deep breathing routine during the immediate postanesthesia period.

The nurse explains to Mr. Forbes that his thinking and response time will be somewhat altered by the effects of the pain medicine but will return to normal once the pain medicine is decreased. The nurse explains that during that time, the nurses will be making decisions about his care that he is unable to make due to the effects of the medication. Examples are when he should turn; when he should turn, cough, and deep breathe; and how much help he will need with getting up. The nurse also tells the Forbeses that on some days, he will feel he is making more progress than others. This is a normal way to feel postoperatively, and he is encouraged to discuss these feelings with the nurses. He tells the nurse, "I'm generally able to cope with difficult times by talking. I'm not the kind of person to keep discouraging feelings inside myself."

This preoperative teaching is crucial to a patient's understanding of surgery. A nurse should be sure to explain reasons for procedures and instructions. If these are taken for granted, the patient may not understand why these activities are needed to reach his goals.

The nurse tells Mr. Forbes he will be "NPO" after midnight. He explains the meaning of the abbreviation and the rationale for not taking fluid for a specified time before surgery. In response to the explanation, Mr. Forbes says, "I'll eat a big dinner tonight since I won't get any breakfast."

Since his operation is scheduled for 7:30 A.M., the night nurses will wake him at 5:00 A.M. so he can shower, shave, and scrub his operative hip before the 6:00 A.M. start of intravenous therapy. At that time, he will also receive an intravenous antibiotic to help prevent infection. His preoperative medication will be given intramuscularly at 6:30 A.M. to induce relaxation and decrease secretions. Mrs. Forbes is told she can come to the hospital at 6:15 A.M. and remain with Mr. Forbes until he is taken into the operating room.

DISCHARGE PLANNING

The nurse asks the Forbeses if they have made advance plans for home care after discharge. Mrs. Forbes says she will care for her husband at home with no forseeable problems. Friends will drive them wherever they need to go (e.g., to the doctor's office and grocery shopping) until Mr. Forbes is able to drive again. The nurse tells them a visiting nurse will talk with them prior to discharge to make plans for a nursing visit when they are at home.

Mrs. Forbes says she has already put away any scatter rugs or other items that might be a hazard while Mr. Forbes is using crutches or a walker in the house. She says they will have to watch the dog since he loves to play with un- usual items and may playfully attack the crutches or walker. Both the Forbeses are surprised when the nurse talks about taking an elevated toilet seat home with them. She again uses the hip model and shows them the rationale for decreasing hip flexion during the first eight weeks of the postoperative period.

Mr. Forbes is given a soft scrub brush, clean pajamas, and instructions to scrub his hip area. In doing the scrub, he continues his active participation in rehabilitation.

PERIOPERATIVE ASSESSMENT

After Mr. Forbes has scrubbed his hip, the perioperative nurse will come to complete an assessment on Mr. Forbes and to begin to develop an operating room patient care plan. He tells the Forbeses about procedures surrounding the actual operation. He tells them that at approximately 6:45 the next morning an operating room orderly with a stretcher will come for Mr. Forbes and take him to the operating room. The first stop will be the holding area immediately outside the surgical suite. Here the orderly will shave Mr. Forbes's hip to remove hair that could harbor bacteria. Mr. Forbes will remain in the holding area until the surgery is ready to begin. Mrs. Forbes will remain with him until he is taken into the operating room.

The nurse tells Mr. Forbes that another nurse will be with him during the surgery and will meet him the next morning in the holding area. The nurse also tells him about the equipment he will see. Mr. Forbes asks, "Can I wear my glasses down there so I can see what's going on?" The nurse tells him his glasses will stay at his bedside since they might get broken in the operating room. He asks about the anesthesia, and the perioperative nurse tells him the anesthesiologist will discuss the type of anesthesia with him later that evening.

When the anesthesiologist visits Mr. Forbes, he discusses the available anesthetic agents and the type of anesthesia that will be used. He talks to Mr. Forbes about the importance of coughing and deep breathing after the procedure, and Mr. Forbes demonstrates his proficiency with the routine. In successfully doing so, he again demonstrates his active participation in the rehabilitation process by preparing himself to function postoperatively. After an explanation and instructions are given to the Forbeses the nurse completes the data collection and begins to develop an individualized plan for Mr. Forbes.

Mr. Forbes has received important information that will assist him to cope with new, anxiety-producing experiences. As he gains new knowledge about the surgery, Mr. Forbes travels further in the rehabilitation process.

OPERATIVE PHASE

The next morning, Mrs. Forbes arrives at 6:15 and stays with Mr. Forbes until he is taken into the surgical suite. The perioperative nurse comes to take him into the operating room. He checks Mr. Forbes's identification band and asks him which hip is to be replaced. He also looks at the patient care plan and asks Mr. Forbes about his limited vision. He says, "My glasses are in the cabinet beside my bed. Since all I'll have to do is the stir-up routine in the recovery room, I won't need them. Things are very blurry, but I'm sleepy anyway, so I won't worry about the things I can't see."

The perioperative nurse assists him from the stretcher to the operating table and remains with him during the induction phase of anesthesia. When he is asleep, the nurse goes into the intraoperative phase of his role as the perioperative nurse. During the surgery, he notes in the assessment portion of the care plan that the surgery was mechanically difficult due to the amount of bony destruction in the hip joint. Therefore, Mr. Forbes and the unit nurses can expect greater than the average amount of pain in the postoperative period.

When Mr. Forbes is transferred into the recovery room, the nurse makes a special point to tell the postanesthesia nurse about the increased mechanical difficulty and also points out the notation on the care plan. The recovery room nurse says he will communicate this information to the unit nurse when the patient is transferred back to his room. The perioperative nurse has participated in the rehabilitation process by assuring both oral and written communication about his assessment to other members of the health care team.

During the recovery process, Mr. Forbes does the turning, coughing, and deep breathing routine quite well when requested to do so by the recovery nurse. The nurse makes a notation on the recovery room notes to that effect, giving feedback about the success of preoperative teaching to the patient's primary nurse.

Before Mr. Forbes is transferred to his room, Mrs. Forbes tells the primary nurse she is concerned that Mr. Forbes may overdo postoperative activity unless the nurses are firm with him. He has normally been a very active man, and "goes full force at anything he does." Since he is so anxious to resume his former active lifestyle, he may try to do too much too soon. The nurse thanks her for the information and explains the postoperative routine used for a patient with a total hip replacement. He reassures the patient's wife that the nurse will advise him not to overdo activity.

POSTOPERATIVE PHASE

On the first postoperative day, the primary nurse involves Mr. Forbes with his morning care. Since his pain is controlled by the medication, the nurse has him assist with his bath. The nurse and patient together plan activities for the following day. The nurse notes these plans in the patient record and on the care plan. By communicating the plans to the patient's wife, the nurse helps relieve the anxieties Mrs. Forbes expressed the preceding day. He involves Mrs. Forbes in turning her husband and also asks her to remind Mr. Forbes to cough and deep breathe at intervals. Thus, the patient's wife becomes more involved in his rehabilitation.

On the second postoperative day, the perioperative nurse comes to visit Mr. Forbes and evaluate his progress. He finds him out of bed in a tilt-back wheelchair, visiting with his wife. Mr. Forbes tells the nurse, "I'm having some pain but not a whole lot—the medicine takes care of it pretty well. I think I'm making real progress being up in the chair. Tomorrow I'm going to begin physical therapy."

Mr. Forbes begins the exercise program with his physical therapist and then goes to the department each morning and afternoon. The therapist has read the nursing assessment, the plan of care, and the notes written by the perioperative and recovery nurses. He is encouraged by Mr. Forbes's progress and independent attitude. He cautions him not to overdo activities and sets a limit on the number of bed exercises the patient should do each hour.

Each succeeding day, Mr. Forbes ambulates a greater distance and is independent with crutches on the 9th postoperative day. Since the wound appears to be healing well, and there are no signs of infection, the surgeon discharges him on the 10th postoperative day.

DISCHARGE INSTRUCTIONS

Both Mr. and Mrs. Forbes can describe and demonstrate the proper technique for home care that they have learned during the hospitalization. The unit nurses have taught them incisional care, use of the elevated toilet seat, the slide-sit maneuver, and techniques for putting on clothes. With their enthusiastic interest, the Forbeses have involved themselves further in the rehabilitation process.

The patient and his wife also have reviewed diabetic care. Both are more comfortable with the disease process since they have discussed it with the diabetic nurse and dietitian. Arrangements have been made for a visiting nurse to check on Mr. Forbes the day after he returns home. Since he lives quite a distance from his surgeon, the nurse will make several visits to check progress in ambulation, assess the incision, and evaluate his diabetic postoperative status.

As Mr. and Mrs. Forbes are leaving the hospital, he tells the nurse he liked everything "except the pain." He says, "If I have to have it done to the other hip, I'll know what to expect. Having the surgery really hasn't been as frightening as I had thought. And, I promise not to overdo with walking and activity at home. I'll follow the doctors' orders and your instructions to the letter."

Mr. Forbes's story shows success in meeting the criteria to achieve the goal of involving the patient, family, or significant others in the rehabilitation process. Both the patient and his wife were involved in planning and implementing his care. Together with the nurses, they set realistic goals and worked to achieve success. Discharge planning that began during the admission process continued throughout the hospital stay. Patient-oriented rehabilitation took place through continual use of the nursing process.

CULTURAL IMPOSITIONS

Not every patient and family or significant others will participate in the rehabilitation process as well as the Forbeses. An example is Mrs. Garcia, a 45-year-old married woman of Mexican-American descent, who enters the hospital for a cholecystectomy. She holds strongly to her cultural heritage and speaks only Spanish, although she does understand a few words of English. Two daughters and one son still live at home and will be able to help Mrs. Garcia after surgery. An English-speaking member of the family plans to remain with Mrs. Garcia during the entire hospitalization.

During the initial nursing history and preoperative visits, the patient tells hospital personnel that she doesn't "want to know anything ahead of time—it's too scary. I just want to have the operation, get well, and go back home." Any attempts by the nurse to talk with her about the surgery are met with resistance. As the nurse explains preoperative and postoperative procedures, the patient turns her head to the wall and will not listen when her children try to interpret the information (see Fig. 14.3).

Differences in goals set by nurses and patients are not uncommon when the care-givers and patients are from different cultural backgrounds. The nurse assumed Mrs. Garcia's anxiety would be alleviated with increased information. However, the patient's statement about advance information being frightening was an important clue to her cultural coping mechanisms. In this instance, providing only necessary information when needed would have served the patient better to meet her

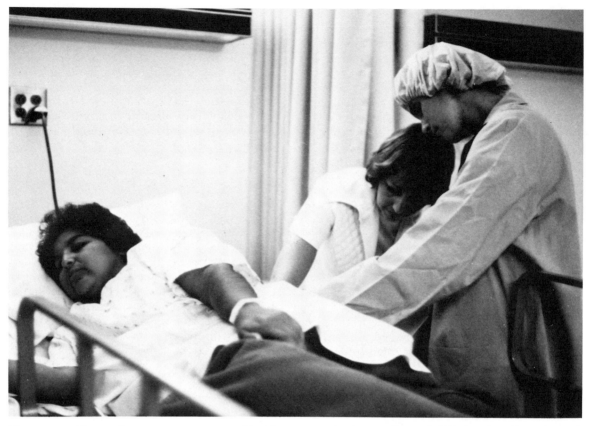

Figure 14.3. *The nurse's preoperative assessment of health status may further complicate rehabilitation of a patient whose culturally oriented coping mechanisms differ from the nurse's.*

stated goal of not receiving advance information.

The nurse calls the clinical nurse specialist in the operating room to discuss the language problem and difficulties with preoperative teaching. The nurse specialist says there is a Spanish-speaking nurse who can be assigned as Mrs. Garcia's perioperative nurse. Although that nurse is unable to make a preoperative visit, the family is relieved to hear that a nurse who speaks the same language will be with Mrs. Garcia in the operating room.

When the perioperative nurse meets Mrs. Garcia just before the surgery, the patient's eyes begin to sparkle as the nurse speaks Spanish with her. Since the nurse has read the patient care plan and has learned of the teach-

ing difficulties with the patient, he again tries to explain the surgery to her. Mrs. Garcia's anxiety seems to diminish a bit prior to the induction of the anesthetic.

The surgery goes without incident until a cholangiogram reveals a retained common-duct stone. Mrs. Garcia returns from the operating room with a T-tube and will need to learn to care for it prior to discharge. The surgeon informs the family about the T-tube and says, "It's OK. She can do it, and you can help her. It will only be for six weeks, then she'll come back and have it out." The family's anxiety increases, and they seek out Mrs. Garcia's primary nurse. He tells them the procedure for caring for the tube at home. They are somewhat relieved by his explanation but still seem anxious. The nurse tells them he will teach them how to help Mrs. Garcia care for the tube.

In the days following surgery, the nurse shows the family and Mrs. Garcia how the tube is clamped and how it is drained. The patient shows revulsion for handling the tube but gradually begins to do so gingerly. Finally, she asks her daughter to ask the nurse why the tube is there. "Why didn't the doctor take it out during the operation? Why do I have to come back to have it out?" The nurse realizes the surgeon has not fully explained the tube's purpose to the patient and family. Using anatomical drawings, he explains the function of the gallbladder and why the tube was left in. After the explanations, the patient and family seem somewhat relieved, but they make no more progress in caring for the tube and incision.

In planning for discharge, the nurse arranges for a home health nurse to visit Mrs. Garcia in her home. In the referral, the primary nurse communicates the anxieties of the patient and family, their adaptation to the postoperative situation, the discharge teaching, and the minimal extent to which the patient and family participated in the rehabilitation process. When the nurse visits the patient at home, he will assess Mrs. Garcia's adaptation to caring for the tube at home. If more teaching is necessary, he will use the teaching in the hospital as a basis for any further information the patient needs to deal with the situation at home.

In Mrs. Garcia's case, the patient and family resisted participating in the rehabilitation process in the way the nurse expected. The patient summed up the hospital experience with the following statement: "The only good thing about it was the nurse who spoke Spanish to me. I can't wait to get home."

Will Mrs. Garcia reach the wellness end of the rehabilitation continuum? Physically, she will attain her goal but not without psychological trauma that will remain with her. Nurses with cultural backgrounds different from their patients need to be acutely aware of indications given by patients that will assist the goal-setting process. Since patients are encouraged to "own" their illnesses and work through the rehabilitation process, their participation can only be successful if assessment and planning take place on cultural as well as physical levels.

Outpatient Rehabilitation

When a patient has outpatient surgery, what role does the perioperative nurse play in rehabilitation? The surgical outpatient is better able to draw on his own resources since the procedure is more minor than most inpatient surgery. However, since there is minimal time to develop a teaching plan for the patient, the type of teaching to assist the patient in his rehabilitation is crucial. Goal setting and beginning discharge teaching are incorporated into the initial assessment process; then they are completed with the patient after the procedure is finished. The nurse needs to feel certain the patient fully understands self-care instructions before he is discharged.

For example, Jim Smith, a 28-year-old construction worker, is having surgery on his right third finger due to a previous injury from a work-related accident. Prior to the surgery, the perioperative nurse demonstrates the correct above-head position and explains the rationale for its use. The patient demonstrates the position and states the correct reasons for keeping his hand in the proper position. The nurse also discusses how long it will be necessary to maintain the position—until he sees the surgeon in the office five days after the surgery. The patient says his girlfriend will look after him, take care of the house, prepare meals, and anything else necessary. He says he'll feel a bit silly keeping his hand in the correct position. The nurse again explains the rationale for the correct position and discusses complications that can happen to the operative hand and arm if the proper position is not maintained.

When Jim's girlfriend comes to pick him up, the nurse again explains the correct position and has the patient demonstrate it and explain

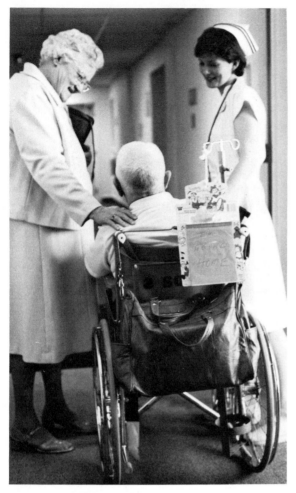

Figure 14.4. Going home is a major milestone in rehabilitation; however, many patients continue to need professional nursing service for full recovery at home.

as he assists the patient with his participation in rehabilitation. Examples of patients having major and minor surgical procedures and appropriate interventions are reviewed. Emphasis is placed on the nursing process, focusing on teaching and communication. Criteria for reaching rehabilitation goals are studied, as well as factors influencing the attainment of the goals (see Fig. 14.4).

References

1. Stryker, Hugh. *Rehabilitative Aspects of Acute and Chronic Nursing Care*, 2nd ed. Philadelphia: W. B. Saunders, 1977.
2. Schickendanze, Ruth H., and Mayhall, Pamela D. *Restorative Nursing in a General Hospital.* Springfield, Ill.: Charles C. Thomas, 1975.

Suggested Readings

DeLoach, Jane Emily. *General Surgical Nursing.* Garden City, N.Y.: Medical Examination Publishing Co., 1979.

Farrell, Jane. "The human side of assessment." *Nurs 80* 10(4):74–75, 1980.

Gordon, Marjory, Sweeney, Mary Anne, and McKeehan, Kathleen. "Nursing diagnosis: Looking at its use in the clinical area." *Am J Nurs* 80(4):672–674, 1980.

Gruendemann, Barbara J., Casterton, Shirley B., Hesterly, Sandra C., Minckley, Barbara B., and Shelter, Mary G. *The Surgical Patient: Behavioral Concepts for the Operating Room Nurse*, 2nd ed. St. Louis: C. V. Mosby, 1977.

Hartman, Mary Ann. "Assessment: One factor in effective client teaching." *Nurs Forum* 18(4):405–414, 1979.

Hartson, David, and Hartson, Kandy M. "The five-minute interview." *AORN J* 31(4):605–608, 1980.

Klos, Don, Cummings, K. Michael, Joyce, Jan, Fraichen, Janet, and Quigley, Anne. "A comparison of two methods of delivering presurgical instructions." *Patient Couns Health Educ* 2(1): 6–13, 1980.

LeMaitre, George D., and Finnegan, Janet A. *The Patient in Surgery: A Guide for Nurses*, 4th ed. Philadelphia: W. B. Saunders, 1980.

its rationale to his friend. Involving the patient in his own rehabilitation, the nurse is also reinforcing the teaching he has done in a limited time.

In this chapter we look at the sixth goal of planning perioperative patient care: For the patient, family, or significant others to participate successfully in the rehabilitation process. We examine the role of the perioperative nurse

Luckmann, Joan, and Sorenson, Daren Geason. *Medical-Surgical Nursing*, 2nd ed. Philadelphia: W. B. Saunders, 1980.

Meisenheimer, Claire Gavin. "Continuing care: The educator's role" *Nurs Admin Q* 4(Spring):17–22, 1980.

Murray, Rosemary, and Kijek, Jean C. *Current Perspectives in Rehabilitation Nursing*, vol. 1. St. Louis: C. V. Mosby, 1979.

Phippen, Mark L. "Nursing assessment of preoperative anxiety." *AORN J* 31(6):1019–1026, 1980.

Price, Mary Readtovich. "Nursing diagnosis: Making a concept come alive." *Am J Nurs* 80(4): 668–671, 1980.

Thorpe, Constance J., and Caprini, Joseph A. "Gallbladder disease: Current trends and treatments." *Am J Nurs* 80(11):2181–2185, 1980.

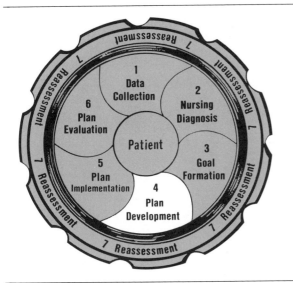

The plan for nursing care prescribes nursing actions to achieve the goals.

Developing the Care Plan

The patient care plan prescribes nursing actions to achieve the goals. Goals have been formulated, and now the plan for patient care must be developed. This chapter discusses the written care plan, its format, what should be included, and then relates it to the operating room care plan and standards of care. An individualized care plan is given as an example of how plans can be developed. Once the plan has been developed, it is communicated to others involved in giving care. Methods for communicating the plan are explored and examples given.

The Written Care Plan

The written care plan provides an outline of the aim of nursing care and prescribes nursing actions that must be performed to achieve the patient goal. The written plan individualizes care because each patient reacts to care in his own way. Patient-centered care is the objective of every nurse, and this necessitates adapting care to meet individual needs of patients. If used systematically, the planning process allows for coordination and continuity of care. The written plan assures that the needed information about each patient is available to the staff. Most care plans are located in a card file on the patient care units at the nurses' station.

Various forms for written care plans have been developed. The form is usually designed by the individual hospital to meet specific needs. As the care for the patient changes, the care plan can be updated or revised. Thus, a complete picture of the patient is available at all times. The written plan should reflect the acuity level of the patient and validate the amount of nursing care needed. The nurse can then make judgments about who will be assigned to provide care to the patient. She must be able to review the written plan and evaluate the effectiveness of care given.

Forms do not need to follow a prescribed format, but it is important that the format be flexible so the information can be easily revised according to the patient's condition. If the plan is not kept up-to-date, the information becomes meaningless, and it can no longer be used to guide care of the patient. Whatever the format, the care plan should be designed so actions can be organized. It should reveal the purpose of planning, the goals developed from the nursing diagnosis, and whether these are long-term or immediate goals. The nursing activities to achieve the goals are incorporated.

A typical care plan on a surgical unit is divided into several sections:

1. Patient history, including illnesses and personal, family, or social history
2. An area for communicating information or problems that all staff members need to be aware of, or appointments for the patient

3. Allergies
4. Teaching needs
5. Tests and procedures
6. Daily laboratory work
7. Nursing care
8. Discharge plans

Provision is also made for the patient's name, age, sex, physician, diagnosis, and other pertinent data. The patient care plan in Fig. 15.1 illustrates the type of information that might be included for a specific patient.

Standards of Care

Based on the *Standards of Perioperative Nursing Practice* (1) and the requirements of the Joint Commission on Accreditation of Hospitals (JCAH), most hospitals have developed standards to guide practice. The standards are based on common problems patients experience when having various types of surgical procedures. Standards of nursing care vary from hospital to hospital, but some common elements are: (1) usual problems; (2) expected outcomes; (3) deadlines; (4) nursing orders; and (5) criteria. One standard might have the components given in Table 15.1. Another standard might look like that given in Table 15.2.

Care Plan for the Perioperative Patient

In addition to the plan of care developed and used by nurses on the surgical unit, the perioperative nurse completes a plan specifically

Table 15.1. *First Example of Nursing Care Standards.*

Usual Problems	Expected Outcome	Nursing Action
Preoperative 1. Patient lacks knowledge about surgical experience and OR nursing care.	1. Patient will verbalize understanding of her surgery prior to receiving preoperative medication.	1. Talk with patient preoperatively and provide supportive teaching. Encourage patient to view preoperative teaching film. Answer patient's questions about what to expect.
2. Potential injury due to transportation to the operating room.	2. Patient arrives safely and comfortably in OR.	2. Assess measures for safe transportation. Document on OR nursing care plan.

8610-112-81D

PORTER MEMORIAL HOSPITAL — PATIENT CARE PLAN

SIGN NAME AFTER EACH ENTRY | PERMANENT RECORD | WRITE WITH BLACK INK (SPACE AVAILABLE ON BACK)

DISCHARGE PLANS (Including referrals, diet, equipment, medications, treatments etc., as needed.)

Addressograph

Date	Problem Number	PROBLEM/Nursing Diagnosis	GOAL/Expected Outcome	Deadline	PLAN/Nursing Orders	Date Revwd. Revised
3/25	1	Knowledge, lack of external resources (human + material)	Patient will verbalize understanding of his preoperative care	Preop	Provide explanations about each phase of the preoperative period. 1) pre-op: NPO, preop meds, IV line, shave, antiseptic scrub, where family can wait, approx. length of surgery 2) intra-op: EKG, BP, Foley catheter, poss. blood transfusion, drains, jaw wiring, trach, etc. 3) post-op: ICU, poss. ventilator, frequent suctioning, turning, coughing, respiratory therapy, pain, meds, dressing change, etc.	

Admission: Date 3/25/82 | Religion Prot. | Surgery & Date Left Hemiglossectomy, Left hemimandibulectomy, Left neck dissection, tracheostomy | Additional Diagnosis | Consulting Physician(s) R. Farnsworth

Hour 3 30 pm | Name (Last) (First) Fischer, Ralph E. | (Male) Female | Age 79 | Admitting Diagnosis/Problem Recurrent carcinoma left lateral tongue and alveolar ridge | Physician C Bates

Figure 15.1. *A preoperative problem that might be found on a patient care plan on the nursing unit.*

Table 15.2. Second Example of Nursing Care Standards.

Usual Problems	Expected Outcomes	Deadlines	Nursing Orders	Criteria
Postoperative 1. Patient's potential for impaired circulation due to kinking of skin flap, pressure on flap, or hematoma.	1. Flap warm and pink with good blanching. Minimal swelling. No kinking of or pressure on flap from affected extremity.	Until pedicle flap separated from chest.	Instruct patient to pull up gently with arm.	1. Skin warm. 2. Color pink. 3. Minimal swelling. 4. No evidence of pressure on skin flap.

for the perioperative period. This plan includes only information relevant to the surgical procedure. The purpose is to communicate with team members in the operating room and provide a guide for continuity and comprehensive care. The care plan which the perioperative nurse designs for the patient is usually separate from those developed on the nursing unit. The focus is on the immediate preoperative period, the intraoperative period, and the immediate postoperative period. It incorporates a brief physical, psychological, and sociocultural assessment. The form then provides space for a care plan to be written. Categories in the form may be patient problems, needs, and nursing diagnosis; objectives and goals; plan and nursing orders; what nursing actions were carried out or implemented; and evaluation.

To develop the plan, a nurse from the operating room sees the patient preoperatively and collects pertinent data. She reviews the patient's chart and unit nursing care plan. In an interview, usually conducted after the patient has been admitted, she gathers information to plan nursing care during the intraoperative period (see Fig. 15.2).

Communicating the Plan

The written care plan is one tool used for communicating information to other members of the health care team. Other forms used by operating room personnel include preoperative checklists and operating room nurse's notes. The operating room care plan provides other members of the team with a current plan for the patient. It follows the unit care plan as closely as possible to assure continuity of care. The plan must be made accessible to the nurses caring for the specific patient. This is usually accomplished by giving the plan of care to the nurses assigned that patient at change-of-shift report, prior to setting up cases for the day, or putting the care plan in the operating room.

PREOPERATIVE CHECKLISTS

Operating room checklists (see Fig. 15.3) are also used to communicate information in the care plan. Upon arrival in the operating room, the nurse can immediately see what nursing actions or patient responses have been checked off or filled in. When the patient is admitted to the room, the nurse checks off appropriate items, such as surgical procedure, verification of patient, emotional status upon admission to operating room, position for surgical procedure, known allergies, and presence of prosthetic devices. The operating room checklist should not take the place of the written care plan. It is a tool for communicating what care has been given and what care is needed, which is an essential part of any plan.

NURSE'S NOTES

Operating room nurse's notes (see Fig. 15.4) are also useful for communicating the plan for care during the perioperative period. The nurse's notes are used to record nursing activities performed, patient outcomes, and evaluation statements. Data recorded before and during surgery are used by the nurse immediately postoperatively in planning post-

Left hemimandibulectomy
Left hemiglossectomy
PROCEDURE: _Left neck dissection & tracheostomy_
SURGEON: _C. Bates_
PRE-OP DIAGNOSIS: _Recurrent Ca left lat. tongue_
PREVIOUS SURGERY: _Laser vaporization lesion tongue_
exc. biopsy alveolar ridge, subtot. colectomy (Ca)
CHRONIC ILLNESS: _bronchitis_

PREVIOUS TRAUMA: _Mod. R nasal septal deviation_

VITAL SIGNS

B/P _160/90_
PULSE _68_
RESPIRATIONS _18_
TEMPERATURE _98.6_
HEIGHT _5' 7"_
WEIGHT _182 #_
COUGH _____ OCCASIONAL FREQUENT DRY PRODUCTIVE
ALLERGIES: _Ethanol (oral intake) ?Penicillin_

CHART REQUIREMENTS

PERMITS: ✓
H & P: ✓
LAB WORK: _CBC, UA, PT PTT, VDRL, SMA15, CT scan, EKG,_
chest x-ray
NPO STATUS: _p 2400_
PRE-OP MEDS: _Vistaril 50 mg, Robinul 0.2 mg, Ancef, Gm T_

TYPE & CROSS ✓ _____ # UNITS _3 units packed RBC's_ ON HOLD

Prev. surg. (cont'd) R cataract extraction
cholecystectomy
hiatal hernia repair

_530 126 20 M79_
Fischer, Ralph E.
C. Bates 03 25 82

INTRAOPERATIVE CARE PLAN

NURSING DIAGNOSIS	GOAL	PLAN	IMPLEMENTATION	EVALUATION

PORTER MEMORIAL HOSPITAL PREOPERATIVE ASSESSMENT FORM
(Adapted from: AJN: Volume 73 #8 pg. 1373)

Figure 15.2. Intraoperative care plan shows data obtained for developing individualized plan of care.

Name/Initial

I. PRE-OP TEACHING:
    ☐ Video ☐ 1:1 ☐ Group ☒ O.R. .... *PC*

II. REQUIRED FOR SURGERY:
    Consent for Surgery signed.................... ☒ Yes ☐ Accurate.......... *PC*
    Special permits signed (i.e. Sterilization).... ☐ Yes ☐ Accurate ☒ NA.... *PC*
    History & Physical .... ☒ On chart ☐ Dictated..... *PC*
                                                  ☐ If none, O.R. notified.....
    Lab report on chart.......................... ☒ Urinalysis ☒ CBC......... *PC*

III. OPTIONAL:
    SMAC 24 on chart............................. ☒ Yes ☐ Not ordered....... *PC*
    EKG Report/strips on chart................... ☐ Yes ☒ Not ordered....... *PC*
    Chest X-ray done............................. ☒ Yes ☐ Not ordered....... *PC*
    Respiratory test records on chart............ ☒ Yes ☐ Not ordered....... *PC*
    Blood ordered................................ ☒ Yes ☐ No ☐ Ready....... *PC*
    Pregnancy test report on chart............... ☐ Yes ☒ Not ordered....... *PC*
    P.T.T.. ☐ Yes ☒ Not ordered....... *PC*

IV. VITAL SIGN/TEST VALUES:
    All within normal limits..................... ☒ Yes ☐ No............... *PC*
    Physician notified of abnormals.............. ☐ Yes ☐ No...............

V. PROCEDURES:
    Naso-gastric tube inserted................... ☒ Yes ☐ Not ordered....... *PC*
    Foley catheter............................... ☒ Yes ☐ Not ordered....... *PC*
    Ted hose/Ace bandages........................ ☐ Yes ☒ Not ordered....... *PC*
    Scrub skin preparation....................... ☒ Yes ☐ Not ordered....... *PC*
    Enema.. ☒ Yes ☐ Not ordered....... *PC*
    Douche....................................... ☐ Yes ☒ Not ordered....... *PC*

VI. DAY OF SURGERY:
    Bath/oral care completed..................... ☒ Yes............... *PC*
    Bobby pins, prosthesis, (contacts) (glasses)
      makeup, jewelry............................ ☒ Removed................. *PC*
    Rings: ☒ Taped on ☒ Valuables envelope ☒ Given to family ☐ None....... *PC*
    Gown on (undergarments off).................. ☒ Yes................. *PC*
    Voided....................................... ☒ Yes _____ Time....... *PC*
    I.D. bracelet on and accurate................ ☒ Yes................. *PC*
    I.D. bracelet on extremity not affected by surg ☒ Yes................. *PC*
    I.V. Record on chart......................... ☒ Yes ☐ NA............. *PC*
    Medication Record/SMC Kardex on chart........ ☒ Yes................. *PC*
    Patient instructed to stay in bed............ ☒ Yes................. *PC*
    Patient instructed not to smoke.............. ☐ Yes ☒ NA............. *PC*
    Side rails up................................ ☒ Yes................. *PC*
    Dentures/partial plate: ☒ Yes ☐ No......... ☐ Left in.............

TPR *98⁶*   BP *160/90*   HT *5'7½"*   WT *182#*

PRE-OPERATIVE MEDICATIONS
Vistaril 50mg   Robinul 0.2mg   Time *7³⁰ am*
Ancef Gm. ī   Time *7³⁰ am*
Allergies *Ethanol (oral intake)*

Comments _____

_____   *530 126 20   M 79*
Addressograph plate on chart ☒ Yes   *Fischer, Ralph E.*
Verification of patient identification with O.R. transport   *C. Bates   03 25 82*
                 (Signature) *Patricia Crum*
To Surgery *3/26/82* *7³⁰ a* *Patricia Crum*
           Date   Time   Signature

Figure 15.3. Preoperative checklist used as a communication tool.

Porter Memorial Hospital / Swedish Medical Center
OPERATIVE RECORD

530 126 20 M79
Fischer, Ralph E.
C. Bates 03 25 82

Addressograph Here

Operative Times

OR # ___4___   Anesthesia Begin 7 45 am   Surgery Began 8 30 am
                Anesthesia Ended 4 00 pm   Surgery Ended 3 45 pm

Anesthesia

Anesthesia: Method ☒ Inhalational ☐ Block/Regional ☐ Local Infiltrate ☐ Spinal ☐ Other _____ ☐ None

Agent ☒ Ethrane ☐ Fluothane ☐ Nitrous/Narcotic ☐ Other _____

Administered By _T. Barry_ _____ MD _____ CRNA

Position and Locations

Patient Position: ☒ Supine ☐ Prone ☐ Jackknife ☐ Lateral ☐ Lithotomy ☐ Other _Egg crate mattress, heel + elbow pads_

Other Item Locations:
1. Safety Strap = =
2. Bovie Plate = ☐
3. Monitor Leads = O
4. Tourniquet = +
   Time On___ Off___ On___ Off___
   Pressure Ck'd - Yes___

Front   Back

5. Temperature Probe
   ☐ Oral ☐ Anal
   ☐ Axil R L
   ☒ Scapula (R) L
   ☐ Other _____
6. ☐ Aquathermia

Diagnosis and Surgery

Preoperative Dx _Recurrent squamous cell Carcinoma, left lateral tongue and alveolar ridge_

Operation _Left hemiglossectomy, left hemimandibulectomy, left neck dissection and tracheostomy_

Persons Present

Postoperative Dx _Same_

Surgeon _C. Bates_ ____ MD Assistant _S. Schell_ ____ MD Assistant _____

Scrub Nurse(s) _J. Parson CST_ Circulating Nurse(s) _M. Long RN CNOR_ Other Persons Present _____

Counts and Signatures

Counts:
Sponge ☒ Correct ☐ Unresolved ☐ N/A
Needle ☒ Correct ☐ Unresolved ☐ N/A
Inst. ☒ Correct ☐ Unresolved ☐ N/A

Final Count:
Circulating Nurse _M. Long RN_ Signature Scrub Nurse _SP_ Initial

If Unresolved, Xray Taken? ☐ Yes ☐ No If No, Explain Below

Drains, Packs and Catheters

Drains: ☐ T-Tube ☐ Penrose ☐ Sump ☐ Chest ☒ NG Tube ☒ Hemovac ☐ Other _____ ☐ None

Drain Location _left neck wound_

Packs: Type _____ Location _____ ☐ None

Urinary Catheter: Type & Size _#16 Foley c̄ 5cc bag_ Inserted By _C Bates MD_ ☐ None

Implants and Prosthetics

Manufacturer _Dow Corning_ Lot/Serial No. _2167/STT 34567_

Type _Silastic trach tube_ Size _#7 fr._ ☐ None

Lab

Services: ☒ Specimen To Lab # of Specimens _2_   ☐ Culture # of Cultures _____ ☒ None
         ☒ Frozen Section ☐ None   Culture Site _____

Charges and Comments

Charges:

Observations and Comments:
Patient states he is comfortable after Transfer to OR bed.

When transferred to RR, no evidence of pressure areas or impaired skin integrity

Patient Discharged To: ☒ RR ___ ICU-CSU ___ Room

660-003-77

Figure 15.4. Operating room record provides continuity of care by linking the preoperative and postoperative periods.

anesthesia care. The data are also used by others involved in giving patient care. Notes are particularly useful if the charting format follows the nursing process. Other methods the nurse uses to communicate information to those involved in the patient's care include reporting, patient care conferences, and multidisciplinary conferences.

REPORTING

Change-of-shift reports usually are given when one shift of nurses comes on and another leaves. It always occurs at the beginning of the shift. This may be in the morning, afternoon, or evening. Information is shared pertaining to equipment, supplies, types of surgery, and patients. The nurse in charge may conduct the report, but in many situations, nurses who have developed care plans on specific patients share the plan with others involved in the care of the patient. This can be done while the group is convened or on an individual basis.

In some operating rooms, the team leader or assistant head nurse for each specialty communicates information about patients to be cared for in each specialty. Other hospitals use tape recorders to transmit information from one shift to another. This has proved successful in many situations because it does not require overlapping time at change-of-shift. The nurse coming on a shift can listen to the report and then relieve the nurse in the operating room. At the same time, she can validate or question any of the information communicated via the recorder. For example, the following information might be communicated relating to the care plan for a patient with a fractured femur:

- Maintain fractured limb in alignment.
- Place trochanter roll along right hip.
- Transfer slowly and gently to OR.
- Examine area described as painful for signs of pressure, increased edema, and skin breakdown.
- Maintain traction with free pull.

At the end of a procedure, the OR nurse transmits information to other nurses in the operating room, recovery room, and patient care unit and to the patient's family. Information is continuously given to carry out, alter, or revise the plan for any patient. The information is provided to various members of the team at points throughout the patient's perioperative experience.

PATIENT CARE CONFERENCE

In some hospitals, the patient care conference has replaced the traditional team conference. However, both focus on an individual patient to provide the best care possible. These conferences can take place before or after surgery.

Conferences prior to the procedure focus on what can be done for the patient. For example, a young teenager is scheduled to have skin grafts. The operating room nurse who did the preoperative assessment found the girl had been badly burned as a child and was having a series of surgeries to alleviate contractures and for cosmetic effects. The nurse decided to have a patient care conference and invited the nurse from the teen unit to participate. Objectives for the conference were that the operating room personnel would be able to:

1. Provide emotional support and comfort during transportation and positioning in the OR.
2. Gain background information that would assist in planning specifically for her care intraoperatively.
3. Plan instruments, supplies, and draping.
4. Prevent infection since areas of the body were without skin covering.

The conference was about 15 minutes long but productive. Other OR nurses who had cared for this patient shared what they had done during surgery that was successful. The unit nurse provided information about her likes and dislikes and what would help in relating to her.

This conference was patient oriented, but other conferences may be disease oriented. For example, a postsurgery conference was held about a patient who had malignant hyperthermia during surgery. The information shared was invaluable when another patient developed the same condition two weeks later.

Patient care conferences provide an opportunity for group discussion by personnel involved in the patient's care and assist in individualizing the care. The staff gains a better understanding of the care they should give. In some instances, policies and procedures are clarified.

The nurse needs to do advanced planning for the conference so it will run smoothly and everyone will gain information beneficial for nursing care. The time for the conference is arranged with the head nurse or nurse in charge of the operating room. The conferences may be conducted at change-of-shift, at a specific time when the specialty nurses are available, or during the regularly scheduled time for education or inservice. Short conferences that last no more than 10–15 minutes are preferable.

When selecting a patient, consider a patient with problems that require some creativity to solve. A patient with an unusual diagnosis such as myesthenia gravis or Gullain-Barré disease or patients on long-term sternal therapy might be interesting to involve the staff in planning for. The nurse might discuss how care for the patient having an elective procedure, such as a cholecystectomy, compares to that for a patient who does not have the condition. New or revised types of surgical procedures are interesting. A patient having a cochlear implant or laser surgery for cervical intraepithelial neoplasia may provide for interesting discussion when planning care.

The nurse will have to prepare for the conference by conducting a preoperative interview and gathering data from the nursing unit and the patient record. In some situations, she may want to review literature specific to the disease or surgical procedure. This will give her added knowledge and provide background for the conference, which will add an educational dimension.

It is well to put some points in writing so the nurse will be able to conduct the conference in an organized manner. She should be sure to start the conference on time. If possible, she should have the group seated in a circle or at tables in an arrangement conducive to group participation. Although members of the group should be encouraged to participate, she should be in control of the discussion. The discussion should center on the patient and topic being presented. Some points will lend themselves to teaching opportunities. She can direct the group to recognize patient problems and develop suitable methods for solving the patient's problem. Because this is a nursing conference, the individualized patient care plan should primarily focus on nursing actions. At the end of the conference, the nurse should review her objectives and obtain feedback about how well they were met. The group should suggest what should be planned for this patient. After the conference, the plan is documented and made available to all participating in the care.

MULTIDISCIPLINARY CONFERENCES

The multidisciplinary conference is common in hospitals. These may focus on one or a group of patients. One such conference might be held weekly for one particular type of patient, for instance, patients having open heart surgery. In the conference, all cases scheduled for surgery that week and all heart surgeries done in the past week are reviewed. Cardiologists, cardiovascular surgeons, and radiologists routinely attend the meeting. Other specialists (e.g., nephrologists, respiratory physicians) attend when the patient case involves their services. Nursing representatives from all areas dealing with the preoperative, intraoperative, and postoperative cardiac patient attend. Support personnel, such as the chaplain, generally are present.

The purpose of presenting the patient case is to increase the quality of care by:

1. Sharing information that will allow better nursing care for the patient (e.g., "Low pain tolerance," "Poor left ventricle," "Intraaortic balloon pump will be in place preoperatively," "Difficult family member")
2. Presenting results of new procedures (angioplasty) and approving new protocols (streptokinase)

3. Providing an opportunity for peer exchange in critically evaluating decisions preoperatively and postoperatively

The physician conference is becoming an increasingly important method for transmitting patient information to members of the team.

Other multidisciplinary conferences may take place on the patient unit prior to surgery and may involve agencies from outside of the hospital, such as Reach to Recovery. This group sends in a volunteer who has had breast surgery to meet with patients scheduled for mastectomy. The volunteer also meets with the nurses to provide information that will be important in planning care. Patients having colostomies need to be referred to the enterostomal therapist, who works with the patient, nurses, and family preoperatively as well as postoperatively. The operating room nurse is a member of the team and attends conferences to share information about the surgical procedure and what will happen to the patient intraoperatively. She also learns about the patient and care given on the nursing unit so she can consider it in planning for the patient during surgery.

Families and patients are involved in some of the conferences because they are considered members of the team. They need to be involved in their care. If they do not understand their illness, the disease process, and what they can and cannot do postoperatively as a result of the surgery, they will not be able to assist in working toward goal achievement. In conferences where the physician, chaplain, dietician, nurses, patient, and family attend, and the plan of care is discussed, agreed upon, and carried out, the patient goals are more likely to be met.

Patient Situation

Even though standards of care are helpful in determining the nursing care plan, each patient requires individualized care. The patient situation used throughout this book illustrates the need for an individualized care plan.

Mr. Fischer, who is scheduled for a possible left hemiglossectomy, left mandibulectomy, and neck dissection, has been seen in his room by the perioperative nurse. She has completed the assessment and collected data pertinent to his procedure. Goals were written, and now the plan is being put into writing.

Communication is one of the most important aspects of Mr. Fischer's care plan because he will not be able to talk postoperatively. Part of the plan is to teach Mr. Fischer alternative methods of communicating, so he can let his family and the nurses know how he is doing. The nurse will show him how to use a magic slate that will be kept by his bed. With the slate, he can write short messages and erase them easily. She also will show him how to use the nurses' call bell. Because he will have a tracheostomy, she will show him hand signals he can use to communicate, and Mr. Fischer tries them out. He will use one finger for yes and two fingers for no. The nurse makes a note to have the other health team members ask him yes or no questions whenever possible. Since Mrs. Fischer cannot drive, the nurse helps Mr. Fischer plan a way to communicate with her by telephone. He will learn how to tap on the mouth piece, with one tap for yes and two taps for no.

With such a complicated surgery, Mr. Fischer does not have a clear idea of all the procedures that will be done. The nurse plans that activities will be explained to him for each phase of his surgery. Examples are:

1. Preoperative activities:
   NPO after midnight
   Preoperative medications
   Intravenous infusion line
   Antiseptic scrub
2. Intraoperative activities:
   Electrocardiogram
   Blood pressure
   Foley catheter
   Possible blood transfusions
   Drains
   Jaw wiring
   Tracheostomy
3. Postoperative activities:
   Intensive care unit
   Possible ventilator
   Frequent suctioning
   Turning
   Respiratory therapy
   Pain medication
   Dressing changes

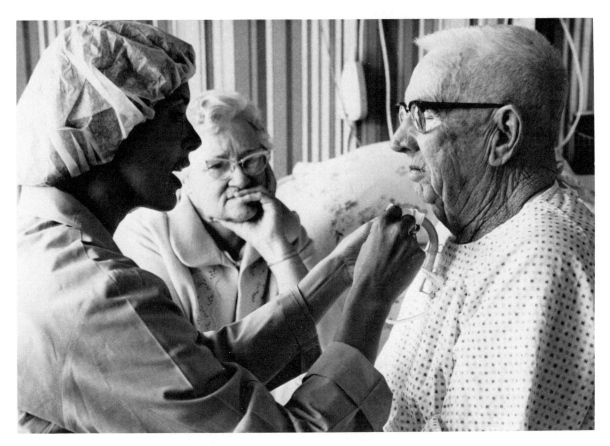

Figure 15.5. The plan is to discuss the tracheostomy tube with the patient prior to surgery.

One of the intraoperative goals is that Mr. Fischer will be free of neuromuscular complications 24 hours postoperatively. The perioperative care plan includes such activities as: (1) using positioning devices on the operating room table to prevent pressure over bony prominences (flotation pad, air mattress pad, or egg crate mattress); (2) placing foam pads on heels and elbows with possible foam ring under buttocks; (3) putting rolled towels under left shoulder as needed; (4) checking with the anesthesiologist and surgeon regarding padding wanted under head and neck; (5) checking with anesthesiologist and surgeon regarding flexion of table or placement of blanket under popliteal space to lessen strain to lower back; (6) asking patient about his level of comfort. All the planned actions are based on data collected about Mr. Fischer during the preoperative assessment.

Postoperatively, the plan addresses Mr. Fischer's respiratory problem. He will have a tracheostomy, which will alter his normal airway. To maintain a patient airway, the nurse will check with the surgeon intraoperatively and have available the type and size of tracheostomy tube that will fit the patient. The recovery room will be notified if a ventilator is necessary. Thus, the equipment will be available and functioning when the patient arrives in the recovery room. For safety, during transportation from the operating room to the recovery room, an ambu bag and oxygen tank will be ready on the patient's bed prior to transfer. A pair of wire cutters will be with patient at all times.

Mr. Fischer is susceptible to respiratory complications because of his history of bronchitis, smoking, and previous exposure to environmental irritants. The plan includes preoperative teaching for coughing, deep breathing, and turning. Mr. Fischer demonstrated these activities preoperatively so the nurse could see that he would be able to do them postoperatively. Preoperatively, the nurse also plans

INTRAOPERATIVE PATIENT CARE PLAN

Mr. Ralph Fischer

NURSING DIAGNOSIS	GOAL	PLAN	IMPLEMENTATION	EVALUATION
PREOPERATIVE Knowledge, lack of external resources (people or material)	Patient will verbalize understanding of his perioperative care prior to administration of preoperative medications.	Provide explanations regarding each phase of perioperative period. 1. Preop: NPO, preop meds, IV line, shave, antiseptic scrub, where family could wait, approximate length of surgery, etc. 2. Intraop: EKG, BP, Foley catheter, possible blood transfusions, drains, jaw wiring, trach etc. 3. Postop: ICU, possible ventilator, frequent suctioning, turning, respiratory therapy, pain meds, dressing change, etc.		
Communication, impaired verbal due to surgical anatomical resection, jaw wiring, tracheostomy.	Patient will be able to communicate postoperatively.	1. Teach patient to use magic slate and nurses call bell 2. Teach patient hand signals (one finger-yes, two fingers-no) 3. Ask patient yes and no questions whenever possible 4. Teach patient to communicate on phone by tapping on mouth piece.		
INTRAOPERATIVE Potential for neuromuscular damage due to required positioning and length of surgical prodecure.	Patient will be free from neuromuscular complications 24 hours postoperatively.	1. Question patient preop re: any ROM limitations or neurosensory problems. 2. Use positional devices on OR table to prevent pressure over bony prominences (i.e., flotation order mattress, egg crate, etc.) 3. Place foam pads on heels and elbows and consider foam ring under buttocks 4. Have rolled towel available for affected shoulder (prn) 5. Check with anesthesiologist and/or surgeon re: padding desired head and neck 6. Check with anesthesiologist and/or surgeon re: flexion of table or placement of blanket under popliteal space to lessen strain to lower back 7. After preliminary positioning ask patient about his level of comfort and adjust accordingly 8. Prior to RR transfer check bony prominences and buttocks for discoloration document findings and communicate abnormal findings to RR		

Figure 15.6. The development of the patient care plan including preoperative and intraoperative nursing diagnoses, goals, and plan for Mr. Fischer.

NURSING DIAGNOSIS	GOAL	PLAN	IMPLEMENTATION	EVALUATION
POSTOPERATIVE				
Respiratory: Alteration in airway (tracheostomy, hemiglossectomy, mandibular fixation.)	Patient will have patent alternative airway until tracheostomy is closed	1. Intraop: have ABG kits available 2. Check with surgeon re: type and size of tracheostomy tube. 3. Notify recovery room if ventilator necessary 4. Have ambu bag and oxygen tank ready on patient bed prior to transport 5. If jaw wired, have wire cutters available for recovery room.		
Increased risk for postop complications due to: 1. History of bronchitis 2. History of smoking 3. Exposure to environmental irritants.	Patient will be free of respiratory complications 48 hours postop. 1. Infection 2. Atelectasis 3. Aspiration	1. Preoperatively teach respiratory exercises (coughing, deep breathing, turning). Have patient return demonstrate and state rationale. 2. Discuss altered breathing pattern via tracheostomy 3. Explain need for frequent suctioning 4. Due to increased risk of aspiration elevate head of bed per physician's orders and monitor closely for signs of respiratory distress during transport. 5. Monitor nasogastric tube for patency and return of gastric secretions.		

Figure 15.7. The development of the patient care plan including postoperative nursing diagnoses, goals, and plan for Mr. Fischer.

to discuss altered breathing patterns due to the tracheostomy and the need for frequent suctioning and coughing (see Fig. 15.5). During transportation immediately postoperatively, she plans to elevate the head of the bed to decrease risk of aspiration or difficult breathing. Figures 15.6–15.7 depict a portion of the care plan for Mr. Fischer.

References

1. *Standards of Perioperative Nursing Practice.* Kansas City: American Nurses' Association and Association of Operating Room Nurses, 1982.

IV

Implementing Perioperative Patient Care

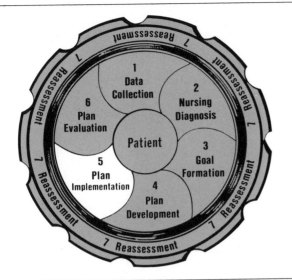

The plan is converted to action.

Implementing Nursing Actions

The third component of the nursing process, implementation, begins when the patient care plan is put into practice and ends when all nursing activities have been carried out and documented. Two important functions are: (1) performing the nursing action and (2) documenting the action performed.

What the nurse does with or for the patient is described as a nursing action. Nursing actions are selected to achieve the specified objectives. They may be dependent or independent. Dependent nursing actions are prescribed by the physician or other members of the health team and are carried out by the nurse. Positioning the patient for surgery, administering medications for patients having local anesthesia, and hemodynamic monitoring are examples of dependent nursing actions. Independent nursing actions are designed and carried out by the nurse. Explaining to the patient what will happen in the operating room, assessing the patient's level of consciousness, and communicating with the patient's family during surgery are independent nursing actions.

Actions may also be shared with other members of the team. Performing sponge, needle, and instrument counts is a shared responsibility. The surgeon participates in the actual counting and shares legal responsibility with the nurse. Nurse and surgeon are both responsible for patient safety in the operating room environment. They jointly monitor apparel, traffic in and out of the operating room, and the containment of contaminants. The Association of Operating Room Nurses has provided examples of general nursing activities as a guide for nurses (1) (Table 16.1).

Specific activities for each patient are developed in the plan of care prior to the patient's arrival in the operating room. For example, Mrs. Cross arrives in the operating room for a breast biopsy and possible subtotal mastectomy. Discovering an arthritic elbow, the nurse notes the need for special padding and extra protection in the care plan and provides it. As part of the plan, the nurse also explains to Mrs. Cross what he is doing in a soft, gentle voice. This relaxes and comforts Mrs. Cross.

Table 16.1. Examples of Nursing Activities in the Perioperative Role.

Preoperative Phase	Intraoperative Phase	Postoperative Phase
Preoperative assessment	*Maintenance of safety*	*Communication of intraoperative information*
Home/clinic	1. Assures that the sponge, needle, and instrument counts are correct	1. Gives patient's name
1. Initiates initial preoperative assessment	2. Positions the patient	2. States type of surgery performed
2. Plans teaching methods appropriate to patient's needs	a. Functional alignment	3. Provides contributing intraoperative factors, i.e., drain, catheters
3. Involves family in interview	b. Exposure of surgical site	4. States physical limitations
Surgical unit	c. Maintenance of position throughout procedure	5. States impairments resulting from surgery
1. Completes preoperative assessment	3. Applies grounding device to patient	6. Reports patient's preoperative level of consciousness
2. Coordinates patient teaching with other nursing staff	4. Provides physical support	7. Communicates necessary equipment needs
3. Explains phases in perioperative period and expectations	*Physiological monitoring*	*Postoperative evaluation*
4. Develops a plan of care	1. Calculates effects on patient of excessive fluid loss	Recovery area
Surgical suite	2. Distinguishes normal from abnormal cardiopulmonary data	1. Determines patient's immediate response to surgical intervention
1. Assesses patient's level of consciousness	3. Reports changes in patient's pulse, respirations, temperature, and blood pressure	Surgical unit
2. Reviews chart	*Psychological monitoring* (prior to induction and if patient conscious)	1. Evaluates effectiveness of nursing care in the OR
3. Identifies patient	1. Provides emotional support to patient	2. Determines patient's level of satisfaction with care given during perioperative period
4. Verifies surgical site	2. Continues to assess patient's emotional status	3. Evaluates products used on patient in the OR
Planning	3. Communicates patient's emotional status to other appropriate members of the health care team	4. Determines patient's psychological status
1. Determines a plan of care	*Nursing management*	5. Assists with discharge planning
Psychological support	1. Provides physical safety for the patient	Home/clinic
1. Tells patient what is happening	2. Maintains aseptic, controlled environment	1. Seeks patient's perception of surgery in terms of the effects of anesthetic agents, impact on body image, distortion, immobilization
2. Determines psychological status	3. Effectively manages human resources	2. Determines family's perceptions of surgery
3. Gives prior warning of noxious stimuli		
4. Stands near/touches patient during procedures/induction		
5. Communicates patient's emotional status to other appropriate members of the health care team		

Continuing to carry out the plan, the nurse puts on antiembolism stockings to aid varicosities that create a potential circulatory problem.

Determinants of Nursing Action

A variety of factors determine the types of nursing actions selected to meet the needs of patients. A philosophy of nursing and underlying values are guides in planning care. Actions will also be influenced by the importance assigned to the patient's problems and the depth to which they have been explored. The amount of involvement with the family and other members of the team will influence activities selected. How the nurse perceives his role will influence the care planned and implemented. The perioperative nurse may choose to focus his scope of practice on the intraoperative phase, giving less attention to the preoperative and postoperative phases. He may do an assessment and evaluation on the unit, or he may expand his practice to include nursing activities in the home, clinic, and physician's office both preoperatively and postoperatively.

Hospital policies and procedures also have a bearing on nursing actions. For instance, if the hospital policy states that families or significant others are not permitted in the holding area, some nurses will follow the policy rigidly without modifying it to meet patient's needs. Other nurses will generally follow the policy but in extenuating circumstances realize that the patient's need can only be met by allowing a family member into the area for a short time to provide emotional support or alleviate fear.

Hospital standards of care provide another guide for nurses. The standards prescribe nursing orders which have been approved to establish the level of care patients receive. Nurses have a responsibility to individualize the standards of care by determining which problems are specific to a certain patient and develop the plan accordingly. In performing an assessment on a patient having a cataract removed, for example, the nurse may determine that the patient is apprehensive and hypertensive. The nursing orders in the standard of care for patients having cataract surgery may indicate that the patient should be allowed to verbalize anxieties, express concerns about the impending surgery, and state knowledge regarding the disease process and expected outcomes of surgery. For hypertension, the orders are to notify the anesthesiologist and take and record baseline blood pressure preoperatively. These nursing orders are used in selecting actions appropriate to each patient.

Other human and material resources are available when determining what nursing actions can be used to achieve the goals. If a patient having palliative surgery for carcinoma of the esophagus is demonstrating a great deal of anger, the nurse may decide that a chaplain or psychiatric clinical specialist should see the patient. If the hospital has neither, the nurse could seek out a social worker or an appropriate volunteer. Nursing actions depend on the types of equipment and supplies accessible within the hospital. If the nurse determines that a patient needs constant cardiac monitoring during transportation to the operating room, the nursing action is to transport the patient with a portable monitor. If this piece of equipment is not available, alternative action would be taken. For example, a nurse skilled in care of the critically ill could accompany the patient. He would carefully assess any observable parameters such as pulse, respiration, and color.

Finally, the nurse's own capabilities determine actions. His knowledge base, communication skills, interest in others, and concern for the patient all play a role. If a nurse has not performed a procedure or is unfamiliar with the task, he is usually unwilling to do it. For instance, a patient is scheduled for a hip fixation. The orthopedic surgeon requests a Chick table. If the nurse has never used this piece of equipment, he will be reluctant to be assigned on the case unless another person who knows how to use the table is also assigned to the same room. Remember two important points regarding nursing capabilities. As a licensed professional, the nurse is legally accountable for his actions. He should inform his supervisor if asked to perform a procedure for which he is not qualified. At the same time, he should take it upon himself to gain more knowledge and learn new skills. Nurses have a responsibility for maintaining competency.

Nursing Capabilities

A sound educational background in nursing is a prerequisite for the specialty of perioperative nursing. The arts, sciences, and humanities broaden understanding and give the nurse additional resources that influence the type of care patients receive.

A perioperative nurse's capabilities are made up of knowledge, skill, and performance. Knowledge is defined as "an oganized body of information, usually factual or procedural, which, if applied makes adequate performance of the job possible" (2:10). Knowledge of perioperative nursing includes a thorough understanding of theories and principles of the science of nursing. It requires the nurse not only to comprehend information but also to have the ability to analyze, synthesize, and apply it to a wide variety of situations. Having knowledge does not guarantee it can be used to perform a skill properly; it simply means the nurse has the information available to make performing the skill possible.

Knowledge specific to the perioperative role includes:

- Nursing process
- Perioperative standards of practice
- Baseline data on patient having surgery
- Cultural differences in patients' responses to surgery
- Principles of asepsis
- Interviewing techniques
- Anatomy and physiology
- Normal laboratory values
- Theories of behavioral psychology

Nursing activities require skills. A skill may be defined as proficient manual, verbal, or mental manipulation of data, things, or people. Manual skills, involving psychomotor activity, range from very simple tasks to complex procedures. They include the basic ability to hold a pencil or pen and write on the operative nurses' notes, as well as the more complicated task of positioning the patient on the operating room table. Verbal skills are used when interviewing a patient and giving an oral report to a surgeon or supervisor. The perioperative nurse uses mental skills when formulating nursing diagnoses, interpreting laboratory values, analyzing patient problems, and determining a plan of action.

Skills for the perioperative role include:

- Identifying the patient on admission to the surgical suite
- Performing a physical assessment
- Establishing rapport with a patient and family
- Coordinating the chaplain's visit to meet with patient and family needs
- Cleansing the patient's skin
- Interpreting laboratory data

The third component of a nurse's capabilities is performance, defined as the execution of an action. Because an individual possesses knowledge and skill does not necessarily mean a nursing action will be performed at the expected level or according to the established procedure. Attitude plays an important role in performance.

Attitude is hard to define, but we can readily see the effect. The nurse who is warm, caring, and friendly, and transmits confidence and cooperation conveys a high level of competence. The nurse's attitude toward a patient in pain can affect his level of tolerance. Combined with knowledge and skill, a caring attitude provides the patient with complete and compassionate support.

Performing competently entails a variety of intangible qualities:

- Self-reliance
- Sensitivity to human needs
- A value system with behavior that is predictable, consistent, and pervasive
- Knowledge of one's own strengths and limitations

- Tolerance of racial, cultural, and religious differences
- Responsibility for one's own behavior

Selecting Nursing Actions for the Perioperative Patient

Nursing actions are consistent with the plan of care and are selected to assist the patient toward goal achievement. For example, the patient who is 6 feet 5 inches tall will need an extension placed on the operating room table to maintain body alignment. The obese patient will need an arm board and other positioning devices to assure body alignment. Both actions are intended to meet the goal of the patient's being free from harm due to positioning.

The activities provide continuity of care for the patient through the preoperative, intraoperative, and postoperative period. Psychological support is an example of a nursing action that demonstrates continuity of care. The patient who demonstrates fear and anxiety about the impending surgery and the operating room requires nursing interventions such as encouraging the patient to express feelings, ask specific questions related to fears, relating to the patient at his level of understanding, and accepting the patient's feelings without being judgmental. The perioperative nurse collaborates with the unit nurse, other team members, and patient and family to plan interventions that will prepare the patient for surgery. Assisting the patient to handle anxiety and fear prior to surgery is the initial goal. Intraoperatively, the nurse provides emotional support by reinforcing the patient's adaptive response to fear, giving realistic reassurance, touching, and explaining what is happening (see Fig. 16.1). Postoperatively, the patient is told the outcome of surgery, and behaviors that promote recovery are reinforced. Psychological support is essential throughout the entire surgical experience because the patient is acutely aware of his surroundings and is constantly evaluating the quality of human interaction.

Nursing actions are selected that demonstrate the nurse's concern for the patient's welfare and also produce the desired effect with a minimum of effort, expense, and waste. Activities that ensure a safe environment might include maintaining asepsis during a procedure; containing and confining soiled sponges, linen, specimens, and instruments; performing equipment checks; and keeping the room temperature and humidity at standard levels.

The judicious use of supplies such as suture, sponges, needles, and drapes demonstrates the nurse's concern for the patient's expenses. Organization of time and planning of activities will save the patient money in operating room charges. By reducing the time the patient is in the operating room, the nurse reduces the time the patient is exposed to the surgical procedure and therefore may reduce the incidence of wound infection.

Nursing actions should reflect the patient's right to individualized care and the preservation of dignity. As stated in Chapter 8, the patient has rights that must be incorporated into the plan of care. These are outlined in the *Patient's Bill of Rights* published by the American Hospital Association (3). The patient has a right to privacy, a right to know what is expected, and a right to refuse treatment. The nurse's role includes patient advocacy. During transfer from the unit to the surgical suite or to the operating room table, the patient's dignity should be preserved by his being covered and provided warmth and comfort. During the surgical preparation, the patient should not be exposed more than necessary. Responding to the patient's questions and explaining procedures are ways of meeting the patient's right to know.

The nurse is only one of the members of the health care team responsible for the patient's welfare during the surgical experience. The interventions employed by nursing must be congruent with therapies and the treatments prescribed by other members of the team. Cooperative effort aids in achieving the patient goal.

For example, the team must work together when a patient goes into a malignant hyper-

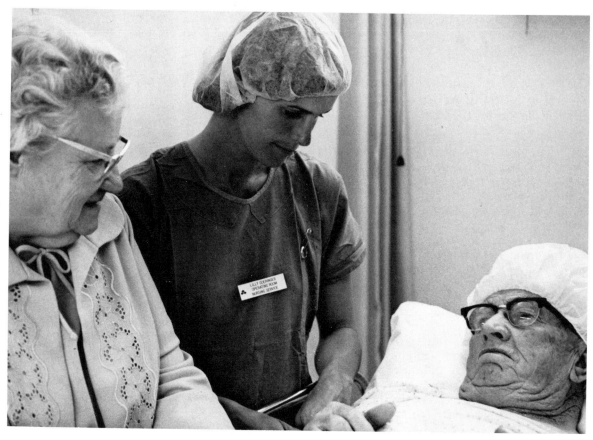

Figure 16.1. The nurse provides emotional support in the holding area.

thermia crisis during the surgical procedure. Nursing actions such as packing the patient in ice and placing a rectal probe for monitoring the temperature are congruent with therapies employed by the anesthesiologist. Hemodynamic monitoring prescribed by the physician entails nursing actions such as continuously taking blood pressures and interpreting and communicating data to the physician so therapeutic measures can be taken.

Responsibility for Directing Patient Care

The assignment of personnel to perform the specified nursing actions takes place in the planning phase and should be incorporated into the patient care plan. As each planned activity is carried out, the registered nurse is responsible and legally accountable. The nurse has the option of personally performing the nursing activity or assigning it to another individual. When supervising another individual, the nurse must be certain the activity can be carried out competently. He also guides activities so the goal will be attained. He should ascertain that the best prepared person is caring for the patient; the person must have appropriate intellectual, interpersonal, and technical skills and the proper educational background. The individual performing the nursing action must be able to make nursing judgments, interpret data, and make decisions about the patient's care.

Once the care has been given, the patient's response is evaluated. This is the responsibility of the nurse assigned the patient. The patient's response can be evaluated during or after care. Methods for monitoring the effects of nursing activities include observation of nurse performance and patient response, comments from the patient and family, and documentation in the patient record.

Documenting Nursing Actions

Documentation is the recording of data specific to an individual patient in the patient record. Both the nursing activity and the patient's response to the nursing activity are recorded. The purpose of documentation is to prove that the care was given. In the past, recording of preoperative and postoperative patient information by unit nurses was for the most part adequate, but recording of information specific to the patient's surgery was sparse. Greater emphasis is now placed on depicting continuity of care through surgery, thus providing a more complete picture of care given by perioperative nurses. Documentation provides a comprehensive review of data about the patient that can readily be retrieved either concurrently or retrospectively. Therefore it can be used in quality assurance to measure effectiveness of nursing care. Furthermore, documentation depicts patterns of care, levels of care, and information for classification of patients for fiscal and administrative accountability. The information can also be used when legal questions arise to verify and validate care provided and accurately reflect patient responses. Accurate reporting of information is a nursing responsibility that demonstrates accountability for nursing actions. Nurses should recognize the importance of their role in assuring the highest level of practice. Finally, the information can be used for research or teaching purposes. In this sense, it becomes part of the body of scientific knowledge for improving the practice of nursing and patient care (see Chapter 24).

The patient record has several places for documenting nursing care and the patient's response to surgery. One is the preoperative checklist where the nurse might record preoperative patient teaching, procedures such as insertion of a Foley catheter or nasogastric tube, and identification of the patient upon admission to the surgical suite. A perioperative nursing care plan is designed specifically for the surgical experience. A well-developed care plan becomes a useful tool for documentation. The operating room record or nurse's notes are a form used to record intraoperative nursing care. It includes such data as the placement of electrocardiograph leads and electrosurgical grounding pads; position of the patient during the procedure; implantable devices; accuracy of sponge, needle, and instrument counts; and other vital information that reflects nursing care provided.

When documenting nursing activities, the perioperative nurse uses the plan of care as a guide. The information recorded should be consistent with the planned activities. These activities must also lead to goal attainment, since the activities were designed with the patient goal in mind. For example, if an intraoperative nursing action was to place the patient in the lithotomy position according to policy and procedure, the goal was that the patient would be free of neuromuscular complications due to positioning. The documentation records what the nurse did and the result:

Nursing actions
- Patient placed in a lithotomy position
- Both lower extremities simultaneously placed in stirrups
- Both lower extremities padded for protection

Patient outcome
- Lower extremities maintained in alignment
- No noticeable dislocation of hips
- No complaints of hip joint pain.

From this, it can be determined that the care was effective in achieving the patient goal.

Nursing activities may not be effective in all situations. Accurate documentation reveals if there was a negative response or if the desired result was not attained. When this occurs, the nurse reassesses the patient and the new data are used to formulate a revised plan of action. The entire process is repeated.

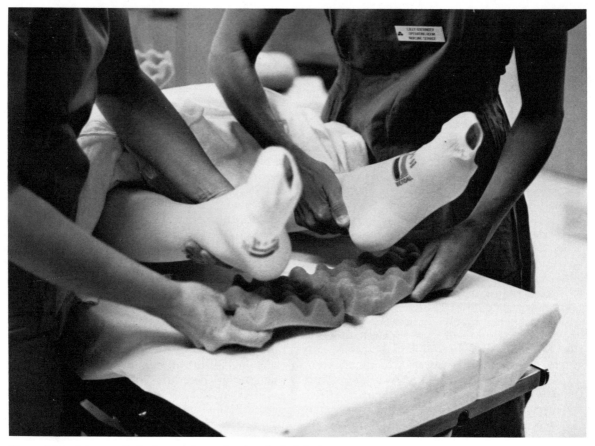

Figure 16.2. Intraoperatively, foam pads are placed under both heels.

Patient Situation

Mr. Fischer is scheduled for a left hemiglossectomy, left hemimandibulectomy, and left neck dissection. Information pertinent to the operating room has been obtained, nursing diagnosis formulated, goals set, and a plan developed. At this point perioperative nurses are putting into action the plan of care which has been individualized for Mr. Fischer (see Figs. 16.3 and 16.4).

One of Mr. Fischer's problems was his lack of knowledge about specific events surrounding the surgical procedure. The perioperative nurse explains to him what will happen. The evening before surgery he will take a shower. In the morning, he should shave as closely as possible because the surgery will involve his face. He should drink no water or fluids from midnight until sometime after

surgery. The nurse explains that he will be given medication that is a drying agent in the morning. The drying agent will decrease the secretions in the mouth, which in turn decreases the potential for aspiration of fluids. He will receive another medication that makes him drowsy. This is to dull his remembrance of the many activities associated with his transportation, his transfer to the operating room table, and his preparation for surgery. The nurse tells Mr. Fischer and his family when he will be taken to the operating room, where the family can wait, and the approximate time he will return to the room.

The perioperative nurse asks Mr. Fischer if he has any questions and then asks him to explain in his own words his understanding of the surgical procedure and anesthesia.

INTRAOPERATIVE PATIENT CARE PLAN

Mr. Ralph Fischer

NURSING DIAGNOSIS	GOAL	PLAN	IMPLEMENTATION	EVALUATION
PREOPERATIVE Knowledge, lack of external resources (people or material).	Patient will verbalize understanding of his perioperative care prior to administration of preoperative medications.	Provide explanations regarding each phase of perioperative period. 1. Preop: NPO, preop meds, IV line, shave, antiseptic scrub, where family could wait, approximate length of surgery, etc. 2. Intraop: ECG, BP, Foley catheter, possible blood transfusions, drains, jaw wiring, trach, etc. 3. Postop: ICU, possible ventilator, frequent suctioning, turning, respiratory therapy, pain meds, dressing change, etc.	• Specific information provided regarding the events surrounding the surgical procedure • Explanations given regarding expectations of the patient and family • Encouraged to express fears and anxieties • Patient explained his understanding of the surgical procedure and anesthesia. • Preoperative instruction regarding postop care: 1-coughing, deep breathing, turning 2-pain 3-drains and tubes 4-IV 5-possible ventilator • Patient demonstrated turning, coughing and deep breathing exercises.	
Communication, impaired verbal due to surgical anatomical resection, jaw wiring, tracheostomy.	Patient will be able to communicate postoperatively.	1. Teach patient to use magic slate and nurses call bell 2. Teach patient hand signals (one finger-yes, two fingers-no) 3. Ask patient yes and no questions whenever possible 4. Teach patient to communicate on phone by tapping on mouth piece.	Nurse conducted preoperative assessment • Rapport was established with patient and wife • Patient taught how to use alternative methods of communicating • Patient and wife return demonstrated use of fingers and phone messages.	
INTRAOPERATIVE Potential for neuromuscular damage due to required positioning and length of surgical procedure.	Patient will be free from neuromuscular complications 24 hours postoperatively.	1. Question patient preop re: any ROM limitations or neurosensory problems. 2. Use positional devices on OR table to prevent pressure over bony prominences (i.e., flotation order mattress, egg crate, etc.) 3. Place foam pads on heels and elbows and consider foam ring under buttocks 4. Have rolled towel available for affected shoulder (prn) 5. Check with anesthesiologist and/or surgeon re: padding desired for head and neck 6. Check with anesthesiologist and/or surgeon re: flexion of table or placement of blanket under popliteal space to lessen strain to lower back 7. After preliminary positioning ask patient about his level of comfort and adjust accordingly. 8. Prior to RR transfer check bony prominences and buttocks for discoloration document findings and communicate abnormal findings to RR	Operating Room: 1. Patient denied ROM limitations preoperatively. 2. Patient placed in supine position with egg crate mattress. 3. Foam pads on both elbows and heels. 4. Rolled towel placed under shoulder. 5. Head and neck slightly extended. 6. O.R. table flexed to lessen strain on lower back during procedure. 7. Patient states he is comfortable. 8. Physical assessment when transferring to recovery room revealed no evidence of pressure areas or impaired skin integrity.	

Figure 16.3. Intraoperative patient care plan including preoperative and intraoperative nursing diagnoses, goals, plans, and implementation for Mr. Fischer.

INTRAOPERATIVE PATIENT CARE PLAN

Mr. Ralph Fischer

NURSING DIAGNOSIS	GOAL	PLAN	IMPLEMENTATION	EVALUATION
POSTOPERATIVE				
Respiratory: Alteration in airway (tracheostomy, hemiglossectomy, mandibular fixation.)	Patient will have patent alternative airway until tracheostomy is closed.	1. Intraop: have ABG kits available 2. Check with surgeon re: type and size of tracheostomy tube. 3. Notify recovery room if ventilator necessary 4. Have ambu bag and oxygen tank ready on patient bed prior to transport 5. If jaw wired, have wire cutters available for recovery room.	Operating Room: 1. Blood drawn for ABG and sent to lab 2. Silastic tracheostomy tube size #7 inserted. Recovery Room: 3. Placed on ventilator per ET tube at 50% FiO₂, 1000 tidal volume, rate 12. 4. Ambu bag at bedside. 5. Wire cutters at bedside.	
Increased risk for postop complications due to: 1. History of bronchitis 2. History of smoking 3. Exposure to environmental irritants	Patient will be free of respiratory complications 48 hours postop. 1. Infection 2. Atelectasis 3. Aspiration	1. Preoperatively teach respiratory exercises (coughing, deep breathing, turning). Have patient return demonstrate and state rationale. 2. Discuss altered breathing pattern via tracheostomy 3. Explain need for frequent suctioning 4. Due to increased risk of aspiration elevate head of bed per physician's orders and monitor closely for signs of respiratory distress during transport. 5. Monitor nasogastric tube for patency and return of gastric secretions.	Note: 1. Preoperatively the nurse conducted an assessment and taught the patient with return demonstration. 2. (see Implementation Problem #1) 3. (see Implementation Problem #1) 4. Head of bed elevated immediately postop and until patient returned to nursing unit. Postop Unit: 1. Nasogastric tube to gravity drainage with scant amount of light green drainage. 2. Complaining of nausea and NG tube being uncomfortable. 3. Patient vomiting and aspirated secretions into lungs. 4. Physician notified.	

Figure 16.4. Intraoperative patient care plan including postoperative nursing diagnosis, goals, plans, and implementation for Mr. Fischer.

Another important aspect of preparing Mr. Fischer for his surgery is the preoperative instruction. The nurse tells Mr. Fischer about coughing, deep breathing, and turning. The nurse then has him demonstrate them in order to evaluate his participation and the potential effectiveness of his actions. The nurse tells him he will have pain, explaining where it will be and why he will have it. The nurse adds that it is important that he ask for pain medication before the pain gets too intense and more difficult to manage. Mr. Fischer will have an intravenous infusion, drains from the operative site, and a nasogastric tube. The nurse explains the reason for these devices and the part they play in the postoperative care. Because Mr. Fischer is having a temporary tracheostomy, he will be unable to speak and will have trouble communicating. The nurse teaches the patient various methods for postoperative communication. A magic slate is one of the ways Mr. Fischer will communicate his needs. He practices writing the word "shot" which means he is having pain. A finger signal is devised where Mr. Fischer can respond to yes and no questions. One finger means yes; two fingers, no. Because his wife will be calling him on the phone he will also tap on the mouthpiece. One tap means yes; two taps, no. The nurse implements the plan developed in Chapter 15 and after teaching it has Mr. Fischer and his wife demonstrate the methods selected. The perioperative nurse documents nursing actions on the patient record as well as the operating room care plan.

One of the intraoperative goals established for Mr. Fischer is that he will be free of neuromuscular complications 24 hours postoperatively. In the op-erating room, the nurses place him in a supine position with an egg crate mattress. Foam pads are put on both elbows and heels with a rolled towel under the shoulder to extend the head and neck slightly. The operating room bed is flexed to decrease strain on the lower back during the procedure. His position is monitored during the procedure, and an evaluation is done by the nurse before Mr. Fischer is transferred to the recovery room. There is no evidence of skin impairment or musculoskeletal complications. The nurse documents the activities performed intraoperatively and the postoperative evaluation.

In the recovery room, the perioperative nurse communicates information about Mr. Fischer, his condition, and needs for special equipment to the recovery room nurse. The nurse then initiates care, placing Mr. Fischer on a ventilator and monitoring physiological and emotional status. When he is discharged from the recovery room, the nurse communicates with the family in the waiting room.

References

1. Association of Operating Room Nurses. "Operating room nursing: Perioperative role." *AORN J* 27:1156, 1978.
2. Hercules, P. R., and Kneedler, J. A. *Certification Series Unit III. Knowledges, Skills, and Content Areas for Study.* Denver: Association of Operating Room Nurses, 1979.
3. *Patient's Bill of Rights.* Chicago: American Hospital Association, 1972.

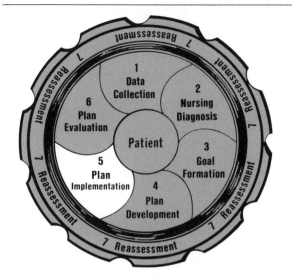

The patient is brought to the operating room safely.

Transporting the Patient

For many patients the preoperative period is a series of frightening and uncomfortable events that can cause extreme anxiety. The trip from the nursing unit to the operating room can be one of these events because the patient is suddenly confronted with the reality of her impending surgery. A critical time, it is the patient's last conscious period before completely surrendering and placing herself in the hands of others.

It is not surprising that patients report feelings of vulnerability, helplessness, and loss of self-esteem during this time. Nurses and orderlies enter the room, strip her of her possessions, dress her in a gown without a back, and strap her to a gurney. Then it is off to the operating room with everybody chatting, smiling, and making small talk. Meanwhile, the patient lies quietly on the gurney, wondering and anticipating.

The process of transporting the patient to the operating room is often viewed as a chore by the nursing staff and delegated to the least skilled worker. A transition between the nursing unit and the operating room, it is often a time when nursing care is neglected. Yet the patient still has physical, psychological, sociocultural, and spiritual needs that must be met. This is a time when the patient needs nursing care.

The purpose of this chapter is to fill the transitional void and assist the nurse in planning for the perioperative nursing care that should be implemented while the patient is being transported to the operating room. It includes a discussion of the closed and open systems of transporting patients and the management of transportation, including the role of the transporter, methods that can be used, and specific patient problems during the transportation. Finally, the scope of nursing activities that should be accomplished from the time the patient leaves the nursing unit to her transferal to the operating room bed are discussed.

Systems for Transporting Patients

There are two types of systems for transporting patients, open and closed. The open method uses a gurney taken from the operating room to the nursing unit and back again. Depending on the type of gurney, this system is less expensive than the closed system and is used in most hospitals. Some objections are made to this system because the gurney leaves the clean area of the operating room and returns with outside contaminants — especially on the wheels.

The closed system is designed to eliminate the transfer of nursing unit contaminants into the operating room. A closed system gurney at the minimum has two transport bases, one for the nursing unit and the other for the operating room, and a bed with a roller support that permits the patient to be moved from one gurney to the other without handling.

The operating room supervisor determines which system of transportation to use. Variables that need to be considered are the cost of implementing each system and whether the physical layout of the operating room will accommodate the closed system. Finally, it is necessary to decide if wheel contamination is a significant factor in the aseptic environment of the operating room, which has not been adequately determined (1).

Management of Transportation

RESPONSIBILITY FOR TRANSPORTATION

Transporting the patient to the operating room is always a *nursing* responsibility. Ideally, an operating room orderly under the supervision of a unit nurse should transport the patient to the operating room. This provides for continued monitoring of the patient by the unit nurse until she is admitted to the operating room and placed under the care of the operating room nurse. This assures continuity of nursing care and communication between nurses.

Unfortunately, the ideal is often impractical if not impossible to achieve. Hospital staffing frequently makes it difficult for the nurse to leave the unit. Likewise, there are few operating rooms that can spare a nurse to transport patients. Consequently, the task is assigned to an orderly. Even though the task is delegated, the operating room supervisor remains responsible and accountable for the welfare of the patient during the transportation period. The operating room supervisor should ensure that the perioperative patient care plan provides guidance to the orderly assigned this task and that he is thoroughly familiar with basic transportation protocol. There are times when it is mandatory for a nurse to assist in transporting the patient. In such cases, an agreement between the nursing unit and the operating room will have to be made as to who will accompany the patient during transport.

THE ROLE OF THE OPERATING ROOM NURSE

The OR nurse can best fulfill her responsibility in assuring safe transportation by making a preoperative assessment and, if necessary, planning for the transportation in the perioperative patient care plan. But if the perioperative patient care plan is to be successful it must be understood by and communicated to the transporter.

Interpreting preoperative assessment data and applying it to the transportation period as well as the intraoperative period can be difficult, but it is not impossible. It is easier if the operating room nurse accepts the idea that the transportation of the surgical patient indeed is within the realm of perioperative nursing.

During the perioperative assessment, the nurse should be alert to patient data that can be used in developing diagnoses, goals, and nursing actions that pertain to transportation. If the nurse focuses on the following assessment factors, formulating a pertinent care plan will be simpler:

1. Age, height, and weight
2. Psychological and emotional status
3. Sensory status, such as poor eyesight or hearing
4. Respiratory status
5. Cardiovascular status
6. Neuromuscular status
7. Presence of medical devices, such as catheters, chest tubes and bottles, and intravenous infusion containers

The case of Mrs. Doe illustrates how to abstract pertinent transportation data from the overall assessment data. Mrs. Doe was admitted to a medium-sized community hospital for a cholecystectomy. The night before surgery, an operating room nurse did a preoperative assessment and collected the following data.

1. 43 years old, 5 feet 5 inches tall, 235 pounds.
2. Alert and oriented. Patient states she is nervous and dreads going to surgery. She said, "I've never been a patient in a hospital before. Where will my husband wait? He's so worried." The patient has slight hand tremors, moist palms, and is slightly tearful during the interview.
3. Has hyperopia and extremely poor eyesight without her eyeglasses. She verbalized concern about not being able to see very well in the recovery room after surgery.
4. States she has a difficult time breathing while lying flat. The operating room nurse placed the patient in dorsal recumbent position and observed labored breathing.
5. Has history of hypertension with control by medication. Bilateral varicosities observed in lower extremities.

6. States she has chronic arthritis in the right shoulder that can cause severe discomfort with weight bearing.
7. No medical devices at the time of assessment. The intravenous infusion will be started in the operating room.

The perioperative nurse used these data to develop a perioperative patient care plan (see Table 17.1).

Many patient care problems may occur during transportation. The astute operating room nurse will be able to identify potential problems and make the appropriate plans.

GOALS OF TRANSPORTATION

The individual assigned the role of transporter, whether she is a nurse or an orderly, has three fundamental goals to meet. These are: (1) to ensure the completion of preoperative actions, (2) to transport the patient safely, and (3) to communicate with the patient and significant others. The first is governed by hospital policy, while the other two are part of the perioperative patient care plan. Although the nursing activities inherent in each of these goals are discussed, the focus is on specific concepts within each goal.

The first goal is to ensure that preoperative actions are completed. This simply means that the transporter needs to determine if the patient is ready for surgery. Often patients come to the operating room with undergarments, dentures, and jewelry. Instances like these are all too common and occur because the transporter did not complete her prescribed duties. The nonnurse transporter is not accountable if a patient arrives in the operating room unprepared because of such things as low potassium or hematocrit. In this case, the unit nurse should have been more astute in her clinical assessment and have alerted the physician and the operating room supervisor before releasing the patient to the transporter. If the transporter observes the patient for jewelry, asks pertinent questions such as, "Are your undergarments removed?" and, "Do you have dentures?" and reviews the preoperative checklist,

Table 17.1. Perioperative Patient Care Plan Depicting Transportation Problems.

Nursing Diagnosis	Patient Goal	Nursing Intervention
Acute moderate situational anxiety secondary to impending surgery.	During transportation, the patient's level of anxiety will not be increased. This will be evidenced by a lack of hand tremors and moist palms.	1. The operating room nurse responsible for the timing of the preoperative medication will call early enough to ensure that Mrs. Doe receives maximum benefit from the medication. 2. The operating room nurse dispatching the orderly will give the following instructions: a. The patient is to be moved from the bed to the gurney with minimal stimulation. b. The patient's husband will be encouraged to accompany her to the holding area for the purpose of providing emotional support. c. During transport, conversation will be kept to a minimum. This will help to provide a quiet environment and enhance the effectiveness of the preoperative medication. 3. The transporter will carry out all instructions and report to the operating room nurse receiving Mrs. Doe concerning her emotional status during transportation.
Potential for mild respiratory distress and discomfort during transportation to the operating room secondary to obesity.	The patient will be transported to the operating room with no respiratory distress or discomfort. This will be evidenced by the absence of labored breathing. The patient will state that she feels comfortable and is not having difficulty breathing.	1. The operating room nurse dispatching the orderly will give the following instructions: a. After the patient is moved to the gurney she will be placed in a sitting position of at least 45 degrees. The orderly will accomplish this by elevating the head of the gurney and by placing a pillow behind Mrs. Doe's back. The orderly will then ask Mrs. Doe if she is comfortable. If she reports difficulty with breathing, adjustments to the position will be made as necessary.
Potential for patient harm during transfer procedures secondary to severe hyperopia.	The patient will be transferred from the bed to the gurney and from the gurney to the operating room bed without harm.	1. The operating room nurse dispatching the orderly will give the following instructions: a. The patient will be allowed to wear her eyeglasses to the operating room. b. The patient will be assisted from the bed to the gurney by the orderly who will gently hold Mrs. Doe's arm and guide her during transfer. 2. The circulating nurse will also gently guide Mrs. Doe from the gurney to the OR bed. After the patient is safely secured on the OR bed, her eyeglasses will be removed. The eyeglasses will accompany Mrs. Doe to the recovery room. This will help Mrs. Doe to adapt to the recovery room environment and routine following surgery.

she is taking the necessary steps to ensure that preoperative actions are completed.

Of primary importance is the next goal: ensuring patient safety during transport. At this time, the patient is vulnerable to extrinsic environmental hazards. For many patients, preoperative medications will cause physiological alterations such as dizziness, weakness, confusion, and sedation. Impaired ability to interpret sensory data may result in an increased susceptibility to accidents. A phenomenal number of accidents occur yearly to patients after they have been medicated.

Communicating with the patient and his significant others is also an important transportation goal. So often the transporter gets caught up in the technical details of the task that the more human elements of this patient care activity are ignored. It can be argued that the ordinary transporter is not qualified to engage in therapeutic communication with sedated and anxious patients, and these arguments are valid. Furthermore, there is merit in the occasional admonition from the operating room supervisor to the transporter that the less the premedicated patient is stimulated, the more effective the medication. Yet communication during the transportation is necessary. Diligent care during transportation can communicate dialogue to the patient and significant others, "You're in good hands." Often the sincere touch and quiet voice says and accomplishes more than a whole list of planned therapeutic interventions. As a rule, the transporter should maintain a quiet atmosphere. Significant others should be encouraged to accompany the patient to the operating room doors and then be shown to the waiting area. On receiving the patient, the operating room supervisor should be told of the whereabouts of significant others. She should then keep them informed of the patient's progress, especially if the combined operative and anesthesia time is over two hours.

METHODS OF TRANSPORTATION

There is a great variety of transportation vehicles on the market, and it can be difficult to determine which type to purchase. The deci-

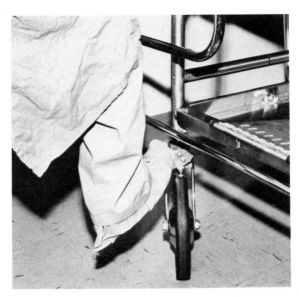

Figure 17.1. The transporter locks the gurney wheel. Photographs in this chapter were taken by David G. Berry, Captain, Army Nurse Corps.

sion should be made by the operating room supervisor after a thorough review of the available products. However, no matter which product is selected there are certain design characteristics that should be considered as essential for each transportation vehicle.

The four-wheeled gurney should be equipped with a braking (locking) device on each wheel and two sets of safety straps, one for over the legs and the other for the torso (see Fig. 17.1). There should also be side rails that can be easily elevated or lowered. The gurney should have six holes for placement of the intravenous standard, two at the head, one on each side, and two at the feet. For transportation of the patient having oxygen therapy, a holding device that will secure the cylinder is convenient. Another requirement is the capability of placing the patient in Trendelenburg, reverse Trendelenburg, and sitting positions with controls that are easy to operate and within quick reach of the transporter. Maneuverability is also an important consideration.

Cribs should be of sufficient size to accommodate children up to four years of age, yet small enough to ensure easy handling. All sides of the crib must be high enough to prevent a standing child from falling. Rails with two elevated positions provide easy access to the patient (see Figs. 17.2 and 17.3). The railing at the head of the crib should be removable in case access to the child's head is necessary. Even though it is difficult to restrain a child, safety straps are important and should be available. Like the adult gurney, an intravenous standard with six holes for placement is necessary. At a minimum, the crib should have the capability of being put into Trendelenburg position (see Fig. 17.4).

Infant care units are used in transporting the compromised neonate and infant (see Fig. 17.5). The unit should provide easy access to the infant, a controlled environment that maintains body temperature, and an oxygen source. The bed portion of the unit should have Trendelenburg capability and there should be a place for securing an intravenous standard.

Another vehicle used for transportation is a surgery lift, which is effective for transporting a comatose patient (see Fig. 17.6). The surgery lift facilitates transfer because it fits under

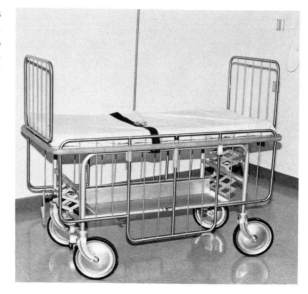

Figure 17.3. A crib with the sides down. Note the safety strap.

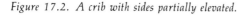

Figure 17.2. A crib with sides partially elevated.

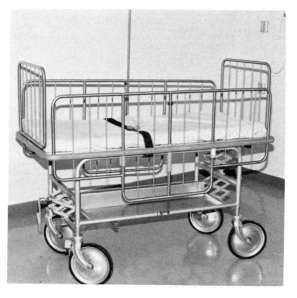

the bed and lowers down over the patient who has been placed on a canvas carrier. The carrier is then attached to the lift with straps. Next the lift is hydraulically elevated enough for the patient to clear the bed and to be moved to the operating room. This device needs to be checked periodically, especially the canvas, which can deteriorate.

The recovery bed can also be used for transporting the patient. It should have the same design characteristics as the gurney except that the bed area should be larger. This is especially important during the postoperative period if the patient becomes hyperactive and begins to toss and turn.

The patient's bed is another possible means of transportation, especially if the patient is unable to be moved. Beds that are intended for transportation should be easy to maneuver. The patient coming to the operating room in a bed must be attended by two transporters, one to push and the other to guide the bed. Unfortunately hospital beds are notorious for having small wheels that have the tendency to get lodged and stuck in crevices, especially when disembarking from an elevator. Electrical patient beds should be checked out by the medical maintenance department and certified as safe before using as a transportation vehicle and plugged into the outlet in the operating room.

The hand-carried litter is not usually used for conveyance, but every operating room should have access to such a device. It can be used to evacuate patients in case of fire or mass casualties. The litter should be sturdy with handles that protrude far enough from the canvas to allow for a firm grip. The canvas that supports the patient must be intact and have no tears. The hand-carried litter should be inspected annually to ensure readiness in case of emergency. Litter transport is not as simple as one would think, and both patient and litter bearer may suffer harm if done incorrectly. Basically, it takes two or four people to carry a litter. The key to a smooth and safe litter transport is teamwork directed by the litter bearer captain. During the two-person carry, the bearer in the rear gives the commands (see Fig. 17.7). During the four-person carry, the bearer in the rear and on the right gives the commands (see Fig. 17.8). There are four basic commands:

Figure 17.4. A crib with the sides down and ends removed.

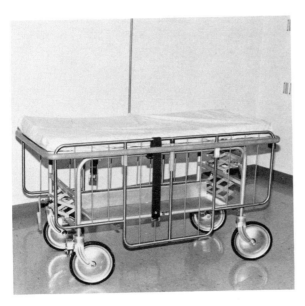

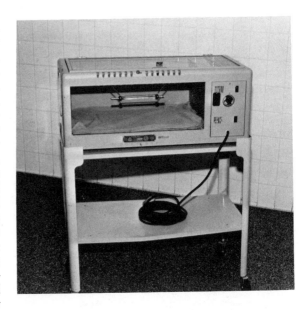

Figure 17.5. An infant care unit. This unit does not contain an oxygen cylinder.

1. Prepare to lift
2. Lift
3. Prepare to lower
4. Lower

Teamwork is important during a litter transport, and a designated individual must be responsible for directing the transport. This is especially crucial because the use of litters is most likely to occur during a mass casualty or fire — times that are prone to confusion.

SAFETY MEASURES

Safety is a priority goal of transportation. Measures to ensure patient safety are quite simple, requiring more common sense than advanced cognitive reasoning. Yet accidents still happen, and hospitals continue to be involved in lawsuits because patients have suffered harm during transportation episodes.

Every individual assigned transporter duties should be thoroughly briefed on the equipment to be used and its safety features. The following are specific safety measures. Due to the importance of safety, many of these measures

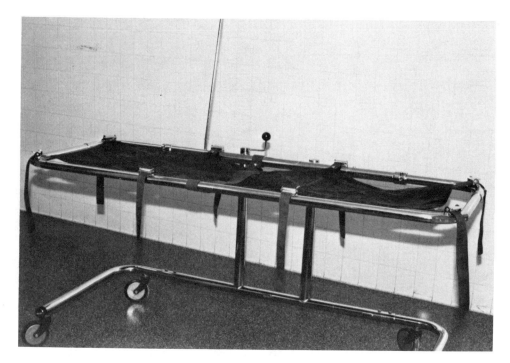

Figure 17.6. A surgical lift.

Figure 17.7. Two transporters preparing to lift a patient. The transporter in the rear gives the commands.

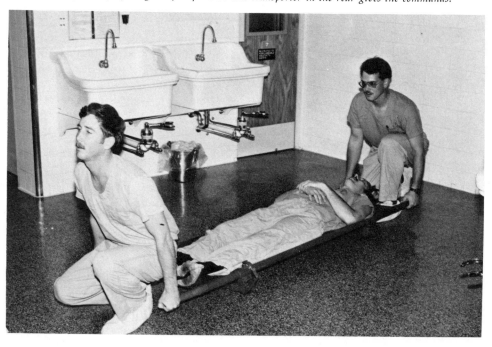

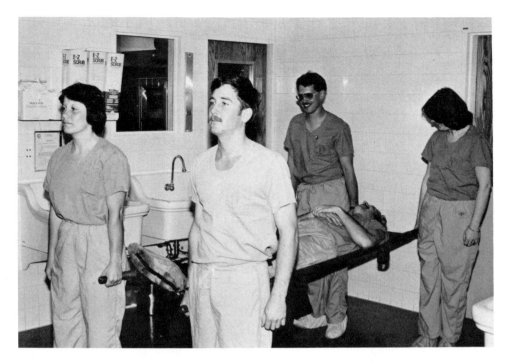

Figure 17.8. Four transporters carrying a patient.

are also discussed in the section, "Scope of Nursing Activities," as tasks that must be accomplished during transportation.

1. Lock (brake) all wheels of transport vehicles prior to transferring patients. If possible, lock the wheels of the patient's hospital bed.
2. Transporters should use their body weight to stabilize the gurney next to the bed by leaning against the gurney during transfer. Likewise, the individual assisting the transporter should use her weight to stabilize the bed next to the gurney.
3. The use of safety straps across the legs and the torso secure the patient and should always be used.
4. If present, the side rails must be elevated.
5. Intravenous infusion containers should be hung on the standard that has been placed at the side of the gurney near the middle or at the foot. This will help to protect the

patient's head in the event the container becomes dislodged.

6. The transporter must ensure that the patient's arms remain at her side or folded across her chest. Elbows that protrude out across the edge of the gurney can be severely damaged if bumped during transportation.
7. The gurney should never be used to push through closed doors. This action is extremely hazardous and can result in trauma to the patient's feet. Doors should be held open so the gurney can be pushed through. If another individual is not present, then the transporter should hold open the door by leaning against it and pull the gurney through with both hands.
8. When turning a corner, extreme caution must be exercised to avoid collision.
9. The operating room supervisor must ensure that routine preventive maintenance is done on all transportation vehicles. There are two critical areas of concern—the brakes and

the side rails. Brakes must stabilize and side rails must lock into position. An unstable side rail can inadvertently release and fall on a patient's arm or hand, causing severe trauma.

If the transporter knows how to operate the equipment, is aware of the possible hazards that can occur during transportation, and exercises common sense, then transportation should be safe. Transporters and those operating transport vehicles are also prone to safety mishaps. Many operating room nurses can attest to this fact, especially the ones that ran over their own feet with heavy gurneys.

SPECIFIC TRANSPORTATION PROBLEMS

It would be ideal if all patients being transported were healthy and able to cooperate fully during the process, but this is not always the case. The transporter often encounters a patient who poses special problems and requires extra care. Of course, the operating room nurse should address these problems in the perioperative patient care plan.

The transporter may encounter these common problems. The patient may have an intravenous solution infusing, an indwelling catheter, or chest tubes and bottles. Patients may be in respiratory distress, in traction, or pregnant. In addition, the preeclamptic and pediatric patient are discussed.

Patients often come to the operating room with intravenous solutions infusing. It is the responsibility of the transporter to protect the infusion system during the transportation episode. The following are guidelines for maintaining the integrity of the infusion.

1. Prior to the transportation, all connections should be checked to ensure that they are secure and tight.
2. Prior to moving the patient to the gurney, the transporter should ensure that the solution tubing is unobstructed and not caught on anything. This will prevent it from being pulled out.
3. Placing the container at the right height will ensure that the flow rate remains steady

during transportation. If it is elevated too high, the rate will increase, and if it is too low the rate will decrease. The unit nurse should adjust the height of the container and check the rate of flow prior to releasing the patient to the transporter.
4. The solution container should be hung at the foot or at the side of the gurney to prevent it from falling on the patient's head if it becomes dislodged during transport (see Fig. 17.9).
5. The transporter should check and ensure that the patient is not lying on the tubing and that it is not kinked, since this will impede the flow of the solution.
6. The transporter must not raise the extremity receiving the infusion above the level of the heart. If this occurs, a negative pressure will be created in the vein, causing air to be drawn into the vein if there are leaks in the infusion system. The result can be an air embolism (2).
7. The transporter must not lower the solution container to the level of the patient because this will cause a backflow of venous blood into the tubing.

When the patient arrives in the operating room, the receiving nurse should inspect the infusion system to determine if it is patent. At this time the transporter should report any mishaps during transportation.

Urinary catheters and drainage bags pose problems because personnel often do not know how to handle them. It is the responsibility of the transporter to ensure that the patient with a catheter has adequate urinary drainage during the transportation. The transporter should check to see that the catheter is secured with tape, brought out over the leg, and connected tightly to the drainage bag tubing. Transporters frequently place the catheter bag on top of the patient's legs and then cover the legs with a sheet. This is thought to prevent embarrassment for the patient, and indeed it might. It is a poor technique, however, and must not be tolerated. The drainage bag should not be placed above the level of the bladder because reflux of urine back into the tubing can occur and become a potential source of urinary tract

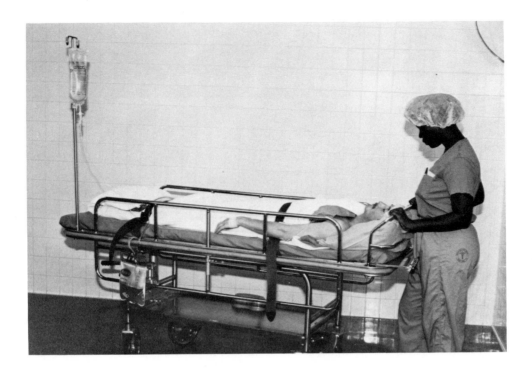

Figure 17.9. The proper way to transport a patient with an intravenous and Foley catheter.

infection (2). All catheters and drainage tubes must be free from kinks, and the drainage bag hung on the side of the gurney during transportation.

Transporting the patient with chest tubes should always be done with a nurse. For the novice transporter, the presence of chest tubes can be a source of anxiety and feeling of "What do I do if the tube becomes disconnected or the bottle breaks?" If the transporter is cautious and follows a few basic rules, problems should be minimal. If the inevitable does occur, however, then there are remedies. If there is a mishap, the physician must be immediately notified.

The primary principle is to keep the chest bottle below the level of the chest and the tubes connected (see Fig. 17.10). If the bottle is elevated above the level of the chest, there can be a reflux of fluid back into the pleural space. If too much fluid enters, the lung might collapse leading to a mediastinal shift. If the bottle is elevated above the level of the chest during transportation, the drainage system will be reestablished if the bottle is lowered. Likewise, if the tubing becomes disconnected, it should be reconnected and personnel should observe the system for proper functioning (2).

Since some chest drainage devices are made of glass, there is the possibility of breakage. If this occurs, it is necessary to prevent air from entering the pleural cavity by immediately clamping the tube if the water seal bottle was *not* bubbling prior to breakage. If the water was bubbling, clamping can cause a tension pneumothorax and an eventual mediastinal shift. Therefore, if the tube is clamped, the nurse should observe the patient for signs of pneumothorax, which include rapid shallow breathing, apprehension, and cyanosis. If the signs of pneumothorax appear, the tube should be unclamped, which will cause air to move in and out resulting in an open pneumothorax and a reduction in pressure (3).

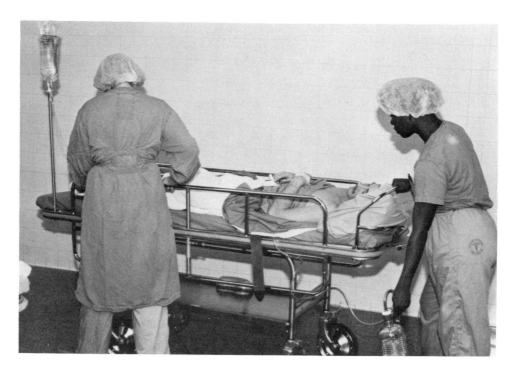

Figure 17.10. *The proper way of transporting a patient with chest tubes and bottles.*

If the transporter inadvertently knocks over the bottle and the water seal is compromised, air can enter the pleural space. This situation can be corrected by placing the bottle upright, which reestablishes the seal. Afterward, the nurse should instruct the patient to take one or two deep breaths, which will force out any air that entered the pleural cavity (2).

There are many nursing implications associated with transporting the patient with chest tubes. The presence of a nurse during transportation is justified when considering the possible complications that might occur with this type of patient.

Many patients come to the operating room without chest tubes, but still have some type of respiratory distress. For these patients, it is necessary to facilitate adequate respiratory effort and comfort. The patient with orthopnea can be helped if she is elevated into a sitting position or pillows are placed behind her back. If the patient is having dyspnea, she should be placed in a position that is most comfortable, which is usually the sitting position. If the sitting position does not produce comfort, however, then leaning forward may lead to relief by causing the patient to use her accessory muscles (2).

The patient in traction can be a problem because the bed is so difficult to maneuver. This is particularly true when the traction apparatus is extensive and cumbersome. A patient may also have to remain in correct body alignment and, if traction is compromised and alignment lost, may experience severe pain. Transporting the patient in traction requires two people, one to maneuver and the other to push. A nurse experienced in orthopedics should accompany the patient to ensure that traction is maintained. If it is lost, then the nurse can apply manual traction until the mechanical is restored. The transporter must know the dimensions of the elevator and operating room doors because not all patient beds with traction devices will fit through these passageways.

Transporting the pregnant patient presents special considerations. Quite often this patient is coming to the operating room for a cesarean section, which may be emergent. She should always be accompanied by a nurse, particularly if in active labor or seriously ill.

The underlying principle when transporting the pregnant patient is getting her to the operating room as quickly and comfortably as possible. Precautions to ensure that the intravenous infusion and urinary catheter remain patent are essential. Another important consideration is positioning of the patient on the gurney. The supine position tends to be uncomfortable for the patient because of the weight of the pregnant uterus on the internal organs. If the patient is encouraged to lay on her left side, respiratory efforts will be easier, and compression of the inferior vena cava by the uterus will be reduced (see Fig. 17.11).

When the patient has preeclampsia or eclampsia, the transportation period is critical. Since this type of patient is prone to seizures, the nurse and transporter need to provide a therapeutic atmosphere with an environment that is not only comfortable but also pleasant. The patient should be protected from noise, bright lights, and other noxious or anxiety-producing stimuli. A padded mouth gag must accompany the patient to the operating room. On the patient's arrival in the operating room, the nurse should check the patient's vital signs, rate of intravenous infusion (especially if there is a magnesium sulfate drip), and the patency of the urinary catheter. Fetal heart tones should also be checked. A suction apparatus and oxygen supply should be readily available in the event of a seizure (4). If a seizure occurs during transportation, the transporter and nurse must take measures to protect the patient from harm. Safety straps should be loose enough to prevent bruising and other trauma, but secure

Figure 17.11. The proper way of transporting the pregnant patient. She is lying on her left side which reduces compression on the inferior vena cava by the uterus.

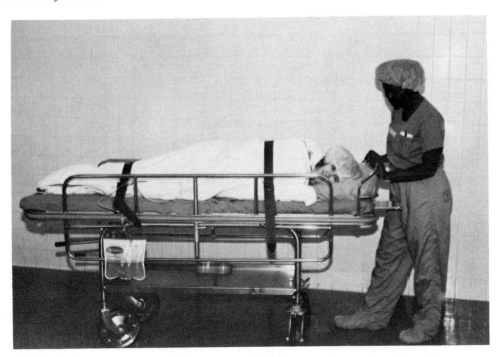

enough to prevent the patient from falling from the narrow gurney. Also, if the gurney has side rails, the patient should be protected from hitting herself on the rails. Following the seizure, transportation must be terminated as soon as possible and the physician immediately notified.

Pediatric patients have distinct and special needs. Children can be extremely unpredictable and therefore vulnerable to possible accident. The correct mode of transportation should be chosen for the child. Nothing is more absurd than attempting to transport a two-year-old on an adult gurney or trying to strap down a hysterical four-year-old child. When premedication is ordered, it should be given far enough in advance to cause the desired effect and allow the child to respond emotionally. In other words, the child should be allowed to cry and then fall asleep. Once the patient is sedated, caution must be taken not to arouse her. A child who has a special toy or blanket should be permitted to bring it to the operating room. It will provide a great deal of comfort and help more than hinder the nurse. The operating room supervisor should consider the possibility of trying alternate methods of transporting the pediatric patient. For the nonsedated patient, walking to the operating room with her parents is acceptable. Likewise, one of the parents should be allowed to carry the emotionally upset child. A special place set aside in the holding area is convenient, and the parents should be encouraged to stay with the child to offer emotional support. No matter what the arrangement, the pediatric patient must never be left alone. There are too many things that can go wrong. This can certainly be attested to by the circulating nurse who left her six-year-old charge while she went to check an instrument card. When she returned the little boy had disappeared. When finally found he said, "I was just looking for the bathroom."

Scope of Nursing Activities

UNIT TO HOLDING AREA

Transporting the patient from the unit to the holding area can be broken down into steps.

These steps are common to all transportation, irrespective of the patient's age or mode of transportation.

1. The nurse should obtain a printed pickup slip from the dispatching nurse or operating room supervisor (see Fig. 17.12). The slip should have the patient's full name, age, unit number, room number, procedure, and operating room number. This will help to eliminate error when picking up the patient.

2. The nurse should obtain the correct transportation vehicle according to patient need. While most patients come to the operating room via gurney, there are those that require a different mode of transportation such as the pediatric patient or patient that is ex-

Figure 17.12. The transporter receives her assignment from the operating room supervisor.

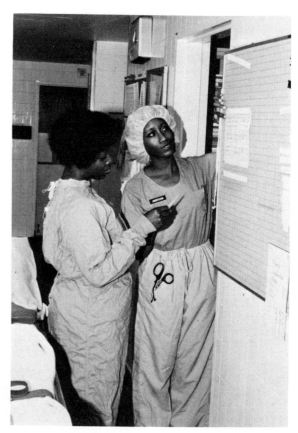

tremely obese and too large to fit on the standard-sized gurney.

3. The nurse should report to the charge nurse on arrival on the nursing unit. The transporter should never approach the patient on the unit without first checking with the nurse. This will help to reduce possible error and enable the unit nurse to assist the transporter in moving the patient to the gurney. Furthermore, the unit nurse will be able to make last minute additions and adjustments to the patient's record (see Fig. 17.13).

4. The nurse should ask the unit nurse or clerk for the patient's record and x-rays. The record and x-ray container must be identified by the patient's name and hospital number. Each hospital will require a variety of forms; however, the following should be included:

- Operative permit form.
- History and physical.
- Physician progress notes.

- Laboratory work. Complete blood count (CBC) and urinalysis are the minimum requirement.
- Nursing notes and patient care plan.
- Electrocardiogram report if the patient is over 40 years of age.
- Tissue report form.
- Report of radiographic examination.

5. The nurse should review the record and preoperative checklist (see Fig. 17.14). It is important the patient receive all ordered preoperative medications prior to being transported. Depending on the type, the medications help to decrease pulmonary and oropharyngeal secretions, assist in obliterating vagal reflexes, allay anxiety, reduce blood pressure and pulse, facilitate a smoother induction of anesthesia, and generally have a sedating and relaxing effect on the patient (5). The transporter can determine if the patient had her medications by checking with the unit nurse. The preoperative

Figure 17.13. The transporter is given the patient's record.

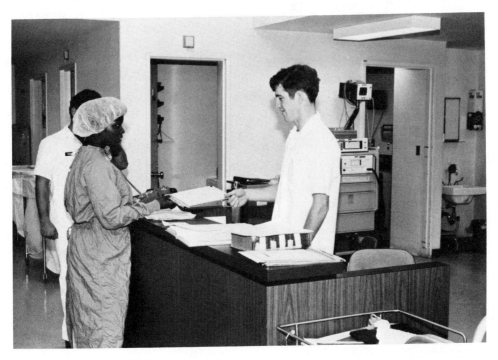

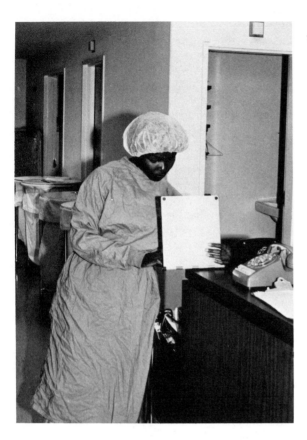

Figure 17.14. The transporter reviews the patient's record.

checklist is a reminder to nursing personnel to complete certain prescribed preoperative nursing activities prior to releasing the patient. The transporter has little excuse to offer if she transports a patient that is not prepared, especially if the preoperative checklist was not completed. A thorough review of the checklist will help to eliminate this possibility.

6. The nurse should enter the patient's room, identify the patient and herself, and tell her what she is going to do. The nurse should ask the unit nurse the location of the patient. Upon arriving in the room, she should check the patient's identity band and ask her name if she is alert and conscious. The nurse should be sure to introduce herself. Nothing can disturb a patient more than to have a complete stranger enter the room and begin a procedure without at least saying hello. The nurse should ensure that the patient's record, pick up slip, and identity band match.

7. The nurse should check the patient to ensure that all personal property, clothing, and prosthesis have been removed (6). If items are found on the patient, the nurse should inform the unit nurse and request that they be removed. It is preferred that all rings be removed. If this is impossible, the ring should be secured with tape. Patients that are wearing hearing aids should be allowed to wear them to the operating room since this will assist the operating room nurse during the identification process and help the patient in understanding and following instructions. Patients with poor eyesight should be permitted to bring their eyeglasses. If they wear their eyeglasses, visual orientation will be maintained and the patient will feel more secure during the transfer process. All clothing should be removed, and the patient covered with a hospital gown. This will prevent soiling of the patient's personal clothing and provide the operating room staff with easy access to the patient's body.

8. The nurse should check and secure all treatment devices such as urinary drainage bags, chest bottles, and intravenous solution containers (6). Securing the treatment devices will help to prevent breakage and protect the patient from harm. Prior to dispatching the transporter, the operating room supervisor should ascertain whether treatment devices are being used on the patient. A preoperative assessment is an excellent way of obtaining this information.

9. The nurse and transporter move the patient from the bed to the gurney (see Fig. 17.15). This step is crucial, because there is high potential for patient harm from a fall. To prevent accidental falling, the gurney must be stabilized against the patient's bed with the wheels of both the bed and gurney locked. The transporter stands so that the gurney is between her and the bed. The unit nurse should be standing so that the bed is between her and the gurney. The patient is then instructed to move from the bed to the gurney. The transporter and nurse lean against the gurney and bed to provide greater stabilization. For patients who cannot

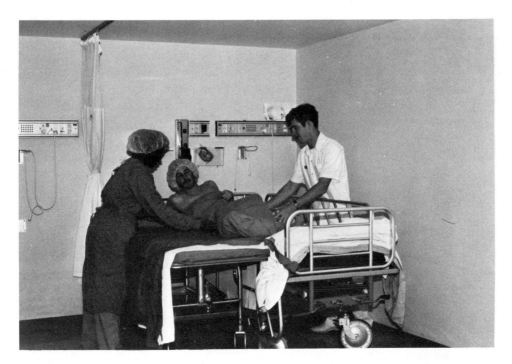

Figure 17.15. Securing the patient with safety straps is important.

easily move from the bed to the gurney, a canvas covered roller can be used or a sheet can be placed under the patient and used to pull the patient onto the gurney. To provide for the patient's modesty, an operating room sheet is placed over the patient prior to transfer. The patient then moves to the gurney while remaining covered with this sheet.

10. After the patient is on the gurney, the nurse should secure her and make her comfortable (6). Following transfer to the gurney, the patient should be covered with the operating room linen, which should be of sufficient quantity to ensure comfort. Restraining straps must be placed over the patient and the gurney side rails elevated. A pillow will enhance patient comfort (see Fig. 17.16).

11. The transporter transports the patient to the operating room (6). The transporter departs from the unit, pushing the patient feet first (see Fig. 17.17). She should avoid swinging the gurney and walking too swiftly as these actions can cause patient disorientation, nau-

sea, and dizziness. Being near the patient's head gives the transporter immediate access to the airway in case of respiratory distress or vomiting. Extreme caution must be exercised when rounding corners, going through doorways, and entering and leaving elevators. The presence of another individual is especially helpful because she can assist in maneuvering the gurney. The nurse should always enter elevators with the patient's head first (see Fig. 17.18). This facilitates patient safety. Also, it is very disturbing for the patient to lie with his head next to the doors that may open and shut a number of times. If feasible, it is desirable to have an elevator restricted to the operating room during transportation periods. This will help to protect the patient from the curious eyes of other passengers, provide for a quieter ride, and decrease transportation time because the transporter will not have to wait for an empty elevator.

12. The transporter releases the patient to the operating room supervisor or other respon-

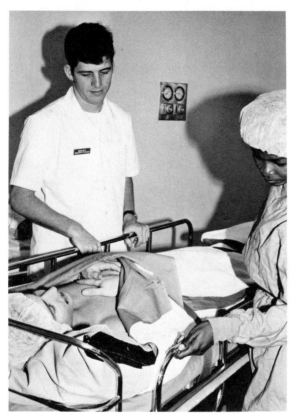

Figure 17.16. *The transporter ensures patient safety by elevating the side rails.*

sible individual. On the patient's arrival in the operating room, the unit nurse should present the chart to the supervisor and communicate pertinent patient information (see Fig. 17.19). If the nurse did not accompany the patient, the transporter should inform the supervisor of any pertinent information concerning transportation.

HOLDING AREA

In some hospitals, the holding area is a separate room in the surgical suite. It is staffed by nurses who care for the surgical patient while the operating room is being prepared. The lighting is usually subdued and there are facilities for shaving, starting intravenous infusions, inserting catheters, and administering medications. There might even be a rocking chair for a frightened child.

This kind of holding area is ideal, but unfortunately is not always the norm. In many hospitals, space and money are at a premium, and areas dedicated for the exclusive purpose of holding patients prior to surgery do not exist. Consequently, the patient arrives in the surgical suite and stays in the hallway until the operating room is ready.

No matter what type of system exists — a separate room or a hallway — the following basic nursing activities must be accomplished for each patient:

Figure 17.17. *On the way to the operating room, the transporter pushes and the nurse guides the gurney.*

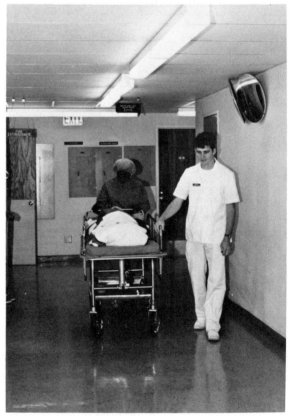

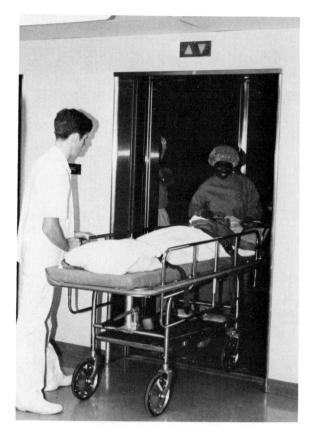

Figure 17.18. Always push the patient head first into an elevator.

1. Identification of the patient
2. Verification of NPO status
3. Verification of allergies
4. Review of the operative permit form
5. Verification of the operative site
6. Review of the clinical record
   a. Complete blood count
   b. Urinalysis
   c. Electrolytes (if ordered)
   d. Electrocardiogram (if ordered)
   e. Radiographic report
   f. History and physical
   g. Nursing notes and patient care plan
7. Preoperative assessment
   a. Initial assessment if not done on the nursing unit by the operating room nurse

b. Reassessment if already done on the nursing unit
8. Update of the perioperative patient care plan or initiation of the care plan
9. Evaluation of that portion of the perioperative patient care plan that pertains to the preoperative period
10. Documentation

If the holding area provides privacy for the patient, nursing activities such as the shave prep can be completed.

All these nursing activities are essential and basic to the perioperative role. Some are self-explanatory, such as identification of the patient and verification of the operative site. Indeed, it is imperative that the right patient be operated on, and the correct operation performed. Review of the laboratory work is another important nursing activity. The nurse is not expected to be a diagnostician, but should have sufficient knowledge to recognize when the data are not within acceptable norms.

Verification of NPO status cannot be done too frequently because of the serious consequences a patient suffers if she aspirates. Some patients will routinely say no to the question, "Have you had anything to eat or drink since midnight?" yet still end up vomiting during induction of anesthesia. They may have felt the one cup of coffee offered by their roommate could do no harm. A technique for eliciting more accurate information is to ask the question in another way, "What did you have for breakfast this morning?" Nurses will be surprised with the answers they get.

Obtaining accurate information about patient allergies can be a trying experience. The first rule is not to trust the data on the record because a notation of NKA (no known allergies) could be misleading. Reconfirmation of a patient's allergy status is important. The nurse should concentrate on allergies and/or sensitivities to pharmacological agents, detergents, bleaches, tape, and suture products. Again, phrasing the question in a particular way may elicit more pertinent information. "Have you ever had iodine on your body before? Did it cause a rash?" "What happens when tape is

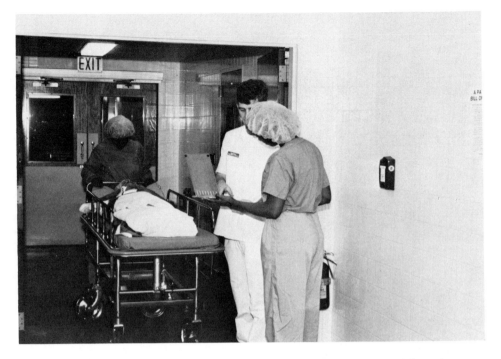

Figure 17.19. The unit nurse gives the OR supervisor the record and communicates pertinent information.

applied to your skin?" "You say you are allergic to penicillin. What happens if you take it?"

Reviewing the operative permit form is a crucial nursing activity that should be regulated by strict hospital policy. Many arguments have occurred in operating rooms because of a disagreement among team members concerning the validity of the operative permit form. Unfortunately, there are a multitude of opinions in the books addressing informed consent, and it is sometimes difficult to find reliable legal guidance. Each hospital should develop a definitive policy concerning surgical consents. This should be a joint effort by the hospital administration, surgical committee, and legal counsel. As a last measure, the board of trustees should review and endorse the policy.

As a general rule of thumb, adults 18 years of age and over who are of sound mind can give informed consent. Those under 18 should have consent given by a legal guardian. An undecipherable signature scribbled by a confused patient may be worthless and should be

approached with suspicion (7). Likewise, consent given by a patient after receiving medication that lowers the degree of alertness and comprehension should be questioned (8). Finally, there are instances when obtaining a consent is impossible because the patient is unconscious. When this happens and the situation is life or death, the "patient may be presumed to have given consent" (9).

In reviewing the consent, the nurse should look for the following:

1. Clear and concise description of the proposed procedure.
2. Identification of the surgeon who will perform the procedure.
3. Signature of the patient. (This should be dated and timed.)
4. Signature of the individual witnessing the patient's signature.
5. Any notations of exceptions to the procedure such as "no photographs are to be taken."

Ideally, the patient will come to the operating room after the operating room nurse has initiated a preoperative assessment and prepared a perioperative patient care plan. The time spent in the holding area can then be used to implement the plan and evaluate its effectiveness. As needed, reassessment should be done to update the plan. There are times, however, when the patient will arrive in the operating room without a prior preoperative assessment or perioperative patient care plan. If this happens, the operating room nurse should immediately initiate a preoperative assessment and patient care plan that at least addresses the essential patient care needs of the intraoperative period.

Documentation is essential throughout the perioperative period. The following example is provided as a guideline for the nurse.

0900: Mrs. Doe arrives in the surgical holding area alert and oriented. According to instructions in the patient care plan, she is sitting at a 45-degree angle on the gurney. There are no signs of respiratory distress. Identity, operative site, and NPO status are verified. Operative permit is in order. Patient denies allergies or sensitivities to pharmacological agents. Mrs. Doe states, "I feel pretty calm, but I wish I would fall asleep." The patient is given a warm blanket and made comfortable in an attempt to induce sedation.

0920: The patient is resting quietly with eyes closed.

It must be mentioned that if the surgical suite hallway is used as a holding area there will be a number of variables that can have a detrimental effect on the patient. Unfortunately, the hallway is not a controlled environment and has a tendency to be chaotic. The patient is parked right in the middle of frenzied activity, subjected to loud and frightening noises, hears incoherent chatter, and views an aseptic panorama that is a far cry from the drama portrayed on television. What must the patient think when she hears all the subdued clinical consultations taking place? In such situations it is imperative for the nurse to support the patient. Certainly the patient advocate role takes on new dimensions, and more time will have to be spent reminding people of the presence of a conscious and anxious patient.

HOLDING AREA TO SURGICAL SUITE

If a formal holding area is available the patient should be kept there until the operating room is prepared. The circulator should not transport the patient to the operating room until the supplies have been opened and the counts taken. It is disturbing to a patient to be whisked into a room, strapped to the bed, and then watch as the circulator frantically plays catch up. Once the patient is in the room, she must be the center of activity and command the highest priority. The trip from the holding area to the operating room should be smooth and relaxed.

SURGICAL SUITE TO OPERATING ROOM BED

When the patient is transferred to the operating room bed, all but two required preoperative nursing activities should have been completed. At this time the nurse identifies the patient one more time and again verifies the surgical site. The patient is then transferred to the operating bed using the same technique employed in transferring her from the unit bed to the gurney. Circumstances of transfer will be modified according to the age and conditions of the patient and mode of transportation. Once the patient is on the operating bed, the nurse should warn her not to move and place a safety strap across her thighs. In addition, comfort measures are implemented, and the patient is prepared for anesthesia according to the standard operating policy of the hospital. Of all times, this is the time for the presence of the operating room nurse.

OPERATING ROOM BED TO POSTANESTHESIA UNIT

The time immediately following surgery can be critical for the patient and therefore must be approached with caution by the OR nurse. Of primary importance is a smooth transfer from the OR bed to the transportation vehicle. If moved too suddenly or roughly the patient may experience a severe drop in blood pressure. Even though surgery is over, the patient is still in a critical condition and may even experience a cardiac or respiratory arrest. The surgical team should be constantly aware of the patient's immediate postoperative vulnerability and alert to possible complications. Quite often this is difficult to do, especially when the procedure has been lengthy and tense, which results in the natural tendency of the team members to become lax in their vigilance.

The usual method of transportation to the postanesthesia unit is on a recovery bed. The actual transfer of the patient from the OR bed to the recovery bed can be accomplished in a variety of ways. The patient is most probably totally immobile and unable to cooperate with the transfer. At a minimum, there should be four individuals transferring the patient: one at the head, one at the feet, and one on each side of the patient. If the patient is exceptionally tall or heavy, more people will be needed for the transfer. During the transfer procedure, the anesthesiologist serves as team leader, gives the transfer commands, and maintains the patient's airway while protecting the head. A lifter sheet that extends from the patient's shoulders to her buttocks is helpful. The individuals on either side of the patient grasp the lifter sheet securely while the individual at the foot of the table grasps the patient's feet. The anesthesiologist should reach under the patient's shoulders while cradling the head. The command to move is then given, and the patient is transferred to the recovery bed. All intravenous lines and tubes coming from the patient's body must be unobstructed prior to transfer. It is quite embarrassing for the nurse as well as detrimental to the patient if a tube is inadvertently pulled out during transfer.

If available, a roller is another device that can be used during transfer. This device is particularly helpful if the patient is obese. Its use requires four people: one at the feet, one at the head, and one at each side. One of the drawbacks with a roller is the necessity of log rolling the patient to her side so that the roller can be placed under her. If the patient is conscious, this extra movement can be frightening and painful.

If a roller or a lifter sheet are not available, the patient can still be moved by four people.

In this type of transfer, the individuals at the sides reach under the patient and grasp one anothers' wrists prior to lifting. The anesthesiologist gives the command, and all lift together. If the patient is heavy, extreme caution must be exercised because the individuals at the sides may lack the strength to lift safely.

The surgical lift can also be used to transfer the patient to the postanesthesia unit. This device is convenient because once the canvas pad is secured to the lift, the patient can be moved smoothly and with a minimum of effort by the surgical team. A drawback with this device, however, is structural stability. If the patient should arrest during transfer to the postanesthesia unit, the surgical lift would not provide enough support to conduct cardiopulmonary resuscitation.

The transfer of children to the postanesthesia unit presents special difficulties. Small children are not small adults. Every precaution must be taken to ensure the child's safety. This can be a challenge when the patient tries to stand up and look for her mother or father. The neonate poses the problem of temperature maintenance. It is advisable to transfer this patient in a prewarmed incubator.

No matter what the transfer method, the circulating nurse should always accompany the patient to the postanesthesia unit. This provides for continuity of care and enables the nurse to assist the anesthesiologist in the care of the patient should the need arise. Also, the circulating nurse will be able to orally report to the postanesthesia nurse what transpired during the preoperative and intraoperative phases of the patient's hospitalization.

POSTANESTHESIA UNIT TO NURSING UNIT

The patient will be released from the postanesthesia unit after she has completely recovered from anesthesia and is cleared by the anesthesiologist. Under normal circumstances, she will be transported to the nursing unit on the recovery bed. Prior to transporting, the postanesthesia nurse should notify the unit nurse that the patient is en route and give a report of her condition. This action will enable the unit nurse to prepare for the patient's arrival and assist in facilitating an efficient transfer episode.

It is crucial that a professional nurse accompany the patient back to the nursing unit. This not only provides for continuity of care but also for skilled nursing care should unexpected complications such as vomiting or hemorrhage arise.

The actual transfer of the patient from the recovery bed to the unit bed is the same as the transfer procedure from the unit bed to the gurney. The only difference is the condition of the patient, who is most likely experiencing pain, is sore, and just not as limber as she was preoperatively. Unless contraindicated, the patient should be encouraged to assist with the transfer. If this is impossible, however, then four people will be needed to move the patient to the bed. The easiest way is to use the bottom sheet of the recovery bed as a lifter. The roller is another option in moving the patient.

The act of transporting the patient from the nursing unit and back again is an important aspect of perioperative care. It takes planning and skill. The patient is vulnerable during this time and may be experiencing any number of discomforts from preoperative anxiety to post-operative pain. The presence of the nurse during the transportation episode will help to alleviate many of these discomforts as well as provide for continuity of nursing care.

References

1. Laufman, H., Ed. *Hospital Special Care Facilities.* New York: Academic Press, 1981.
2. Luckmann, J., and Sorensen, K. C. *Medical-Surgical Nursing.* Philadelphia: W. B. Saunders, 1974.
3. Morgan, C. V., Jr., and Orcutt, T. W. "The care and feeding of chest tubes." *Am J Nurs* 72(February):305, 1972.
4. Fitzpatrick, E., Reeder, S. R., and Mastroniannie, L., Jr. *Maternity Nursing*, 12th ed. Philadelphia: J. B. Lippincott, 1971.
5. Le Maitre, G. D., and Finnegan, J. A. *The Patient in Surgery*, 3rd. ed. Philadelphia: W. B. Saunders, 1975.
6. *Soldier's Manual: Operating Room Specialist*, FM8-9121/2, Washington, D.C.: Department of the Army Headquarters, August 1977.
7. Regan, W. A. "OR nursing law." *AORN J* 31 (June):1225, 1980.
8. Regan, W. A. "OR nursing law." *AORN J* 33 (May):1135, 1981.
9. Regan, W. A. "OR nursing law." *AORN J* 32 (November):781, 1980.

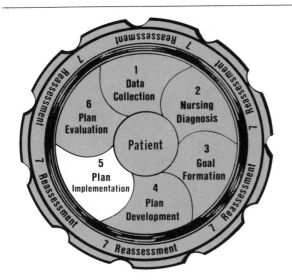

The nurse assists the patient in coping with anxiety.

Psychological Support

For patients, surgery may have an intense psychological impact. For the adolescent with bone cancer who must have a leg amputated, it can have psychological implications for body image. For an older patient, it may confirm the diagnosis of a terminal illness. For the frightened child crying in the holding area, it may be the psychological trauma of separation from parents for the first time. On the other hand, surgery may also have positive implications. A patient may be able to look forward to a better quality of life because of the correction of a physical problem as simple as a hernia that has been causing discomfort or loss of function. Even the illusion of youth may be recaptured through a softening of the visible signs of aging. Whatever the reasons for the surgery, when the patient comes to the surgical suite, he has a need for emotional support.

In the preoperative assessment, the nurse assesses the patient's mental health status, evaluating the patient's level of anxiety about his surgery and his coping methods. In the care plan, the nurse considers psychological problems and plans nursing actions for them. For example, a 42-year-old woman is having a breast biopsy under local anesthesia. In a brief conversation with her outside the operating room, the nurse discovers she is more concerned about the possible finding of cancer than the immediate procedure. The nurse touches her hand gently and reminds her that the vast majority of breast lumps are found to be benign. During the procedure, the nurse attempts to sustain the atmosphere of quiet confidence by explaining everything that is being done in a calm and reassuring voice.

Preoperative Assessment

From the time the patient arrives in the operating room until he is asleep, he needs psychological support. Although the contact between nurse and patient may be brief, it should be meaningful to both. The greatest cure for fear is trust. If the nurse is personable and friendly and conveys a caring, supportive attitude when he first meets the patient, the patient will usually be calm and less frightened.

Nurses are taught that the patient has a right to know, and they often assume that the more a patient knows about his surgery the better. Nurses believe that the greater the patient's knowledge, the lower his anxiety will be. This is not true for all patients at all times. Just as they have a right to know, they have a right *not* to know. Dodge (1) found that simple explanations are not necessarily effective in reducing anxiety. In this study, nurses and patients agreed that it was important for patients to be informed about what was wrong with them, how long their illness might last, and how they could participate in their own care. They disagreed, however, about whether patients always wanted to know how serious their ailment was, their chances of recovery, the likelihood of recurrence, and the expected results of surgery. The nurses were more concerned that patients have a clear idea of what was happening to them. Patients were not as concerned about what was happening as they were about how it would affect them.

In planning for psychological support, the nurse needs to be as careful to individualize care as he is in planning for physiological needs. Completing a mental health assessment, as described in Chapter 5, helps ascertain how much information an individual patient wants and how he will receive it. A few patients will be calm and confident enought to hear everything said and will even ask questions. Many will be so anxious that they can absorb little information and may respond better to a general comment and sympathetic touch. It is the nurse's responsibility to know the best kind of psychological support to offer each patient.

Psychological support is not as easy to prescribe as physiological nursing activities. If a patient's blood pressure drops rapidly, the nurse knows what action to take, but he cannot as readily measure anxiety levels, self-esteem, or coping skills. Offering the appropriate support depends on the nurse's knowledge of emotinal reactions to surgery, his sensitivity to others, empathy, and common courtesy. Psychological support will be a blend of all these and should be provided throughout the patient's surgery.

The mental health assessment should be done on the unit when the nurse has time to probe the patient's attitudes toward his surgery and assess and reinforce his coping mechanisms. If the nurse only has an opportunity to see the patient briefly in the holding area, there will not be enough time to do a complete assessment. The nurse can, however, review the patient's chart for observations about the patient's emotional status by the unit nurse or the perioperative nurse who performed the preoperative assessment on the unit. Even though there is not always enough time to perform a complete assessment, the nurse can reassess the plans for psychological support made during the preoperative interview to see if they are still valid.

Holding area practices vary from institution to institution. In some, the patient is kept in the holding area only until the operating room is ready and then transferred. In other institutions, the holding area is where the preoperative shave is done, the preoperative medication given, intravenous infusion started, and other preparation completed. Whatever the procedure, this is an excellent opportunity to provide reassurance and emotional support. The nurse should explain what he is doing, keep the room quiet, and demonstrate competence.

In many hospitals, the patient's family or significant others may stay with him in the holding area until he is transferred to the surgical suite. Having the family with him as long as possible may help alleviate fear and apprehension.

If there is any delay in the schedule, the nurse should inform the patient as well as his family. When the patient is transferred to the operating room suite, the staff should create as calm and quiet an atmosphere as possible. Patients who overhear staff conversations may misinterpret them. The nurse should eliminate unnecessary noise and activity around the desk area that could disturb the patient entering or leaving the operating room. Lounge doors should be kept shut to decrease noise in the corridor.

Intraoperative Care

Upon admission to the surgical suite, the patient should be greeted by a nurse who is warm and friendly. The nurse should call him by name, and tell him who he is, so he will know that someone cares.

The nurse should introduce the patient to the other members of the team as he is being transferred to the operating table. This act of common courtesy may make the environment less alien. Patients may also feel more secure if they witness the nurse checking their identity, the procedure to be performed, and the surgical consent form (see Fig. 18.1). The surgical patient faces physiological insult, that is, a personal threat, and the nurse's responsibility is to reassure him (2).

Another factor in psychological stress is whether the patient sees his surgeon immediately preoperatively. Dyk and Sutherland (3) emphasize the patient's need for emotional guidance and rapport with his surgeon. In a study of colostomy patients, they found that the patient's anxiety and fears in some cases escalated to confusion, panic, or despair if they had not seen the surgeon. Patients want to know the surgeon is there in the operating room because it gives them a feeling of protection. If they do not see the surgeon, they become more threatened. If a physician other than the primary physician does the surgery,

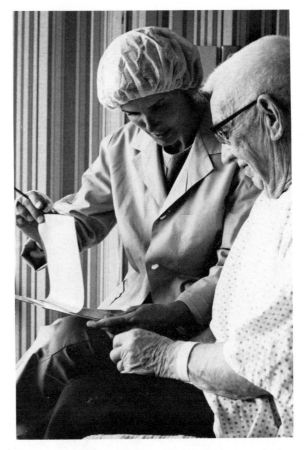

Figure 18.1. The perioperative nurse checks the patient's identity, consent form, and validates with him the surgical procedure to be performed. This gives the patient a feeling of security.

it is critical that the patient knows who is doing the surgery and actually sees the surgeon before the anesthetic is given.

As the patient is moved onto the operating bed, the nurse should explain that it is cold and hard. The word "bed" may sound less threatening than the traditional "table." Also the nurse should explain that because the bed is narrow a safety strap will be placed over his thighs to secure him. The nurse should continue to describe what is happening until the anesthesia is given. If the patient is receiving a local anesthetic, the nurse continues to explain procedures throughout the intraoperative period. These explanations usually focus on stimuli the patient receives or activities that affect him directly.

When the patient first arrives in the operating room, he is usually lying flat on his back, limiting his range of vision, and his arms and legs are firmly secured at his side or on an armboard (see Fig. 18.2). This in itself can be a frightening experience: The patient is secured to a table or bed, not even able to scratch his nose, and he may feel that the bed is so narrow that he could easily fall if he dozed or went to sleep. The nurse can reassure the patient by telling him the bed is narrow, but the safety strap will secure him, and that he will remain by the patient's side when he goes to sleep. The nurse can leave the arm not being used for the intravenous infusion loose at the patient's side. The patient can then check the edges of the table in reference to his body, scratch his nose, and hold on if this makes him feel more secure. The nurse should think about how he would feel in the patient's place and show empathy. This will relax the patient and provide a sense of safety and security. A gentle touch or a holding of the hand is comforting.

While the patient is on the operating room table, prior to being given anesthesia, the nurses and other members of the team have the responsibility for maintaining an atmosphere that will assist in alleviating fear and anxiety.

Hearing is the last of the senses to leave the patient when he is anesthetized and the first to return. There is evidence that patients not only hear comments while they are under anesthesia but remember them. Chance comments of the surgical team may even have an effect on the patient's recovery. Unnecessary noise does not create an atmosphere of trust, calmness, and security. Movements in the room should be kept to a minimum, and in last-minute activities, the nurse should attempt to ensure that supplies, instruments, or equipment are not dropped. He should do counts quietly. Room preparation should be done with a minimum of noise and disturbance. Opening supplies

Figure 18.2. The patient is experiencing anxiety because of the narrow bed. The perioperative nurse assures him that he will be secure with the safety strap over his thighs and that the nurse will be with him when he goes to sleep.

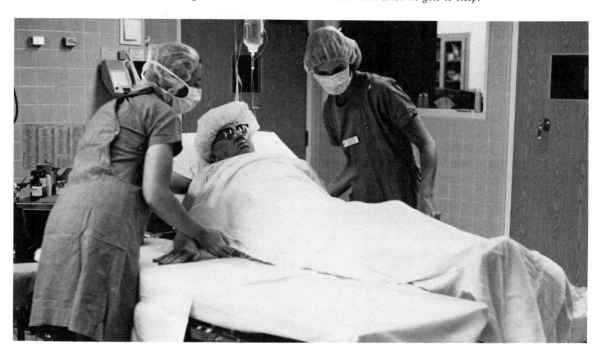

after the patient is on the table may prevent anxiety because the patient will not see the setup when he is transferred. On the other hand, the nurse may not be able to remain by the patient's side because of the need to prepare for the case. In some institutions, the patient is placed on the operating room table in the corridor, and the patient and table are transferred to the operating room. The room can be fully prepared and the patient attended to the entire time prior to induction. Other hospitals set up the room prior to the patient's arrival and transfer the patient from a stretcher to the table in the operating room. No matter which practice is used, the nurse's primary concern is for the patient. It should be kept in mind that any activity or noise tends to heighten the patient's anxiety.

Overhead operating lights should be kept off until the patient is asleep. If local anesthesia is used, the lights are turned on after the patient is draped. The lights should be in place and focused on the incision site rather than in the patient's eyes.

While attaching electrodes for cardiac monitoring, blood pressure cuffs, or electrosurgical grounding pads, the nurse should briefly explain what he is doing and how it affects the patient. The patient lying on the table is dependent on the nurse to keep him oriented to what is happening. For the patient who is dependent on a hearing aid, physical contact is important. Removal of dentures, eyeglasses, and hearing aids creates a feeling of helplessness (see Fig. 18.3). They should be left in place until the last possible moment to decrease the patient's anxiety and make him feel safer in this frightening environment.

Conversation at the scrub sink can cause anxiety. The patient hears that the nurse or surgeon only had four hours sleep last night. He wonders if he wants them involved in his surgery. Laughing and joking give the patient the impression that his surgery is not taken seriously. He may believe his hernia repair is risky and he might not come out of the anesthesia. The woman having open heart surgery is distressed when she hears the nurse asking about the saw blades. She sees herself as a piece of lumber at a construction site. The

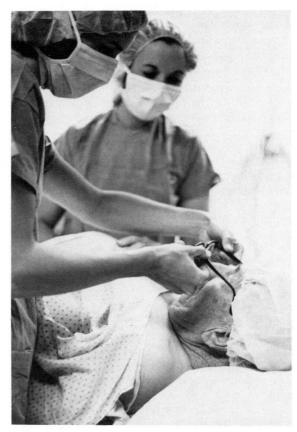

Figure 18.3. The nurse removes the patient's glasses at the last possible minute. This patient's glasses remained with him until induction.

tone of the operating room and the staff should be calm and reassuring.

The nurse should remain close to the patient as anesthesia is administered. Touching the arm, holding the hand, and speaking softly all give the patient a feeling of support and reassurance. Some patients respond to a calm voice saying, "Close your eyes and think of something pleasant," "Have a pleasant fantasy," "Listen to the music and have a beautiful dream." These suggestions help relax the patient and contribute to an uneventful induction. Touch is supportive, but the nurse should realize that he can also communicate reassurance through his tone of voice, inflection, pauses, facial expressions, and body gestures.

Once the patient is asleep, the nurse's role as an advocate continues. He should ensure that the patient's modesty and dignity are preserved. If the patient has expressed concern about the number of people in the room, only essential personnel should be permitted. If persons other than the immediate team are to be present, permission should be obtained from the patient and surgeon prior to surgery.

Immediately after surgery, while the patient is emerging from anesthesia, the nurse should again speak to the patient, calling him by name. He should stay close to the patient while he is transferred to the stretcher and transported to the recovery room.

SPECIAL AGE GROUPS

Teenagers

Teenagers having surgery have special needs for psychological support. They experience different types of problems than the adult. Regardless of the kind of surgery, their focus is on body image, disfiguration, and mutilation. They are aware of their appearance and how they look in contrast to their peers or current media idol. They are concerned with being whole, with all body parts intact.

Independence is another important concept for them. They are striving to attain their individuality and their identity and when faced with the possibility of surgery they become very ambivalent. They try to be brave but cannot always pull it off. Their behavior is inconsistent in that one minute they are demonstrating responsibility and maturity and the next they are completely the opposite.

Cesarean section can be a traumatic experience even for adult patients because many women believe it represents a failure to deliver "normally." The cesarean patient may come to surgery with heightened levels of anxiety due to an exhausting labor and apprehensions about the procedure. For the pregnant teenager, the experience may seem even more overwhelming. Often she has not had the opportunity to attend childbirth education classes. If she is unmarried or the pregnancy is unplanned, she may be facing difficulties beyond the physical rigors of labor and delivery. To a young pa-

tient, the threat of disfigurement from the cesarean incision may be even more disturbing than it is for an adult. Her coping mechanisms may be exhausted, and she may be facing surgery in a state of panic and regression.

Explaining the reasons for the cesarean section and how long it lasts may help reinforce coping skills. The nurse should gently explain what is being done at every step. He should reassure the patient and encourage her to express her feelings. In some hospitals, the father or a significant other may be allowed into the operating room during a cesarean section to provide support. If no visitors are allowed, the nurse will need to provide comfort and support.

Between 90 percent and 94 percent of all teenagers keep their babies (4). When this is the case, the nurse will want to do what he can at delivery to promote bonding between mother and infant. If the teenager is awake when the baby is delivered, he should show her the baby and tell her the sex, color of hair, and most of all the baby's condition. This will help her accept the reality of the birth.

Teenagers having abortions are also in need of special emotional support in the operating room. Due to the circumstances of the pregnancy, they may feel ambivalent and defensive about their decision. They will be acutely aware of how they are treated by the staff and sensitive to signs of rejection. The nurse can assist them to cope by showing acceptance, support, and a nonjudgmental attitude (4).

Children

The child having surgery also requires special emotional support. The operating room can be especially frightening to a child. For the child under four, separation from his parents may be the most traumatic aspect of the procedure. He may never have faced a threatening experience without a parent. In addition, his ability to understand what is happening is limited. With these patients, explanations of what will happen during surgery have little meaning. The nurse can provide support best by holding them or rocking them. Letting the child take a special toy or blanket into the operating room may help calm and distract him.

Schoolage children will have a better understanding of surgery and may benefit from preoperative teaching that includes a tour of the operating room. In some hospitals, nurses take children into the operating room the day before surgery to show them the table, the anesthesia machine, and the mask used to put them to sleep. The next day when they are admitted for their surgery, they are not as frightened and seem to be able to cope with the separation from their parents.

The child's admission to the operating room may go more smoothly if the room is ready before he is brought in so he does not have to watch instruments being prepared and so he does not have to wait for induction. Coordinating his arrival from the holding area with that of the surgeon and anesthesiologist will also minimize the waiting. When the child arrives, the nurse should be prepared to direct his full attention to him. Call him by name, be warm and friendly, and talk to him quietly.

Before induction, it is a good idea to allow the child to sit up, to hold him, or to have him lie on the operating table with the nurse close by and without restraints. Removing clothing can be threatening to children, especially underpants for little boys. The gown and underpants can be left on until after the child is asleep. A quiet atmosphere is especially important for children because loud talking and clashing instruments may provoke fantasies about what will be done to them.

For induction, the anesthetic may be started and the child then placed on the operating room table and restrained as he progresses through the stages of anesthesia. The nurse gently holds the child and talks in a soothing voice while he is going under. Alternatively, the anesthesiologist may talk soothingly while the nurse gently holds the child's hand, then his arms, and finally restrains him until he has arrived at the desired anesthesia plane. The straps are then placed securely to protect him during the procedure.

Older children may be offered choices in how they are induced. They might be asked whether they want to go to sleep with a needle or by breathing through a mask. Whatever choice they make, it should be carried out.

Most children can be put to sleep relatively easily with a mask. The smell of the gas is much more tolerable than it was in the past. Some anesthesiologists use pleasant-smelling extracts such as peppermint or spearmint inside the mask. The child is offered another choice in which smell he prefers. The anesthesiologist encourages the child to breathe deeply and watch the balloon blowing up (5). This involves him in the induction process and helps take his mind off what is happening. If the child already has an intravenous infusion line prior to being brought to the operating room, obviously that will be the desired route for administering the anesthetic.

LOCAL ANESTHESIA

The patient who is awake during surgery has a different perspective from the patient having general anesthesia. He does not fear going to sleep and never waking up again, as do some patients having general anesthesia. He may, however, be apprehensive about what he will see and hear. The operating room nurse may have responsibility for monitoring the physiological and the psychological status of the patient. The patient's anxiety level should be constantly monitored. For example, the awake patient having a nasal reconstruction may have complete confidence in his surgeon, but the drapes over his head, the heat generated by the drapes and overhead lights, the pressure on his face by the surgeon doing the procedure, and the grating and rasping noises all cause anxiety. The nurse can assess how the anxiety is affecting the patient by monitoring his vital signs. Respirations will increase, becoming rapid and more shallow. The pulse will accelerate, color may change, and perspiring will occur. The nurse needs to validate that the patient is feeling anxious because other factors such as medication may cause the same symptoms as anxiety. Muscle cramps, nausea, muscle tenseness, tremor, and facial and body rigidity may indicate a high level of anxiety. Psychological manifestations of anxiety include increased self-awareness, self-consciousness, heightened perception of the surroundings, and at times distraction.

Once the nurse obtains data signifying anxiety, he can intervene by asking the patient how to help him deal with his feelings of concern. The nurse may decide to report his observations to the surgeon and administer medication that has a tranquilizing effect. A caring nurse-patient relationship in which the patient feels comfortable sharing his thoughts will alleviate some of the fear. To provide this type of support, the nurse must:

• Accept the patient's dependency without feeling threatened by it
• Give warmth and friendliness without demanding gratitude
• Adjust to continual and sometimes unexpected change
• Use empathy in gaining insight into the patient's needs without overidentifying with his problems

The nurse must be an accepting listener who creates the opportunity for the patient to talk, and he must demonstrate a sincere interest through his actions.

During a local anesthesia procedure, as during any procedure, the atmosphere in the room is important. The noise level should be kept to a minimum. The traffic in and out of the room should be limited. Conversation must be played down. Focus is on the patient. The nurse should try to place himself in the patient's place and see the surgery through his eyes. Other members of the team, such as the radiologist, pathologist, and consulting physician should be alerted to the fact that the patient is awake.

The nurse should ask the patient if he is comfortable. A pillow may ease discomfort from positioning. Drapes should be positioned to provide adequate ventilation around the patient's face so he can breathe comfortably.

Some patients want to see what the surgeon is doing, but others do not. The nurse should ask them if they want to watch. A middle-aged nursing educator who was having a mass removed from her right palm asked to have her head propped so she could observe. "One must take advantage of every learning opportunity," she commented. Another patient

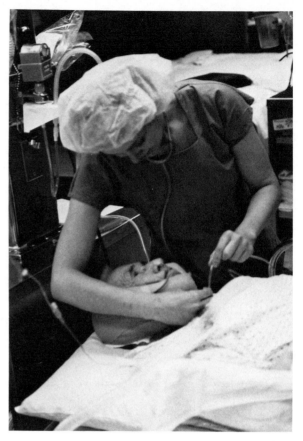

Figure 18.4. The nurse calls the patient by name as he emerges from the anesthetic.

was curious enough to stare at the operating light, watching his hernia repair in the reflected light surface. For the patient who is not so inquisitive, a screen can be used to separate the operative site from his field of vision.

Postoperative Care

When the patient is transferred to the recovery room or unit, the perioperative nurse should report significant psychological data to the nursing staff. For example, if the patient was resistant and fought during induction, he may wake up in the recovery room the same way. Or if the patient went to sleep crying, his concerns may surface again postoperatively. A patient may have requested his dentures as soon as he awakens, and the recovery room staff should be alerted to this. Another patient may be depressed regarding a mastectomy. The recovery room nursing staff will need to provide emotional support to all patients as they awaken (see Fig. 18.4).

The family is included in psychological support as it is in other aspects of the care plan. While the patient is in surgery, family members or friends are anxiously waiting to hear about their loved one. The nurse who has a sense of commitment to the patient and his family will stay in contact with them either by going to the waiting room, sending a message, or telephoning. All he needs to say is, "The surgery is still in progress," "The surgery is taking a little longer than you were told because we were held up and started later," or "Your husband is in the recovery room." If there is a crisis, and the family must be told the surgery was not successful or a malignancy was found, the nurse may accompany the physician and follow up by having the chaplain present.

Providing psychological support and monitoring the emotional status of patients during the intraoperative period is an important nursing activity. Preoperative preparation of patients has an impact on their behavior during surgery. Patients who have had an opportunity to work through their fears and have found coping mechanisms for handling their anxieties are more relaxed when they arrive in the operating room than patients who have not. They also recover more quickly and with fewer complications. Psychological support and therapeutic measures are critical to the well-being of the surgical patient. All persons deserve to be treated in a warm, caring manner. Every patient coming to the operating room is someone's loved one. The nurse should ask himself, "How would I want a nurse to care for my loved one?"

References

1. Dodge, J. S. "What patients should be told: Patients' and nurses' beliefs." *Am J Nurs* 72(October): 1182, 1972.
2. Field, L. W. "Identifying the psychological aspects of the surgical patient." *AORN J* 17(January):86, 1973.
3. Dyk, R. B., and Sutherland, A. M., "Adaptation of the spouse and other family members to the colostomy patient." *Cancer* 9(January-February): 124, 1956.
4. Foote, J. A. "Special needs of the teenage Cesarean patients." *AORN J* 34(November):855, 1981.
5. Gatch, G. "Caring for children needing anesthesia." *AORN J* 35(February):219, 1982.

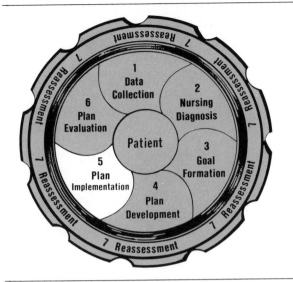

The figure shows a circular diagram with numbered segments: 1 Data Collection, 2 Nursing Diagnosis, 3 Goal Formation, 4 Plan Development, 5 Plan Implementation, 6 Plan Evaluation, with "Patient" at the center, surrounded by "7 Reassessment" around the outer ring.

The nurse continually measures the patient's physical status.

Physiological Monitoring

Understanding body systems and how they are affected by surgery provides a scientific basis for implementing intraoperative care. A comprehensive knowledge of anatomy and physiology of major organ systems, the musculoskeletal system, and the mobility of joints allows the nurse to conduct a preoperative assessment that quickly focuses on an individual patient's problems. With this information, she can draw up a thorough and efficient care plan targeted for these specific problems. During surgery, this background will allow the nurse not only to carry out the plan systematically but also to respond quickly and authoritatively to changes in the patient's status. Moreover, she will be prepared to react promptly and calmly to such surgical crises as cardiac arrest and malignant hyperthermia.

This chapter focuses on three major organ systems, outlining how they are affected by surgery, and providing specific measures for intraoperative monitoring. Emphasis is on the cardiac, respiratory, and renal systems because they have the most far-reaching effects on the patient's surgical outcome. As crucial as these systems are, it is important not to neglect the others. Therefore, a brief overview of the physiological responses of the gastrointestinal, endocrine, integumentary, and musculoskeletal systems is given. Alterations in any organ system affect all the others. The heart and lungs, to function efficiently, depend on the renal system to filter metabolites from the bloodstream adequately. The gastrointestinal system provides the nutrients that fuel metabolism. Disturbances in endocrine secretions may interfere with the functioning of the major organs. The surgical incision traumatizes skin and muscle, calling on the body's resources to aid in healing. The organ systems are interdependent. What affects one will, to some extent, affect all.

Important information about the physiological effects of surgery is given in other chapters throughout the text as well. Chapter 10 on fluid and electrolyte balance provides helpful background for monitoring the respiratory, gastrointestinal, and renal systems. Similarly, Chapter 22 on positioning has implications for the musculoskeletal, neurological, and integumentary systems. For further information on the skin, refer to Chapters 12 and 13 on skin integrity and infection.

The type of physiological monitoring done in the intraoperative period depends a great deal on how the nurse sees herself as a professional. Some nurses are satisfied with a minimal background in anatomy and physiology. They believe the sole responsibility for monitoring belongs to other team members, such as the surgeon and anesthesiologist. Others realize that the broader and deeper their knowledge, the better equipped they are to meet the needs of the patient and participate as a colleague on the health care team. There are few more important times for nurses to be patient advocates. During surgery, stimuli such as anesthetic agents and the surgical procedure cause physiological responses that necessitate intervention. Patients are more vulnerable at this time than at any other time during their hospitalization. During surgery the patient depends entirely on the skilled observation and care given by the OR team.

Positioning is one example of an intraoperative nursing activity that results in ongoing monitoring throughout the procedure. In positioning the body for surgery, the nurse must rely on her knowledge of anatomy and physiology; anesthetized patients cannot tell her which positions are painful or cause numbness. The nurse must be aware that positioning involves not only the musculoskeletal system but all body systems. Merely elevating a leg or turning a patient's body will have effects throughout the body. The experienced nurse anticipates these effects and the problems they may cause because she knows the systems so well. Continuous monitoring throughout the procedure enables the nurse to detect problems before they become serious and intervene with appropriate nursing actions.

Although a nurse's specific responsibilities for monitoring will vary from institution to institution and according to the type of surgery, it will prove useful to the nurse to have specific knowledge regarding her responsibility to monitor the physiological responses of the patient and to implement nursing interventions.

Monitoring the Cardiovascular System

CIRCULATORY PHYSIOLOGY

The primary function of the cardiovascular system is transport. Oxygen is taken through the blood vessels to the cells and exchanged for carbon dioxide; metabolites are delivered to the kidneys; hormones are channeled to where they are needed; and antibodies and bacteria-fighting white cells are deployed to infection sites. Essential to the body's homeostasis, the circulatory system is nevertheless dependent on the body's other major organ systems—respiratory, digestive, and renal. When one is thrown out of balance, all will be affected.

The circulatory system can be divided into two subsystems: the blood circulatory system and the lymphatic system. The first includes the blood and its components, the heart, the blood vessels, and the capillaries; lymphatic structures include the lymph fluid, the lymph nodes, and lymph vessels.

The outstanding structure is the heart, a hollow, four-chambered muscular organ that acts as a pump for the circulatory system. The heart muscle, enclosed in the pericardial sac, occupies the lower portion of the mediastinal cavity between the lungs and anterior to the esophagus and descending aorta.

The heart wall consists of three layers. The exterior layer, or epicardium, is a serous layer containing connective tissue and stored fats. The middle layer, the myocardium, is the muscle body responsible for heart contraction. The endocardium, the internal layer, lines the cavities, valves, and vessels of the heart.

The heart is divided lengthwise by a septum into right and left halves, both containing an upper chamber, or atrium, and lower chamber, or ventricle. The atria are the smaller receiving chambers for the blood, which is pumped from here into the ventricles. Deoxygenated blood flows into the right atrium from the inferior and superior vena cavae and the coronary sinus. Blood is then pumped through the tricuspid valve into the right ventricle. The right ventricle contracts to pump blood out of the heart through the semilunar valve through the pulmonary artery to the lungs and eventually into the lung capillaries. This is the pulmonary circulatory system.

The oxygen-carbon dioxide exchange takes place in the capillary beds of the lungs. The oxygenated blood flows from the lungs via the four pulmonary veins into the left atrium. Blood leaves the left atrium through the mitral valve into the left ventricle.

The left ventricle is a highly muscular chamber with walls three times as thick as the right ventricle. The powerful pumping force of the left ventricle circulates oxygenated blood out of the heart through the aortic valve into the aorta and from there to all body parts except the lungs.

Within the heart are four valves designed to prevent regurgitation or back flow of blood so it may be pumped forward during the cardiac pumping cycle. The heart valves are membranous structures, one type being the atrioventricular (AV) valve, and the other the semilunar valve. The AV valves located between the atria and the ventricles are composed of thin leaflets of endocardium. The tricuspid, or right atrioventricular valve, prevents regurgitation of blood from the right ventricle into the right atrium during ventricular contraction.

The tricuspid valve has three irregular leafs or cusps composed mainly of fibrous tissue. The mitral or left atrioventricular valve allows blood to move from the left atrium to the left ventricle but resists the back flow of blood into the left atrium during ventricular contraction. The mitral valve, a bicuspid valve, is thicker than the other valves and stronger to resist the forceful contractions of the left ventricle. Seventy percent of the blood from the atria will flow into the ventricles as the AV valves open; the remaining 30 percent is pumped in during atrial contraction. This contraction is called the atrial kick and is significant in forcing the remaining blood to the left heart.

The semilunar valves are pocketlike structures located at the outlets of both right and left ventricles. The valves perform a similar function to that of the AV valves. They permit blood to flow forward into the pulmonary artery and aorta but resist the back flow into the ventricles during contraction.

Heart Sounds
Characteristic normal heart sounds are vibrations caused by closure of the valves, which in turn bulge from the back flow of blood during ventricular contraction. The first heart sound or "lub" is heard when the atrioventricular valves close, causing the walls of the ventricles to vibrate from the back flow of blood against the AV valves. The second heart sound or "dub" results from the vibration on the pulmonary artery, the aorta, and to some degree, the ventricles as the semilunar valves close, again causing back flow toward the ventricles.

The Cardiac Cycle
The cardiac cycle is the sequence of events from one cardiac contraction to the next contraction. The cycles are initiated by the electrical conduction system of the heart. The initial electrical impulse is generated by the sinoatrial (SA) node located in the posterior wall of the right atrium near the opening of the superior vena cava. This is the heart's pacemaker, sending the impulse to contract the atria. The impulse is conducted to the AV node located in the lower right wall (septum) between the atria, where it is delayed before passing into

the ventricles. The electrochemical impulse passes through the bundle of His in the AV node into the ventricles, which contain the conductive pathways known as the left and right bundles and Purkinje fibers. This current in the ventricles causes depolarization of the tissues, which contracts the cardiac muscle fibers.

The cardiac cycle consists of two distinct periods: diastole, the period of ventricular relaxation and filling, and systole, the period of ventricular contraction and emptying. During the periods of diastole and systole, the heart valves react to the changes in the blood pressures within the ventricles by opening and closing. During diastole, the semilunar valves close passively when ventricular pressure falls below pulmonary artery and aortic pressure and blood attempts to flow back.

The electrocardiogram (ECG) records the electrical activity of the heart, displaying P, Q, R, S, and T waves. The P wave is caused by the spread of depolarization through the muscles of the atria when the atria contract and atrial pressure rises. Following the P wave is the QRS complex, depicting the depolarization of the ventricles and the onset of ventricular systole. The QRS complex is followed by the T wave, which indicates ventricular repolarization. The T wave occurs prior to the end of ventricular contractions as ventricular fibers begin relaxing.

Regulation of Cardiac Function

Cardiac output is the blood volume ejected by the left ventricle per minute. This value is usually determined in liters per minute using the following formula: cardiac output equals stroke volume (volume of blood ejected by the ventricle with each heart beat) times heart rate. The normal stroke volume, usually referring to the left ventricular output, for the average adult is 70–80 ml. The heart rate for the average adult is 80 beats per minute. Therefore, the normal cardiac output calculated for the average adult is 5–6 liters per minute.

The cardiac output increases proportionally as the heart rate increases to 90 beats per minute. If the rate increases from 90 to 140 beats per minute, the stroke volume decreases proportionally, keeping the cardiac output at the same volume per minute. The reason for a diminished stroke volume is that the ventricles have less filling time during diastole. When the heart rate exceeds 140 beats per minute, the stroke volume decreases faster than the heart rate. Therefore, the cardiac output will continue to decrease with increased heart rates above 140 beats per minute.

One major factor affecting stroke volume is the amount of blood flowing into the heart from the venous system, or the preload. The heart must adapt itself to the continual fluctuations in volume returned. A second determinant of stroke volume is the force of ventricular contraction or contractility as it adjusts to sudden alterations in venous return to the heart or to the peripheral resistance to ejection or the afterload, which is the third major factor. (6)

The heart has an autoregulatory mechanism that alters the force of ventricular contractions to accommodate fluctuations of venous return or cardiac output resistance. This is called the Frank Starling law of the heart. The law involves the striated and cardiac muscle, which may be likened to a spring. Within certain limits, the recoil (contraction) of a fiber will be proportional to how far it is stretched. That is, the force of muscular contraction is determined by the initial length of a muscle fiber, as long as the fiber is not stretched beyond its physiological limit. Therefore, within physiological limits, all blood returning to the heart via the venous system will be pumped out of the heart without allowing excessive damming of the blood in the veins.

Two sets of autonomic nervous fibers also affect cardiac pumping. The first is the vagus nerve containing parasympathetic fibers. The second is sympathetic fibers called cardiac accelerator, or augmentor, nerves. These nerves affect cardiac function in two ways: (1) by altering the heart rate and (2) by changing the contractile force of the myocardium.

One function of the vagus nerve is inhibition of the heart, especially during rest. Vagal stimulation and parasympathetic fibers slow the heart rate and diminish its contractile force. The left vagus nerve innervates the AV node, atrial muscle, and bundle of His. The right vagus nerve supplies the SA node and atrial muscle. The vagus stimulators not only weaken contractions but also delay the speed of electrical impulse transmission through the heart to the ventricles. Therefore, vigorous or continuous vagal stimulation can result in temporary heart block or ventricular arrest.

The augmentor nerves or sympathetic fibers innervate not only the conduction system and myocardium of the atrium, but the ventricles as well. There is greater innervation by sympathetic fibers of the heart compared to parasympathetic fibers. The sympathetic fibers accelerate nervous transmission throughout the heart and strengthen the atrial and ventricular contractions. During stress, the sympathetic or augmentor nerves can increase the force of myocardial contractions up to 250 percent.

Chemical Regulation of the Heart
The following chemical compounds or ions have marked effects on cardiac function.

1. Acetylcholine: This mediator substance is secreted by all parasympathetic nerve endings including the vagus nerve.
2. Catecholamines: Two catecholamines, norepinephrine and epinephrine, found naturally in the body, produce a positive inotropic effect to increase the vigor of myocardial contractions and the heart rate.
3. Potassium ions: Proper intracellular and extracellular concentrations of these ions are needed for maintaining resting membrane potential. Excess extracellular or serum potassium (hyperkalemia) results in decreased action potential of heart muscle cells, cardiac irritability, cardiac dilation, bradycardia, and weak cardiac contractions. The atria, AV node, and the ventricles are depressed. ECG changes following hyperkalemia are a prolonged P-R interval, low P waves, sinoatrial block, tenting T waves, intraventricular block and widening of QRS complex, abnormal S-T segment shifts, and

ventricular fibrillation and standstill with elevated concentrations. In hypokalemia there is less amplitude of the T wave with prominence of the Q wave. (7)
4. Calcium ions: Normal serum calcium is required for myocardial contractions. An increase in extracellular concentrations causes the heart to go into spastic contractions. Calcium deficiency weakens cardiac contractility. In hypercalcemia, ECG changes include short Q-T intervals and increased amplitude of the T wave beginning immediately after the end of the QRS complex. Hypocalcemia lengthens the S-T segment and Q-T interval.

Blood Pressure
Systemic circulation contains 75 percent of the blood volume and refers to the circulation to all the body cells except the lungs. The structures of the systemic circulation are the arterial and venous vessels delivering blood to and from organs and cells to meet maximum metabolic demands. The arteries carry 2–5 liters of blood per minute under high pressure, which the vessel walls resist due to their structural composition.

From the last branch of the arterial system, arteries branch into arterioles. Arterioles have strong muscular walls with the capacity to close or dilate the vessel by several times its regular diameter. This permits alterations in blood flow in response to metabolic demands. The alterations of flow and pressure at this level have a major effect on central pressures. The arterioles branch into thin-walled vessels called capillaries. It is at this capillary level that the metabolic exchanges occur between blood and interstitial spaces. Reversing the process, blood flows from the capillaries to the venules and then to the veins. Compared to the arteries, veins are thin-walled and less muscular. Veins transport blood back to the heart, dilating and contracting to alter blood flow and central pressures.

Blood pressure is numerically equal to the blood flow (cardiac output) multiplied by peripheral resistance. This is the circulatory force that perfuses the body with blood. Normally, the blood pressure is altered in response to circulatory changes at the local site, nervous intervention, and humoral regulation.

Locally, blood flow to tissues responds to specific needs for nutrients such as oxygen, glucose, fatty acids, and amino acids. Other factors, such as the need for heat loss or conservation, blood pH circulating in the brain, and circulating wastes to the kidney can increase or decrease blood flow.

The nervous system has direct control in regulating blood pressure and blood flow by stimulating contraction of the muscle walls of arterioles. Sympathetic vasomotor fibers to the blood vessels alter resistance and therefore blood pressure. The vasomotor center in the upper two-thirds of the brain's medulla and lower third of the pons also activate peripheral vasoconstriction.

The vasomotor center in the brain receives input about circulatory changes via receptors called baroreceptors, which are sensitive to stretching in the artery walls. They are located primarily in the carotid sinuses and the aortic arch. Stimulation of these receptors will alter heart rate and vessel tone.

The anterior hypothalamus is responsible for altering blood pressure in the regulation of temperature. Skin vessels dilate or constrict depending on the need for heat loss or retention.

Hormones and chemical substances in the blood are responsible for humoral regulation of blood pressure. These include aldosterone, norepinephrine, epinephrine, angiotensin, vasopressin, serotonin, histamine, and prostaglandins.

The Lymphatic System

The lymphatic system is a network of lymphatic capillaries leading to a series of larger lymphatic vessels. The lymphatic vessels circulate the clear fluid called lymph. The function of this system is to drain and filter tissue fluid and to circulate lymphocytes, globulin, and antibodies. These substances are manufactured in the lymph nodes, small bodies located at intervals in the lymphatic circulatory course. In addition, the lymphatic system returns vital proteins to the circulation that have leaked out of the systemic blood flow through the capillaries.

Body Responses to Surgical Intervention

The potential circulatory responses to anesthetic agents are oultined in Table 19.5.

INTRAOPERATIVE STIMULI THAT AFFECT THE CARDIOVASCULAR SYSTEM

Positioning

During surgery, the patient's circulatory function depends on how she is positioned. The following outline describes the circulatory effects of each surgical position. Positioning to maintain circulatory homeostasis is discussed in Table 19.1.

Supine position (dorsal recumbent)
1. Mean arterial blood pressure, heart rate, and peripheral resistance decrease.
2. Cardiac output and stroke volume increase.
3. Systolic blood pressure remains the same, but diastolic pressure is decreased; therefore the pulse pressure is greater.
4. There is venous pooling in the lower extremities due to reduction of venous pressure.

Prone position (and modifications)
1. There are few cardiovascular problems if the patient is positioned properly.
2. Venous return is reduced as a result of venous pooling in lower extremities induced by anesthesia.
3. If the patient is improperly positioned, pressure on the inferior vena cava and femoral veins will reduce venous return and cause hypotension. Alternative avenues of circulation do not provide adequate cardiac return. The pressure of the venous plexus on the vertebral column will increase three to five times with pressure exerted on the inferior vena cava and therefore increase intraoperative hemorrhage.
4. Obese patients do not tolerate prone positioning because of potential hypotension or hypoxia due to pressure on the vasculature.
5. When a prone-positioned patient's head is

Table 19.1. Positioning to Maintain Cardiovascular Homeostasis.

Potential Problem	Nursing Activity	Monitoring and Evaluation
Supine Position		
Decrease in blood pressure, heart rate, and peripheral resistance, especially during induction of anesthesia.	Apply ECG electrode. Provide anesthesia with adequate fluid replacement prn. Elevate lower extremities slightly to aid in venous return. (Do not place in Trendelenburg's position.) Insert urinary catheter to assess renal perfusion.	Monitor blood pressure by cuff or invasive technique. Monitor ECG for rate and rhythm prn. Observe for signs of inadequate tissue perfusion, e.g., cyanosis, edema, mottling, clammy skin. Monitor urine output and maintain at 30 cc to 60 cc's per hour minimum.
Venous pooling in extremities due to reduction of venous pressure.	Apply antithromboembolism hose or bandages prn. Elevate lower extremities slightly.	Observe lower extremities for edema. Prevent rolling of hose or bandages to produce a torniquet effect. Ask patient about comfort of the hose, wraps, or elevation of extremities.
Prone Position		
Venous pooling in extremities due to reduction of venous pressure. Pressure on great vessels due to improper positioning, reducing venous return. Increase in central venous pressure, increasing surgical venous bleeding.	Position patient on chest rolls so the abdominal contents hang freely.	Assess abdomen after positioning to determine if there is excessive pressure. Monitor central venous pressure if applicable.
Pressure on carotid sinus can cause hypotension and arrhythmias when head is turned to the extreme left or right. Positioning devices are used to immobilize the head, neck, or shoulders.	Prevent hyperextension of the neck, especially to the extreme right or left. Avoid pressure on carotid sinus, especially when using immobilizing devices.	Assess patient for pressure points prior to draping. Assess head position and maintain in good anatomical alignment. Monitor blood pressure and ECG.
Diminished blood flow to any portion of head, especially eyes, ears, nose, or lips due to excessive pressure.	Provide supporting positioning devices that will alleviate pressure, e.g., donuts, foam, head rests. Prevent any pressure on eyes.	Assess head structures for pressure, diminished perfusion, etc.
Head elevated Position		
Venous pooling in extremities due to reduction of venous pressure. Hypotension due to hypovelemia is more difficult to compensate for while in upright position and can add to circulatory insult.	Provide adequate fluid replacement with anesthesia. Assess blood loss and urine output continuously.	Maintain fluid input. Monitor ECG, blood pressure, and central venous pressure prn.

turned to one side, pressure on the carotid sinus can cause hypotension and arrhythmias.

6. Diminished blood flow to and from any part of the head can result from pressure or hyperextension in the prone position.

Head elevated position
1. Diminished cardiac return from the lower extremities can decrease cardiac output. (a)

Lack of muscle tone from anesthesia combined with increased gravitational force causes severe venous pooling. (b) Intermittent positive pressure breathing can impede venous return from the inferior vena cava.

2. Gravity aids venous return of blood above the heart and impedes upward circulating blood flow. In the upright position brain stem perfusion can decrease due to gravity, and blood accumulates in the lower depend-

ent extremities. In the healthy anesthetized patient, compensatory mechanisms accommodate for gravitational shifts.

3. In the seated patient, hypotension due to hypovolemia or unplanned hypotension should be avoided due to increased demand on the cardiovascular system as it compensates for these physiological changes.

Trendelenburg's position (head down)
1. Blood pressure is usually increased.
2. Cerebral vascular pooling occurs, raising hydrostatic pressure of cerebral spinal fluid. This further impedes cerebral blood flow and can cause stagnant cerebral hypoxia.
3. Patients with heart disease tolerate this position poorly due to increased vascular load to the heart from lower extremities.
4. Glaucoma is aggravated due to increased cerebral blood volume.
5. This position provides better surgical exposure by reducing blood to surgical sites such as the lower abdomen and pelvis. Surgical blood loss is also decreased.
6. Neck veins engorge, facilitating intravenous catheter insertion.
7. Cyanosis to the face secondary to venous engorgement hinders adequate assessment of circulatory and respiratory status during anesthesia.

Lateral decubitus position
1. There is little change in cardiac output.
2. Venous return is not altered.
3. Blood flow to the extremities is not altered if the patient is positioned properly. (1)

General Anesthesia Agents
Each anesthetic agent, combined with preoperative medication, directly influences cardiac function. For specific cardiovascular alterations related to medications or anesthetic agents, refer to Table 19.5.

Inhalation anesthetic agents depress myocardial contractility, but in the healthy patient this depression is offset by increased sympathetic drive. Three other more important ways anesthetic agents affect the circulation are by altering the heart rate, the afterload, and the preload. During anesthesia, cardiac output de-

pends on the heart rate up to a limit, beyond which the output falls again. Dilatation of the vessels either by reduction of sympathetic tone or by direct effect on the smooth muscle may raise cardiac output despite a fall in blood pressure, provided the filling pressure is maintained. (2)

Any situation increasing myocardial effort and oxygen demand during anesthesia and surgery can exacerbate existing problems for the patient. In patients with any compromised cardiovascular functioning, such as ischemic heart disease and hypertension, this situation can be extremely harmful. Although most anesthetic agents reduce myocardial work and oxygen demand, several surgical events initiate powerful sympathetic response that increases heart rate and arterial blood pressure and, therefore, myocardial workload. These stimuli include surgical manipulations of structures in the abdomen and chest, traction on the mesentery, mechanical stimulation of the gall bladder and urinary bladder, and splitting the sternum.

Regional and Local Anesthesia
Regional and local anesthesia may be preferable to general anesthesia, especially in the patient with compromised cardiovascular function. Spinal, subarachnoid, or epidural blocks have the advantages of not requiring intubation, blocking afferent impulses that cause sympathetic responses from surgical stimuli, and provide the patient with a more stable and painless recovery. Hypotension is a risk because the anesthetic blocks nervous intervention to the arterial system. With adequate fluid maintenance and pressure monitoring, however, the complications of hypotension can be minimized.

Hypotension at the time the block takes effect can be a hazard to the hypertensive patient because the control of arterial pressure changes is diminished. The hypertensive patient's response to pressoramines is unpredictable, making hypertension more difficult to manage. The patient's response to blocking agents containing epinephrine must be monitored carefully. This is especially true with hypertensive patients or patients with known cardiac disease.

Induction of Anesthesia

Circulatory instability can be the single most dangerous risk as the patient makes the transition from wakefulness to the anesthetized state, particularly in the patient with hypertension or ischemic heart disease. Two causes of hypotensive episodes are: the pharmacological effects of anesthetic agents and the inhibition of sympathetic nervous activity and the loss of baroreceptor control of arterial pressure that results from loss of consciousness.

With the exception of ketamine, all intravenous anesthetic agents can cause arterial pressure to fall by 20–30 percent in the normal patient. With the same dose to the hypertensive patient, a drop by 50 percent or more can be seen. This major alteration in arterial blood pressure causes myocardial ischemia when the diastolic arterial pressure is decreased to a critical value for any given patient. Therefore, the key principle in managing induction is to avoid sudden arterial hypotension by slowly administering the minimum dose of any agent that will induce loss of consciousness.

Laryngoscopy and Endotracheal Intubation

Laryngoscopy and intubation are performed under light anesthesia and full muscle relaxation, and can be associated with sympathetic nervous activation. The procedures can increase arterial pressure by 20–30 mm Hg and increase the heart rate by 15–20 beats per minute. The normal patient and even the patient with ischemic heart disease can tolerate these changes without further myocardial ischemia. The patient who is most at risk during laryngoscopy and intubation is the untreated hypertensive patient. The same stimulus during laryngoscopy and intubation can cause systolic increases from 140 (after induction) to 250 mm Hg and heart rate increases from 70 to 110 beats per minute. The result of these physiological responses can be subendocardial ischemia and a myriad of other complications. (8)

It would be easy to conclude, therefore, that known hypertensive patients should be maintained on their antihypertensive regimen until the day of surgery. But because most antihypertensive agents are short-acting, and most patients are restricted by NPO orders prior to surgery, the effects of the antihypertensive treatment will be diminished. These patients may have periods of hypertension during surgery and during recovery, which is the greatest concern.

Controlled Hypotension

Controlled hypotension may be initiated for specific procedures in which blood loss may be difficult to control. These include head and neck surgery; neurosurgical operations, especially for aneurysms and vascular tumors; vascular cancer operations; pelvic exenterations; portacaval shunts; and major orthopedic surgery, such as disarticulation procedures. The purpose of controlled hypotension is to decrease blood loss and the need for transfusion, to diminish oozing, and ultimately to reduce the amount of anesthetics used. The condition is achieved pharmacologically. Nitroprusside is often the drug of choice, although hexamethonium chloride and trimethaphan camsylate may also be employed.

Controlled hypotension produces various cardiac physiological responses. Coronary perfusion remains adequate, and there is no permanent myocardial damage as long as the blood pressure is not allowed to fall below 60 torr. Nitroprusside does not alter cardiac output if blood pressure is maintained at 80 torr.

As with any prolonged state of hypotension, controlled hypotension can cause morbidity and mortality. The most common complications are (5):

- Cerebral thrombosis and hypoxia
- Reactionary hemorrhage
- Renal failure, oliguria, and anuria
- Coronary thrombosis, cardiac failure, and cardiac arrest
- Thromboembolism
- Delayed awakening
- Persistent hypotension

Induced Hypothermia

Total body hypothermia allows increased operating time when circulation to vital organs is occluded or compromised. Cooling can be induced by several methods. Surface cooling is achieved by the tub method, a hypothermia blanket, heat exchanger, and topically applied cold solutions. Chilled solutions may be infused intravenously or administered by gastric or rectal lavage. The body temperature is maintained at 28–30°C. Controlled hyperventilation with 100 percent oxygen continues during surgery as the concentration of anesthesia is diminished.

As the body temperature drops, physiological changes ensue. The rate of oxygen consumption falls, and the solubility of carbon dioxide in the blood increases. Blood serum electrolytes are not significantly altered during and after cooling. If the body temperature is dropped to 25°C, the heart rate, coronary flow, and oxygen uptake of the heart decrease by 50 percent. If shivering is prevented, the cardiac output decreases. Blood flow to the brain, kidney, and splanchnic regions decreases as the temperature declines. For every degree centigrade below 37°C, there is a 5 percent decrease in the mean arterial pressure. Cerebral oxygen consumption decreases, and the cerebral spinal fluid pressure falls. The time it takes gross irreparable damage to occur to vital organs is extended to 15 minutes during cardiac arrest if the temperature is reduced to 25°C.

Managed and monitored properly, controlled hypothermia provides adequate tissue perfusion during surgery. Prolonged hypothermia can mask cerebral compression and signs of infection. Localized necrosis of the skin is an additional risk.

PATHOLOGIES THAT AFFECT CIRCULATORY PHYSIOLOGICAL RESPONSES

Aortic Valve Disease

Aortic stenosis or narrowing of the aortic valve increases left ventricular systolic pressure with eventual hypertrophy of the left ventricle. As the lesion progresses, pressure gradients across the valve increase, raising the pressure in the left atrium and pulmonary vessels. Pulmonary congestion and edema can occur, and coronary and cerebral insufficiency are not uncommon. Symptoms include dizziness, syncope, angina pectorus, fatigue, and palpitations.

Patients with mild to moderate aortic stenosis tolerate anesthesia, provided specific precautions are taken. In patients with chronic heart failure, arterial blood pressure is maintained with increased peripheral vascular resistance and a lower cardiac output.

Vasodilation and myocardial depression produced by an anesthetic may severely compromise cardiac function. Therefore, these drugs must be administered with great care and in smaller doses than usual. Acute hypotension and hypoxemia are of particular importance whenever coronary artery disease complicates aortic valve lesions.

Massive releases of catecholamines during endotracheal intubation and surgical stimulation can cause left ventricular failure or circulatory collapse. Tachycardia may impair cardiac function during induction of anesthesia. Thus it is extremely important to maintain adequate anesthesia levels during surgery to control sympathetic responses.

Aortic insufficiency means a pathologic aortic valve fails to close after systole. With the increased pulse pressure, the left ventricle hypertrophies and dilates. Pulmonary edema and congestion, cerebral insufficiency, dizziness, pulsating headaches, and coronary insufficiency can occur.

Patients with free aortic regurgitation and low diastolic pressures are vulnerable to both a drop in arterial blood pressure and rhythm changes. Coronary filling may be sharply decreased due to a reduction in diastolic pressure. Prompt volume replacement can prevent hypovolemia and hypotension secondary to vasodilation from anesthesia.

Mitral Valve Disease

Often associated with rheumatoid disease, mitral stenosis is a narrowing of the mitral valve that impedes blood flow from the left atrium to the left ventricle during diastole. The stenosis raises left atrial pressure as well as pulmonary artery and right ventricular systolic pressures. The right ventricle is affected by the low output, but often the left ventricle is not affected. Clinical symptoms include dyspnea, orthopnea, pulmonary edema, hemoptysis, pulmonary infection fibrosis, and atrial fibrillation.

Digitalis and diuretics are often prescribed for patients with mitral stenosis. These also affect physiological responses. Hypokalemia and hypovolemia should be avoided because hypotension and arrhythmias may be life-threatening, particularly during anesthesia induction. Anesthetic agents, especially halothane, may cause vasodilation and myocardial depression, which complicate the already low output.

Coronary Artery Disease

Patients with coronary artery disease have a diminished blood flow to the myocardium related to their myocardial oxygen demand. Any increase in demand, therefore, can bring on myocardial ischemia and infarction. Tachycardia and hypertension raise myocardial oxygen consumption. During anesthesia and surgery, hypertension from increased sympathetic stimulation should be treated by deepening the anesthesia level. Severe hypotension with a drop in diastolic pressure compromises coronary artery perfusion.

POTENTIAL COMPLICATIONS OF CIRCULATORY FUNCTION

Any situation that interferes with circulatory function can precipitate a medical emergency. Cardiac function is sensitive to two major chemical alterations—hypercarbia and endogenic catecholamine release in response to surgery and anesthesia. From these, many complications can ensue. Potential complications are described in Table 19.2.

MONITORING THE PATIENT'S CARDIAC RESPONSES

Monitoring the patient's cardiac vascular responses during surgery is an effort of the whole surgical team. Sound clinical judgment, observation, and medical devices are all employed in a continuous assessment of cardiac status. Data are collected on: respiratory function, clinical laboratory values, blood pressure, electrocardiograph responses, arterial blood gases, central venous pressure (CVP), pulmonary artery pressures, pulmonary artery wedge pressure, urinary output, mucous membranes, skin coloring, and color of blood at the surgical field. Lack of proper monitoring during surgery ultimately leads to poor management of the patient's altered physiological status.

The nurse may have primary responsibility for monitoring during local anesthesia cases, and she may assist anesthetists in their role as primary monitors during general anesthesia cases. Initial data are collected in a preoperative assessment. Laboratory values of hemoglobin, hematocrit, white blood cell count, red blood cell count, pH, potassium, sodium, and arterial blood gases if drawn should be evaluated. Vital signs are noted preoperatively to provide a baseline for alterations during surgery. Preoperative mentation should be assessed as an indicator of circulation to the brain. Urinary output indicates the quality of renal function and tissue perfusion. The patient's skin coloring and any diaphoresis indicate tissue perfusion, especially to the mucous membranes and extremities. Edema, distended neck veins, pulmonary congestion, and hypertension can signal cardiovascular disturbances, including circulatory overload and ventricular heart failure.

The patient may offer information about her current or historical cardiac status, such as angina, heart palpitations, dyspnea on exertion, orthopnea, orthostatic hypotension, radiating jaw or arm pain, history of rheumatic fever, and family history. Lifestyle, including diet, obesity, smoking, stress response levels, and exercise can all give insight into potential cardiac responses during surgery.

Other important elements in the preoperative assessment include the presence of any disease states directly affecting cardiac physiological responses. These may include diabetes, hypertension, hyperthyroidism, pheochromocytoma, coronary artery diseases, valvular heart disease, and respiratory pathology. Acute trauma can directly affect fluid volume levels and cardiac functioning intraoperatively.

Table 19.2. Potential Circulatory Complications.

Potential Complications	Possible Causes
Hypotension resulting in decreased tissue perfusion	narcotics anesthesia, especially during induction hypoxia reflexes surgical manipulation restricting venous return positioning hemorrhage adrenocortical insufficiency heart disease transfusion reaction air embolism
Hypertension, increasing myocardial oxygen consumption	pain hypoxia hypercapnia hypervolemia reflex stimulation increased intracranial pressure pheochromocytoma medications, including ketamine, vasopressor amines, succinylcholine, and light anesthesia catecholamine response to stress
Cardiac arrhythmia causing ischemia of vital organs, congestive heart failure, pulmonary edema, intrathoracic thrombosis with embolism, myocardial infarction, and cardiac arrest	anesthetic agents intubation anoxia duration of surgery positioning alcoholism digitalis toxicity fluid-electrolyte imbalance organic heart diseases congenital heart defects coronary artery disease hypertension

Cardiac arrest following asystole	many complex etiologic factors.
	hypoxia and hypercarbia are the underlying factors.
	primary factors potentiating the problem:
	    electrocution
	    coronary occlusion
	    isoproterenol overdose
	    any cause of respiratory failure:
	        airway obstruction
	        central nervous system depression
	        neuromuscular failure
	Potential causes:
	    flail chest
	    pneumothorax
	    massive atelectasis
	    acute pulmonary embolism
	    congestive heart failure
	    overwhelming pneumonia
	    Gram-negative septicemia
	    lung burns
	    carbon monoxide poisoning

Table 19.2. (Continued)

Potential Complications	Possible Causes
	massive blood loss
	susceptible patients:
	geriatric patients
	pediatric patients
	patients with:
	arrhythmias
	heart block
	digitalis toxicity
	myocardial infarction
	congestive heart failure
	fluid-electrolyte imbalance
	massive hemorrhage
	heart surgery
Low cardiac output	cardiac tamponade
	massive hemorrhage
Hypercapnia	obesity
	chronic lung disease
	inappropriate method of anesthesia
Hyperkalemia	rapid administration of cold blood
	excessive potassium administration
	trauma
	burns
	renal failure
Direct cardiac stimulation to the heart causing cardiac arrest	any intracardiac catheter or electrode placement
Coronary occlusion	embolus
	thrombus
	ligation
	contrast media directly injected into cardiovascular system.
Overdose of drugs causing cardiac arrest	cardiac glycosides
	catecholamines
	anesthetic drugs
Disseminated intravascular coagulation (DIC) in later stages of circulatory failure	sepsis
	prolonged bleeding
	any situation that releases tissue materials into the circulation that induce blood coagulation and platelet aggregation, e.g., prostate surgery

Adapted from Snow, J. C. *Manual of Anesthesia*. Boston: Little, Brown and Co., 1977.

Intraoperative Monitoring

Monitoring may begin with the use of a precordial stethoscope to monitor heart rate, rhythm, and heart sounds via auscultation. An esophageal stethoscope may be inserted by the anesthesiologist to obtain more direct monitoring.

Doppler monitoring amplifies blood circulation or arterial pulsation during procedures on patients whose blood pressure or pulse may be inaudible or difficult to obtain. These include infants, obese patients, and any patient the anesthesiologist judges to need continuous Doppler monitoring.

The topical Doppler probe is usually applied at the radial pulse site. Conductive jelly or cream aids in transmission of emitted waves from the blood circulation to the electrical conduction cord. This is translated into audible sounds.

The sphygmomanometer provides indirect measurement of systolic and diastolic blood pressures. These values can provide limited information about the vitality of the heart, its functional pumping efficiency, and the status of circulation.

Proper placement of the cuff ensures accurate readings. The cuff should be wide enough to cover two-thirds of the upper arm: if it is narrower, the results will be high; if it is wider, the results are low. The center of the inflatable bag should be placed directly over the brachial artery, above the antecubital fossa.

The ECG is the only means of monitoring the electrical activity of the heart. A preoperative ECG should be done on all patients 35 years and over or on any younger patient when indicated.

ECG pads should be applied prior to induction of anesthesia with adequate inspection of the skin surface. Avoid placing pads over bony prominences, scarred tissue, rashes, or pooled solutions. If the patient is excessively hairy, a wet shave may be indicated. Standard ECG leads I and II are more often employed with ECG lead placement of left arm, left leg, right arm. Lead placement should not interfere with the surgical prep or surgical field.

The ECG provides a continuous display of electrical activity that can be seen by the whole surgical team. Heart rate is often displayed on a digital readout, and most monitors are equipped with a device for drawing permanent tracings. ECG monitoring allows you to assess cardiac activity continuously, especially during the crucial stages of induction of anesthesia, intubation, and beginning of surgical stimulation.

ECG monitoring provides for early recognition of arrhythmias, conduction deficits, myocardial ischemia, and myocardial infarction as well as the effects of anesthetic agents, cardiac drugs, and electrolyte imbalance. Tachycardia, bradycardia, extra systole, S-T depression, and inverted T wave indicating inadequate coronary artery perfusion are all represented immediately on the electrocardioscope. During cardiac arrest, the ventricular asystole and ventricular fibrillation can be differentiated. Although the ECG does not indicate heart failure, it may give warning signs. Limitations in the use of the ECG are that it cannot monitor hemodynamic events or the efficiency and force of contraction of the myocardium, and it cannot evaluate cardiac output. For detection and management of cardiac arrhythmias during surgery see Table 19.3.

Invasive Monitoring

For this type of monitoring, a catheter is placed into a blood vessel, heart chamber, or cerebral spinal fluid space. The system can be open or closed to atmospheric pressure. Often a transducer and amplifier are employed. The transducer contains a sensitive diaphragm displaced by pressure changes from the patient's circulation. This is converted into electrical activity by the transducer's electrical circuit and is displayed on a monitor screen.

Direct or invasive measurement of arterial blood pressure is done by percutaneous or cutdown arterial cannulation. The radial artery is the usual site, but brachial and femoral arteries can be employed. Prior to cannulation of the artery, Allen's test is performed to assess whether there is adequate collateral circulation to the hand. This indicates that tissues will be perfused while the catheter is in place.

One advantage of direct arterial blood pressure measurement is accurate detection of moment-to-moment variations in intraarterial blood pressure even before the patient becomes symptomatic. The surgical team can then intervene immediately to compensate for fluctuations in pressure that could be life-threatening. Another advantage is that access into the arterial circulation allows continuous arterial blood gas samples to be taken. Analysis of the blood gases PO_2, PCO_2, pH, and bicarbonate provide information about tissue perfusion.

Patients who benefit most from direct arterial line cannulation include the critically ill, those in cardiogenic shock, trauma victims, cardiac surgery patients, and patients receiving hypothermic or hypotensive anesthesia.

Nursing responsibilities during surgery for setup and insertion of arterial line monitoring devices vary with the institution. Nurses familiar with the setup of fluid administration, intraflow, transducer, and monitoring devices can provide more comprehensive care. Likewise, trouble-shooting is more effective when there is a broader understanding of monitoring arterial line tracings.

Arterial line pressure is represented on an oscilloscope that traces the arterial wave form. Systole is represented on the screen by a sharp ascent of the wave form, and diastole is represented by a more gradual descent. The descent is interrupted by the dicrotic notch, representing the closure of the aortic valve. Wave form variations denote cardiac pathology, alterations in cardiac output, changes in peripheral vascular resistance, and artifacts in the monitoring system. Significant values interpreted from arterial line pressures are:

1. Systolic pressures: Pressure of the vascular system during ventricular contraction.
2. Diastolic pressure: Pressure of the vascular system during ventricular filling.
3. Mean blood pressure: Average pressure in the peripheral arterial system during the entire cardiac cycle. This is the most important blood pressure value obtained during cardiac arrhythmias and during periods of increased vascular resistance.
4. Pulse pressure: The pressure difference between systolic and diastolic pressures.

Dampening or distortion of the wave form is caused by a mechanical obstruction in the indwelling catheter. The obstruction can be due to backblocking, clot formation, wedging of the catheter tip against a vessel wall, or bubbles trapped anywhere between the diaphragm of the transducer and the pressure source. This dampened wave form is displayed as a significant decrease in systolic pressures and an increase in the diastolic pressure, decreasing the pulse pressure. The dicrotic notch is also lost on the tracing.

Invasive monitoring of CVP assesses right heart competence. Measuring pressures exerted by venous return to the right heart indicates the ability of the right side of the heart effectively to manage this venous return. A catheter is inserted either into the median cubital vein, external jugular vein, or subclavian vein and threaded up to the superior vena cava. Insertion poses the risks of causing a pneumothorax, so a chest x-ray is required to confirm the placement of the catheter.

CVP monitoring can help determine if the patient's hemodynamic failure is a result of hemorrhage or heart failure. Hemorrhage is associated with a fall in CVP, whereas an increased CVP can indicate heart failure. CVP essentially measures preload, or the amount of blood brought to the heart. The normal range is 3–10 cm H_2O. Monitoring equipment includes a manometer on which the zero level is equal to the position of the right atrium. CVP monitoring may be indicated in elderly patients, patients in whom massive blood transfusion or fluid administration is expected with the risk of overhydration, cardiac patients, trauma victims, patients with major intraoperative blood loss, patients with questionable volume status, patients in the upright position during surgery, and open heart surgery patients with pheochromocytoma.

There are drawbacks to limiting hemodynamic monitoring to the CVP values. CVP cannot monitor pulmonary wedge pressure, myocardial contractility, the ability of the heart to pump, or the afterload (the resistance against which the heart pumps). CVP measures only the preload of the right heart. The right heart pumps blood into the pulmonic circulation and not the systemic circulation. Although both sides of the heart can be affected by altered hemodynamic states, systemic complications may occur before affecting CVP. It is essential, then, to monitor left side heart function simultaneously in patients with any alteration in hemodynamic status or with multisystem disease.

Pulmonary artery and wedge pressure are measured by the Swan-Ganz catheter, which provides direct invasive monitoring of the pressures of the left side of the heart. The Swan-Ganz catheter is inserted into a median cubital vein or subclavian vein and advanced by the circulatory blood through the heart to rest in the right ventricle. Catheter placement is visualized by fluoroscopy in conjunction with ECG monitoring.

Table 19.3. Management of Cardiac Arrhythmia.

Arrhythmia	Potential Causes	Treatment	Comments
Sinus tachycardia: heart rate 100–160 beats/minute	Stress, exercise, fever, anemia, hemorrhage, hypoxia, hypotension, hyperthyroidism, heart failure, epinephrine administration, atrophy	Treat and correct underlying nausea.	Administer digitalis for heart failure.
Sinus bradycardia: normal sinus rate 40–60 beats/minute	Elderly patients, athletes Patients with history of myxedema, obstructive jaundice, increased intracranial pressure Manipulation during surgery such as pressure on carotid sinus, eye muscle surgery, vagal stimulation Occurs during anesthesia with halothane, narcotics, and succinylcholine IV administration	Atropine isoproterenol, cardiac pacing.	Hypotension occurs when there is decreased cardiac output.
Premature atrial contractions (PACs)	Patients with a history of heavy intake of coffee, tobacco, and alcohol Digitalis toxicity Anesthesia of any type Myocardial ischemia, infarction, or chronic lung disease	Treat underlying causes, sedation PRN, quinidine.	Difficult to detect on electrocardioscopes. But can be expected when periods of irregularity are present between QRS complexes. Diagnosis is made from palpation of radial pulse in conjunction with the ECG. Observed in healthy and unhealthy hearts.
Paroxysmal atrial tachycardia (PAT): atrial rate 150–250 beats/minute		Vagal stimulation (Carotid massage-Valsalva maneuver). Vasopressors, digitalis propranolol, atrial pacing.	Observed in healthy and unhealthy hearts. Rapid succession of abnormal P waves. 1:1 ventricular response.
Atrial flutter: atrial rate 250–350 beats/minute	Organic cardiac diseases	Digitalis, low energy D/C countershock.	ECG shows P waves replaced by flutter waves, and therefore, the baseline shows a sawtooth appearance.
Atrial fibrillation: P waves not visible; QRS complex occurs irregularly; P waves replaced by T waves at a rate of 400–600 beats/minute	Occurs in rheumatic mitral valvular disease, coronary artery disease, hyperthyroidism	Digitalis therapy to slow heart rate. Digoxin to slow heart rate during surgery if atrial fibrillation is of sudden onset. D/C countershock for persistent atrial fibrillation. Quinidine or procainamide given	Diagnosis derived from deficit of apex and radial pulse. Pulse is irregular Because of diminished diastolic filling time, there is a decreased cardiac output. The result is a diminished organ tissue perfusion, potential for congestive heart disease, hepatic and renal insufficiency. Atrial stasis and thrombus formation with subsequent

Table 19.3. (*Continued*)

Arrhythmia	Potential Causes	Treatment	Comments
		to maintain normal sinus rhythm during or after cardioversion.	emboli to vital organs and extremities can occur.
Complete heartblock (third-degree heart block)	Organic heart disease	Isoproterenol, cardiac pacemaker.	Make preparations for pace-maker insertion. All impulses to ventricles are not being transmitted. P waves and QRS waves are in total dissociation from each other. Atria and ventricles contract independently of each other.
Right bundle branch block	May be found in normal hearts, congenital defects, coronary artery disease, hypertension, heart valve disease	Temporary pacing may be required prior to surgery.	Damage to a branch of bundle of His. Rhythm is regular. QRS complex is wide and notched. T wave is deflected opposite.
Premature ventricular contractions (PVCs)	Actual heart disease, medications, metabolic disturbances, unknown causes	Oxygenation of lungs. Lidocaine. Treatment of under-lying causes (hypoxia, light or deep anesthesia, etc.). Management of digitalis toxicity. Procainamide. Quinidine.	Multifocal PVCs may precipitate ventricular fibrillation. Most common arrhythmia. Bigeminy PVCs occurring with every second contraction. Trigeminy PVCs occurring with every third contraction.
Ventricular tachycardia: bizarre ECG; irregular QRS complexes; P waves unrecognizable	Severe ischemia of cardiac muscle, digitalis toxicity, fluid/electrolyte imbalance, anoxia, heart block during Adams-Stokes episodes, overdose of catecholamines	Sedation, lidocaine, procainamide, DC countershock, diphenylhydantoin. Hyperventilation with oxygen during surgery.	May precipitate ventricular fibrillation. Impulses are generated from ectopic focus from lower chambers of the heart. Rapid thready pulse, distant heart sounds, decreased blood pressure, narrow pulse pressure. Do not vagal stimulate as this does not decrease heart rate. Digitalis may lead to ventricular fibrillation.
Ventricular fibrillation (cardiac arrest)	Ischemia to the heart; precipitating arrhythmias listed above	Cardiac arrest and cardiopulmonary resuscitative measures. Electrical defibrillation, sodium bicarbonate, etc.	Most serious of all arrhythmias. Irregular movements of ventricles. Impulses are sporadic and uncontrolled. Ventricular contractions are ineffective. Ventricular asystole, cardiac failure, and death are the outcomes if intervention is not immediate.

Adapted from Snow, J.C. *Manual of Anesthesia.* Boston: Little, Brown and Co., 1977.

There are four external lumens of the Swan-Ganz catheter:

1. Proximal lumen: The opening lies in the right atrium and is used to measure CVP and provide an injection port for fluids and iced solutions to measure cardiac outputs.
2. Distal lumen: This is attached to a transducer to monitor pulmonary artery pressures as it rests floating in the right ventricle or pulmonary artery. When the balloon is inflated, it travels and wedges in the pulmonary artery, where the distal lumen will measure pulmonary capillary wedge pressure.
3. Balloon: This lumen provides direct access to the balloon located at the distal portion of the Swan-Ganz catheter. When momentarily inflated, the balloon will migrate and wedge into the pulmonary artery, allowing for indirect pressure monitoring of the left ventricle. This pressure is known as the pulmonary capillary wedge pressure.
4. Thermistor: This lumen inserts directly into a computer to calculate cardiac output. The thermistor is located at the distal tip of the Swan-Ganz catheter resting in the right ventricle.

The Swan-Ganz catheter provides pulmonary artery (PA) pressures including systolic, diastolic, mean, and mean pulmonary capillary wedge pressures (PCWP). Normal values are:

- PAD = 8–15 mm Hg
- PCWP = 6–12 mm Hg

The PA diastolic and PCWP are indications of left ventricular-end diastolic pressure (LVEDP), which is the pressure in the left ventricle prior to contraction. PCWP is indicative of left ventricular pressure because it measures the unobstructed flow from the pulmonary arteries, capillaries, left atrium, and left ventricle during diastole while the mitral valve is open just prior to contraction of the ventricles.

PCWP values can be used essentially in the same way as CVP values are used to determine right heart functioning. Low PCWP indicates a decreased volume, and the patient needs more fluids. If the PCWP and PA pressures are elevated, the patient could be in cardiogenic shock, and overhydrated. She may need less fluids or a diuretic. It is important to remember that during heart failure left ventricular pressures rise first as blood remains in the left ventricle after failure to eject the existing volume during systole. Therefore, an elevated left ventricular and diastolic pressure can be an early indicator of heart failure.

During surgery, cardiac output is measured infrequently due to present difficulties with technique. If cardiac output measurements are performed, the thermodilution technique will often be employed. A known quantity of cold solution is administered into the distal lumen of the Swan-Ganz catheter located in the right atrium. The resulting change in blood temperature is then detected by the thermistor resting in the pulmonary artery. Cardiac output is inversely proportional to the integral temperature change. This change is communicated via the fourth lumen inserted into a computer that calculates cardiac output and displays it on a digital readout. Table 19.4 is a trouble-shooting chart for invasive pressure monitoring.

Monitoring the Respiratory System

RESPIRATORY PHYSIOLOGY

A basic review of the normal physiology of the respiratory system may be helpful in understanding the patient's physiological response to surgery. Respiration, simply put, is the transport of oxygen from the atmosphere to the cells with an exchange for carbon dioxide. Oxygen enters the body and carbon dioxide leaves the body via the respiratory passageways. In a person who is breathing normally, inspiration is the flow of atmospheric air containing oxygen and other gases through the respiratory passages to the alveoli. Expiration is the flow of oxygen and gaseous body wastes, including carbon dioxide from the alveoli, through the respiratory passages, to the atmosphere.

Table 19.4. Trouble-Shooting for Invasive Pressure Monitoring.

Problem/Complication	Causes	Precautions	Solutions
Arrhythmias such as premature atrial contractions (PACs) and premature ventricular contractions (PVCs)	Irritation of valves and endocardium by the catheter. Knotting of the catheter. Return of catheter from pulmonary artery to right ventricle.	Monitor ECG Have resuscitation equipment available at all times.	Examine catheter for defects or kinks prior to insertion. Adhere external lumen to skin by suturing and taped pressure dressing. Avoid extensive manipulation.
Infection at insertion Thrombophlebitis Hemorrhage Disconnection	Irritation at site. Break in aseptic technique. Inadequate connection by tape or suture.	Assess insertion site frequently for any signs of inflammation and hemorrhage at site or on dressing.	Lubricate catheter with saline or water before insertion. Change dressings, stopcocks, and tubing daily using aseptic technique. Avoid overmanipulation and repeated punctures of tissues during insertion of catheter.
Pulmonary artery perforation from Swan-Ganz catheter	Pulmonary hypertension. Overinflation or prolonged inflation of balloon in pulmonary artery. Migration of balloon into smaller arteries.	Inflate balloon slowly and only long enough to determine wedge pressure. Do not overinflate the balloon.	Stop inflation of balloon and do not reinflate. Monitor vital signs, ECG.
Inability to balance monitor	Damaged transducer. Inappropriate connection to amplifier. Defective dome.	Balance dome before attaching intraflow. Attach proper transducer to desired amplifier.	Change dome, transducer. Check connection to amplifier.
Drifting	Insufficient warm-up time.	Allow for sufficient warm-up time.	
False low reading	Dampened wave forms. Incorrectly balanced transducer. Air trapped in the system. Rapid flushing of system.		Rebalance transducer. Evacuate air. Tighten connections.
Discrepancy between cuff pressure and direct line pressure	Direct pressures most often are more accurate. In the hypotensive patient, decreased cardiac output and vasoconstriction make cuff pressure inaudible.		Use direct arterial line pressure to determine blood pressure.
Dampened pressures	Air in system. Blood in transducer. Clot in the system. Malpositioning. Occlusion or kinking of tubing.		Evacuate air from system. Change transducers and kinked tubing. Reposition catheter by manipulation. Secure catheter.
Sudden change in tracing configuration	Catheters dislodged. Transducer needs rebalancing and calibrating. Transducer not at right atrium level. Transducer connections loosened.		Reinsert catheter prn. Recalibrate transducer. Adjust transducer to level of right atrium. Tighten all connections.

The respiratory passages, through which the air flows, perform several functions. As air enters the body through the nose it is warmed, moistened, and filtered. Much less air enters the body through the mouth, and it receives less conditioning prior to entering the lungs. Air passes through the nose, mouth, and pharynx entering the trachea via the opening provided by the epiglottis. The epiglottis functions to close off the opening of the trachea to solids or liquids passing through the pharynx to the esophagus. During the cough reflex, the epiglottis closes in response to foreign matter irritating the lower respiratory passages. Air is trapped in the lungs, and the abdominal muscles then contract using other respiratory muscles to expel this air forcefully. Air and the foreign matter are expelled past the epiglottis, which now opens.

As air flows past the epiglottis during inspiration, it enters the larynx and vocal cords. There vibrating structures are responsible for phonation. Phonation takes place during the expiratory phase of respiration as the expired air flows between the margins of the laterally vibrating cords.

Continuing along the respiratory pathway, inspired air flows through the trachea. The trachea, or "wind pipe," is a tubular structure 4–5 inches long supported by cartilaginous rings separated by fibrous muscle tissue. It functions as a passageway for air to reach the lungs. The trachea is lined with a beating, ciliated mucous-coated epithelium that also aids in mobilizing small foreign matter toward the pharynx.

Splitting from the distal portion of the trachea are two primary bronchi or bronchial tubes, each of which supplies oxygen to one of the lungs. They differ significantly in structure. The right main stem bronchus is shorter, wider, and takes a more vertical course than the left bronchus. This is significant because foreign bodies and endotracheal tubes usually enter the right bronchus rather than the left.

The primary right and left bronchus continue to branch into thousands of air passages called bronchial tubes. These tubes continue to subdivide, and their final microscopic divisions are called alveolar ducts. Each alveolar duct terminates with alveolar sacs that re-semble grape clusters. The alveolar sacs are composed of singular cavities called alveoli. A highly developed network of capillaries surrounds each alveoli. It is at this point that the gaseous exchange between blood and inhaled air transpires.

The lungs, which contain the bronchi, the bronchioles, and alveoli, are two cone-shaped organs occupying the left and right thorax from the diaphram to 1.5 inches above the clavicle. The lungs expand and contract with the upward and downward movement of the diaphragm to lengthen or shorten the thoracic cavity.

The thorax expands and contracts by two mechanical forces. The first is the contraction and descent of the diaphragm, causing the chest to expand and the lungs to distend as they fill with inspired air. The second force is the elevation or depression of the ribs to increase or decrease the anterior-posterior diameters of the chest cavity. Diaphragmatic breathing, or normal breathing, is characterized by deep, quiet inspirations and expirations accompanied by relaxation and contraction of abdominal muscles. Costal breathing, on the other hand, is shallow, characterized by upward and outward movement of the chest using external intercostal and scalene muscles. Inspiration is characterized by the *active* contraction of the inspiratory muscles, allowing air to enter and distend the lungs. Expiration is a *passive* activity caused by the elastic recoil of the lungs and thorax to return to their prior resting state.

Intrathoracic pressures vary with inspiration and expiration as air flows from an area of lesser pressure to an area of greater pressure. During inspiration, intrapleural pressure becomes slightly less than atmospheric pressure. This negative intrapleural pressure causes air to move inward toward the lung. During normal expiration, the intrapleural pressure rises to about + 3 mm Hg, and air then flows outward through the respiratory passageways.

This passive outward flow of air from the lungs is directly related to the lung's elastic recoil. Several factors influence the lung's ability to recoil. The first is elastic fibers of the lung, which are continually stretched and thus attempting to shorten. The second factor is the surface tension between air and fluid in the alveoli, which requires energy to overcome. Surface tension is broken down by surfactant, a lipoprotein excreted by the alveolar epithelium into the alveoli. This reduces the muscular effort needed to expand and deflate the lungs. Expandability of the lungs and thorax is known as compliance.

The ultimate goal of respiration is maintaining adequate concentrations of oxygen, carbon dioxide, and hydrogen ions in body fluids. The body has neural and chemical receptors regulating these gaseous concentrations. The respiratory center is a group of neurons located in the reticular substance of the medulla oblongata and the pons in the brain. Nerve impulses from the medulla are conducted via the phrenic nerve to stimulate diaphragmatic contraction. Changes in pH and carbon dioxide are sensed by chemoreceptors in the medulla. An increase of the $PaCO_2$ will increase cerebral spinal fluid pressure, positive hydrogen ion concentration, and decrease pH. The decreased pH stimulates the central receptors in the medulla to increase the respiration rate. This is a physiological response to rid the body of excess carbon dioxide via expiration to maintain homeostasis.

Chemoreceptors sensitive to oxygen, carbon dioxide, and positive hydrogen ion concentration levels in the body fluids are also located outside the central nervous system in the carotid bodies and aortic bodies. The carotid bodies, located in the bifurcation of the common carotid artery, transmit nerve impulses via the glossopharyngeal nerve to the medulla. The aortic bodies, located in the arch of the aorta, transmit impulses via the vagus nerve to the medulla. Although these chemoreceptors respond to changes in concentrations of oxygen, carbon dioxide, and positive hydrogen ion levels in the blood stream, the PCO_2 has the greatest effect on regulating the respiratory response.

INTRAOPERATIVE STIMULI THAT AFFECT THE RESPIRATORY SYSTEM

During the patient's surgical experience, a vast number of integrated stimuli alter physiological status. Each body system, including the respiratory system, is directly affected by these stimuli to produce multiple body responses.

Anesthesia

Prior to the day of surgery, the anesthesiologist will assess the physical and mental status of the patient to determine the preoperative medication to use. Preoperative medication is given prior to the induction of anesthetic agents primarily to decrease tension and anxiety and provide a smoother anesthetic induction, maintenance, and emergence. The medication also minimizes side effects of anesthetic agents, such as salivation, bradycardia, and vomiting. The preferred drugs are the narcotic analgesics used in conjunction with an anticholinergic agent.

Preoperative medications directly affect respiratory functions. Therapeutic doses of most narcotic analgesics depress all phases of respiratory activity, including rate, minute volume, and tidal exchange. Irregular and periodic breathing as a result of the narcotic agent reduces the responsiveness of the brain stem's respiratory centers to increases of PCO_2. The narcotic analgesics also depress pontine and medullary centers, which regulate respiratory rhythm and response to electrical stimulation. In addition to depressing the respiratory center, the most important effects of the narcotic analgesics are to release histamine, depress the cough reflex, and dry secretions.

Anticholinergic medications are administered to alter specific respiratory activities. Most provide mild respiratory stimulation, decrease the incidence of laryngospasm, and most important, decrease bronchial secretions. The flow sheet of anesthetic agents (Table 19.5) gives an overview of respiratory responses to the most common anesthetic agents used intraoperatively.

Inhalation anesthetic agents are delivered to the lungs with each respiration. Larger concentrations of the agent are administered initially to provide a more rapid induction. Then maintenance levels of the anesthetic agent can be employed sooner (2). During the first stage of anesthesia, respiratory responses remain mostly unaffected. In the second stage of anesthesia, respirations are irregular in rate and depth. Laryngeal, pharyngeal, and swal-

Table 19.5. Flow Sheet for Anesthetic Agents

Agent	Route of Administration	Induction	Elimination	Nervous System	Respiratory System	Cardiovascular System
Halothane (Fluothane) volatile liquid	Inhaled—calibrated vaporized with O_2 and N_2O	3–8 min. smooth	90% via lung metabolized and excreted in urine	Cerebral depression; parasympathetic stimulation.	Progressively depress respiration; decrease in tidal volume; nonirritating; bronchial dilation; pharyngeal-laryngeal reflexes rapidly obtunded	Bradycardia; depresses myocardium; decreases cardiac output; decreases blood pressure.
Enflurane (Ethrane) volatile liquid	Inhaled—calibrated vaporized with O_2 and N_2O	3–8 min. smooth	Most via lungs; unchanged metabolites in urine	Cerebral depression; muscle irritability and twitching; EEG changes with low $PaCO_2$ sympathetic depression.	Respiratory depression dose related and progressive; laryngeal pharyngeal reflexes rapidly obtunded; sweet odor; no bronchodilatory effect	Mild hypotension.
Isoflurane (Forane)	Inhaled—calibrated vaporized with O_2 and N_2O	7–10 min. can produce coughing, breath-holding, laryngospasm	Exhaled via the lungs relatively unchanged	Increases cerebral blood flow with transient rise in cerebral spinal fluid pressure (reversed by hyperventilation).	Pungent odor; pharyngeal-laryngeal reflexes rapidly obtunded; profound respiratory depressant; respirations must be monitored closely and supported when necessary. Tidal volume decreases, respiratory is unchanged.	Decreases blood pressure, heart rate stable. Heart rhythm is stable. Cardiac output is stable.
Gases Nitrous Oxide-N_2O (1772) (1884)	Inhalation with O_2	2–3 min.	Unchanged via lungs	Mild cerebral depression.	Nil with 20% O_2.	Nil with 20% O_2.
Injectables Sodium pentothal (1934)	IV with O_2 relaxants and analgesics	15–45 sec.	Detoxified by liver, muscle tissue, and blood enzymes	Reflexes active, parasympathetic predominate, cerebral depression.	Dose related resp. depression bronchial tone.	Depression of myocardium; cardiac output decreases.
Dissociative agents Innovar (droperidol)	IV	5–8 min.	Metabolized and excreted in urine	Marked tranquillity without	Patient may forget to breathe.	Generally stable.

Other	Muscle Relaxation	Contraindications	Advantages and Uses	Disadvantages and Complications	Emergence
Decreases metabolic rate.	Poor to fair	Myocardial insufficiency; recent M.I.; known liver disease; obstetrics; halothane exposure in last three months; known maligant hyperthermia candidates.	Nonflammable, potent, smooth induction recovery; safe for pediatric use, preferred for asthmatic patients.	Expensive; narrow margin of safety; arrhythmias common; cannot use with epinephrine type drugs; "halothane hepatitis", 1/10,000—56% mortality; postop shivering.	15–20 min.
Decreases metabolic rate.	Dose dependent; potentiates non-depolarizing relaxants	History of seizures	Rapid, smooth induction and recovery; non-flammable, some muscle relaxation.	Postop shivering; CNS irritability	5–15 min.
	Muscle relaxation adequate for intraabdominal operations; muscle relaxants are markedly potentiated; most profound with nondepolarizing type.	Known sensitivity to halogenated agents; obstetrical patients; children under age 2.	Nonflammable, some muscle relaxation, minimal cardiac insult, potent. repeated doses are safe. minimal amount metabolized by body, therefore safer for use by personnel.	Expensive, hypotension, respiratory depression, some arrhythmias, shivering, nausea, vomiting, postoperative ileus, elevation of white blood count Increased blood loss during abortions.	Rapid 5–15 min.
	None	None	Potentiates other anesthetics, analgesics and sedatives, rapid, pleasant induction and recovery, good analgesic	Weak agent, unconscious state not obtainable without hypoxia.	2–3 min.
Depresses adrenals.	None	Hemorrhage and shock; cardiac insufficiency; asthma; metabolic and electrolyte disturbance; porphyria; Addison's; acidosis; hypothyroidism.	Pleasant, rapid induction and recovery, non-flammable, Rx convulsions	Cannot be reclaimed like inhalation agents; phlebitis at injection site; postop shivering-true thermal reaction; hypnotic only—no analgesia or relaxation.	2–10 min. 1st dose
	None			Both agents given together to produce effect may be combined	Rare hallucinations; no muscle relaxation.	3–6 hours duration (possible carryover to 24 hours)

Table 19.5. (Continued)

Agent	Route of Administration	Induction	Elimination	Nervous System	Respiratory System	Cardiovascular System
Fentanyl	IV	1–5 min.		somnolence; subcortical action. Indifference to pain.	Marked depression.	Not significant; mild bradycardia.
Ketamine	IV or IM	1 min.	Detoxified by liver	Profound analgesia, sensorium appears disconnected but not comatose.	Minimal depression; reflexes intact.	Blood pressure and heart rate increase.
Muscle relaxants O-tubocurarine IV (non-depolarizing) (1935)	IV	2–3 min.	Renal and biliary unchanged	None at clinical doses	Dose related paralysis of resp. muscles, increased bronchial tone due to histamine release possible	Non significant
Succinylcholine (depolarizing) (1906) (1951)	IV or IM Not reversible	1 min.	Hydrolyzed by plasma psuedo-cholinesterase	Nil	Paralysis of resp. muscles	Bradycardia extrasystoles not uncommon

Other	Muscle Relaxation	Contraindications	Advantages and Uses	Disadvantages and Complications	Emergence
			With N$_2$O and relaxants, pleasant induction and recovery, profound analgesia without cardiac and cortical depression, analgesia extends into post-op period, vascular stability. few arrhythmias, pt. can cooperate during procedure, some amnesia.	Tone of intercostal muscles— stiff chest, weak, emetic, respiratory depression.	30–60 min. cumulative duration
	Tone increases	Cerebral vascular disease or brain tumors; hypertensive disease; psychiatric disturbances; thyroid medication	For superficial (non-visceral pain) diagnostic procedures, infants and children; bronchial disease, burn Rx	Hypertension; vivid dreams during emergence; patients require *quiet* recovery room, to visceral analgesia no relaxation; spontaneous movement common.	5–10 min. duration
	Good on striated muscle	Myasthenia gravis; severe renal disease; electrolyte imbalance.	Acts by competitive inhibition of neuromuscular junction; prevents acetylcholine from reaching receptor sites. Good relaxation at light anesthesia levels; no tolerance to repeated usage; reversal possible with neostigmine diagnosis of myasthenia gravis, Rx tetany.	Histamine release possible cumulative effect, respiration must be supported, masks signs of levels of consciousness— danger of the "awake" paralyzed patient	20–60 min. duration
Increases spinal fluid and intra-ocular pressure		Family history of complications, burn cases, intra-ocular surgery.	Acts by causing a persistent depolarization at motor end plates, short-acting.	Muscle fasciculation and pain; prolonged effect due to psuedo-cholinesterase deficiency; large doses may lead to secondary non-depolarizing block, malignant hyperthermia; masks level of conciousness.	2–3 min duration

lowing reflexes are obtunded in the lower levels of this second stage. During stage three, there are four planes of anesthesia. The respiration response display can include the onset of a regular pattern of breathing to cessation of breathing altogether. During the first plane, inspiration is longer than expiration. The second plane is characterized by decreased intercostal muscle activity (thoracic respirations), and reflexes of the vocal cords and laryngospasm begin to disappear. It is in this plane that the respiratory response to skin incision disappears. Strength of intercostal muscles decreases in the third plane, and the diaphragm weakens. Abdominal respirations are separate from the intercostal respirations. Inspiration is shorter than expirations, and some patients, especially men, display only diaphragmatic respiration. At the fourth plane, intercostal muscles are paralyzed, and spontaneous respirations cease. As anesthesia deepens, respiratory activity reduces until breathing stops. Stage four of anesthesia occurs only in error. It is in this stage that respiration has ceased and circulatory failure ensues (3).

The respiratory effects of spinal and epidural blocks are much less dramatic than the effects of a generalized inhalation anesthetic. A spinal block depresses respirations centrally and peripherally. Total respiratory cessation is likely when there are gross errors in techniques and dosages. If respiratory failure occurs despite proper technique, it is likely to be due to inadequate circulation in the brain stem resulting from a severe hypotensive response (2). Characteristically, respirations during spinal and epidural anesthesia are quiet and unlabored. Most often, there will be only minimal changes in tidal volume or ventilatory function.

Blood gas tensions show minimal changes from normal values during spinal and epidural blocks. Quiet respirations are a result of involvement of the diaphragm and the fifth to ninth intercostal muscles. During high spinal anesthesia, involving the intercostal nerves, there is complete relaxation of the abdominal walls. This aids in the descent of the diaphragm and abdominal contents during inspiration.

Positioning

Surgical positioning during the intraoperative phase directly affects the respiratory systems. Specific alterations of respiratory function depend on the position used. The following outline relates respiratory effects to the position of the anesthetized patient. Nursing activities for positioning the patient are described in Table 19.6.

Supine position (dorsal recumbent)
1. Compromised respiratory function.
2. Decreased vital capacity compared with the erect position.
3. No great alteration in anterior and upward excursion of chest during inspiration.
4. Decreased diaphragmatic excursion because the contents of the abdominal viscera are now located against the upper wall of the abdomen.
5. More even distribution of ventilation from apex to base of lung.

Prone position (and modifications)
1. Respiratory system is most vulnerable in prone position.
2. Body weight against abdominal wall limits diaphragmatic movement so increased airway pressure is needed to ventilate.
3. Limits tidal volume.
4. If patient is improperly positioned, there is hypoventilation if the abdominal wall is not free to expand. The entire back will rise with inflation of the lungs, creating continual movement of the surgical field.
5. If the patient is positioned so there is unrestricted abdominal movement with respiration with support of thorax and pelvis, then compliance, tidal volume, oxygen concentration and positive end expiratory pressure will not be greatly altered.

Head elevated position
1. Unimpaired respiratory movements.
2. Downward displacement of abdominal contents, resulting in freer diaphragmatic movement.
3. Ventilation of the base of the lungs.
4. Minimal restriction of the ventral expansion of anterior chest wall.
5. Potential reduction in the diffusing capacity

of oxygen because of perfusion of upper regions of the lungs.

6. Potential ventilatory insufficiency and respiratory acidosis during use of general anesthesia and muscle relaxants. The surgeon may require presence of spontaneous respirations as indicator of brain stem function. In addition, when hyperventilation is chosen as a method to decrease intracranial pressure, spontaneous ventilatory drive is lost as PCO_2 is decreased. Therefore, hypoventilation will lead to respiratory acidosis. The use of judicious mechanical hyperventilation can be used to correct hyperventilation.

Trendelenburg's position (head down)

1. Potential for respiratory embarrassment secondary to restricted diaphragmatic movement due to impingement of viscera, increasing the potential for atelectasis.
2. Once the patient is returned to the horizontal plane, potential for aspiration pneumonia resulting from an accumulation of gastric contents in the hypopharynx.
3. Suprisingly minimal impairment of respiratory function as shown in blood gases, pH measurement, respiratory rates, and minute volume, but mechanical ventilatory assistance is encouraged.
4. Reduced vital capacity with greatest changes in elderly and obese patients.
5. Increased lateral pressure enhancing fluid transudation into alveoli. The patient may display pulmonary congestion and edema.

Lateral decubitus position

1. Compromised respiratory function due to weight of body on lower chest.
2. Restricted movement of chest.
3. Limited movement of diaphragm as a result of flexion of lower limbs toward the abdomen.
4. Difficulty in controlling aspirations of secretions from the affected lung to the unaffected lung.
5. When anesthetized patient is breathing spontaneously, the dependent lung has better ventilation at the expense of the lower lung.
   a. The lower hemidiaphragm has greater range of contractility due to the abdomi-

nal viscera pushing the diaphragm higher into the thorax and thus increasing ventilation.
   b. Both perfusion and ventilation of lower lung are increased in the spontaneously breathing patient.
6. When paralyzed patient is being artificially ventilated:
   a. The upper lung assumes greater compliance and ventilation increases due to less pressure from abdominal contents and diaphragm to be overcome and due to the vascular bed being much less distended.
   b. Tidal volume is increased (1).

Surgical Procedure

Although surgery has general effects on the respiratory system, there will also be direct effects if the surgical incision is near the diaphragm. The greatest alterations in the mechanics of respiration are seen after procedures involving the upper abdomen. The effects are substantially less after thoracic and lower abdominal procedures and minimal after peripheral procedures (4).

Functional changes include decreased tidal volume, vital capacity, and functional residual capacity. The reduced function is greatest during the first 24 to 48 hours postoperatively. Decreased vital capacity and tidal volume are often a result of splinting the respiratory muscles. Pain relief through systemic, epidural, or intercostal blocks does not allow vital capacity to increase to the preoperative state. Possible reasons for this alteration in respiratory function are distention of the bowel, residual pneumoperitoneum from the surgical procedure, and surgical trauma to the expiratory muscles.

In most nonthoracic operations, the surgery itself has no intraoperative effect on $PaCO_2$ or pH values. Minor alterations in $PaCO_2$ are usually attributed to residual anesthetic agents and preoperative narcotics. On the other hand, postoperative alterations in PaO_2 are usually significant due to alveolar collapse.

Many surgeons believe a transverse upper abdominal incision causes fewer pulmonary complications than vertical abdominal incisions. In a study by Williams and Brenavitz compar-

Table 19.6. Positioning to Enhance Respiratory Function.

Patient Problem	Nursing Activities	Monitoring and Evaluation
Supine		
Potential airway obstruction in chin-down position; head pillows can aggravate the problem, especially in the premedicated patient.	Maintain airway; position head to decrease chin-to-chest angle; do not use head pillows, especially with premedicated children.	Assess respiratory rate, rhythm, and chest expansion; respirations should be quiet and unlabored.
Difficulty with chest expansion because base of lungs is no longer in dependent position and abdominal contents push against the diaphragm; seen especially with obesity, chronic obstructive pulmonary disease, pregnancy, and abdominal distention.	Place in Trendelenburg's position or flex at waist elevation; provide more pillows prn; provide supplemental oxygen in the awake patient, respirator assisted ventilation for the unconscious patient.	Assess chest expansion; inquire about patient's comfort and respiratory status.
Prone		
Hypoventilation due to abdominal and chest wall resisting movement during inspiration of gases; surgical field may move as the upper back moves with ventilation.	Place chest rolls under thorax and pelvis so abdominal movement is unrestrained. Do not use draw sheet over chest because this creates a sling that has a binder effect on abdominal and respiratory movement.	Inspiration shall be achieved without movement of upper back.
Trendelenburg's		
Decreased vital capacity; decreased lung volume; decreased compliance; increased pulmonary blood volume; predisposition to atelectasis and hypoxemia; patients with mitral stenosis already have increased left pulmonary artery pressure and increased pulmonary blood pressure; they tolerate this position poorly; endotracheal tube can be displaced into right main stem bronchus during positioning.	Assist anesthetist with intubation and ventilation prn; assist with endotracheal positioning prn; maintain airway in awake patient; administer oxygen.	Monitor placement of endotracheal tube by breath sounds and chest movement; monitor respirations; monitor ECG for hypoxia-induced arrhythmias. Monitor arterial blood gases, central venous pressure, and pulmonary artery pressure in the severely compromised patient during extended surgery.
Head elevated		
Air embolism; symptoms are: Change in Doppler tones Alterations in heart sounds Decreased blood pressure Ventricular arrhythmias Onset of strong spontaneous ventilation Heart murmur of variable pitch	Prevent by: Assisting with Doppler positioning to amplify circulatory flow Maintaining patency and functioning of left atrial pressure monitoring line Treat by: Providing jugular decompression to prevent further entry of air Assisting with irrigation of incision to submerge, detect, and occlude entry of air into blood vessel Providing vasopressive drips prn per physician's orders to increase blood pressure Administering lidocaine prn per physician's orders to treat cardiac arrhythmias Assisting with aspiration of air via LAP line.	Monitor: Doppler LAP line ECG Respiration Blood pressure by cuff
Respiratory acid-base imbalance due to hypoventilation	Assist anesthetist to maintain mechanical hyperventilation.	Assess patient for spontaneous ventilatory drive as a result of

Table 19.6. (*Continued*)

Patient Problem	Nursing Activities	Monitoring and Evaluation
		increased PCO_2. Monitor ECG for arrhythmias; draw periodic blood gases.
Lateral decubitus		

Risks to dependent lung: flooding of tracheobronchial tree with drainage (blood, irrigant, purulence)	Assist anesthetist with insertion of bronchial blocking tubes; provide adequate suctioning at the field.	Assist anesthetist with monitoring respiratory status.
		Monitor
		  Lung sounds for fluid accumulation
		  ECG
		  Oxygenation of blood by noting blood color at surgical site

Atelectasis from hypoventilation	Assist with inserting endotracheal tube; provide adequate endotracheal suctioning; position patient so lower lung expansion is not restricted by tape or positioning devices.	Assess breath sounds after tube placement; monitor blood gases; check blood color at incision; assess chest movement for adequate expansion.

ing vertical and transverse incisions, no significant differences could be found for vital capacity, tidal volume, functional residual capacity, maximal breathing capacity, or PaO_2 (4).

Maintenance of Airway

Establishing and maintaining a patent airway usually precedes any other intraoperative activity. As anesthesia is administered and the patient approaches unconsciousness, a well-fitted face mask is applied. Tilting the head backward displaces the mandible and helps keep the airway open. Preoxygenation with 100 percent oxygen for at least two minutes helps to diminish hypoxia. The relaxed mandibular muscles and submandibular tissues allow for hyperextension of the head and the mandible, easing insertion of the endotracheal tube with a laryngoscope.

Once in place, the endotracheal tube may create the following physiological alterations:

1. Since inspired air may be inadequately conditioned, filtered, warmed, and humidified, there can be irritation to the pulmonary membrane.
2. Mucous secretion may increase.
3. There is a potential for bacterial infection.

4. Aphonia occurs because the vocal cords are bypassed.
5. Misplacing the endotracheal tube into one bronchus at the level of the carina can lead to obstruction and atelectasis of the non-ventilated lung.
6. Nasal intubation can cause specific complications: (a) epistaxis; (b) submucosal dissection; (c) dislodging a nasal polyp to the lung, causing obstruction or potential for infection (5).

PATHOLOGIES THAT AFFECT THE RESPIRATORY RESPONSES

Obesity

Obese patients are susceptible to many medical problems intraoperatively. Respiration is one that requires special attention. Many obese patients cannot comfortably maintain a dorsal recumbent position due to decreased inspiratory capacity. Functional residual capacity is decreased. When they are in the supine position, the alveolar oxygen and tension gradient are increased significantly. Decreased lung compliance is a direct result of adipose tissue surrounding the chest.

Intubation is often difficult because these patients have a limited range of motion. Ventilation following intubation may also be difficult. A hiatal hernia, common to obese patients, also complicates effective respiratory functioning if there is a significant amount of gas in the stomach.

Chronic Obstructive Pulmonary Disease (COPD)
COPD includes respiratory disorders in which air flow within the lung is obstructed. Examples are chronic bronchitis, emphysema, and asthma. Chronic bronchitis is irreversible and progressive, often preceding or accompanying pulmonary emphysema. Pathologic changes of chronic bronchitis include inflammation of the bronchial wall with hypertrophy and hyperplasia of mucous secretions, bronchial glands, and mucosal goblet cells. Cilia are lost, accompanied by scarring and distortion of the bronchiole wall. Chronic bronchitis is associated with a chronic or recurrent cough.

Asthma is a condition of recurrent labored respirations associated with recurrent obstruction of the bronchi. Bronchial obstructions are frequently caused by allergen sensitivities. Emotional crises can also cause asthmatic attacks. There is an increase in the contraction of smooth muscle and hypersecretion of mucus. The mucus is characteristically tenacious.

Emphysema is a chronic anatomical disorder occurring in patients with chronic bronchitis and asthma. Heavy smoking is the most significant cause of emphysema and COPD, with air pollution and occupational hazards also contributing. In emphysema, the alveoli and walls of the lungs are distended, thin, and deteriorated. The lungs are large, relatively bloodless, and pale, and they collapse with difficulty. Patients exhibit clubbing of the fingers.

Physical assessment of the patient with COPD reveals other symptoms such as an increased anterior-posterior diameter with restriction in the lateral motion of the rib cage. There is decreased diaphragmatic excursion, and wheezes and rhonchi are noted on inspiration and expiration. Expiration and forced expiratory time are prolonged. Cyanosis, edema, and distended neck veins are present. Hypoxia exists as a result of severe ventilation-perfusion inequalities in the lung. Respiratory centers are less sensitive to increases in carbon dioxide

tension due to the accumulation of bicarbonate in the cerebrospinal fluid. With the administration of oxygen to relieve hypoxia, further respiratory depression can ensue.

POTENTIAL COMPLICATIONS OF RESPIRATORY FUNCTION

Any situation interfering with adequate ventilation can lead to a true medical emergency and requires immediate rectification. In the operating room, any number of factors can lead to an altered response in respiratory function. Potential complications and their causes are outlined in Table 19.7.

MONITORING THE PATIENT'S RESPIRATORY RESPONSES

The operating room nurse continually assists the anesthesiologist in assessing the patient's respiratory status in the intraoperative phase. The nursing activities in Table 19.6 and 19.8 may be performed to maintain or enhance respiratory functioning.

Monitoring the Renal System

RENAL PHYSIOLOGY

The primary organs of the genitourinary system are the kidneys. Their primary functions are twofold: the elimination of the end products of protein metabolism (primarily urea), and regulation of body water and its constituents. These functions are accomplished by the formation and excretion of urine. Once the urine is formed in the kidneys it is transported through the ureters to the bladder where it is stored and eventually excreted from the body.

A cross-section of the kidney shows a darkened center known as the medulla and a pale outer portion called the cortex. It is within the cortex of each kidney that nearly 2.4 million nephrons are contained.

The nephron is the primary working component of kidneys. The three components of the nephron are: the glomerulus, which filters the blood; Bowman's capsule, which houses the

Table 19.7. *Potential Complications of Respiratory Functions.*

Potential Complications	Possible Causes
Laryngeal spasm	Any irritant to the tracheal bronchial tree can cause laryngospasm, e.g., secretions, endotracheal tubes, suctioning; the irritability threshold is decreased in smokers and COPD patients.
Improper and uncorrected placement of the endotracheal tube	Intubation into right main stem bronchus; atelectasis and hypoxia of the nonintubated lung result.
Inadequate lung expansion	Causes include: Disease process, such as emphysema, atelectasis, and pneumothorax Improper positioning in the lateral and prone positions, decreasing expansion of the lungs
Obstructed ventilation	Causes are secretions, foreign bodies, cuff inflated over endotracheal tube, tumor, or existing pathology.
Respiratory depression	Preoperative medications (especially narcotic analgesics) may have this effect.
Difficulty with intubation or failure to accomplish intubation	Causes may include spinal fusion; tumor; facial fracture limiting mandibular movement, usually in conjunction with facial fracture or oral surgery; nasal intubation; arthritis of the cervical vertebrae or temporal mandibular joint; and stenosis due to pathology, congenital anomaly, or radiation therapy.
Aspiration leading to Mendelson's syndrome (pulmonary edema and bronchospasm)	Contributing factors are: Accumulation of oral secretions or blood in the oral pharynx Regurgitation during anesthesia, which may be more likely if the patient is in Trendelenburg's position or prone or if on ventilatory assistance Predisposing conditions, including obesity, hiatal hernia, abdominal distention, pregnancy, and esophageal stenosis or tumor Patient who has eaten recently Patient with potentially full stomach due to delayed gastric activity from trauma, obstruction, or recent myocardial infarction

glomerulus and channels the fluid to the renal tubule, the third component.

The blood to be filtered by the capillaries within the glomerulus enters through the afferent arteriole and leaves through the efferent arteriole. The thin walls of the arterioles of the glomerulus filter the blood to allow a protein-free plasma to pass into Bowman's capsule. This passive filtering process occurs as a result of fluid diffusing under pressure through the capillaries into Bowman's capsule.

The rate of flow from these capillaries, termed the glomerulus filtration rate, is ultimately dependent upon the blood pressure and circulating blood volume. Although nearly 1,200 ml of blood will be filtered through the kidneys in a minute, only 125 ml of glomerular filtrate will leave the glomerulus and enter Bowman's capsule.

Obviously 125 ml/minute cannot be converted into urine and excreted by the bladder without dehydrating the circulatory system. A significant amount of this plasma is reabsorbed within the renal tubules. These are subdivided into three sections: the proximal tubule, the loop of Henle, and the distal tubule. Of the 125 ml of plasma that leaves the glomerulus, approximately 1 ml of plasma will eventually be excreted as urine. The three sections of the tubules reabsorb different substances within the plasma filtrate. Among the components of the end products of metabolism that may be filtered from the nephron include urea, creatinine, uric acid, urates, and sodium, potassium, chloride, and hydrogen ions.

Reabsorbtion rates can be significantly altered by the physiological status of the body. Hormones can greatly change excretion and reabsorbtion of fluids within the nephron. If body fluid levels are low, or if blood flow to the kidney is diminished, antidiuretic hormone (ADH) is excreted to stimulate reabsorbtion within the distal tubule. The result is a lesser but more concentrated amount of urine.

Table 19.8. Intraoperative Monitoring.

Nursing Activities	Rationale
Preoperative (prior to induction) Assess respiratory status and maintain respiratory function. Maintain patent airway. Provide O$_2$ for transport if indicated. Keep patient's head up.	Preoperative medication depresses respiratory function. Transporting patients, with pillows, can obstruct the airway due to chin-down position, especially pediatric patients. Supplemental oxygen may be needed for existing pathology, especially heart disease and lung disease.
Intraoperative Maintain airway in awake patient. Provide supplemental O$_2$ via nasal cannula. Keep head elevated when possible and prevent chin from dropping down. Remind patient to deep breathe. Assist the anesthetist with establishing and maintaining an airway. Observe patient's respiratory response during induction for rate; depth; rhythm; coloration of tissues, especially the mucosa; and cardiac rate and rhythm in response to tissue perfusion.	Respirations are depressed due to medications or shock. Obstructions due to positioning impair respiratory functions (eg, chin-down, tongue relaxed). Apnea occurs from decreased respiratory drive from oxygen administration. Respiratory rate, character, and function are altered during induction of anesthesia.
Assist the anesthetist with endotracheal intubation. For oral-tracheal intubation: Assist with visualization of the cords by retracting the cheek and applying pressure prn. Prevent aspiration of stomach contents during induction or extubation, especially in high-risk patients. Position patient for greatest ease of intubation, minimizing risk of regurgitation and aspiration. Tilting head up reduces chance of passive regurgitation but makes aspiration inevitable if regurgitation occurs. Intubation is more difficult. Head is tilted down if regurgitation occurs. Emesis will flow out of mouth. Potential for passive regurgitation is increased. Lateral position with head tilted down provides greatest protection of airway from aspiration, especially after extubation. Increases difficulty of intubation. Apply cricoid pressure, palpate cricoid with thumb and second finger. When patient is unconscious apply firm pressure. *Maintain this pressure until tube is in place and cuff is inflated.* If vomiting occurs, release pressure to prevent esophageal rupture. Provide suctioning.	Skinfolds, adipose tissue, and mustache hairs can obstruct cord visualization. Cricoid pressure allows the cords to be more easily seen. Aspiration of stomach contents into the lungs causes aspiration pneumonitis and Mendelson's syndrome. Gastric contents with a pH lower than 2.5 cause chemical burn to the tracheobronchial tree, producing bronchospasm and exudation and increasing lung fluid. Exudation in turn causes a ventilation perfusion problem and fluid shift, leading to hypoxia, trachycardia, and hypotension. This is followed by infiltration of polymorphs and phagocytes, destroying normal lung tissue. Morbidity and mortality are greatest when gastric contents have a pH below 2.5. This occludes esophagus and prevents aspiration of stomach contents into lungs. This is done to evacuate secretions, blood, and emesis from oral, pharyngeal, and tracheal passages.
Assist the anesthetist with awake nasal intubation. Determine patient's history of hypertension, blood dyscrasias, anticoagulation therapy, and nasal septal deformity. Provide emotional support. Restrain patient, especially upper extremities. Assist anesthetist with topical nasal anesthetic. Assist anesthetist with intubation.	These patients have an increased incidence of severe nasal bleeding after nasal intubation. Nasal intubation for awake patients is emotionally and physically traumatic. It stimulates coughing and sneezing reflexes, and the patient may resist intubation efforts.

Secretion at the tubular level can also involve substances not related to reabsorbtion. The most outstanding is the hydrogen ion that is abundant in the body during the acidotic state. The proximal tubules will secrete hydrogen ions from the blood in a compensatory effort to eliminate acids from the blood. Initially, however, the respiratory system responds more quickly in an attempt to establish homeostasis of the pH within the blood, but over an extended period of time, the kidneys are more effective in the elimination of the hydrogen ions.

Another hormone significant in the regulation of kidney function is aldosterone. Aldosterone affects sodium reabsorbtion from the filtered plasma within the renal tubules. For example, sodium will be reabsorbed during states of dehydration due to perspiration and salt loss.

Once the urine is formed in the nephron, the collecting tubules will carry urine from several nephrons that will eventually flow from the cortex into the medulla, forming the renal pelvis—an extension of the ureter.

There are two ureters, one per kidney. These tubes carry urine from the kidney to the posterior wall of the bladder.

PHYSIOLOGICAL RESPONSES TO SURGERY

Surgery alters renal function in all patients, whether they have an existing renal problem or not. In this section, we discuss the effects of surgery on patients with and without prior renal insufficiency, suggest factors for the nurse to assess preoperatively, and describe renal monitoring during the procedure.

Patients without existing renal insufficiency will nevertheless have changes in their renal functioning caused by surgery. Most patients will be underhydrated because they have been NPO for at least 8 hours before surgery, and intravenous fluid replacement may have been inadequate. The fluid deficit will be even more severe in patients who have had vomiting, diarrhea, and nasogastric suctioning. Appendectomy patients, especially children, are likely to be dehydrated because they may have had nausea, vomiting, and diarrhea for 24 hours or more. Because they have lost the ability to concentrate the urine, elderly patients may come to the operating room with a fluid and electrolyte imbalance (see Chapter 10).

During surgery, hypotension from blood loss affects renal function. Deprived of blood flow, the kidneys will not receive sufficient nutrients, and the blood will not be filtered adequately. Wastes will accumulate in the bloodstream, as they will in the kidneys themselves, since the circulation may not be adequate to filter their blood supply. The buildup of wastes engenders a systemic response.

Certain agents administered during surgery may have a toxic effect on the kidneys, causing intratubular precipitation and possibly acute renal failure. Contrast media, such as agents used for cholangiograms and arteriograms, can have this effect. Diabetic patients are especially at risk for contrast dye reactions. Diuretics cause sodium loss and can result in acute tubular necrosis. Mannitol, for example, causes rapid sodium concentration and excretion.

Drugs the patient is already taking or those given intraoperatively may cause a hypersensitive reaction that may result in acute renal failure. For example, phenytoin (Dilantin) can cause a kidney inflammation.

Urinary tract infections may either arise or be aggravated during surgery. Existing urinary infections must be controlled before patients are brought to surgery. If they are not caught, they may be spread to other parts of the body during the operation. During surgery, infections may be brought on by surgical manipulation of the urethra, cystoscopy, or insertion of a Foley catheter.

Patients with known kidney disease need special precautions before surgery. Underlying renal impairment can be expected in patients with hypertension, diabetes, and heart disease. Care must be taken not to overload these patients with fluids or create an electrolyte imbalance, metabolic acidosis, or hyperkalemia. The anesthetist will avoid using anesthetic agents and preoperative medications that are excreted by the kidneys, since these can aggravate the situation.

PREOPERATIVE NURSING ASSESSMENT

During the preoperative interview, the nurse should consider the following points in assessing the possible effects of the surgical procedure on the patient's renal system:

1. From the patient's chart, the nurse notes:
   a. Serum creatinine level
   b. Results of urine culture
   c. Daily weights
   d. Input and output
   e. Central venous pressure
   f. Sodium and potassium serum levels
   g. Electrocardiograph reading

2. Does the patient have known renal disease? The presenting symptoms are protein in the urine, edema, increased BUN (blood urea nitrogen) and creatinine levels, hypertension, and abnormal electrolyte levels.

3. Other symptoms of an acute or chronic renal condition are small kidneys from atrophy or a congenital problem; a history of kidney transplant, nephrectomy, or end-stage renal disease; uremic symptoms or anemia; chronic renal disease; suppressed red blood cell formation; and hemolyzing of red blood cells in the glomerulus.

4. Ask the patient about the nature of the renal lesion. Is it a glomerular lesion? a vascular lesion? a tubular problem? This may indicate whether she will receive medical or surgical treatment.

5. Determine the level of renal function from 24-hour creatinine tests, which measure the glomerular filtration rate.

6. From the nature of the patient's problem and the type of surgery, the nurse may be able to determine the likelihood of the patient's need for further treatment such as dialysis. For example, if the patient has been in surgery many hours without output, she may need to be dialyzed.

MONITORING RENAL FUNCTION

Urinary output provides a method of assessing not only renal function during surgery, but also cardiovascular function, tissue perfusion, and hydration of the body. Inserting an indwelling Foley catheter prior to or at the time of surgery is a common and simple method of obtaining data for renal assessment. With the catheter, urine output can be measured hourly, and as the value approaches 40–60 ml/hour, tissue perfusion and fluid replacement can be assumed adequate. A normal kidney excretes excess fluid volume to restore fluid and electrolyte balance.

A Foley catheter should always be inserted in patients who will have long surgeries with anticipated fluid volume replacement or transfusion of blood components. If the surgery is extended for any reason, assess the patient for bladder distention. If the bladder is distended, a Foley catheter should be inserted to prevent bladder rupture or reflux into the renal pelvis. Ureteral catheters provide anatomical landmarks during abdominal surgery. This can be invaluable when previous surgical scars or intraperitoneal adhesions prevent adequate visualization of the ureters. The ureteral catheters help the surgeon to avoid inadvertent ligation or incision of the ureters.

Ureteral catheters also provide for direct measurement of urinary output and renal function of individual kidneys. This is especially helpful in patients with impaired renal function or only one kidney.

Infection is always a risk with ureteral or urethral catheters, and the surgeon may decide that the risk outweighs the benefits of direct measurement from a ureteral catheter. Or prophylactic antibiotics may be administered before and during surgery, especially when there has been a traumatic catheterization. Mefoxin is currently the antibiotic of choice to combat bacteria introduced into the bloodstream via a venous sinus traumatized during catheterization.

Nurses on the patient's unit should have assessed and recorded the urinary output at least hourly and documented the results on a flow sheet.

The urine's color indicates several variations in renal physiological response. Some pharmacologic agents such as vitamins can tint the urine orange. Some foods such as asparagus cloud the urine or alter the odor. These signs should not be confused with the symptoms of urinary tract infection. Observations are validated by noting the results of urine analysis.

Blood in the urine is always significant, and the nurse should notify the surgeon and anesthesiologist when this happens during the procedure. During massive transfusion and cardiopulmonary bypass, for example, hemolysis occurs, leading to the excretion of blood components in the urine. Perforation of the bladder or ureters during peritoneal and suprapubic surgery can cause blood components to appear in the urine. It is important to note the color and rate of the blood appearing in the urine. Is there frank bleeding? Is the urine slightly pink? Are there clots? Is the color dark brown? As part of intraoperative monitoring, the nurse checks for accurate labeling of collection receptacles.

As with all body systems, renal physiological responses should be continuously monitored. From her preoperative assessment and intraoperative observations, the nurse can provide crucial information to the surgeon and other team members.

Monitoring Other Body Systems

GASTROINTESTINAL SYSTEM MONITORING

The digestive tract or alimentary canal is a hollow muscular tube that extends from the mouth to the anus. It includes the mouth, pharynx, esophagus, stomach, small intestine, large intestine, colon, rectum, and anus. The principal function is the provision of the body with fluids, nutrients, and electrolytes. The secondary function of the tract is to dispose of the waste residues from the digestive process. Only the wastes of the digestive system are eliminated from it; wastes of body metabolism are excreted by other routes. The digestive tract secretes electrolytes and enzymes, which it uses to break down the raw materials ingested. It then moves the ingested products at the appropriate rate to ensure complete digestion of the food and absorption of the end products into the bloodstream.

Preoperatively, the surgical patient is ordered to take nothing by mouth to allow any food or fluid in the digestive tract to move through. In most abdominal procedures affecting the gastrointestinal tract, a nasogastric tube is inserted prior to the procedure to prevent aspiration. Until clear fluid remains, enemas are ordered to evacuate the bowel. This makes the inside lumen of the bowel clear and as bacteria-free as possible.

Preoperative teaching is aimed at preparing the patient to do postoperative exercises, deep breathing, and ambulation as soon as possible to avert potential complications by returning the gastric system to normal functioning. Responses of the digestive system during surgery depend on the method of anesthesia, type of surgical procedure, preoperative medications, and existing pathology. Nausea and vomiting, responses by the awake patient, may be caused by hypertension during spinal anesthesia; hypoxia secondary to respiratory inadequacy; anxiety and tension; administration of narcotics, especially morphine and meperidine hydrochloride (Demerol); parasympathetic overactivity during spinal anesthesia with subsequent vagal stimulation; and surgical manipulation of the gastrointestinal tract. Biliary colic can occur in the awake patient as a result of morphine administration.

The nurse's responsibility during surgery is to measure and assess output from the nasogastric tube. Contents should be assessed for amount, color, and presence of frank bleeding or coffee-ground emesis. Because electrolyte imbalance can occur secondary to nasogastric suctioning, serum electrolytes should be routinely evaluated (see Chapter 10). Gastric distention can impede surgical exposure during intraabdominal procedures. Delayed gastric emptying, paralytic ileus, obstruction for any reason, and lack of adequate anesthetic relaxation can contribute to distention.

Paralytic ileus, a postoperative complication, is caused by a lack of peristaltic activity. Caused by a reflex paralysis, it occurs following abdominal surgery. During the operative procedure, the bowel may be handled extensively, causing it to cease functioning for a period of time. Usually paralytic ileus is treated postoperatively by aspirating gastric secretions via the nasogastric tube until the bowel begins to function. In more severe cases of obstruction, surgical treatment may be necessary.

During surgery, rectal tube insertion may be required to aid in evacuation of lower gastrointestinal contents. This may occur on some types of colon surgery, hemorrhoidectomy, or sigmoidoscopy, or in some instances, presurgical cleansing of the colon was inadequate.

ENDOCRINE SYSTEM MONITORING

The endocrine system is responsible for generalized and long-lasting control and communication of body states. The system is composed of the eight endocrine glands: the islet of Langerhans in the pancreas, the gonads, adrenal, hypophysis or pituitary, thyroid, parathyroid, thymus, and pineal. All the endocrine glands have unique and independent functions, but they are also interdependent. For example, the release of hormones from one gland influences the release from another.

The term *hormone* means "to set in motion." The glands secrete hormones that govern many aspects of our lives. For example, the pituitary gland secretes thyrotropic (thyroid-stimulating) hormone (TSH), which stimulates the thyroid gland. The pituitary also secretes somatotropic hormone (STH) and gonadotropic hormones (LH, FSH, and LTH). STH stimulates growth, while gonadotropin affects maturity and functioning of primary and secondary sex organs. The thyroid gland secretes hormones that stimulate metabolism and lower plasma calcium and phosphates. The parathyroid's secretions affect calcium and phosphorus metabolism. The adrenal gland secretes hormones that affect ability to deal with stress and govern certain secondary sex characteristics. The islet of Langerhans secretes insulin, which promotes the metabolism of carbohydrates. The thymus, situated in the mediastinal cavity, reaches full development in early childhood. Its function is unknown. The function of the pineal gland, which is in the brain, is also unknown.

The endocrine system is a complex network affecting physiological responses. Surgery is often required to remove pathologic endocrine glands. Types of surgical procedures are thyroidectomy, parathyroid gland resection, unilateral and bilateral adrenalectomy, and hypophysectomy. During such procedures, specific monitoring activities should be employed to anticipate altered physiological responses. Guidelines for monitoring responses specific to the endocrine system are given in Table 19.9.

One example of an endocrine disorder is diabetes in which the diabetic has a high propensity for infection. The surgical wound takes longer to heal because of the slow regeneration of the vascular system, and the skin is more likely to break down. In addition, the patient with diabetes has the usual treatment regimen interrupted because diet is temporarily changed and insulin dosage readjusted.

The preoperative goal is to regulate the patient's diabetes before taking her to the operating room, so these patients may have to be in the hospital several days prior to their surgery. If the patient requires emergency surgery, she will need constant monitoring of vital signs, frequent laboratory studies, and vigilant nursing observation.

For nonemergent cases, the typical preoperative preparation includes no food, water, or insulin by mouth. Usually, the surgery is scheduled in the early morning. A blood sugar test is taken and reported to the surgeon within one hour before the surgery. The blood sugar level assists the anesthesiologist in determining the type of intravenous fluid to start prior to induction. While the patient is in surgery, monitoring depends on the severity of the diabetes. The mild diabetic may not need glucose until immediately postoperatively in the recovery room. The moderate or severe diabetic will require an intravenous infusion of glucose and possibly the addition of insulin during the surgical procedure.

Nursing activities include constant monitoring of the patient's positioning and pressure areas to prevent any skin breakdown. It also involves ECG monitoring and taking vital signs. If blood sugars are taken intraoperatively, the nurse will assist in obtaining the specimens. Accurate intake and output of fluid should be recorded. Postoperatively, the goal is to stabilize the patient's condition, reestablish control of the diabetes, and prevent any possibility of infection.

In summary, the endocrine system plays a major role in the patient's response to surgery, whether a gland is being surgically removed or a body system is being operated on that affects the functioning of the endocrine system.

Patients who have endocrine disorders have many problems. Surgical intervention is only one method of treatment and then only for pathology in certain glands. Many patients who have endocrine disorders also have surgery on other body systems such as musculoskeletal, gastrointestinal, and cardiovascular. A complete review of postoperative complications must be undertaken.

INTEGUMENTARY SYSTEM MONITORING

The integumentary system, or skin, which covers the entire external area of the body, is considered an organ. The skin can be divided into two distinct layers, the epidermis and the dermis (or corium). The epidermis is the outer layer composed of epithelial tissues that are continuously replaced. Melanin, black or dark brown pigment, is found in this layer. The deeper layer, or dermis, is composed of fibrous connective tissues. Within the dermis layers are nerve endings, sweat glands, and hair follicle roots. The circulation of blood flow to the skin is greatest in this layer.

The skin has four major functions: sensation, protection from the environment, temperature regulation, and excretion. The operating room nurse can directly or indirectly monitor physiological responses through changes in the integumentary system. Physiology of the skin is discussed more thoroughly in Chapter 12.

Sensation
Alert patients are sensitive to heat, pressure, pain, and touch. Patients alert the nurse to stimuli that are causing skin sensations through verbal and nonverbal cues. Whenever possible, it is desirable to ascertain what is comfortable for a patient prior to induction of anesthesia because this can indicate potential pressure points during surgery. Because sensation is diminished during anesthesia, a thorough nursing preoperative assessment of the patient's integumentary and skeletal muscle status should be done (see Chapter 22).

Protection
The skin protects body structures from harmful chemical agents and mechanical injury. The skin also prevents excessive loss of fluids and electrolytes.

Foreign substances that endanger the integrity of the skin can lead to complications, such as infection, fluid and electrolyte loss, pain, and death. Skin preparation solutions used in the operating room can protect or injure the skin. If the patient is hypersensitive to solutions, tissue reaction and breakdown can occur. Alternative solutions must be employed to avoid potential problems. Povidone-iodine solutions can be irritating to sensitive skin, the eye, and conjunctiva. Alcohol solutions are irritating to mucous membranes. Debilitated patients, such as the elderly, dehydrated patients, and chronic renal failure patients, need additional protection from solutions, pressure, and excessive manipulation. Burn patients lose protection from invasion by bacteria and mechanical and chemical elements, and they lack a means to control fluid and electrolyte loss. Special intervention is required.

Temperature Regulation
The skin is directly responsible for eliminating or conserving heat. As the body temperature increases, blood vessels in the skin dilate to allow more blood to circulate superficially, resulting in heat loss. In contrast, when the body temperature is decreased, blood vessels constrict to decrease the exposure of blood to the surface. This, in turn, conserves heat. Evaporation of sweat from the skin surfaces also causes body heat loss.

Heat loss or heat production directly affects the patient's physiological responses to surgery. The metabolic oxygen need is increased or

Table 19.9. Guidelines for Monitoring Responses Specific to the Endocrine System

Procedure/Pathology	General Considerations	Nursing Activities
Parathyroidectomy	Hypercalcemia Kidney stone formations with impaired renal ECG abnormalities Hypovolemia secondary to nausea, vomiting, polyuria, anorexia.	Continuously monitor ECG and vital signs. In severe hypovolemia invasive pressure monitoring such as CVP or arterial lines may be necessary. Monitor intake and output. Renal function should be continuously assessed. If pneumothorax results from mediastinal exploration, a chest x-ray will be required as well as chest tubes, instruments and suction equipment.
Pheochromocytoma-tumor of chromaffin cells of sympathoadrenal system (predominately adrenal medulla)	Excessive secretion of epinephrine and norepinephrine Severe hypertension Ventricular arrhythmias Alpha-blocking drugs, such as phentolamine (Regitine), given preoperatively Beta blockers given for arrhythmias Hypovolemia Nipride infusion for hypertension	Invasive hemodynamic pressure monitoring Continuous ECG monitoring to identify and treat arrhythmias. Monitor arterial blood gases Assess and maintain renal function
Adrenalectomy/Adrenal cortical tumors, metastatic breast tumors, various pathologic states affecting adrenal functioning	Hyperaldosteronism with conservation of sodium and hyperexcretion of sodium via the kidneys. Hypokalemia Muscle weakness, tetany ECG abnormalities and ventricular arrhythmias Hypervolemia from increased sodium conservation Hypertension with ensuing cardiovascular complications, i.e., cardiomegaly, congestive heart failure, stroke and renal dysfunction.	Continuous invasive hemodynamic pressure monitoring Monitoring serum electrolytes Monitoring arterial blood gases Assess and maintain renal function
Thyroidectomy	Retrosternal goiter can compress trachea and alter trachea and alter respiratory function. Tracheal deviation may present intubation difficulties. Awake intubation or tracheostomy may be the method of choice. Bilateral recurrent laryngeal nerve dissection can necessitate a tracheostomy.	If tracheostomy necessary, have instrumentation and tracheostomy tubes accessible. Assist anesthesia with intubation. See Table 19.8.
Hyperthyroidism (Thyrotoxicosis)	Severe alterations of circulatory and metabolic functioning are often present. Uncontrolled, the condition can lead to a thyroid storm. Circulatory Responses: 1. Tachycardia, atrial fibrillation, ventricular irritability 2. Cardiomegaly, increased systolic blood pressure, congestive heart failure Metabolic Responses: 1. Increased temperature 2. Increased metabolic rate 3. Increased oxygen consumption 4. Weight loss	Comprehensive cardiovascular monitoring of the patient. 1. Electrocardiograph (ECG) 2. Central venous pressure (CVP) 3. Arterial line for hemodynamic monitoring 4. Temperature 5. Respiration Continuously assess physiological limits. Use small endotracheal tubes when patient awake for intubation. If tracheostomy is necessary, have instruments and tracheostomy tubes accessible.

Table 19.9. (Continued)

Procedure/Pathology	General Considerations	Nursing Activities

	5. Vomiting
	6. Diarrhea
	Neurologic Responses:
	  1. Anxiety
	  2. Agitation
	  3. Nervousness
	Ophthalmologic Changes:
	  1. Exophthalmos
	Respiratory Changes:
	  1. Hyperventilation
	  2. Potential for respiratory obstruction
	    due to glandular enlargement.	

decreased by 13 percent for every 1°C lost or gained. In the pediatric patient or the patient with compromised cardiopulmonary function, heat loss leads directly to morbidity and mortality. The postoperative patient with a body temperature of 36°C or less can tolerate a brief period of hypothermia with little clinical risk. But untreated hypothermia and shivering are hazardous.

Shivering induced by heat loss or by certain inhalation anesthetics increases tissue oxygen demand by 400–500 percent. Minute ventilation is increased, and cardiac output must also increase to maintain aerobic metabolism. If cardiopulmonary compensation is inadequate to meet the increased demand, aerobic cellular metabolism occurs, resulting in metabolic acidosis. Vital organs, including the brain and heart, may suffer tissue ischemia. The shivering patient with intrinsic cardiopulmonary disease may go into respiratory and cardiac arrest.

Maintenance of body temperature preoperatively and intraoperatively is the key to preventing postoperative hypothermia. A significant amount of heat is lost preoperatively due to transport to the OR, preoperative medications causing vasodilation, and induction of anesthesia, causing further vasodilation. Low ambient operating room temperatures often contribute to heat loss.

Nursing activities to prevent heat loss perioperatively include:

- Provide warm thermal blankets prior to induction of anesthesia.

- Use warm prepping solutions and irrigations.
- Administer warmed intravenous fluids in the high-risk patient.
- Administer only warmed blood.
- Use aquathermia heating pads on high-risk patients and during surgeries with significant surface exposure and fluid loss.
- Use portable heat lamps as needed.
- Keep overhead lights on the patient when possible.
- Only expose surface tissues when necessary for surgery.
- Cover infants' heads with stockinette caps since much heat is lost from the head surface.
- After dressings are applied, provide additional warmed blankets.

Whenever possible, administer oxygen and gases that are heated and humidified. Then the body will not have to expend energy to warm and humidify the inspired gases.

Assessment of the integumentary system provides information about:

- Hyperthermia: Patient is flushed, skin is warm and diaphoretic.
- Hypothermia: Skin is pale, mottled, and cold to touch; moderate cyanosis.
- Hypertension: Skin is flushed.
- Hypotension: Respiratory disturbance, cyanosis, or pallor.
- Biliary obstruction: Jaundiced (yellow) skin.

The surgical patient's skin can be monitored in a variety of ways intraoperatively, and for all patients having anesthesia it should be monitored immediately postoperatively. An esophageal thermometer is an accurate monitoring mechanism. The thermometer should be positioned in the lower mediastinum below the pulmonary veins between the heart and the descending portion of the aorta. These temperatures will represent core temperatures or temperatures of the central circulation.

Tympanic membrane probes are a very accurate means of recording temperature of blood flowing to the brain. These temperatures are significant because they parallel core temperatures and also reflect sudden temperature changes. Tympanic perforation is always a risk, and tympanic membrane temperature monitoring should never be used in patients with intrinsic tympanic disease or previous ear surgery.

Rectal temperature monitoring is less accurate because it reflects only peripheral body temperatures. It does not measure core temperature consistently because the probes are positioned far from the body core temperatures and the thermoregulating centers in the brain.

Topical noninvasive temperature devices also do not truly reflect thermal core temperatures. They are useful in reflecting patterns of temperature. Measurement of skin temperature is actually much less than core temperatures.

Excretion

The skin has a minor excretory function. Approximately 4–8 gm of carbon dioxide are excreted per day by this organ. During the intraoperative period the nurse must recognize that because of other physiological responses to the anesthesia and surgical procedure, the loss of wastes through the skin may increase (see Chapter 10).

Observation of the skin color, texture, and dryness is an ongoing assessment activity performed intraoperatively. The color of the patient's nails should also be evaluated throughout the procedure. Based on the preoperative baseline assessment, the perioperative nurse will be able to detect changes occurring during the operative period such as reddened areas, rashes, burns, excoriations, cyanosis, and temperature changes. Continuously monitoring of the integumentary system allows the nurse to be aware of the physiological responses to surgery and enables her to implement appropriate actions.

MUSCULOSKELETAL SYSTEM MONITORING

The musculoskeletal system includes bones, joints, muscles, and related connective tissue. The skeletal system serves as a protection to vital organs and soft tissues. It supports and provides a framework for the entire body. Red blood cells are manufactured in the bone marrow, and the bone is a storage area for mineral salts such as calcium and phosphorus.

The muscular system makes up to 40–50 percent of the body's weight. There are three types of muscle: cardiac, smooth, and striated. The involuntary cardiac muscle is found only in the heart, whereas the smooth muscle, which is also involuntary, is found in hollow structures such as the digestive tract, blood vessels, and the urinary bladder. These are controlled by the autonomic nervous system. Striated muscle is voluntary and is a combination of muscle and connective tissue. These muscles are almost always attached to bones.

Striated muscle gives the human body its shape and holds it in its distinctive upright position. Through an intricate relationship with the nervous system, muscle cells convert chemical energy into the mechanical effort needed to propel the body forward and perform both fine and gross motor movements.

Elongated myofibrils are the basic muscle cells, arranged in bundles. Longitudinal sections of the myofibrils, called sarcomeres, are the basic unit of contraction. Sarcomeres are made up of the proteins actin and myosin, which are believed to cause contractions through their interactions.

Muscle contraction stems from a finely tuned relationship between muscle cells and motor nerve axons. Axons may serve one or many muscle fibers, determining how fine or how large the movements will be. For example, in a finger, one axon may be connected to one muscle fiber, whereas in a leg muscle, one axon may serve many fibers. The connection between the axon and muscle fiber on the cell membrane is the myoneural junction.

Contraction is a result of electrical and chemical events transpiring at this junction. An electrical impulse sent from the brain along the nerve to the myoneural junction releases acetylcholine. This substance causes depolarization of the cell membrane and a chemical reaction leading to contraction.

Energy for muscle contraction is provided by the breakdown of adenosine triphosphate (ATP) into adenosine diphosphate (ADP) and free phosphate ions. To replenish the rapidly utilized ATP, creatine phosphate and ADP are converted to creatine and ATP by the enzyme phosphokinase.

Intraoperative monitoring of the musculoskeletal system includes activities associated with positioning and the patient and anesthesia. In Chapter 22, positioning and its effects on the musculoskeletal system are reviewed. During the operative procedure, the nurse must continue to ascertain that the patient's body is in physiological alignment and that there is no undue pressure being exerted on the patient by members of the team, equipment, and draping materials. Anesthesia and its effects on the musculoskeletal system are discussed in Chapter 11.

Malignant hyperthermia (MH), a complication affecting the skeletal muscle, is not a common crisis, but it can be averted. MH is an often fatal hypermetabolic syndrome induced by certain exhalation agents and depolarizing skeletal muscle relaxants. This pharmacogenic disease is one of the most common causes of anesthetic-induced deaths in America. It is estimated that 1 per 10,000 to 1 per 15,000 persons in a normal hospital population are affected.

Triggering agents in susceptible individuals are halothane, succinylcholine, and to a lesser extent ether, ethrane, some local anesthetics, curare, and pavulon. The primary site affected by these agents is for the most part unknown, but the disease is postulated to be myogenic, neurogenic, and endocrinogenic, with a general derangement of cell membrane structure and function. Malignant hyperthermia is therefore multifocal in etiology.

MH is an inherited disease with 50 percent or more of the offspring affected. Although it is not specific to gender, according to some reports, more men than women are affected. Pediatric patients appear to be more susceptible but patients affected by MH have been reported from age 18 months to 78 years. Malignant hyperthermia has been documented throughout the United States, with the Midwest having a greater incidence. MH does not necessarily occur with the first or initial exposure to the triggering agents. Initial onset has been recorded after the 14th anesthetic. Most alarming is that, if not treated with dantrolene sodium (Dantrium), there is a 57–70 percent fatality rate.

Essentially, malignant hyperthermia occurs when susceptible muscle, exposed to certain triggering agents, becomes unable to control levels of intramyoplasmic calcium released from the sarcoplasmic reticulum. The result is an increased and sustained level of ionized calcium in the myoplasm of the skeletal muscle.

The onset of symptoms is a cascade of events, and it is difficult to differentiate primary from secondary symptoms. Signs are a result of the response to increased myoplasmic calcium and sustained muscle contractions. Skeletal muscle oxygen consumption and temperature rise with an eventual increase in body oxygen consumption and temperature. Heat is the byproduct of metabolism, chemical reactions, and friction from the activity of the muscle cells abutting each other. This warms the local extracellular fluid, which in turn warms the blood. There is a central venous desaturation, and central venous and arterial hypercarbia. Metabolic acidosis is a result of increased lactic acid production, whereas respiratory acidosis is a result of increased production of carbon dioxide and the inability of the lungs to exhaust the elevated levels. Increased levels of potassium, myoglobin, and creatine phosphokinase (CPK) circulate in the bloodstream as a result of membrane dysfunction. The hyperkalemia aggravates underlying respiratory and metabolic acidosis, and most important, increases cardiac irritability. Myoglobinuria will result in acute renal failure. Later signs include pulmonary edema, muscle edema, coma, paralysis, coagulation defects, disseminated intravascular coagulation, left heart failure, and peripheral limb ischemia resulting in gangrene.

Often, the initial symptom will be muscle rigidity, especially of jaw masseter muscles with the injection of succinylcholine, evolving to generalized muscle fasciculations. It is important to recognize these as symptoms and not a result of undermedication, because 90 percent of patients who display muscle rigidity to succinylcholine have malignant hyperthermia. The onset of symptoms can be multifocal. There is sudden unexplained inappropriate tachycardia with tachypnea and spontaneous ventilation despite the anesthetist's attempts to control ventilation. The blood pressure is unstable. Arrhythmias, usually ventricular and multifocal, are a result of sympathetic hyperactivity, an increase in serum potassium, or both. There is dark blood on the surgical field despite adequate inspired oxygen. The skin shows cyanotic mottling and profuse sweating. There is an initial slow then rapid rise in temperature, sustained as high as 108°F (42.7°C) or more.

Patients susceptible to MH can at times be identified in a preoperative assessment. These individuals have a high incidence of muscle abnormalities including ptosis, kyphoscoliosis, squinting, winged scapula, pectus excavation, large soft muscle masses, and hypermobility of joints such as fingers and hips. They display muscle rigidity during crisis and may have a family history of sudden death during or after anesthesia.

Either before or after the crisis, diagnosis is confirmed by muscle biopsy, usually from the inner thigh. The muscle is exposed to caffein and halogenated agents. In those susceptible to malignant hyperthermia, tissue will display microscope hypercontractibility, and diagnosis will be confirmed.

Some general comments about the malignant hyperthermia crisis when it occurs in the operating room are important.

1. Malignant hyperthermia is one of the crisis situations that may occur in the operating room. Prompt recognition and intervention are critical to clinical success.

2. Malignant hyperthermia can develop as late as 24 hours after surgery. Incidence is 1 in every 14,000 operations. Mortality is 60 percent.
3. Certain drugs, such as succinylcholine (Anectine), curare, pancuronium (Pavulon), and halothane are recognized as capable of precipitating MH in susceptible individuals.
4. There are a variety of theories for the etiology and pathophysiology of MH. Stress and undisclosed anxiety may play a significant role.
5. Preparation of presurgical dantrolene sodium administration for susceptible individuals: adult—100 mg four times daily for three days; children—2.2 mg/kg of body weight in divided doses per day.
6. Dantrolene sodium preparation: reconstitute with sterile water; shake until solution is clear. Available in 20-mg vials; 36 vials cost $960; shelf life is 24 months (1981).

Medications used for reversing the crisis include:

- Chlorpromazine 25 mg
- Dantrolene sodium 20-mg vials
- Furosemide (Lasix) 40 mg
- Glucose 50 percent (Bristoject)
- Heparin 10 ml
- Insulin regular 50 units/ml
- KC1 40 mEq
- Mannitol 500 ml 20 percent
- Methylprednisolone (Solu-Medrol) 1 gm
- Sodium bicarbonate 5 percent
- Procainamide 1 gm
- Hydrocortisone sodium succinate (Solu-Cortef) 200 mg
- Diazepam 10 mg.

These medications should be available at all times.

The actions for the prescribed medications should be written into a procedure or protocol along with the medication for referral at the time needed (Fig. 19.1).

Signs and Symptoms
1. Cardiovascular desaturation
2. Cardiovascular and arterial hypercarbia
3. Metabolic acidosis
4. Respiratory acidosis
5. Hyperkalemia
6. Elevated CPK
7. Tachycardia
8. Arrhythmias
9. Profuse sweating
10. Unstable blood pressure
11. Cyanotic mottling of skin
12. Tachypnea, spontaneous ventilation
13. Dark blood in surgical field despite adequate inspired oxygen
14. Fever, rapid rise in temperature (1°F per minute)
15. Rigidity, profound shivering, muscle fasciculations

At Onset
1. Stop anesthesia and surgery immediately as mechanical stimulation worsens event.
2. Change rubber goods and anesthesia machine.
3. Hyperventilate with 100% oxygen.
4. Administer medication: dantrolene sodium, procainamide, droperidol, corticosteroids, furosemide, mannitol.
5. Initiate cooling with intravenous iced solution and surface cooling with ice and hypothermia blanket until core temperature returns to 38°C. Apply ice packs to great vessels: femoral, axillary, head, and neck.
6. Reverse acidosis and hyperkalemia.
7. Secure monitoring lines: central venous pressure and arterial line.
8. Monitor ECG, urinary output, blood gases, electrolytes.
9. Maintain adequate urine output.
10. Record events on established forms: ECG, temperature, heart rate, blood pressure, central venous pressure, arterial line, urine output, skin color (see Fig. 19.2).
11. Monitor patient carefully for at least 24 hours. Smoldering is a late complication. The patient appears to respond to therapy but underlying cellular disorder smolders; therefore, symptoms recur. Renewed therapy is necessary to terminate the syndrome entirely.

Figure 19.1. Signs and symptoms associated with malignant hyperthermia and emergency treatment regime. (Prepared for use at Porter Memorial Hospital, Denver, 1981, by Donna Bernklau, Robin Knapp, Paulette Rutter, and Cynthia Yanick, operating room nurses.)

Drug	*Action*
Chlorpromazine	Controls agitation, decreases shivering, causes vasodilation.
Dantrolene sodium	For management of the fulminant hypermetabolism of skeletal muscle in MH crisis.
Dantrolene sodium	Also a direct-acting skeletal muscle relaxant, which reduces muscle rigidity by preventing release of calcium from the sacroplasmic reticulum into the myoplasm. It restores normal muscle function and terminates the progressive acidosis and heat production.
Furosemide (Lasix)	Ensures adequate urine output.
Mannitol	Provides renal support.
Solu-Medrol	Stabilizes cell membranes.
Sodium bicarbonate	Reverses acidosis.
Procainamide	Increases calcium reuptake; management of arrhythmias.
Hydrocortisone (Solu-Cortef)	Reduces edema.
Diazepam	Causes a rapid fall in temperature and amnesia.
Insulin and glucose	Used to treat hyperkalemia; mix 10 units of regular insulin in 50 percent glucose to decrease serum potassium by taking it into intracellular spaces.

Some operating rooms have established policies to provide direction to the staff when a crisis occurs. They have assembled equipment and supplies that are readily accessible. Recording sheets may assist the nurse to document events during the emergency situation. An example is provided in Fig. 19.2.

In summary, malignant hyperthermia is a sudden onset of pharmacogenic crisis that requires immediate medical and nursing inter-

MALIGNANT HYPERTHERMIA RECORDING SHEET

RECORDER:

TIME - ONSET OF SYMPTOMS:

INITIAL SIGNS AND SYMPTOMS:

ABG's DRAWN	K's DRAWN	Iced Saline Given	Dantrolene	Thorazine	Lasix	Glucose 50%	Kcl	Mannitol	Na Bicarb	Pronestyl	Solu Medrol	Solu Cortef	Temp	Lidocaine	Valium

FOLEY INSERTED BY	TIME	N G TUBE INSERTED	RECTAL TEMP. PROBE INSERTED	ANES TUBES CHANGED	SODA LIME CHANGED	ICE PLACEMENT	OTHER COOLING

MISC. COMMENTS.

Developed for use at Porter Memorial Hospital, 1981
By: Donna Bernklau, RN, Paulette Rutter, RN, Robin Knapp, RN

Figure 19.2. Malignant hyperthermia recording sheet. Developed at Porter Memorial Hospital, Denver, by Robin Knapp.

vention. Although it occurs rarely, the pre-operative indicators are often overlooked. Therefore, it is essential that complete pre-operative assessments be done with in-depth histories about previous anesthetic complications and even family background before anesthesia is administered. The nurse's role is to assist in data collection and to monitor during the intraoperative procedure. Once the crisis occurs, the team works together to reverse the crisis. If treated promptly and accurately, the patient will survive without residual muscular problems.

References

1. Martin, J. T. *Positioning in Anesthesia and Surgery.* Philadelphia: W. B. Saunders, 1978.
2. Churchill-Davidson, N. C., ed. *A Practice of Anesthesia,* 4th ed. Philadelphia: W. B. Saunders, 1978.
3. Dripps, R. D., Eckenhoff, J. E., Vandam, L. D. *Introduction to Anesthesia,* 5th ed. Philadelphia: W. B. Saunders, 1977.
4. Cheney, F. W. "Effects of surgery on pulmonary function." In D. G. Hershey, ed. *Refresher Courses in Anesthesiology,* vol. 6. Chicago: American Society of Anesthesiology, 1978.
5. Snow, J. C. *Manual of Anesthesia.* Boston: Little, Brown and Co., 1977.
6. Reed, Charles C. *Cardiopulmonary Perfusion.* Houston: Texas Medical Press, Inc., 1975.
7. Winsor, Travis. "Electrolyte abnormalities and the electrocardiogram." *JAMA* 203:5, 1968.
8. Prys-Roberts, C., and Melocke, R. "Management of anesthesia in patients with hypertension or ischemic heart disease." *Internat Anes Clin* 18:181, 1980.

Suggested Readings

Bull, S. "Vascular pressures and critical care management." *Nurs Clin North Am* 16:225, 1981.

Dienes, R. S., Jr. Inadvertent hypothermia in the operating room. *Plast Reconstruc Surg* 67:253, 1981.

Dobbs, G. "The prevention and treatment of Mendelson's syndrome." *Curr Rev Nurse Anesthet Lesson* 6. 4:44, 1981.

Guyton, A. C. *Basic Human Physiology: Normal Function and Mechanisms of Disease,* 2nd ed. Philadelphia: W. B. Saunders, 1977.

Hardy, J. D. *Complications in Surgery and Their Management,* 4th ed. Philadelphia: W. B. Saunders, 1981.

Hercules, P. R., Lekwart, F. J., and Fenton, M. V. *Pulmonary Restriction and Obstruction.* Chicago: Year Book Medical Publishers, 1979.

Jacob, S. W., and Francone, C. A. *Elements of Anatomy and Physiology.* Philadelphia: W. B. Saunders, 1976.

Lalli, S. M. "The complete Swan-Ganz." *RN* 41:64, 1978.

Lees, O. E., Kim, Y. D., Macnamara, T. E. "Noninvasive determination of core temperature during anesthesia." *South Med J* 73:1322, 1973.

Rhodes, M. J., Gruendemann, B. J., and Ballinger, W. F. *Alexanders' Care of the Patient in Surgery,* 6th ed. St. Louis: C. V. Mosby, 1978.

Smith, R. N. "Invasive pressure monitoring." *Am J Nurs* 78:1514, 1978.

Woods, S. L. "Monitoring pulmonary artery pressures." *Am J Nurs* 76:1765, 1976.

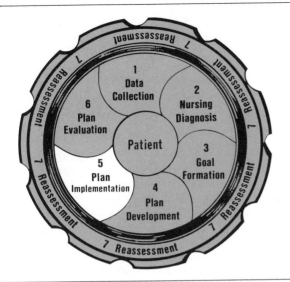

The nurse uses instruments and equipment appropriately.

Instruments and Equipment

The function and use of instruments and equipment in the operating room is a large part of the body of knowledge for the experienced operating room nurse. It is essential for students and beginning registered nurse practitioners to systematically learn this information in order to give knowledgeable, safe, professional nursing care to the patient during the intraoperative phase of the perioperative experience. Knowledge of equipment and instruments gained from other areas of nursing experience can be applied and used in providing nursing care in the operating room.

The professional nurse in the operating room functions primarily in the role of circulating nurse, although to function with total professional knowledge and expertise in this role the circulating nurse must have a complete understanding of the scrub person's role. Most professional nurses will speak enthusiastically about the role of scrubbing; many state they prefer this area although it is a technical role. Both positions require extensive knowledge in the realm of instrument and equipment use for the care of the patient.

In this chapter some of the pieces of equipment and instruments commonly used in the care of the patient in the operating room are discussed. This list is not all-inclusive by any means. The pieces of equipment and instruments commonly used in some of the specialty services are also mentioned. The patient is followed as he moves through the operating room, beginning with his transfer to the operating room table and ending when he is removed from the table at the completion of the surgery. How the circulating nurse and scrub person use the equipment and instruments is discussed. Since the principal role of the nurse in the operating room is as the circulating nurse, let us begin with the essential equipment used by the circulating nurse.

Equipment

The nurse should become familiar with all the equipment in the operating room itself (see Fig. 20.1). This can be accomplished by moving it about, cleaning it, and raising and lowering the surgical table and Mayo stand. Switches can be turned off and on once the nurse safely knows how they are used. Handling the equipment is important. This familiarizes the nurse with everything he will be required to work with in the performance of his duties.

OPERATING ROOM TABLE

The operating room table is expensive, complex, and an essential piece of equipment used for all surgical procedures (Fig. 20.2). It has been specifically designed to meet the needs of the surgical patient. There are several types of operating room tables available, such as general surgical, orthopedic, and urological.

It is essential that the circulating nurse be proficient in the manipulation of this piece of

Figure 20.1. A basic operating room showing the variety of equipment the nurse uses in care of the patient intraoperatively, with the surgical table as the center of activity.

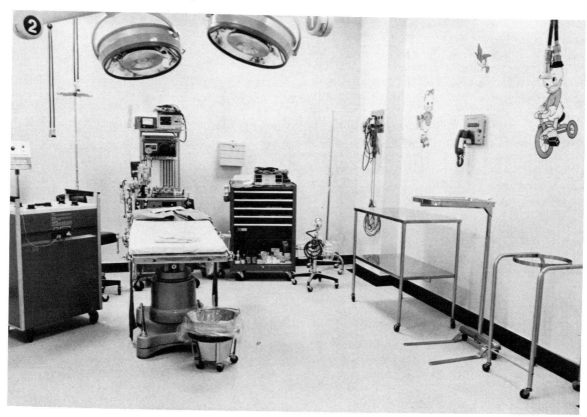

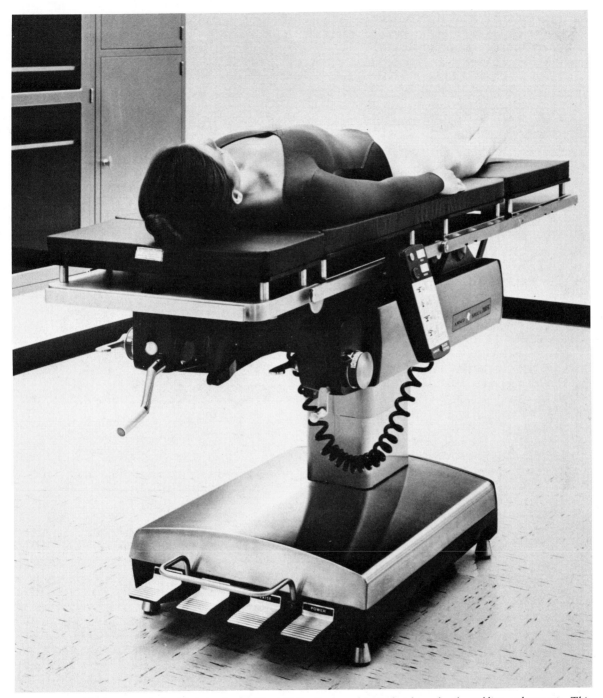

Figure 20.2. *The basic surgical table in supine position. Notice the tunnel immediately under the padding and supports. This tunnel allows for the placement of x-ray cassettes under the patient during surgery for intraoperative x-rays. The push button control panel for changing the table's position is located on the right side of the table. (Photograph courtesy of AMSCO/ American Sterilizer Company, Erie, Penn. 16512.)*

equipment if he is to safely position the patient. The nurse must be familiar with all parts of the table and accessories available.

Prior to the patient's arrival in the operating room, the table should be checked for cleanliness and completeness according to the procedure scheduled. Attachments should be readily available depending on position anticipated—stirrups for the patient to be placed in lithotomy position or the table extension for the patient who is 6 feet 6 inches tall. Padding for the accessories may be necessary and should be readily available for the protection of the patient. As most modern operating room tables are electrically operated, it is necessary to perform an electrical safety check including all cords and plugs prior to use.

It is the circulating nurse's responsibility to be sure that the table is locked in place prior to moving the patient from the gurney to the table. It is essential that the safety strap is securely in position once the patient is on the table (see Fig. 20.3).

Most surgical tables have been designed to allow x-rays to be taken during the operative procedure (see Fig. 20.2). The tops are penetrable by the x-rays, and a tunnel beneath this holds the needed film or cassette in a variety of positions.

These tables are versatile and can be arranged for the numerous positions required for operative procedures, such as Trendelenburg, lateral (see Fig. 20.4), lithotomy (see Fig. 20.5), jackknife (see Fig. 20.6), or just a slight left or right tilt to the top and others. Knowledge of the control box (see Fig. 20.2) is essential to assist with positioning of the patient. The nurse may also be asked to make adjustments to the table and patient position during the intraoperative period.

Many parts of the table are removable with specialized attachments; for example, the head section may be removed to allow the insertion of a head rest for the craniotomy patient. Again it is the nurse's responsibility to know all the parts, how to remove them, and to add attachments quickly and safely. It is recommended that the nurse new to the operating room setting be thoroughly oriented to this equipment and be allowed time in which to

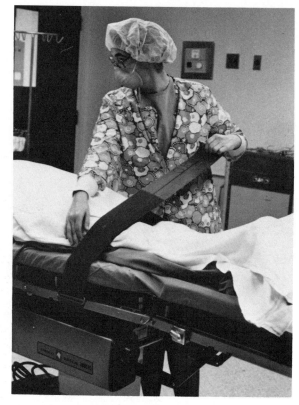

Figure 20.3. The safety belt being placed and secured over the patient on the operating room table.

practice the numerous positions and to remove and attach all accessories.

STERILIZERS

One of the first pieces of equipment used daily by the operating room personnel for most surgical procedures is the sterilizer. Most operating rooms today have at least the flash steam sterilizer within the operating room suite (see Fig. 20.7). Those hospitals on the Friessen concept, where the SPD (Supply, Processing, and Distribution) Department sets up case carts of all sterile equipment, may have only flash emergency sterilizers within the department, with all other sterilization equipment in SPD. It is essential to understand the principles of sterilization, including the operation of this equipment. Modern equip-

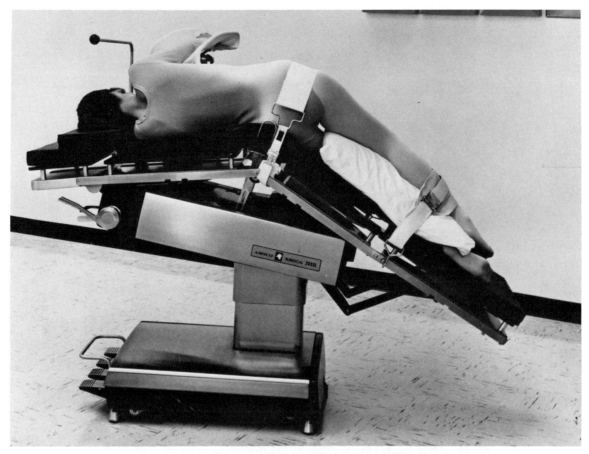

Figure 20.4. Lateral position demonstrating the break in the table at the midpoint along with a general reverse Trendelenburg slant to the table. Safety straps and arm rest are in position. (Photograph courtesy of AMSCO/American Sterilizer Company, Erie, Penn. 16512.)

ment can be computerized and automatically programmed (see Fig. 20.8). The term *flash* is a misnomer used in reference to the emergency sterilizer. This autoclave is used for emergencies — an instrument needs sterilization for a surgery in progress, or unexpected equipment is needed, or an essential instrument becomes contaminated. The basic principles of the flash sterilizer are the same as with all other steam sterilizers. As this sterilizer can be operated without the drying cycle, less time is necessary to complete the cycle.

A monitoring system of graphs provides a permanent daily record of temperature during all cycles. This graph provides a visual demonstration of the chamber temperature. These graphs are kept on file as documentation of proper sterilization.

The flash sterilizer is used for quick sterilization of instruments at high speed, reaching 270°F for rapid sterilization of unwrapped supplies. Steam under pressure floods the chamber to create the needed temperature and then holds the temperature at 270°F for not less than three minutes. The time necessary for reaching the temperature at the beginning of the cycle plus the time necessary to exhaust the steam after completion of the sterilization

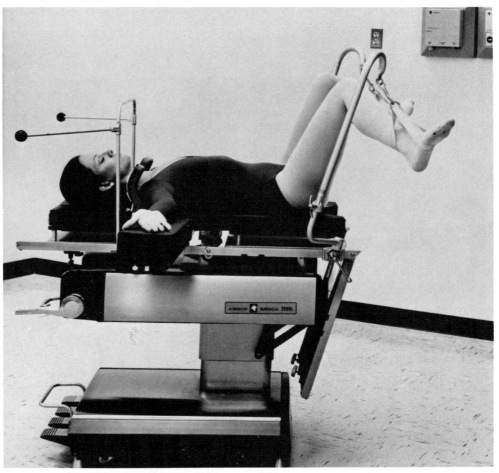

Figure 20.5. Lithotomy position demonstrating the use of the cane stirrup attachments, anesthesia screen at the patient's head, and the folding down of the foot end of the table. (Photograph courtesy of AMSCO/American Sterilizer Company, Erie, Penn. 16512.)

extend this flash cycle to approximately six to seven minutes. It is essential that whenever an item is removed from the sterilizer the operator check the graph to be absolutely certain the correct sterilization temperature was reached.

Care must be used in transporting the sterilized, unwrapped equipment to the point of use in order to maintain sterility. Because of the danger of contamination, this system should be used for emergencies only. It is always a better aseptic technique to use wrapped presterilized items.

SUCTION

Suction equipment in the operating room is essential for safe patient care. This equipment must be checked and in good working order prior to the patient's arrival (see Fig. 20.9).

There must be at least two sets of suction apparatus in the room ready to go. The anesthesiologist uses one to assist in maintaining the patient's airway by removing the accumulation of any secretions. This equipment must be available to him throughout the procedure. In suctioning, he uses either a Yankauer tonsil tip or a suction catheter. While the airway or endotracheal tube is in place the suction catheter is used. After these are removed at the end of the procedure, the tonsil sunction is more useful.

A second or even a third setup may be used by the surgeon or the assistant at the operative site. The suction here is used to remove blood, secretions, or irrigating solutions to maintain visual contact at the point where the surgeon is working. Should hemorrhage occur, it is essential to quickly find the point of bleeding so it can be controlled. The bleeding point has to be seen before it can be clamped.

The suction must always be readily available. Once the patient has been draped at the begin-

ning of the procedure, the scrub person brings to the operative site the sterile suction tubing with tip. Often the surgeon will attach and arrange these as the scrub person brings up the Mayo stand and the circulating nurse brings in the back table and basins.

The distal end of the suction tubing will be passed off the field to the circulating nurse who will then attach them to the appropriate unit and turn them on.

MONITORS

Monitoring the patient during the operative procedure has become standard practice during all operative procedures. In the past, operating

Figure 20.6. *Modified jackknife position demonstrating all joints of the table being used. Notice that the head piece has been removed and inserted at the foot to extend the table at this point. The table base is in a general Trendelenburg mode. (Photograph courtesy of AMSCO/American Sterilizer Company, Erie, Penn. 16512.)*

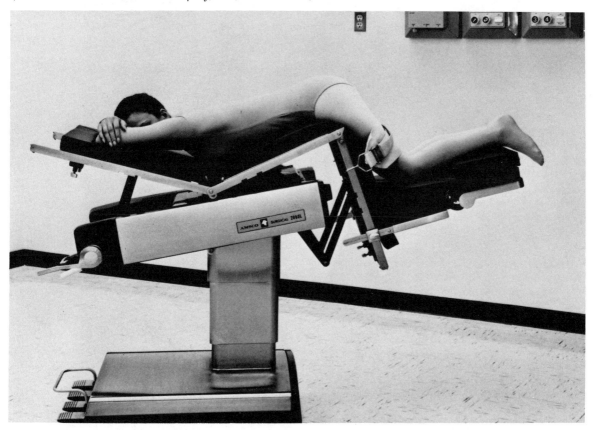

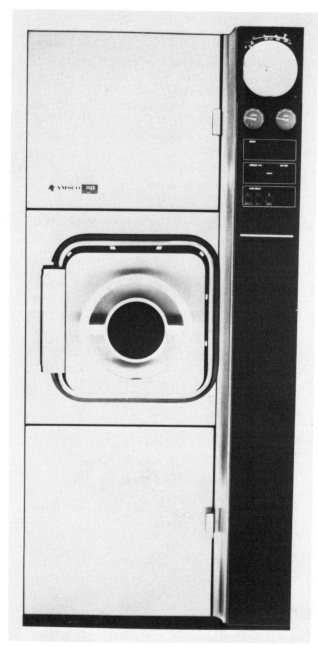

Figure 20.7. The new AMSCO 2025 computerized emergency sterilizer with "flash" cycle. (Photograph courtesy of AMSCO/American Sterilizer Company, Erie, Penn. 16512.)

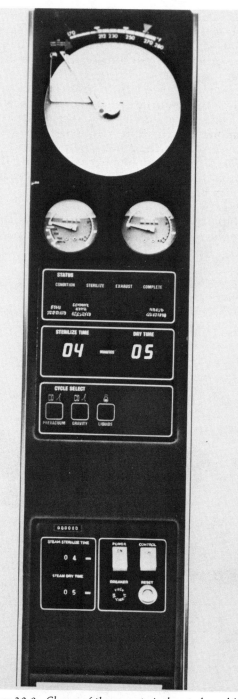

Figure 20.8. Closeup of the computerized control panel for the AMSCO 2025 sterilizer. The mechanism for marking the autoclave graph is a part of this panel. (Photograph courtesy of AMSCO/American Sterilizer Company, Erie, Penn. 16512.)

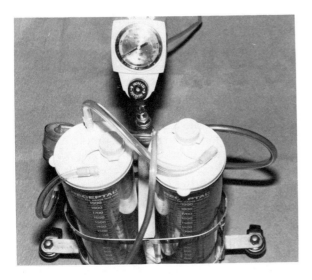

Figure 20.9. A basic double container floor suction unit used for surgery. This must be checked and in working order prior to the patient's arrival.

room nurses were not greatly involved in this area. Today, however, expertise in monitoring is becoming more essential.

In basic cardiac monitoring, although under the guidance of the anesthesiologist, the operating room nurse may be responsible for anything from applying the leads to actual interpretation. Interpretation is becoming more essential as operating rooms become more involved in the area of outpatient surgery and the care of local patients, where an anesthesiologist may or may not be present (see Fig. 20.10).

As the operating room nurse's experience, knowledge, and skill increase, he will become involved in increasingly more complex patient care activities. With this there will be more complex monitoring systems employed to follow the patient's full status throughout the procedure. The circulating nurse may be assisting with many of these procedures.

The basic monitoring system used is the electrocardiograph (ECG). This records the electrical forces produced by the heart as it beats. An ECG oscilloscope of some type is used. Leads are attached to the patient to pick up these forces and transfer them in the form of a wave tracing on the oscilloscope screen or read-out graph paper.

Two leads are essential to pick up these forces, with a third applied as a grounding wire (see Fig. 20.11). These electrodes are placed on the patient's chest or extremities. The pads used are available pregelled and disposable and will snap on to the lead wires. The clarity of the tracing on the scope depends on the proper placement of these leads.

Basically, there is a relationship between the wave displayed on the scope or paper strip and the cardiac anatomy and physiology at that moment. It is essential to know the various waves, intervals, and complexes, and what is normal and what is abnormal based on the pattern presented. Knowledge of the relationship of the P wave, QR interval, the QRS complex and the total width of the pattern are necessary for interpretation.

It is not the intent of this chapter to present the information necessary to interpret this pattern and the great variety of rhythms and arrhythmias that can occur. A course in basic arrhythmias is helpful to the operating room nurse and many are offered by the American

Figure 20.10. An example of a basic cardiac monitor used intraoperatively. The type shown also has digital read-out of pulse and alarm systems that can be set to specific levels to alert personnel to possible problems.

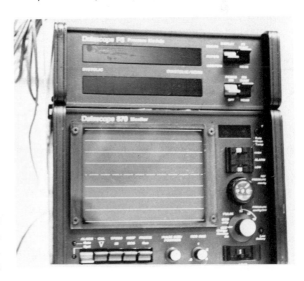

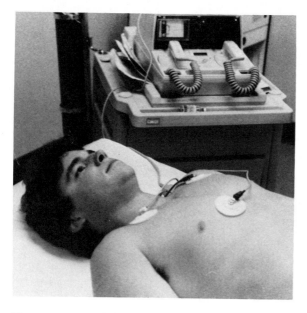

Figure 20.11. Placement of the electrodes is crucial in obtaining accurate PQRST patterns. (Photograph courtesy of Physio-Control Corp., Redmond, Wash. 98052.)

Heart Association in the Advance Cardiac Life Support courses and other groups. Many hospitals also offer such courses for their critical care nurses. As operating room nurses are critical care nurses, they should be included in these courses.

There are numerous types of ECG monitors available, some with just the basic oscilloscope screen and others that include displays of heart beat and blood pressure. Some are put out as a total lifesaving system seen in the LifePak System (see Fig. 20.12) in combination with a defibrillator.

EMERGENCY EQUIPMENT

Any patient, whether under general anesthesia or local block, can react adversely, at any time, to any of the medications, the stress of the procedure, or hemorrhage during the intraoperative phase. General anesthesia has a certain level of morbidity even for the patient in good condition having elective surgery. The team must also be prepared for the patient known to be a poor surgical risk. A cardiac or respiratory arrest can occur with any given patient at any moment during the intraoperative period.

For the total protection of the surgical patient, it is imperative that the surgical team know intimately the emergency equipment available in their particular suite. When a critical situation occurs the response must be swift and efficient in order to be lifesaving.

Where is the equipment located? The nurse should find it on the first day in the operating room and review the policy and procedure established for the department. Most operating rooms have established an emergency *crash* cart so that everything that is needed for cardiac and respiratory arrest is together in one spot and on wheels that can be moved quickly to the patient's side (see Fig. 20.13).

Usually the defibrillator and monitor are plugged in when the cart is in its home spot to recharge batteries. They must be unplugged before attempting to move the cart to the patient's side.

The nurse should know the emergency call signals established for the department, where they are located, and how to activate them. These signals may include a call light or buzzer which should remain on until enough people have gathered to care for the patient.

The cardiac monitor is an integral part of the crash cart. The solitary monitor has already been reviewed.

The cardiac defibrillator is a necessary piece of equipment during emergencies. The defibrillator provides an electrical force that can be applied to the patient's chest at the time of cardiac arrest. This force can stimulate the heart muscle to contract. The force can also be used to abolish ventricular fibrillation.

Defibrillation was first used internally on the heart muscle by Bech in 1947. This method has now progressed to external application to stop ventricular fibrillation. To be most effective defibrillation should be done in the first minute of arrest. With every passing minute the patient has less chance of survival.

The defibrillator is basically a condenser of stored electrical energy that can be discharged when needed. Today's equipment can be small, portable, and combined with a cardiac monitor as seen in the LifePak 6 (see Fig. 20.12).

To apply this electrical force to the patient, two metal paddles with conductive gel are used. The paddles are placed on the patient in a manner whereby the electrical current will pass through the heart. The placement of the paddles is crucial. One can be placed to the right of the sternum at the third interspace and the other on the anterior wall below the apex of the heart. The paddles must have skin contact. Pressing firmly on the paddles will provide good contact.

The operator must be careful not to touch the electrodes, the patient, or the metal on the bed or the electrical current will flow directly to him and he will also be jolted. Everyone caring for the patient at this time must avoid contact with the patient and these elements at the moment of electrical stimulation.

During the moment of defibrillation, the cardiac monitor and oxygen to the patient should be turned off to prevent explosions. The level of the electrical current at this time is generally about 300 W/second.

After use it is essential that the equipment, including the paddles, be cleaned properly.

Figure 20.12. The LifePak 6 is a combination defibrillator and cardiac monitor found on many emergency carts. The external paddles are left attached and in full view ready for use. (Photograph courtesy of Physio-Control Corp., Redmond, Wash. 98052.)

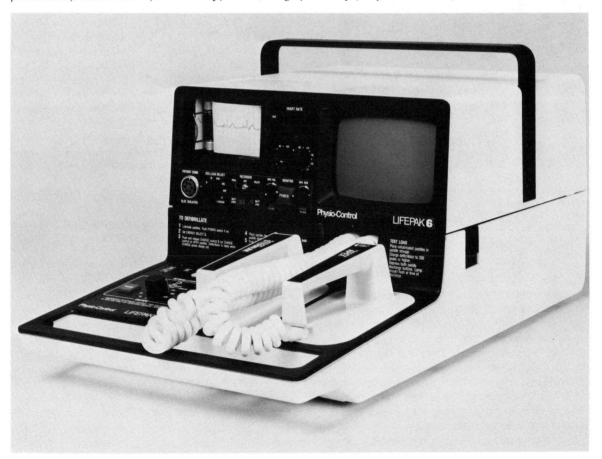

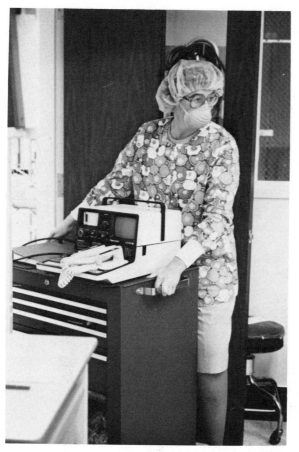

to respond and breathe on his own. Some patients may respond slowly and continue to need ventilatory assistance, particularly during transportation from the operating room to the postanesthesia recovery room. Other patients may purposefully be kept heavily sedated in the immediate postoperative phase with continued intubation and attachment to automatic ventilating equipment. Again the ventilation bag is essential to transport such patients from one place to another. This bag is used in emergency situations throughout the hospital where the patient's respirations need to be maintained.

ELECTROSURGICAL EQUIPMENT

Today more and more complex electrical equipment is being used in the operating room to provide care to the patient during the intraoperative experience. It is essential that those using this equipment have a basic understanding of electricity and how it works. It is not the intent of this chapter to cover the physics of electricity; there are several articles that provide this explanation for operating room nurses (see "Suggested Readings").

Orientation to surgery should include instruction, demonstration, and return demon-

Figure 20.13. A typical emergency cart is painted red and has several drawers that contain all the necessary medications, syringes, needles, IV solutions, and tubes. The defibrillator and paddles with monitor sit on top for ease in accessibility. This cart must be checked daily for completeness.

Figure 20.14. The Laerdal ventilation reservoir bag and mask can be used to maintain the patient's respirations during emergency situations or transport of ventilator-dependent patients. (Photograph courtesy of Laerdal Medical Corp., Armonk, N.Y. 10504.)

The conductive gel used on the paddles must be removed carefully to prevent a metal oxide from forming which could interfere with the electrical flow in later use of the equipment.

Another piece of equipment generally found on the emergency cart is a ventilation bag (see Fig. 20.14). During the procedure with the patient under general anesthesia the patient's respirations are maintained by the anesthesiologist using automatic ventilating equipment. Once the procedure is completed and the drugs of anesthesia are reversed, the patient begins

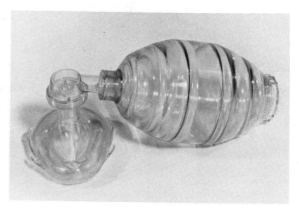

stration of all electrical units found in the operating room. Written instructions should be available from the manufacturer. Written instructions on or with the equipment are most helpful.

Any electrical unit can be hazardous to both the patient and the staff. Safety precautions must be meticulously followed for the well-being of all involved with the procedure, the patient being the prime concern.

All equipment should be checked prior to use to ensure that it is in good working order. All the cords and plugs should be checked for exposed wires or frays in the insulation. If defects are found, this equipment should not be used. The alarm system should be checked not only for that equipment but also the general alarm system within the suite. Damaged units or equipment not running properly should never be used. Faulty equipment should be reported, labeled, and removed immediately. A preventive maintenance program is essential for all electrical equipment. An ongoing program of this nature is mandatory in all hospitals.

Tightly wrapped cords damage the insulation and the wiring. Running over the electrical cords with other equipment can also damage the cords. Three pronged plugs are required for all electrical equipment used, with larger explosion-proof plugs being required in the operating room. The nurse has a legal responsibility for the proper functioning of equipment attached to the patient. All safety checks must be completed prior to the entry of the patient into the operating room.

Use of electrical equipment should be included as part of the documentation done in the operating room. Because of this, electrosurgical equipment needs to be numbered so that name and number of the equipment can be entered on the patient's chart.

The prime piece of electrical equipment that is used for most patients in surgery today is the *electrocautery unit*. It is called by several different names, the most prominent being "Bovie" after Dr. F. Bovie who in the 1920s was one of the prime developers of the present electrocautery system (see Fig. 20.15).

The electrocautery unit uses a high fre-

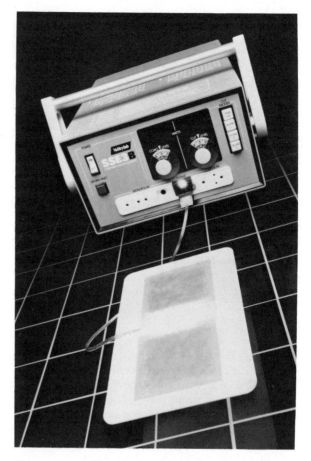

Figure 20.15. The Valleylab SSEE3B unit is an example of recent solid-state electrosurgical units that have been developed. The different currents are controlled by the dials. Notice the pregelled disposable ground dispersion plate in the foreground. (Photograph courtesy of Valleylab, Inc., Boulder, Col. 80301.)

quency electrical force to cauterize bleeding vessels to maintain hemostasis. By changing the current this electrical flow can also be used as a cutting edge, i.e., as a scalpel. The cauterization current is used most frequently.

The controlled electrical current is passed from the main transformer to the patient via a sterile pencil attached to the equipment by a wire. A switch on most pencils controls the current flow (Fig. 20.16). These items can be either disposable or reusable and may be resterilized by either steam or gas. Some makes of electrocautery are controlled by a foot

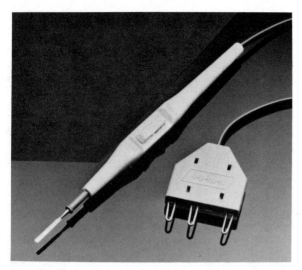

Figure 20.16. *The Valleylab disposable hand-switching water resistant pencil. (Photograph courtesy of Valleylab, Inc, Boulder, Col. 80301.)*

switch. The unit is then controlled by the foot of the surgeon as the current is needed.

With the advent of modern technology this equipment is now converting to solid-state units. Solid-state allows for pinpoint coagulation. Since the module is a smaller, more compact unit, it occupies less space and is more mobile than the larger, older units.

The numbered dials on the unit do not reflect the actual voltage delivered. They represent the range of power. If the surgeon asks for continued increase in the power because he is not obtaining the desired results, the nurse should check the total system to make sure that contact is being made. To continue to increase the power is extremely dangerous to the patient and is a point of negligence in nursing care.

To complete this circuit safely, a ground dispersion plate or pad must be in contact with the patient's skin with appropriate lubrication (see Fig. 20.15). This returns or drains the electrical current back to the electrocautery unit. If this complete circuit is not functioning properly, burning can occur at any point of contact to the patient. Proper placement of the grounding pad is a key to the safety of the

patient. Any fleshy part of the body is appropriate. Bony areas should be avoided.

DOCTOR'S PREFERENCE CARDS

There are many different types of surgeries that can be performed. The same procedure can be performed using different techniques depending on the surgeon's preference based on his education and experience. In one operating room a particular procedure may be performed in as many different modes as there are surgeons performing that type of procedure.

In order to assist in efficiency and organization, nurses have developed *doctor's preference cards*. There should be a card for each procedure that a surgeon performs, and the only constant is that change will occur. The process of developing and updating these cards is continuous to keep up with changes.

These cards contain vital information for the nurses caring for the patient and must be a part of the care plan. All this information needs to be reviewed prior to the patient's arrival. The cards are necessary to gather the appropriate supplies and also to list the areas and type of suture the surgeon will use throughout the procedure.

They do not take the place of good professional nursing knowledge but do assist with specific care that the surgeon will order. Preference cards are basically standing orders of the surgeon and, combined with the nursing care plan formulated by the operating room nurse, provide individualized care for the patient. The nurse should be prepared for the unexpected and know his patient completely. He should have a well-organized nursing care plan and follow it. For the beginning practitioner or one not familiar with a particular surgeon, it is most helpful to have these cards posted in a convenient location during the procedure for easy reference.

Instruments

The patient has arrived and the monitors are in place. The circulating nurse has assisted the anesthesiologist with the induction of general anesthesia. Position has been established, initial counts performed, and skin prep completed. The patient is draped, and the suction and electrocautery have been attached. It is time to begin the surgery.

At this point the focus is on the scrub person and the preparation needed to provide the appropriate instruments and supplies to the surgeon.

Unfortunately there is no standard nomenclature for the instruments used in surgery. The names change not only from region to region, but also from hospital to hospital and manufacturer to manufacturer. What any particular operating room team may call their instruments depends greatly on the surgeons and where they were educated.

Instruments are constructed of a high grade of stainless steel in a variety of qualities. The 400 series has excellent qualities for surgical instruments including some noncorrosive characteristics and good tensile strength. Surgical instruments are made by highly trained technicians in several areas of the world including Pakistan, Germany, and the United States. Although delicate, they can withstand innu-

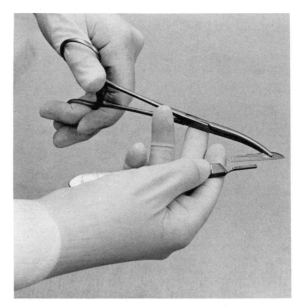

Figure 20.18. Use a clamp to assemble the knife blade and handle, to prevent cuts.

merable sterilization cycles if handled and used properly.

Each instrument, by its design, is made to do a particular job and function in a particular fashion and should be used only for that purpose. There are four basic types of instruments — cutting (sharps), clamps, grasping, and retractors (see Chapter 11).

Prior to the actual surgery a certain amount of instrument preparation must occur. Even the instruments for a short, relatively simple procedure require preparation because a small set still has many instruments, such as can be seen in the minor set (see Fig. 20.17). Disposable knife blades need to be placed on knife handles (see Fig. 20.18). Sponges are placed on sponge sticks (see Fig. 20.19) and used in deep incisions to absorb body fluids. Peanuts (K-Ds, or pushers) are placed on clamps (see Fig. 20.20) and are used in dissection of tissue. Sutures can also be placed on a clamp for use as a tie (see Fig. 20.21). Sutures and needle packages are opened and the needles are placed on needle holders (see Fig. 20.22).

Whether the surgeon is right or left handed is known by checking the doctor's preference

Figure 20.17. A minor set contains numerous instruments of various types. It is essential that the operating room nurse know the instruments and their uses.

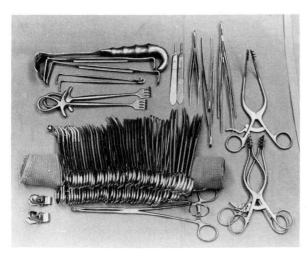

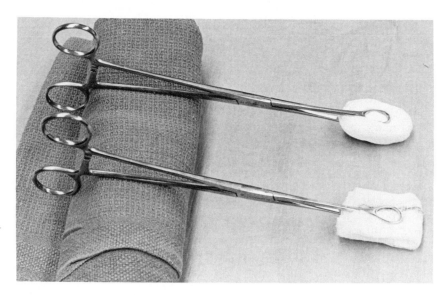

Figure 20.19. *Sponges used on sponge sticks must be radiopaque and a part of the sponge count. The 4 × 4 is folded and then placed in the sponge stick, which is then closed.*

card. The needles on the needle holder need to be adjusted accordingly (see Fig. 20.23).

Many operating rooms have developed *basic back table* and *Mayo stand setups*. A basic back table and Mayo stand setup for instruments can be very helpful to the beginning practitioner in the operating room. Laying the instruments on the back table in a specified manner will assist the scrub person in locating the various instruments, as they are needed, throughout the surgery. There is no specific design that is better than another, but it is helpful to use only one basic setup during the learning process (see Fig. 20.24). The basic setup can be adapted to accommodate all the instrumentations that are needed for the variety of surgical procedures performed.

Instrument counts necessitate the use of organized basic back table and Mayo stand setup to facilitate counting. If each person who scrubs has his own placement, the counting time will be extended and unorganized.

Basic setups are also very helpful at those times when the circulating nurse and scrub person need to be relieved, such as at shift changes. The individuals taking over will then know where instruments are on the setup and

Figure 20.20. *Peanuts are placed at the end of a Mayo (Kelly) clamp with a small portion beyond the tip of the clamp. This is used to gently push and separate tissue during dissection.*

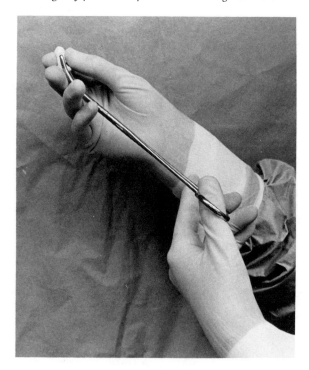

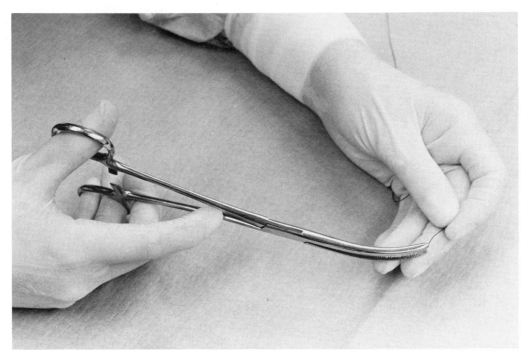

Figure 20.21. Place one end of the suture in the tip of the clamp which is then closed. Different types of clamps may be used for this, such as Mayo, right angled, or tonsil clamps.

the transition will be smoother. There is nothing so frustrating to the surgeons as to have the relieving scrub person or circulating nurse unable to find an instrument in the setup that they have already used.

During the setting up time, the scrub person must be observant of all the instruments in the set to be used. Are they working properly? Each instrument must be checked prior to use on the patient. Most instrument sets today are probably selected and put together by someone other than the nursing team in the operating room. Hospitals on the Friessen concept have the instruments put together in another department.

The instruments are checked at the time they are put together, but it is still the ultimate responsibility of the nursing team in the operating room, at the point of use on the patient, to perform the final safety check on all instruments and equipment used.

The Mayo stand and back table are now ready, as is the patient and surgeon. The Mayo stand and back table are moved into place (see Fig. 20.25). The Bovie cord and suction are put into position and attached. Sponges are up, and the surgeon puts out his hand to receive the first instrument.

The first items to be passed are those necessary to make the incision. Instruments do the work of the surgeon and are an extension of his hands. They come in all different sizes and shapes with each one having a particular job to do.

For the incision, a surgical knife, or scalpel, is needed. The scalpel has two parts: the handle and disposable blade. There are several sizes and shapes of both blades and handles. Since the scalpel's basic function is to cut, care must be observed whenever the knife is being handled by anyone on the team as the blade is razor sharp. The nurse should always know where the knife or knives are — on the back table, Mayo stand, or in use.

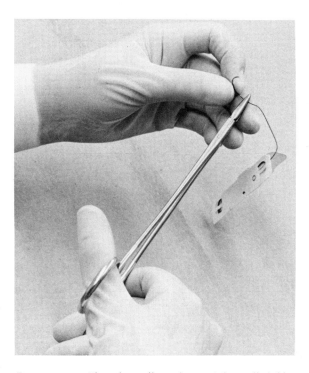

Figure 20.22. Place the needle in the tip of the needle holder approximately a third of the way down the shaft of the needle from the junction where the suture is attached. The point of the needle is toward the scrub person.

The nurse passes the scalpel to the surgeon handle first with the blade down, in position to make the incision. This move must be deliberate and in a manner to avoid cutting the surgeon or self. The scrub person's hand should be above the cutting edge as demonstrated in Fig. 20.26. At this same moment the assistant will also need clamps to assist in the control of bleeding. This is the fundamental job of all clamps; hemostasis. They make surgery possible by preventing and controlling the loss of blood. They come in a variety of shapes and lengths (see Fig. 20.27). On the skin, subcutaneous tissue, and underlying tissues, shorter instruments are needed in comparison to those necessary in operating deeply within the patient such as kidney and thoracic surgery.

The nurse places the clamp firmly into the assistant's hand in a position of use. The clamp should be closed with the rings of the handle being firmly, yet lightly, snapped into the palm

leaving the curve and point free to be applied to the tissue. Hold the clamp by the box lock as it is passed (see Fig. 20.28). The assistant may want a clamp in each hand and, depending on the procedure, he may want many until the incision is completed.

The nurse should practice handing the instruments ahead of time with both hands. Left-handed people may find using both hands for passing easier than right-handed people. Scrubbing will be easier if the nurse can learn to pass instruments with either hand and at the same time — one to the surgeon and the other to the assistant. This motion is the same for all clamps, be they short or long, delicate and fine, or thick and heavy, pointed, angled, straight, or curved.

The surgeon may wish to cauterize the bleeding vessel that has been clamped at this point (see Fig. 20.29). Or he may tie these points off, and he will need a strand of suture material (see Fig. 20.30). If he ties the vessel the ends of the suture need to be cut. Immediately after passing the tie, the nurse should have a suture scissor ready for him.

There are many types of scissors, each with their own specific function and level of delicacy. The nurse should know the differences between the various scissors. A delicate scissor meant to cut tissue must never be used as a suture scissor, and it is up to the scrub person to see that this is done (see Fig. 20.31). There are a variety of tips, blades, curves, and angles available.

The suture scissor is straight and can be seen at the 7 o'clock position in Fig. 20.31. Scissors come in lengths from 4 to 14 inches. The scrub person needs to select a length suitable to the immediate need. The surgeon working on the subcutaneous tissue can use 7¼-inch scissors, the most frequently used size. This clamp-tie-cut suture process may continue in series until all the bleeding has been controlled.

Suture scissors should always be available as they will be used throughout the procedure. It is also helpful to the scrub person to have a second pair of suture scissors available in order to cut and prepare sutures while the surgeon uses the other pair.

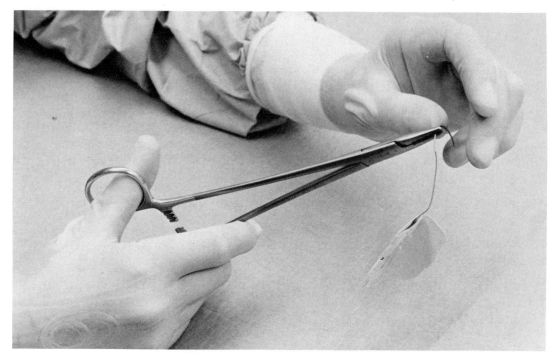

Figure 20.23. For the left-handed surgeon, the right-handed nurse can load the needle normally and then nearly turn the needle over. The left-handed scrub person performs these maneuvers in reverse order.

Figure 20.24. A demonstration of a basic back table setup after all the instruments have been prepared for surgery.

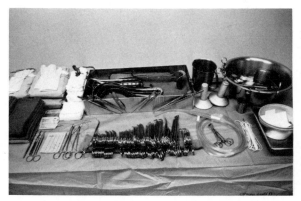

Figure 20.25. The scrub person slides the Mayo stand in over the patient's feet, being careful that the tray does not come in contact with the patient's feet. The circulating nurse moves the back table and other equipment into place.

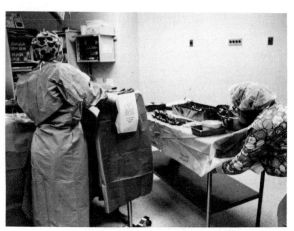

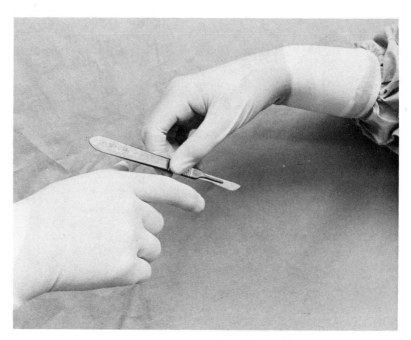

Figure 20.26. Hand the scalpel in position of use with the blade edge down to come in contact with the patient's skin. Always use caution when handling the scalpel to avoid cutting anyone.

Figure 20.27. Basic clamps come in a variety of shapes (straight or curved) and lengths. They can have heavy or fine tips, as seen in the first two clamps on the left.

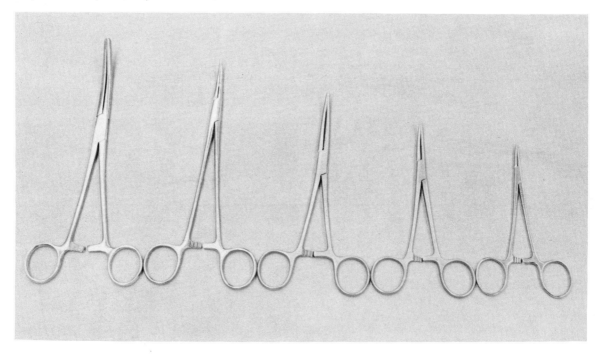

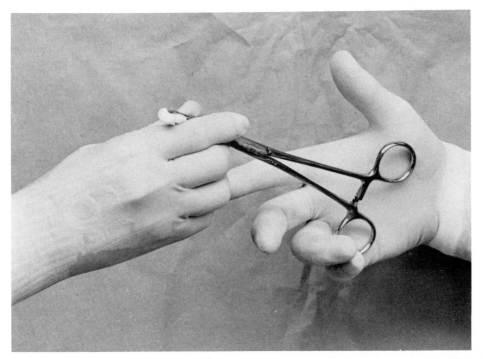

Figure 20.28. This clamp holds a peanut, but the basic motion for passing a clamp (whether curved, straight, angled, short, long, or with or without sponges) remains the same.

Figure 20.29. Pass the cautery pencil as the surgeon will use it.

Figure 20.30. Hold the suture material out to the surgeon. Come in and under his extended fingers, and up as he grasps the suture.

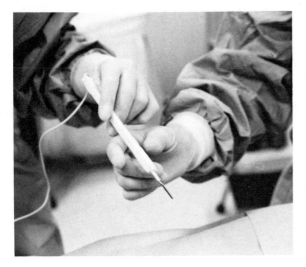

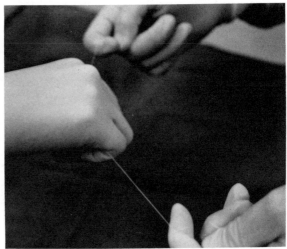

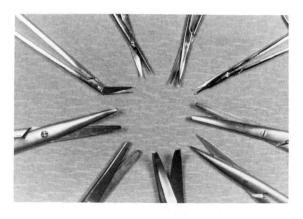

Figure 20.31. *Scissors come with a variety of tips, blades, curves and angles with each meant for a specific job in surgery. The four in the top of the picture are fine and delicate and used for vascular, eye, ear, and plastic surgeries.*

Another instrument used during the incision may be simple pick-ups with teeth to grasp, or pick up tissue, as the surgery proceeds. Tissue forceps are constructed with one and two teeth, or with multiple teeth, or plain with no teeth. The types with one and two teeth are most frequently used (see Fig. 20.32*A*). Pick-ups come in various lengths, widths, and points with each type used for a variety of tissues (Fig. 20.32*B*).

As the surgery proceeds, the subcutaneous tissue will need to be pushed or gently pulled aside. The assistant will need retractors for this. Retractors come in a variety of shapes and sizes and may be hand held or self-retaining. One frequently used at this point in surgery is the Army-Navy retractor (see Fig. 20-33) or a small size Richardson retractor (see Fig. 20.34). Other types of retractors available are rakes with either sharp or dull prongs (see Fig. 20.35), and self-retaining of many styles and sizes (see Fig. 20.36).

Figure 20.32. A, *Pick-ups are passed to the surgeon in a position to be used. Remember this point about all instruments and this will tell you how to pass them. B, Pick-ups come in a variety of types and sizes. Notice that some have teeth and others are plain.*

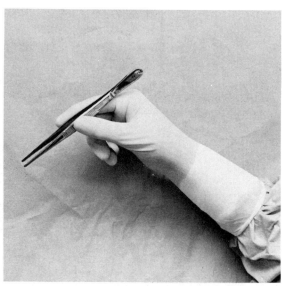

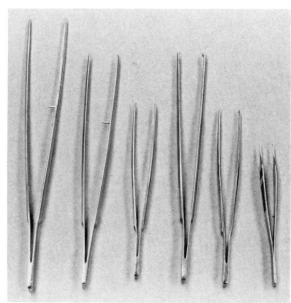

A

B

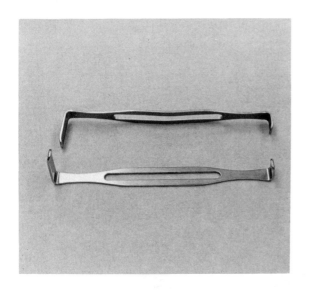

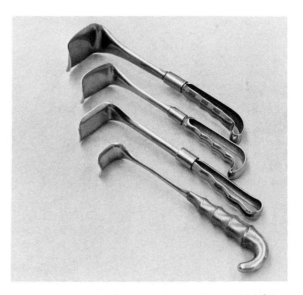

Figure 20.33. The Army-Navy retractor is hand held and generally used in pairs. Notice that it is double ended with different size blades.

Figure 20.34. Richardson retractors come in a variety of sizes to hold back various depths of tissue. They can be used singly or in pairs.

Figure 20.35. Rake retractors with sharp and dull prongs are generally used in pairs and are hand held.

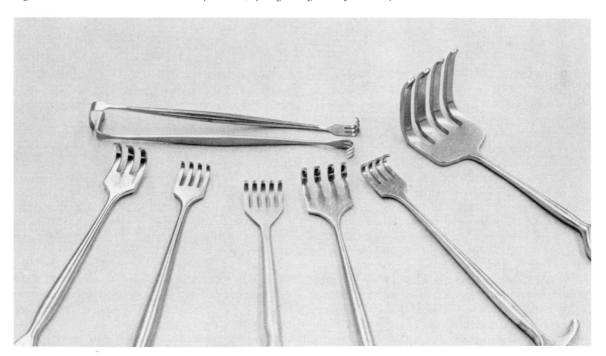

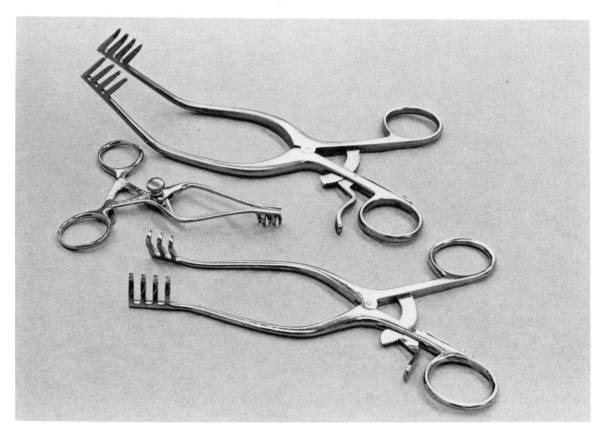

Figure 20.36. Self-retaining retractors are not hand held but have ratchets, springs, or locks to hold them in position.

These instruments should be handed to the surgeon in position of use. Richardson and Deavers have handles and are self-explanatory, but some, such as the Army-Navy retractor in Fig. 20.34, are double-ended. The end to be inserted into the patient depends on the size of the job to be accomplished. Judgment is necessary, and by watching what the surgeon is doing the scrub person can anticipate the need.

At this point in basic abdominal surgery the fascia and muscle need to be penetrated and bypassed. This is done in the same manner as with the subcuticular layer. A suture may be necessary at any one of these points.

Use of sutures and needles is a vast subject with several books published by the various suture manufacturers. These books cover the subject in great detail and should be read by the serious students of operating room nursing.

Sutures are basically used to hold the tissue together during wound healing or to control hemorrhage by tying off bleeding vessels. Surgical needles are designed to carry the suture through tissue with minimal trauma. Both suture and needles are available presterilized in easy to open packages.

There are numerous types of sutures that are used at various times during the surgery. Suture can be absorbable such as chromic or plain catgut and some synthetic materials or nonabsorbable such as silk, cotton, and nylons of all types.

Most needles used today are disposable. They come in a variety of sizes and shapes with various points and eyes, each with their own particular use. Needles and sutures are also available as one continuous unit, the swedged-on or atraumatic needle. Here the suture has been previously attached to the eyeless needle by the manufacturer.

There is a sequence of use to the suture, and each doctor has a preference on what and where to use the various needles and sutures. This should be listed on his preference card— what will be used during the incision and entry, the main portion of the procedure, and the closure.

It takes time and practice to be able to assemble the correct suture with the appropriate needle and have it ready for the surgeon when needed. For the surgeon to use this combination of suture and needle, a needle holder is necessary (see Fig. 20.37). Needle holders come in a variety of shapes and sizes for use at various times and types of surgeries.

The needle holder goes into the surgeon's hand as any clamp would, but attention must be paid to the direction of the needle. It must be in position of use and the suture material should not be allowed to bunch up in the surgeon's hand (see Fig. 20.38).

The peritoneum is the last layer to go through before entry into the abdominal cavity. Both the surgeon and assistant may use a pick-up with teeth to lift the peritoneum so it is not lying against any organ beneath it (see Fig. 20.32). The surgeon will need a clean knife to nick this structure to make a hole. He will then need a Metzenbaum scissor, a delicate tissue scissor (Fig. 20.39), to cut the peritoneum. At this point he will explore the cavity. Small loose 4 × 4 sponges should be removed from the

Figure 20.37. Needle holders have short stubby jaws in comparison to clamps. They are made specifically to hold needles firmly. They come in a variety of shapes and sizes to fit the sizes and shapes of needles plus the variety of procedures to be performed.

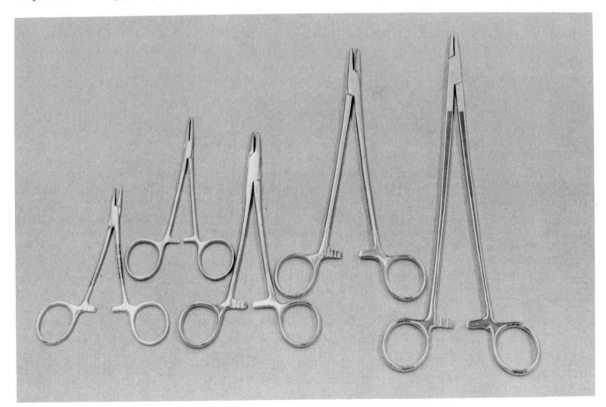

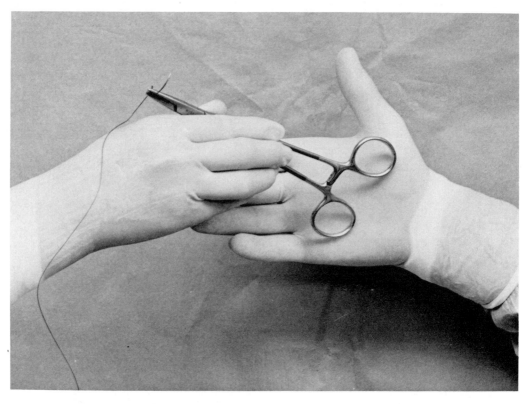

Figure 20.38. Needle holder loaded with atraumatic suture being passed to a right-handed surgeon. Notice that the suture material is over the scrub person's hand hanging free.

operative site at this point and should be used now only on a sponge stick.

A self-retaining Balfour retractor will be inserted (see Fig. 20.40). Laparotomy sponges may be placed along the sides of the incision to protect the tissue.

Once this entry into the patient has been completed, innumerable types of surgery can be performed. In abdominal surgery, a splenectomy, cholecystectomy, or numerous gastric and gastrointestinal surgeries can be performed. For gastric and gastrointestinal surgery, a whole new approach has been developed to perform these surgeries: i.e., stapling.

GASTROINTESTINAL SURGERY

A technique originally developed in Russia to mechanically suture tissue has been advanced further here in the United States. As surgeons have gained experience in the use of these instruments, there has been a significant change in performing procedures requiring ligation and division, anastomosis, resection and closure (see Figs. 20.41–20.45).

This method has gained popularity due to reduction of edema which generally occurs with handling of tissue. The B shape of the inserted staple allows circulation to pass through the tissue at the staple line to the cut edge. The staples are made of a nonreactive type metal that minimizes reaction and infection. These staples are available in preloaded sterile cartridges that are attached to the instrument just prior to being used by the surgeon.

These devices have significantly reduced the amount of time necessary to perform an anastomosis, resection, etc., meaning less handling

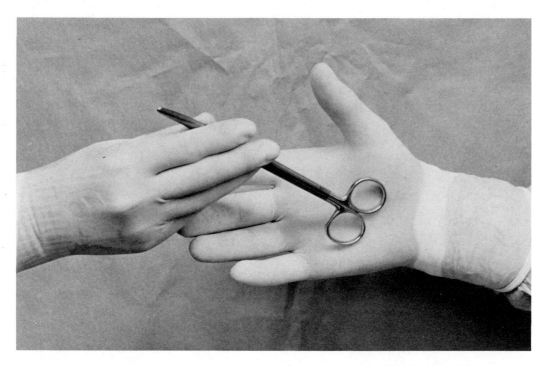

Figure 20.39. *The scissor is placed in the hand as a hemostat is passed. A little snap or flip of the wrist, just at the moment of contact, is helpful. The scissor is firmly in place and the surgeon knows this without moving his eyes from the surgical site.*

of tissue, less edema, and also a decrease in the length of time a patient is under the effects of anesthesia.

The devices shown in the figures are metal and reusable; however, disposable, preloaded, one-time implements are also available, as are disposable skin guns.

Figure 20.40. *The Balfour retractor has two parts, the retractor and blade.*

GYNECOLOGICAL SURGERY

Another series of surgeries within the abdomen are those performed by gynecologists on women patients of all ages. The most frequent procedure performed in this specialty is the D and C (dilatation and curettage) for diagnostic studies of the lining of the uterus, or retained placenta after deliveries and for termination of a pregnancy (Fig. 20.46).

Some of the specialized equipment used in this area include stirrups of some type, as many of these patients are placed in lithotomy

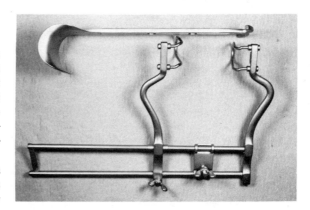

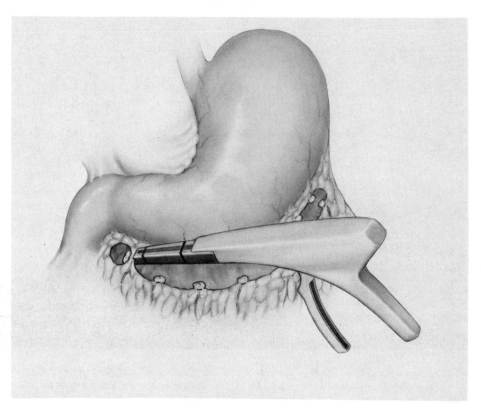

Figure 20.41. The LDS™ Model is shown during a Billroth II gastrectomy procedure. The stomach is being mobilized using the LDS™ to ligate and divide the omental vessels. The jaws of the LDS™ are slipped around the vessel and fat to be divided and fired. Two staples ligate the vessel; simultaneously, a knife in the LDS™ divides the vessel between the staples. (Photograph and caption courtesy of United States Surgical Corporation © USSC 1974, 1975, 1980.) We acknowledge the use in this work of certain copyrighted materials which have been reprinted with permission of United States Surgical Corporation as indicated by: © USSC 1981. These materials are copyrighted © United States Surgical Corporation 1981, All Rights Reserved, and may not be reproduced in any form or by any means.

position where the patient's legs are raised and abducted to expose the perineal region (see Fig. 20.5). The stirrups must be level and at the proper height for the individual patient. The patient's back must be well supported with buttocks flush with the break in the table. It is essential that the patient's legs and feet go into these stirrups simultaneously to prevent stress and damage to the patient's

hips. Having two people available at this time is ideal with each person gently raising a leg at the same time and placing the foot into the strap of the stirrups. It is essential that the strap is flat in all areas of contact with the foot. At the conclusion of the procedure it is vital that the patient's feet are carefully removed from the stirrups and the legs gently and slowly lowered together. To do this rapidly

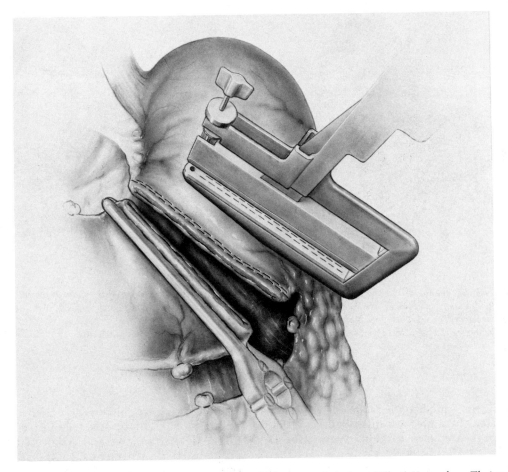

Figure 20.42. The TA 90™ is shown as it is being used to close the gastric pouch during a Billroth II procedure. The jaws of the TA 90™ are slipped around the stomach at the level of transection. The pin is screwed into place, the jaws are tightened, and the staples fired. Before removing the instrument, a clamp is placed on the specimen side and transected using the TA 90™ edge as a cutting guide.(© USSC 1974, 1975, 1980.)

could cause a sudden drop in the patient's blood pressure. Lowering the legs one at a time can place undue strain on the patient's back and hips with a possibility of dislocation occurring. The vacuum curettage unit (see Fig. 20.47) is used for aspiration of the contents of the uterus. This has become an accepted, safe method of terminating early pregnancies. It is used in conjunction with a D and C set of instruments. Sterile disposable cannulas and aspirating tubes are connected to the machine. A gauze sleeve attached to the inside of the primary bottle, at the end of the aspirating tube, will contain the specimen which is then sent for laboratory examination.

Another common procedure requiring special equipment is laparoscopy for endoscopic visualization of the pelvic cavity. A small in-

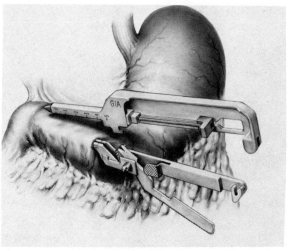
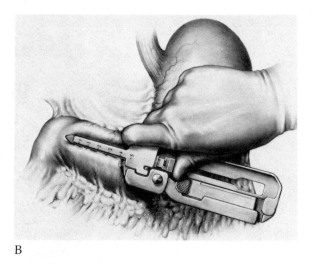

Figure 20.43. A, the GIA™ model of Autosuture is used to incise the stomach and secure hemostasis of the cut edges in one application. A stab wound is made into the gastric wall at the level for the gastrostomy. One fork of the GIA™ is inserted into the lumen of the stomach and the other fork is placed on the serosal surface. B, demonstrates the second step, the closure of the GIA™ and firing of the staples. Two double staggered hemostatic staple lines have now been placed in the gastric edges. (© USSC 1974, 1975, 1980).

cision at the umbilicus is made. The telescope is inserted through a cannula (see Fig. 20.48). Fiberoptics are used for lumination (see Fig. 20.49).

The pelvic organs are examined for diagnostic confirmation or for minor operative procedures. The operative procedures are performed through the laparoscope. A second small incision is made or the acorn cannula is inserted into the uterine cervix to allow for manipulation of the uterus for better exposure. Biopsy of suspicious tissue can be done. Reproductive sterilization by incising and cauterizing the fallopian tubes can be accomplished. Many times this procedure is performed to rule out suspected problems and thereby avoid unnecessary surgery.

In order to distinguish the various organs in the area, it is necessary to instill a gas into the abdominal cavity for distention. The gas best suited for this is carbon dioxide, and in an average size adult about 3 liters are used. An insufflation apparatus and sterile attachments are necessary to deliver the gas intraabdominally (see Fig. 20.49). A sterile Verres needle is inserted abdominally and connected to polyethylene tubing attached to the insufflator. The carbon dioxide flows into the patient at about 1 liter/minute. Gauges on the insufflator indicate the amount of gas ejected into the cavity and are carefully monitored by the surgeon and circulating nurse. It is important that all pieces of the set fit snugly to prevent leakage of the gas during the procedure. Fogging of the lens is common during this procedure. Dipping the lens in a warm solution can keep this to a minimum.

PLASTIC SURGERY

The beginning practitioner in the operating room will also find specialized equipment in the area of plastic surgery. This branch of surgery deals with trauma patients, those with congenital problems, carcinoma, and psychoplastic surgeries. It is not restricted to any

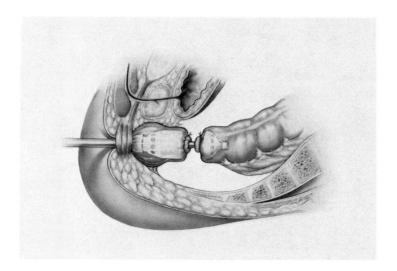

A

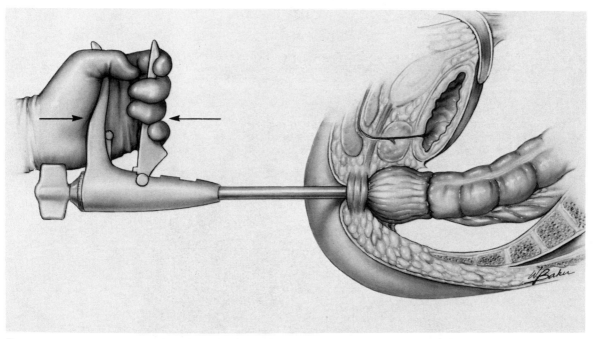

B

Figure 20.44. A, *In a low anterior resection EEA™ is used to perform the anastomosis. The EEA™ is introduced into the anus and advanced to the level of the purse string. The EEA™ is opened and the anvil is introduced into the proximal colon with the rectal purse string suture being tied. B, Ensure that the tissue is snug against the cartridge and anvil to reduce the possibility of bunching or overlapping as the tissue is approximated. Check that all tissue layers are incorporated within the loading unit prior to firing the staples. The EEA™ is closed and the staples fired. A circular double staggered row of staples joins the bowel, and simultaneously, the circular blade in the instrument cuts the stoma. (© USSC 1974, 1975, 1980).*

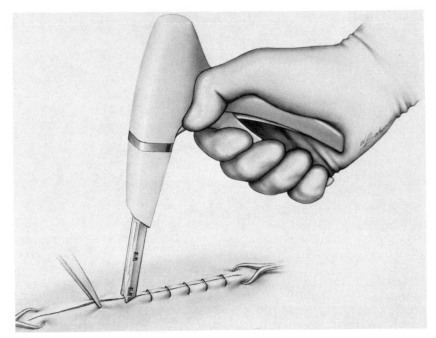

Figure 20.45. *The SFS™ model of Autosuture is used during skin closure. The cartridge tip rests lightly on the skin as the staples are placed by partially squeezing the handle. The staples are spaced at normal intervals for skin closure. (© USSC 1974, 1975, 1980).*

Figure 20.46. *A basic D & C set. In the lower right-hand corner is the weighted vaginal speculum put into position first. On the left, proceeding left to right, are shown Hagar dilators used to dilate the cervix. Uterine sound is used to measure the depth of the uterine cavity. Four curettes are used to scrape the wall of the internal uterine cavity to obtain specimen for diagnostic studies.*

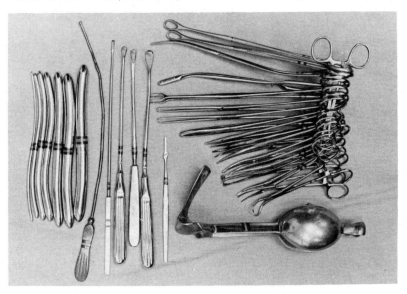

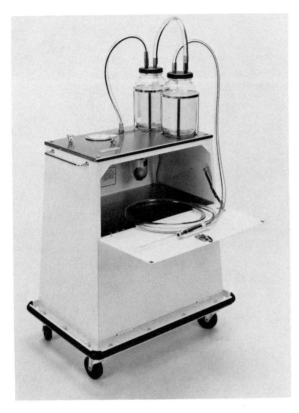

Figure 20.47. *The Berkeley VC-2 System with dual collection bottles. The tubing and cannula displayed on the open door are disposable and are available presterilized. (Photograph courtesy of Cooper Medical Devices Corp., Berkeley Bio-Engineering Division, San Leandro, CA.)*

particular anatomical area. This type of surgery deals first with restoration of function and second with appearance.

This specialty evolved out of the need to move and handle tissue gently and with technical exactness. The instruments are fine and delicate (see Fig. 20.50) as are the sutures and needles. Many of these procedures can be performed under local anesthesia.

What is done can often be visualized. Photographs are most helpful to the surgeon. The location of the incision is critical, and he may wish to sketch it out with the use of methylene blue marking pen.

Frequently used equipment in this specialty are dermatomes for grafting of tissue, gen-

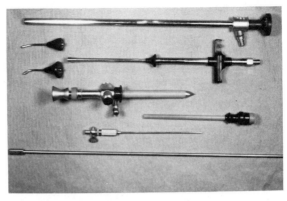

Figure 20.48. *The laparoscope allows for visualization of the pelvic cavity. As there are many pieces to a laparoscope setup, a checklist can be helpful to ensure the inclusion of all items and to check the total system during the setup process.*

erally from one part of the patient to another. These grafts can be removed by simple razor or knife, but generally dermatomes are used. These can be adjusted so various thicknesses of skin can be acquired. The split-thickness graft includes the entire epidermis and dermis (see Fig. 20.51).

Once the graft has been obtained, it should be kept in a moist, saline sponge or, if the edges tend to curl, placed on the bottom of a pan with the moist sponge over it. Every precaution should be taken to prevent dropping

Figure 20.49. *The insufflator contains CO_2 and delivers it intraabdominally via sterile tubing and Verres needle. Gauges on the panel indicate the amount ejected into the cavity.*

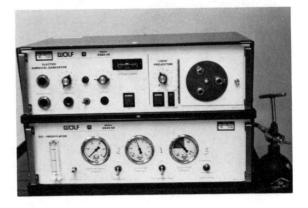

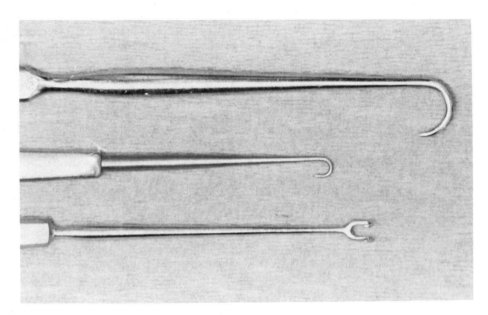

Figure 20.50. Skin hooks of various sizes are used to gently retract or elevate the skin. Notice the extremely small and fine hooks on these instruments.

Figure 20.51. A, The air-powered Brown dermatome is a popular type of dermatome used in obtaining skin grafts. Presterile, disposable, one-time-use blades are available. B, Padget dermatome is a manual instrument. The white tape displayed is attached to the drum and used to receive the skin graft as it is cut. The blade comes presterile and is disposable.

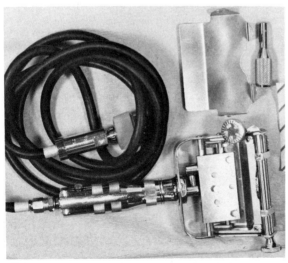

A

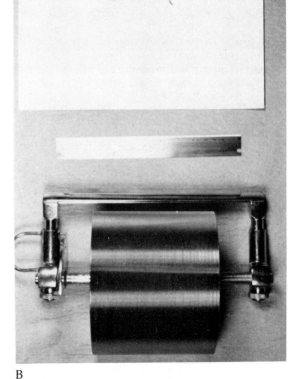

B

it. A small graft can be expanded to cover a larger area by multiple slits in the graft. This can be done automatically by passing the graft on a carrier through a skin mesher which uniformly places the slits. A variety of sizes are available which determine the expansion of the graft.

Seldom does the surgeon in this specialty have an assistant; therefore, the scrub person is the assistant. In this role the nurse will be suctioning, retracting tissue, cutting suture, and using the cautery under the doctor's supervision. While performing these activities, arm or hand support prevents any shaking motion.

ORTHOPEDIC SURGERY

Orthopedic surgery basically deals with bony structures of the body and requires completely different instruments and equipment from general surgery. The most frequent diagnosis in this area is fractures, with the goal of orthopedic surgery being to control pain and reestablish the patient's mobility. The type of treatment employed depends on the patient's condition, position of the fracture, bone healing capacity, and the dangers of infection.

For most orthopedic surgeries the general surgical table, with the patient in supine position, is all that is necessary. For the patient with a fractured hip or femur, a specially designed orthopedic table can provide traction and good alignment intraoperatively (see Figs. 20.52 and 20.53). These tables are equipped with x-ray shelves and cassette holders to allow for x-rays or fluoroscopic examination during the procedure (see Fig. 20.54).

Fracture tables are heavy and awkward to move and require two people to move and assemble. Once it is in position in the operating room, the nurse locks the table in place. This table can be used for many positions, each requiring different extensions. It is helpful to have each piece labeled and stored in an organized fashion for ease in accessibility and attachment.

It is essential that members of the orthopedic surgical team have a full understanding of the fracture table prior to use. What parts are needed, where they go, and how they are attached are all crucial problems that team members must be able to handle accurately and safely. As the electrocautery unit is used a great deal in orthopedic surgery, the metal parts of the fracture table that come in contact with the patient must be well padded to protect the patient from burns. The manufacturers of this equipment have brochures and extensive inservice programs available in the safe use of these tables. For hand and arm surgery, a side table extension or attachment can be slid into place on the regular surgery table.

Pneumatic tourniquets are generally used for all extremity surgery. They restrict the venous blood flow but do not totally prevent the arterial flow, allowing a clear view of the operative site (see Fig. 20.55). Care must be observed in the use of the tourniquet.

The cuff is applied far enough away from the incision site so it will not be in the way, and the area where it is to be applied is padded with sheet cotton. The padding must be kept smooth, as a wrinkle can cause skin or nerve damage. In a correctly sized cuff, there is an overlapping of the ends by 2–3 inches.

The nurse checks the gauge prior to use to be sure it is running properly and accurately. The surgeon will determine the pressure setting. The time that the tourniquet goes up must be documented on either the operating room nurse's notes or the anesthesia record. The surgeon should be informed of the length of time the tourniquet has been on at regular intervals during the surgery.

Instruments in orthopedics include periosteal elevators, bone holding clamps, bone cutting instruments (osteotomes, ronguers, curettes), drills, and miscellaneous others such as mallets and screwdrivers (see Figs. 20.56–20.61). These instruments allow the surgeon to align the bone fragments, cut and reshape the bone, and drill holes for the application of hardware to be held by screws fixing the fracture in place for healing.

Basic to patient care in orthopedic surgery is the use of plaster of paris as casting material. The purpose of this material is to immobilize the fracture site after bone alignment has been attained by either closed or open reduction. Prior to application of the plaster, the

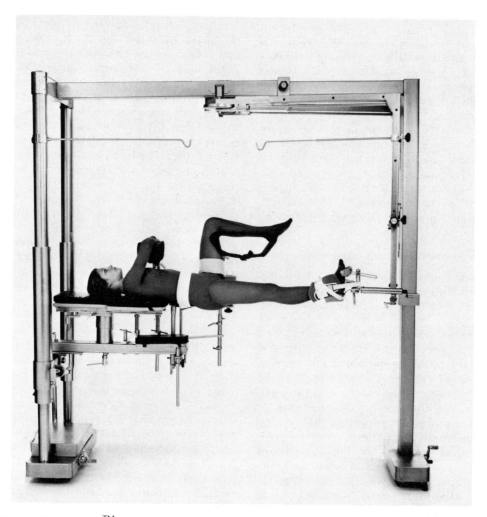

Figure 20.52. Chick-Langren™ *table setup for right hip pinning procedure. Patient is supine with the affected leg secured in traction and the nonaffected leg raised and abducted in the Well Leg Support Assembly. Cantilever table design and overhead suspension of leg spars allow easy access for mobile image intensifier placement. (Photograph courtesy of Chick® Orthopedic, Parke-Davis Orthopedic Division, Greenwood, S.C.)*

incision site will be dressed. The doctor will then pad the extremity or area to be casted with stockinette and sheet wadding to protect the patient's skin.

There are different types of plaster, some slow drying and some fast drying. The surgeon will determine which type to use. The plaster comes in dry rolls or splints that are immersed in water for application. A small bucket with water is needed. The plaster roll is dropped end first into the water. When the bubbles stop, the roll is ready to be removed from the water. The nurse squeezes the excess water from the roll by pushing both ends toward the middle. The nurse hands the roll to the doctor with the end pulled out so he can immediately begin to apply it. The plaster is very pliable and the doctor can mold it to fit the patient.

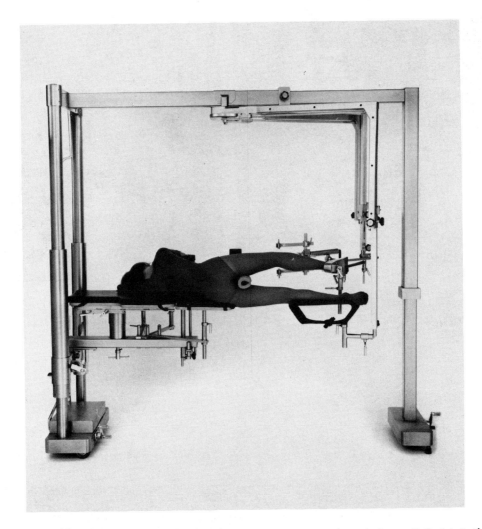

Figure 20.53. Chick-Langren™ table setup for closed/intramedullary nailing of the right femur. Patient is in the lateral decubitus position with nonaffected leg resting on the Well Leg Basket. The setup includes a 90-degree traction bow to accommodate either a Steinman pin or Kirshner wire. (Photograph courtesy of Chick® Orthopedic, Davis Orthopedic Division, Greenwood, S.C.)

Drying occurs quickly and the plaster solidifies, although not completely for several hours. Pillows under the extremity during the drying period will help to prevent indentations of the soft material.

Procedures in orthopedics can be very complex and may require additional background and specialization. Knowledge of prostheses and their very specialized instrumentation, as in total hip replacement and Harrington Rod spinal procedures, is necessary. The laminar air flow units may be used during these procedures.

AIR-POWERED EQUIPMENT

Air-powered equipment includes a variety of drills and saws used in several surgical special-

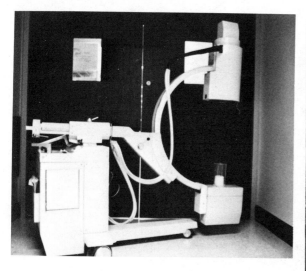

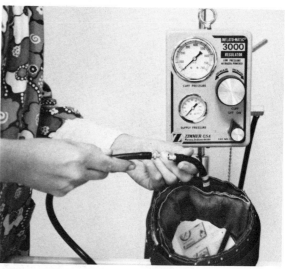

Figure 20.54. The C-Arm is a fluoroscopic imaging system which presents real-time images on a television monitor. This system is most frequently used intraoperatively on orthopedic procedures, particularly with the fractured hip patient.

Figure 20.55. Pneumatic Tourniquet is generally used in surgeries of the arms and legs. The cuff comes in a variety of sizes to match the extremity—larger for the male patient and surgery of the leg, smaller for children and surgery of the arm.

Figure 20.56. Periosteal Elevators, one-quarter-inch to one-inch wide, are used on the bone to scrape back the periosteal tissue, the outermost layer of the bone.

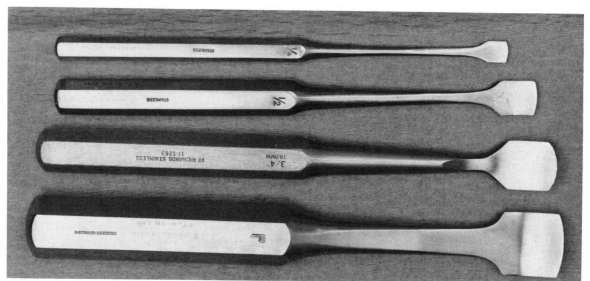

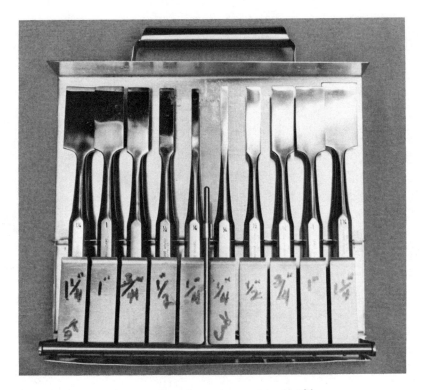

Figure 20.57. Osteotomes can be curved or straight and come in a variety of widths.

Figure 20.58. Osteotomes are used with a mallet to cut into the bone.

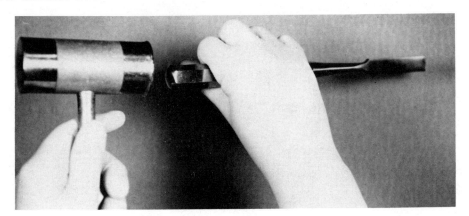

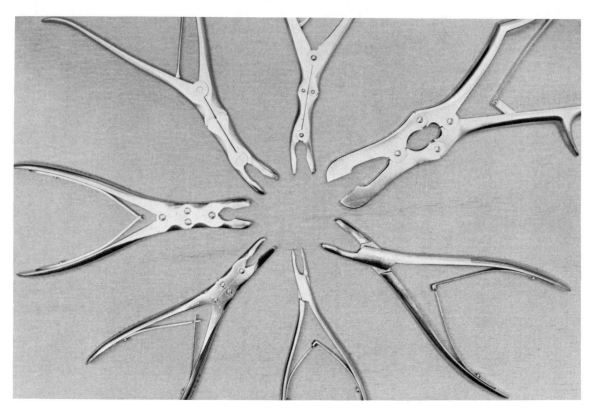

Figure 20.59. Rongeurs are used for biting into the bone. They are double or single action (two single-action ronguers are at the 4 and 6 o'clock positions with all the others being double actioned). The biting cup size also comes in various sizes and angles.

Figure 20.60. Curettes are used to scrape the bone tissue; they have different size cups and are available in a variety of angles and lengths.

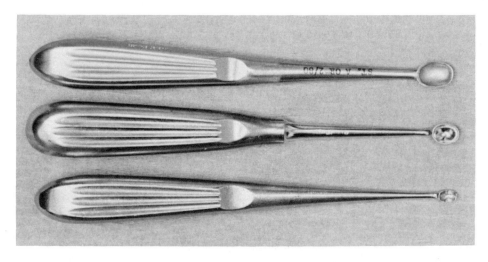

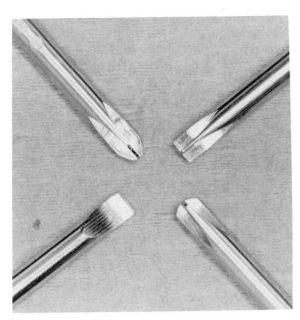

Figure 20.61. *Screw drivers are used to put the screws in place when fixating the fracture.*

ties for jobs related to sculpting, cutting, and repairing bony tissue. In 1961 the first powered drills were developed by Dr. Hall, a dentist. Prior to this, these techniques were performed by hand—a tedious procedure (see Fig. 20.62).

It was soon realized that powered equipment could reduce operative time and trauma to tissue dramatically. This, in turn, meant that the patient was under anesthesia for a shorter period. Today these drills are used in many specialties besides dentistry; orthopedics and neurosurgery are the most frequent, but they are also being used in maxillary facial, oto-microsurgery, and even heart surgery with the splitting of the sternum.

The power is obtained with the use of air or nitrogen under pressure. This compressed air can be stored in large portable type C tanks using a pressure gauge to control the flow at specified pounds per square inch (psi) (see Fig. 20.63). Or the compressed air can be piped into the operating suite in the same manner the suction vacuum, nitrous oxide, and oxygen are delivered. This type is controlled by a wall unit that acts as the pressure gauge and con-

Figure 20.62. *Until 1961 hand drilling was the only method available to the orthopedic surgeon and neurosurgeon. These drills are still available but are seldom used.*

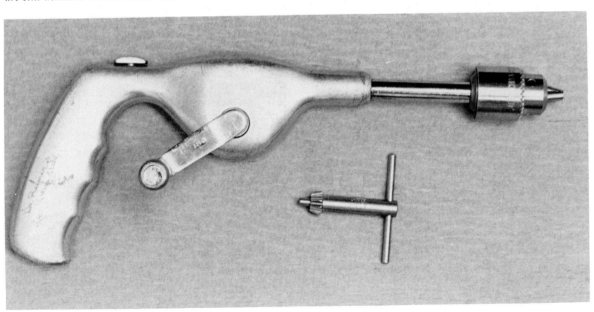

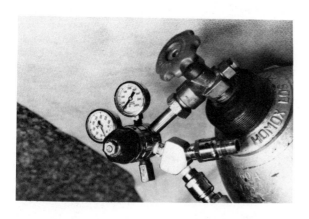

Figure 20.63. Air pressure determines the speed (rpm) of the air-powered equipment. When tanks of compressed air are used, they must be checked prior to the surgery to make sure that they contain sufficient air to complete the procedure. (Photograph courtesy of 3M Surgical Products Division, St. Paul, Minn. 55144.)

trols the flow delivering specific pounds of pressure. Special high-power hoses are used to connect the source of the power with the drill (see Fig. 20.64).

The pounds of pressure needed to drive the motor change with the job expected of the equipment. For microdrills, such as those used in otomicrosurgery, 80–90 psi is appropriate. For sculpting or cutting hard, large bones, a larger drill system of 110 psi with up to 20,000 rpm is used (see Fig. 24.65).

These drills are precision instruments and should be handled as such. Care is necessary in putting them together correctly and cleaning and oiling them after a procedure. The manufacturer's recommendations must be followed for sterilization. This equipment is never immersed in any liquid. Fluid will penetrate the interior of the drill and cause extensive rusting and damage necessitating expensive repairs and downtime. With rust accumulation, the motor will freeze up. There is danger to the patient, anger for the surgeon, and frustration for the nurses when a drill freezes during an operative procedure.

There are many attachments to each drill, with different ones being used at various

Figure 20.64. A, High-pressure hoses are sterilized with all air-powered equipment. These hoses deliver the compressed air to the equipment and allow for the exhaust. B, When attaching the air hose to the equipment, the fit should be snug, and the equipment tested prior to use on the patient. (Photograph courtesy of 3M Surgical Products Division, St. Paul, Minn. 55144.)

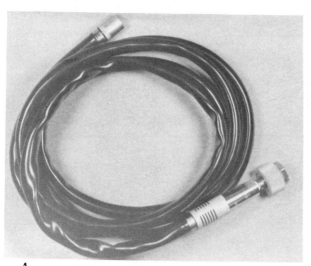

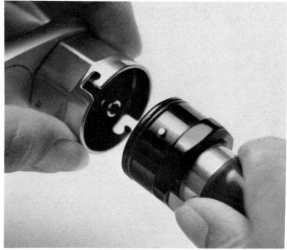

A

B

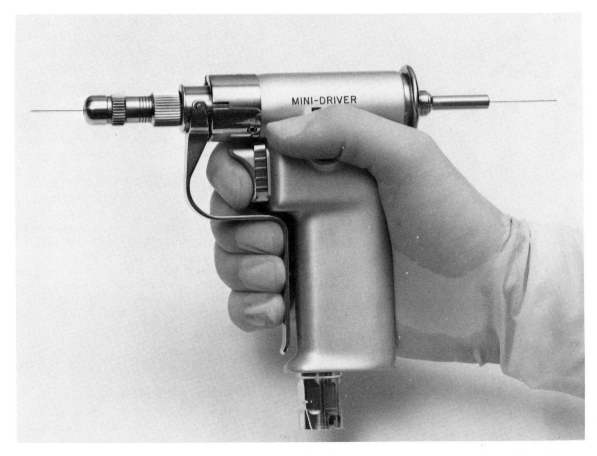

Figure 20.65. This 3M K111 Mini Driver is an example of modern air-powered equipment available to the surgeon. This is set up with the Swanson K-wire chuck attachment with K-wire in place. Normal operating pressure is 90–110 psi. (Photograph courtesy of 3M Surgical Products Division, St. Paul, Minn. 55144).

points in a procedure for a variety of jobs (see Fig. 20.66). A hole or several holes need to be drilled for the placement of a metal plate to hold the fracture together for healing. Here drill points, screw, and screw driver will be needed (see Fig. 20.67). Removing, reshaping, and reaming of bone at the knee or hip joint for placement of a total joint prosthesis require saws and blades of various sizes and shapes. Forward and reverse modes of speed are necessary for some of these activities. During a craniotomy, burr holes are drilled through the cranium and cut to eventually lift

a section of this bone out and away to allow for surgery on the brain.

There are three types of chucks that can be placed on the main drill body (see Fig. 20.68). Each chuck accepts other accessories, allowing for greater versatility of each piece of air-powered equipment. The pieces must match the chuck on the drill in order to use the motor's drive power.

There are several manufacturers of air-powered drills. All have extensive inservice programs in the care, handling, and operation of this equipment. This service needs to be

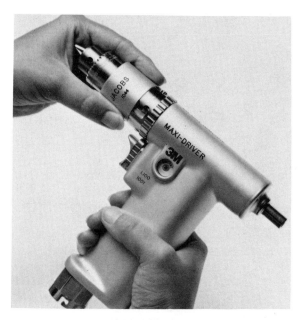

Figure 20.66. A Jacobs Chuck is being inserted into the 3M Maxi Driver. It is inserted into the handpiece opening. Snap the parts together until the release ring secures the chuck. To remove the chuck rotate the release ring and pull it out of the chuck. (Photograph and directions courtesy of 3M Surgical Products Division, St. Paul, Minn. 55144.)

used and presented frequently for initial instruction, to assist new staff members, and to remind everyone on at least a yearly basis that these are precision instruments that require a certain amount of care. With this care they will give good service and last a long time.

NEUROSURGERY

Closely related to orthopedics, neurosurgery has many bony structures removed or penetrated to reach the main structures of the nervous system. To reach the brain, a flap of bone from the cranium has to be removed or burr holes made through it. To reach the spinal cord, vertebra from the spinal column may be partially removed.

Many surgeries in this specialty are complex. Examples include suboccipital craniectomy, intracranial aneurysm, and acoustic neuroma with possible use of microneurosurgical prin-

ciples. The nurse functioning in this area is highly specialized and has extensive knowledge of neuroanatomy and the use of a multitude of highly specialized neurosurgical instruments. The beginning practitioner should be familiar with the equipment and instrumentation basic to this specialty.

One of the most frequently performed procedures is the laminectomy. This may be performed by either an orthopedist or a neurosurgeon depending on the diagnosis, the patient's selection, and the surgeon's expertise. In this procedure one or more of the vertebral laminae are removed to expose the spinal cord. This procedure is done most frequently for herniated disk and can be done at various levels of the spinal column, from cervical to lumbar, with the patient in prone, sitting, or lateral position. Lumbar laminectomies are the most common. The patient is usually prone, but some surgeons prefer the patient in the lateral position.

The standard surgery table is used for neurosurgery, but numerous attachments are added

Figure 20.67. The AMSCO Hall Orthairtome II is a multipurpose orthopedic drill capable of driving taps, screws, pins, and wires.(Photograph courtesy of AMSCO/Hall Surgical, Santa Barbara, Calif.)

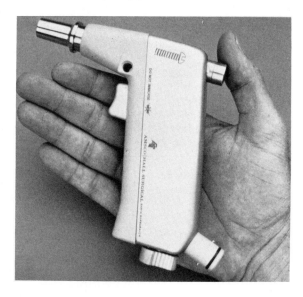

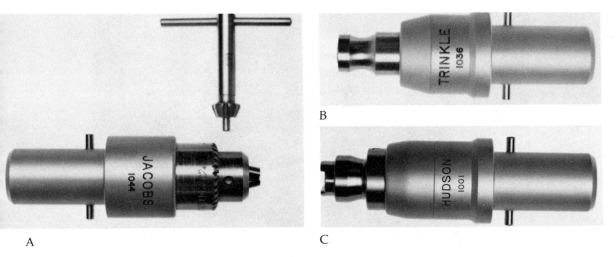

Figure 20.68. A, The L110 Jacobs Chuck for the 3M Maxi Driver is for use in driving up to one-quarter-inch pins, straight shank twist drills, to intramedullary reamers. Use the chuck key to loosen or tighten the chuck. B, The L112 Trinkle chuck is used in driving twist drills with trinkle arbors, or in powering automatic screwdrivers with trinkle arbors. The sleeve is retracted to accept drill or screwdriver fully. C, The Hudson Chuck is used during intramedullary reaming. The sleeve is retracted to accept a Hudson arbor or reamer. Release the sleeve to secure the attachment. (Photographs and caption courtesy of 3M Surgical Products Division, St. Paul, Minn. 55144.)

for the various surgeries. For the patient scheduled for lumbar laminectomy, rubber rolls or a frame are used to maintain the patient's position yet allow for continued ventilation (see Fig. 20.69). The type preferred by the surgeon should be listed on the doctor's preference card and should be ready on the operating room table when the patient arrives. The patient will be anesthetized and intubated on the stretcher and then turned and rolled over onto the operating room table and frame. Extra people are necessary to move the patient safely without injury to patient or staff. Extra padding may be needed. Care is necessary with the patient's arms and hands so they are moved in a physiologically sound manner and placed on well-padded arm boards. On the male patient it is essential that the external genitalia are in no way compromised by the frame or table due to this position.

The instruments used for this procedure are a basic neurosurgical set plus special laminectomy instruments which include currettes and ronguers of various types, periosteal elevators, and nerve root retractors (see Figs. 20.70–20.72).

Basic to all types of neurosurgery is the cautery unit for the control of hemorrhage. Along with the regular cautery machine, the neurosurgeon will use a bipolar coagulation unit with forceps (see Fig. 20.73). The unit isolates the current output with very little leakage at the forcep tip, allowing its use close to vital structures without damaging them. As it is a bipolar cautery unit, a grounding plate is not necessary.

For many neurosurgical procedures on the cranium, a head rest is essential. There are several types available that can be adapted for use in a variety of patient positions. To use the head rest, the head section to the standard surgery table needs to be removed. The prongs of the head rest will fit into the head section of the surgery table (see Fig. 20.74).

For surgeries of the head and neck, the standard Mayo stand is not suitable; it is not large enough for the instruments needed. Special neurosurgical overhead tables have been developed of which the Mayfield is one (see Fig. 20.75). This is placed over the patient and draped to include it in the sterile field. In place, this table is much higher than the Mayo

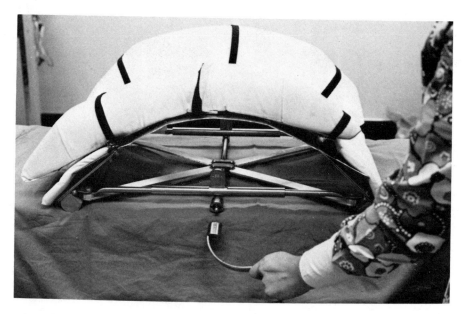

Figure 20.69. *The Wilson Convex Frame is used in position by the lumbar laminectomy patient in a prone position. The frame can be raised or lowered using the handle shown.*

Figure 20.70. *Kerrison Rongeurs are specifically designed to facilitate the removal of lamina bone during a lumbar laminectomy. A variety of angled jaws are available.*

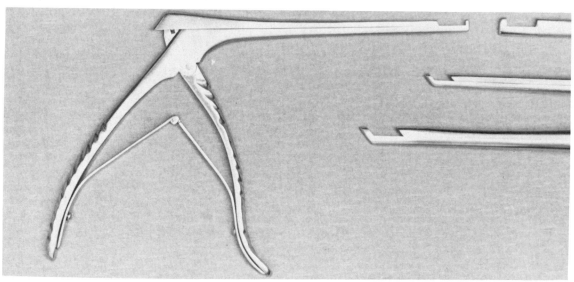

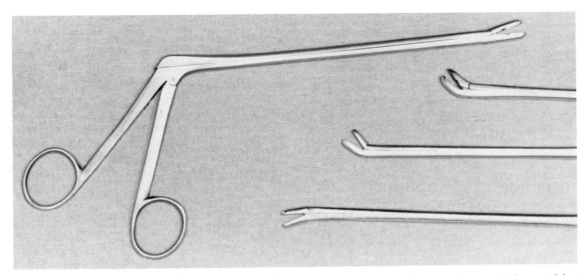

Figure 20.71. Pituitary rongeurs come in various cup sizes and angles. They can be used to remove herniated disk material during laminectomies or to biopsy brain or tumor tissue. Depending on the cup size, they can be used for macro or micro surgery.

Figure 20.72. Nerve root retractors are specifically designed to gently move the nerves coming directly out of the spinal cord.

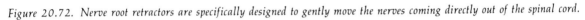

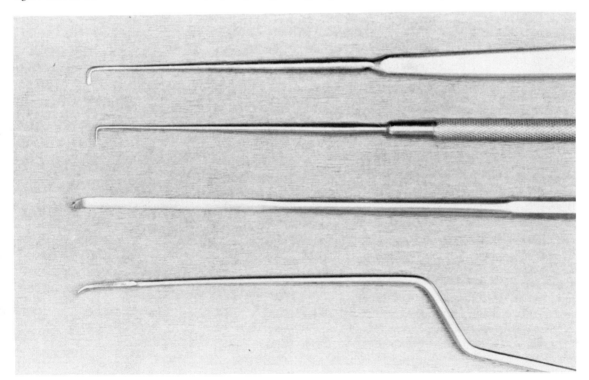

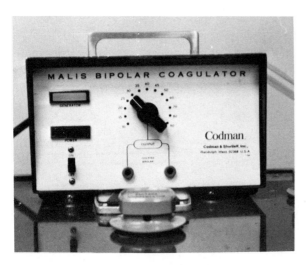

Figure 20.73. The bipolar coagulation unit isolates completely the output of current between the tips of the cautery forceps. This allows the use of the coagulation current in close proximity to vital structures without damage to them.

stand, and the scrub person will need a long high lift to stand on in order to reach everything. Once it has been draped off, the scrub person will move the necessary instruments onto it.

Basic to any craniotomy procedure is the air-powered equipment used to penetrate and remove parts of the cranium. The 3M Craniotome (see Fig. 20.76) is the latest development in this area and has numerous attachments, including the perforator which is used to penetrate the skull. The perforator can be replaced with a blade and dura guard to cut the bone flap. This is also interchangeable with a wire-pass drill bit which is used when the bone flap is replaced at the closure and wired into place.

These few pieces of equipment are only a sample of the innumerable ones being used in neurosurgery today. There are many changes occurring as microneurosurgery develops with the use of microscope, video screens, and new microsurgical instruments. The nursing specialist learns to handle these skillfully after many additional hours of study and practice beyond the beginning practitioner.

OPHTHALMIC SURGERY

The human eye is an extraordinary organ in the body. It provides one of the most precious senses we have, sight. A great deal of progress has been made in the last 30 years in eye surgery.

Think of the anatomy of the eye and remember how small and delicate the eye and all its parts are. The instruments used for surgery in this area match this anatomy and are small, fine, and delicate, as well as expensive. Special care is needed in the handling of these instruments (see Fig. 20.77).

Before handling these instruments the scrub person and surgeons should wash their gloved hands to remove any powder that could be on them. Grains of powder could cause granulomas or other healing problems that could be devastating to the eye. At first glance, because they are so small and delicate, eye instruments appear very different from basic surgical instruments. On closer examination, it can be seen that they are similar. There are scalpels, clamps, forceps of various types, scissors, and needle holders.

Figure 20.74. The Gardner headrest is a three-point skeletal traction device used in numerous craniotomies. It provides stability to the patient's head during surgery.

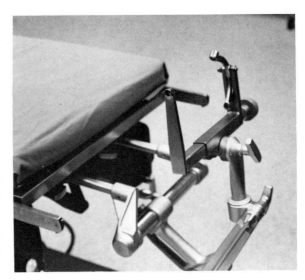

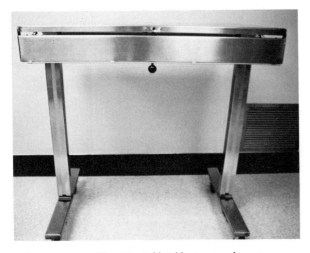

Figure 20.75. The Mayfield table is extra large to accommodate the numerous instruments necessary for intracranial procedures. The height of the table allows it to be positioned over the patient in a sitting position.

Unlike other instruments, these instruments should not be handled by the points or tips, but they must still be handed to the surgeon in position of use. This is doubly important as most procedures in ophthalmic surgery are performed through the operative microscope, and the surgeon will generally not take his eyes away from the scope to see what the scrub person is doing. Every time he looks away from the scope his eyes must adjust and refocus, and to look back through the scope requires another adjustment.

The operative microscope has made many eye surgeries possible and greatly facilitates the more common ones such as cataract extraction. These microscopes are also used in ear, plastic, neuro, and vascular surgeries.

These scopes can either be on a rolling stand or mounted on a ceiling rack (see Figs. 20.78 and 20.79). When moving the microscope on the stand, great care must be taken since it tends to be top heavy and can tip over. The head and arms of the scope must be kept in, close to the center post with the head over the longest arm of the foot piece, and moved slowly. Touching the lens will cause smudging. The microscope lens should be cleaned only with lens paper and special lens solution.

These microscopes are used to illuminate and magnify the operative site. By having better view of the site, greater delicacy and finesse of procedure can be performed. The lens system can be adjusted during the procedure from 6 to 40 times in power, without adjusting the height of the scope from the operative site.

Many microscopes can accommodate an observer arm, which is an additional lens attached to the microscope head to allow the assistant, scrub person, or the circulating nurse to visualize the progress of the surgery.

When not in use, the microscopes should be covered to prevent dust from accumulating on the lens and other delicate parts. The ceiling mounted scopes can and should be removed from the mounting when not in use and placed in the padded box provided by the manufacturer.

In using the small fine instruments for eye surgery under the miscroscope, the surgeon must use equally as fine motions on the delicate, small anatomy where he is working. This takes great concentration on his part. It is essential that the environment around him be

Figure 20.76. The 3M Craniatome can be used for burr holes when attached to the perforator. Remove the perforator and to the remaining motor add the neurotome blade and dura guard which can be used to carve out bone to facilitate exposure of the brain. (Photograph courtesy of 3M Surgical Products Division, St. Paul, Minn. 55144.)

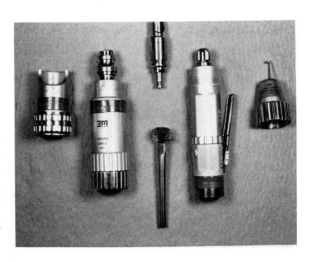

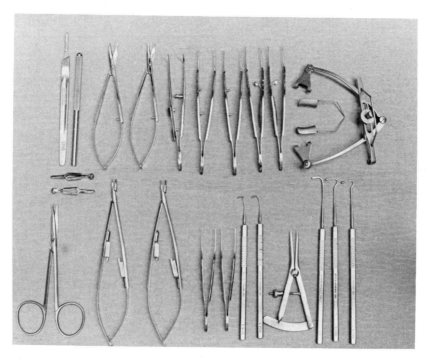

Figure 20.77. This basic cataract set demonstrates the delicate design of eye instruments. These instruments must be gently and carefully handled at all times.

conducive for this. A quiet atmosphere must be planned, including no phone calls or use of any intercommunication system. Talking and traffic must be kept to a minimum.

One of the most common eye surgeries is cataract extraction. Today there are several techniques that can be used: intracapsular extraction using the cryoextractor, the extracapsular method, artificial lens implantation, or phacoemulsification using ultrasonic energy to fragment the inner lens material with aspiration.

Figure 20.80 shows the cryosurgical system. This is a nonelectrical system that uses nitrous oxide as a controlled, rapid cooling agent. The temperatures can drop to −80°C. Control is by foot pedal and can be operated by the surgeon during the procedure. There are a variety of cryoprobes of different angles that are available. Dual tanks of nitrous oxide are attached to the backside of the console and table.

When the surgeon depresses the pedal, nitrous oxide is released causing rapid cooling of the probe. By releasing the pedal, defrosting automatically occurs. The temperature can be adjusted by regulating the pressure of the gas flow. This is done by the circulating nurse turning the labeled control knob on the front of the console.

This element is used in cataract surgery at the point of removal of the lens. After the incision has been made and the lens exposed, a cryoprobe is used to touch the lens, freezing it almost instantaneously. This solidifies the lens material allowing for easy removal from the eye through the incision. The principle of cryosurgery is also useful in gynecology, otolaryngoscopy, and proctology.

OTOMICROSURGERY

The anatomy and physiology of hearing is complex, and much of it is contained within a

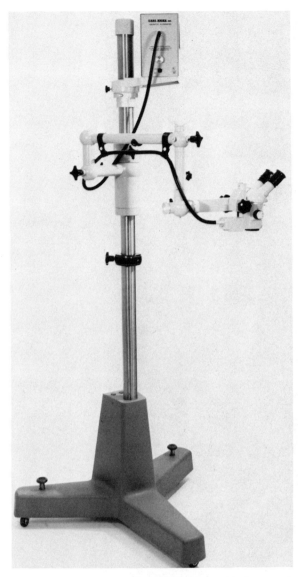

Figure 20.78. The Zeiss OPM 1 with moveable floor stand. Since the invention of the operative microscope, microsurgical procedures have spread to various surgical disciplines. (Photograph courtesy of the Karl Zeiss, Inc., New York, N.Y. 10018.)

very small bony anatomical area. The instruments and equipment used in this specialty reflect this anatomy. The instruments of otomicrosurgery are smaller than those for ophthalmic surgery (see Fig. 20.81).

Part of the complexity in ear surgery is due to the tiny operative field that is involved with surgery through an ear speculum (see Fig. 20.82) and the use of the operative microscope for illumination and magnification (see Figs. 20.78 and 20.79). It is a unique specialty. It cannot be easily mastered but the student needs, and can develop, a general awareness of otomicrosurgery as performed in today's operating room. Close teamwork is required in this area.

Otomicrosurgery requires very tiny delicate instruments which can tolerate very little abuse (see Fig. 20.83). Great care must be taken to protect them. There are several types of metal boxes available for these instruments. These instruments should be stored and sterilized in such a box to protect them from damage. These metal boxes are also useful in protecting delicate eye instruments (see Fig. 20.84).

Great care must be taken with these instruments so that they are not dropped, dumped together, or subject to rough handling. Because of the very fine picks, scalpels, and curettes on the instruments and the tiny cups on the alligator forceps of various shapes and sizes, very little force is needed to fracture these delicate instruments.

With these tiny instruments, it is essential that the scrub person have good eyesight as it is difficult to distinguish differences in the minute tips of the ear instruments. Some of the instruments may be engraved on the handle with distinctive marks to assist the scrub person. Special instrument wipe material is available to clean them during surgery. A toothbrush is also helpful.

As in eye surgery, the atmosphere in the suite is an essential element. All must be in readiness when the patient and surgeon arrive to prevent any unnecessary activity or noise. Telephone and any other intercom system should be turned off and not used. This could disturb the surgeon at the moment he is performing a delicate move. Each move must be precise, and noise can cause an unnecessary, unwanted motion.

As with eye surgery, the gloves of the scrub person and surgeons need to be washed prior to handling the sterilized instruments. Powder can act as a foreign body in the wound. If

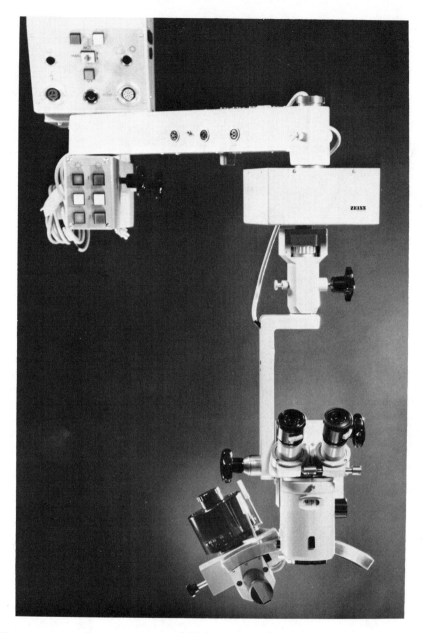

Figure 20.79. There are a variety of support systems available for mounting the operative microscope, with the latest addition being the ceiling mounted. This design allows total freedom of movement around the operating table. (Photograph courtesy of the Karl Zeiss, Inc., New York, N.Y. 10018.)

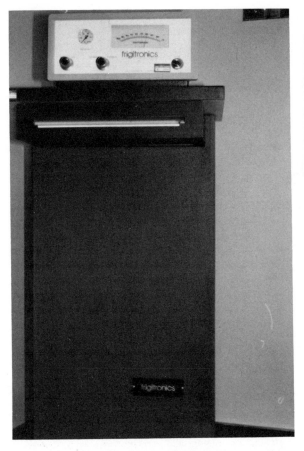

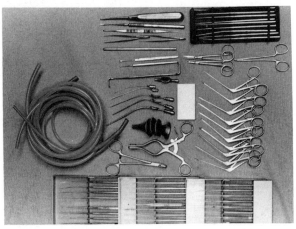

Figure 20.81. The development of these delicate instruments for ear surgery, coupled with the use of the operative microscope, allows the surgeon to perform numerous surgeries of the ear.

Figure 20.80. Frigitronic Cryoextractor use in cataract extraction for the removal of the lens by freezing the tissue. Small probes are used to deliver the freezing nitrous oxide to the lens.

Figure 20.82. In performing ear surgery the surgeon works through an ear speculum. The Shea speculum holder secures the speculum in place and maintains its position, allowing a free second hand for the surgeon.

unwashed and washed gloves are compared under a microscope the amount of powder and lint that can cling to the unwashed gloves can be seen. Both items can be transferred to the instruments and into the wound, causing problems for the patient.

The scrub person must hand the instruments in a method usable by the surgeon. This can be difficult as the operative site will not be readily visible. An observation arm on the microscope is helpful for both the circulating nurse and scrub person.

After the surgeon has received an instrument, he may wish the scrub person to guide his hands back into the line of his microscope

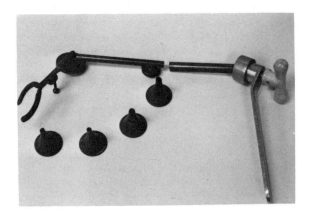

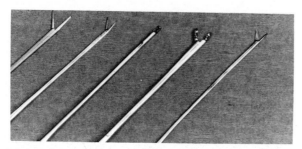

Figure 20.83. *The tips of some of the ear instruments are very small and difficult for the scrub person to see. Notice the cups and scissors.*

vision. For the surgeon to remove his eyes from the scope necessitates refocusing back and forth to the scope's magnification.

As the inner ear structures are surrounded by bone, it is often necessary to use drills of various sizes and shapes. The earliest drills used in the area were modifications of dental drills. Two common drills used in this area today are the Micro Drill and the Shea Drill (see Figs. 20.85 and 20.86).

The drill points are very small and are of various types and sizes: diamond burrs, cross-cutting burrs, and polishing burrs.

ENDOSCOPY

Endoscopy is the visualization of a body cavity that allows for inspection of its contents and walls. It can be as simple as reviewing the eye grounds and ear canal during a basic physical examination. It can be as complex as intraoperative nephroscopy or retrograde cholangiopancreatography. The procedures of endoscopy are major tools for diagnostic studies and are becoming methods for treatment in many specialties.

The equipment used in this area has greatly changed since the first endoscope was developed in 1806 by the German Bozzini. The first instrument was a simple metal tube with reflective candle light using a hand mirror. Today the rigid metal scopes are still being used but with many refinements over the original.

Great strides were made in endoscopy as the science of electricity became refined. Edison's

light bulb allowed for the development of light carriers being placed in the scopes. Lamm's discovery of fiberoptics in 1930 brought further progress in lighting systems. Fiberoptics uses multiple microscopic glass fibers, wrapped in a sheath, which allow light to travel through them without distortion (see Fig. 20.87).

Developments in optics have also influenced endoscopy. In 1879 Nitze developed the first telescope to be used for visualization of a deep internal cavity such as the bladder. This telescope used several small lenses separated by larger air spaces. Recently this system has been reversed by Harold Hopkins in England using larger glass rods and small air spaces. This new system allows for greater resolution and magnification with wider field of vision. Resolution is the clarity of detail that can be seen. Because of this the best feature has become the ability to take still and motion pictures allowing for detailed observation and examination of areas of concern.

Many endoscopic procedures can be performed in the physician's office or on an outpatient basis in the hospital. We are concerned here with those procedures most likely to be performed in the operating room, be they

Figure 20.84. *Storage and sterilization of any of the delicate instruments such as those of ear surgery are greatly facilitated by these metal boxes.*

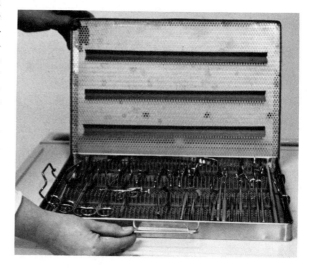

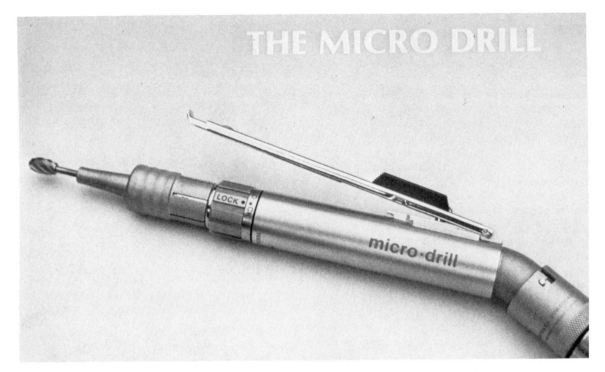

THE MICRO DRILL

Figure 20.85. The AMSCO Hall Micro Drill drives a variety of burs for sculpting bone and can be utilized on ear surgery. (Photograph courtesy of AMSCO/Hall Surgical, Santa Barbara, Calif.)

Figure 20.86. The Shea Drill is another popular drill used in ear surgery.

Figure 20.87. Fiberoptic illumination is crucial in endoscopic procedures.

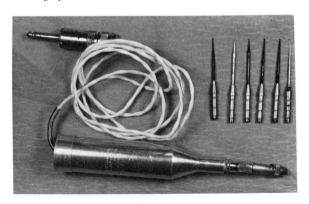

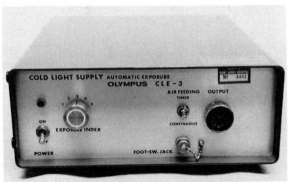

under general or local anesthesia. Some operating rooms have an area set aside for such procedures, an endoscopic room or the "cysto" room for urological procedures.

Some endoscopic procedures can be performed through natural openings such as bronchoscopy, cystoscopy, and colonoscopy. Others are performed through small incisions such as the arthroscopy and laparoscopy. Still others are done during major surgical procedures such as the choledochoscopy and nephroscopy.

Bronchoscopy is an example of the first group and is used to inspect the trachea, main stem of the bronchus, and smaller bronchi. This procedure can also be performed to remove a foreign body, such as a peanut or pin, or other type of obstruction to the airway. It is sometimes used for deep suctioning in patients with atelectasis.

Small biopsies or brushings can be taken of suspicious areas of the bronchial tree (see Fig. 20.88), or bronchial washings can be performed by inserting 5–10 cc of saline followed by suctioning. A good suction flow is essential during this procedure. A Luken's tube (see Fig. 20.89) can be attached to the suction tubing to gather specimens which are then sent to the laboratory for cytological examination. Fractional studies of the bronchial tree

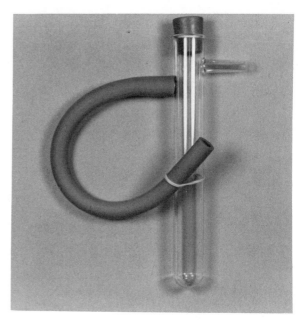

Figure 20.89. The Luken's Tube is attached to the suctioning system used in bronchoscopy to collect specimens for cytologic examination.

necessitate multiple specimens. The locations of these specimens need to be carefully labeled and documented by the circulating nurse.

Bronchoscopy can be performed in many different modes: the patient may be under local or general anesthesia, the patient's position may be supine or sitting, the bronchoscope may be rigid or flexible. The combination used depends on the doctor and his expertise with the equipment and the type of study to be performed. The rigid bronchoscope (see Fig. 20.90) is inserted as a laryngoscope would be in the mouth, nasopharynx, then past the vocal cords into the trachea and on into the bronchial tree. Inspection occurs as insertion takes place. The doctor views the area directly without the use of a telescope. The flexible bronchoscope may be inserted in the same manner or through the nose. The nasal insertion is preferred by many doctors and patients. Vision here is through a series of minute lenses (see Fig. 20.91).

Under local anesthesia, patient cooperation is necessary. Meticulous preoperative prepara-

Figure 20.88. The small biopsy cup and brush used in some endoscopic procedures to obtain specimens.

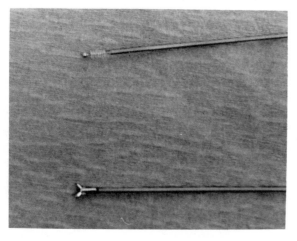

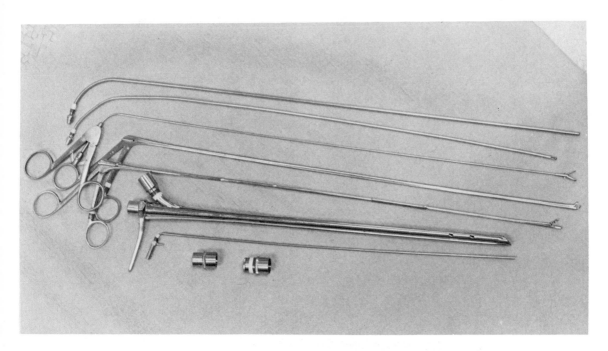

Figure 20.90. *The rigid bronchoscope comes in various sizes. It is basically a hollow tube that provides direct visualization of the area being inspected. Illumination is provided by fiberoptics. Long rigid suction cannulas are essential to remove any secretions.*

Figure 20.91. *The flexible, narrow diameter bronchoscope with movable tip has greatly facilitated and extended the type of examinations now possible of the bronchial tree.*

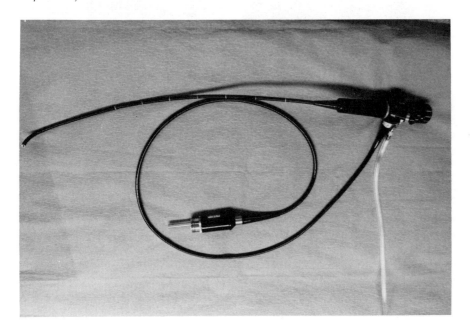

tion of the patient is essential. This preparation can make the difference between a successful and an unsuccessful procedure. As the patient's airway is involved in the examination, anxiety can be very high. Reassurance throughout the procedure is necessary. Patients prefer the thin flexible scopes as they eliminate most of the discomfort.

This procedure at best is a clean procedure. Rigid scopes should be sterilized between patients. The flexible fiberoptic scopes should be well cleaned and disinfected with an appropriate germicide. Many hospitals use povidone-iodine or glutaraldehyde for these scopes. They must all be rinsed extremely well after use of these solutions (see Fig. 20.92). The manufacturer's instructions must be followed care-

Figure 20.92. Proper cleaning of the flexible scope between procedures is essential.

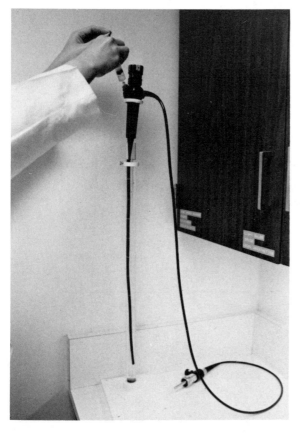

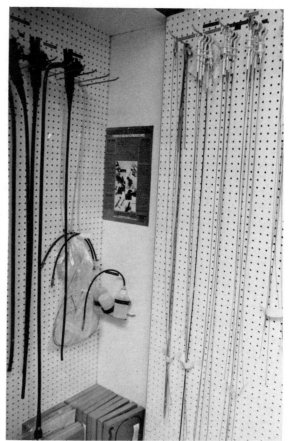

Figure 20.93. Storage of any of the flexible scopes is greatly facilitated by a cabinet where the scopes and flexible biopsy forceps can hang free.

fully. Storage of flexible scopes can be greatly facilitated by a special storage cabinet that allows them to hang full length. This prevents bending and kinking of the scopes and possible breakage to the fiberoptic glass rods or damage to the delicate lens system (see Fig. 20.93).

Another frequently performed endoscopic procedure is *cystoscopy*. The urologist performs this procedure to visualize the interior of the urinary bladder and adjacent structures to assist him in diagnosing a variety of urinary tract pathologies. Simple cystoscopy takes only minutes to complete.

The cystoscope is composed of an interchangeable fiberoptic telescope with various sheaths (see Fig. 20.94). A fiberoptic light source and cord will be needed to activate the lighting system. The cystoscope also contains a system of entry for irrigation solution which is necessary to distend the bladder for visualization of the bladder wall. Introduction of the cystoscope is through the urethra. Lubrication on the sheath facilitates the passing of this instrument.

This procedure can be performed on a standard operating room table with the patient in modified lithotomy position, but most operating rooms have a separate "Cysto Room" which contains a special urology table. This table is adapted to contain and drain all the solution necessary during the procedure. The table also allows for x-rays to be taken for retrograde and other studies.

Another urological endoscopic procedure is the *transurethral resection*. This procedure is done through the scope for the removal of hypertrophy or malignant prostatic tissue or tumor of the bladder neck of slight to moderate size with the use of a resectoscope and cutting electrodes. There are several types of scopes that can be used for this procedure, depending upon the surgeon's preference.

These scopes are complex and delicate, using the basic principles of cystoscopy. They are composed of telescope sheaths, obturators, cutting electrodes, and the working element which provides the motion to the cutting loops.

High-frequency current is passed from the electrocautery unit to the insulated cutting loops. All the precautions necessary for the use of the electrocautery unit need to be followed meticulously during the procedure.

Copious amounts of irrigating solution will be used during this procedure. Neither distilled water nor saline are used for this procedure. Since water is hypotonic and saline disperses the coagulating current, glycine or sorbital is used. With this solution being used, it must be remembered that water is an excellent conductor of electricity. The care of the patient must reflect the danger of this element, and the surgical team must also be cautious for their own safety. The field needs to be kept as dry as possible.

Catheter drainage for most urological procedures is desirable postoperatively. The circulating nurse should be prepared for this with a variety of Foley catheters of various types and sizes.

Figure 20.94. The cystoscope is a very delicate multilensed telescope used to visualize the bladder wall. It is available in various Foley sizes and angles to the lens. The lens at the top of the picture is 30 degrees and the second one is straightforward. The sheaths and obturator are displayed at the bottom of the picture.

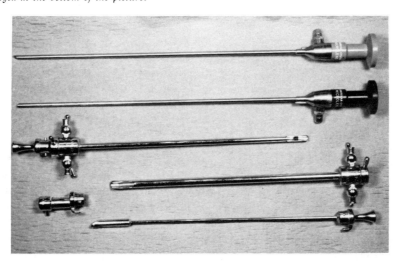

Major operative procedures can use endoscopy, as seen with the use of the choledochoscope during a cholecystectomy. The same instrument can be used during a ureterolithotomy for visualization further into the ureter or into the kidney pelvis. In both instances retained calculi are generally being sought.

Via a small incision in the common bile duct, a right-angled 40-mm choledochoscope is inserted into the hollow viscus. The duct must be expanded to see the interior—the same principle as in cystoscopy of the urinary bladder. The choledochoscope has two basic components: the fiberoptic telescope for visualization and the cannula pathway for delivery of the irrigation solution.

Because the duct is so small, irrigation under pressure is necessary. Normal saline in a plastic bag is preferred because a pressure cuff can be slipped over the bag. The pressure cuff can maintain 300 mm Hg on the body during the procedure. The choledochoscope is attached via sterile tubing to the irrigating solution hung on an intravenous standard. The pressure exerted is sufficient to dilate the duct for visualization and flush out the area.

When a stone is spotted, the scope is grasped and removed with a Randall stone forcep. After removal the area is visualized again with the scope. A full flushing with irrigation solution is done to wash out any bits of calculi. This sounds simple but, indeed, can be tedious and time-consuming.

If visualization further than 40 mm is needed, 60-mm choledochoscopes are available, although seldom used. Some surgeons may use a Fogarty balloon catheter (biliary) or Dormier stone baskets for removal of stones. Flushing is necessary after their use also. A biopsy forcep or brush can also be inserted through the choledochoscope to obtain tissue specimens for histological and cytological examination. A separate sterile field should be set up for this instrumentation to protect the telescope and other parts from inadvertent abuse, such as placing heavy instruments on top of them.

An individual checklist for endoscopic procedures is helpful, particularly for laparoscopy and choledocoscopy where many small pieces, sterile and unsterile, are needed. These checklists will maintain everyone's sanity plus provide efficient, safe patient care. Gentleness is the key to handling all telescopes and fiberoptics.

PACEMAKERS

Pacemakers are necessary when the heart can no longer sustain sufficient beats, as in heart block or arrhythmias with failure of the heart's conductive system. With decreased heart rate, there is a decrease in the amount of oxygen to the heart and brain.

Pacemakers were first implanted in the early 1950s. Today, there are basically two types of pacemakers used for this artificial stimulation of the heart muscle: fixed rate and demand rate. The fixed rate is just that. It is set at a certain rate, for example 70 beats per minute, and stimulates every heart beat. The demand type fires off only when necessary and uses the patient's own ability to beat or not to beat, which will trigger the demand pacemaker into action.

Initially this procedure needs to be performed under fluoroscopy for correct placement of the electrode in the heart muscle. Placement is crucial, as a common problem for these patients is displacement of the electrode (see Fig. 20.95). Time needs to be taken at the point of insertion for proper testing with the Pacing Systems Analyzer (PSA). The PSA is a computer used to test the electrode placement and pacemaker. It assists in finding the best position for the electrode in the heart muscle.

Is the myocardium at the point of contact appropriate? Is it sufficiently sensitive to the stimulation? The testing also assists in determining the specific type of generator appropriate for this patient. The circulating nurse may be asked to use this device. If this is the policy at your hospital, complete knowledge and familiarity with the PSA is necessary before attempting to use it. Pacemaker companies are very willing to present detailed inservices of their equipment. There are many changes and improvements occurring in this field. When the patient is scheduled for battery change only, fluoroscopy is not necessary as

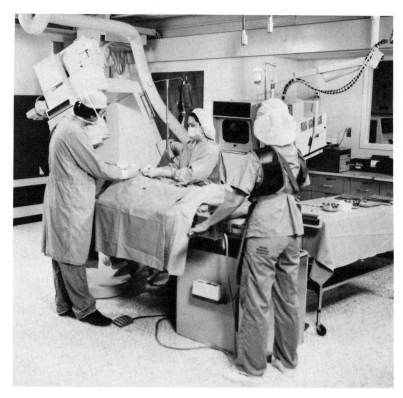

Figure 20.95. The Fluoricon intensifier imaging system utilized during pacemaker insertions for proper placement of cardiac leads. (Photograph courtesy of General Electric Medical Systems Division, Milwaukee, Wis. 63201.)

the electrode is already in place, although placement may be tested.

Today's pacemakers are also programmable, and the functions can be tailored to each patient's specific needs. The established program can be changed as the patient's condition changes. This decreases the need for additional operative procedures to change the pacemaker. The new lithium-powered pacemakers have greater longevity, which again has decreased the number of procedures necessary to sustain the patient (see Fig. 20.96). This procedure may be performed in either the operating room or a special procedures room of the radiology department.

A temporary pacemaker may be used for a period of time in the patient with heart block, prior to surgical implantation to stabilize the patient. This can also be used after myocardial infarct to stabilize rhythm or during drug therapy for arrhythmias.

Most of these procedures are performed under local anesthesia or with standby for general anesthesia. The emergency cart with defibrillator and drugs needs to be readily available. The ECG monitor should be in place along with intravenous solution and oxygen available.

Some of the basic instruments and equipment of surgery as used by the circulating nurse and scrub person are discussed. A few from specialty areas such as orthopedic, neurosurgery, otomicrosurgery, and endoscopy are also covered.

Although many instruments and pieces of

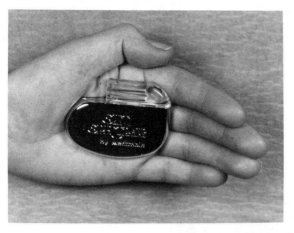

Figure 20.96. *The Medtronic Spectrax™ programmable pacemaker weighs 45 gm and is only 10 mm thin. (Courtesy of Medtronic, Inc., Minneapolis Minn. 55440.)*

operating room is necessary—whether that experience is for one month or twenty years. Innovative procedures are constantly being developed, and there are always improvements and new developments in instruments and equipment used in the operating room.

One last piece of equipment needs to be discussed as surgery is completed. The dressing is in place and the patient is ready to be transferred back to the gurney for transportation to the postanesthesia room. The Robinson roller (see Fig. 20.97) is very helpful in moving the patient, still under the effects of general anesthesia, from the operating room table to the gurney.

Suggested Readings

Aldridge, L. L. "Electrosurgical safety: A continuing concern." *D & G Gown Gloves* 1:11, 1976 (Davis & Geck, American Cyanamide Co.).

American Heart Association. *Advanced Cardiac Life Support.* Dallas: AHA, 1980.

Brooks, S. *Fundamentals of Operating Room Nursing.* St. Louis: C. V. Mosby, 1975.

equipment are covered, many others that the beginning operating room practitioner will encounter are not. This is an immense area of knowledge, and this chapter presents only an introduction to the subject. Continued investigation throughout one's experience in the

Figure 20.97. *The roller is a very helpful piece of equipment in moving the unconscious patient. It moves the patient gently and safely, plus assists the surgery team by preventing muscle strains when moving the patient.*

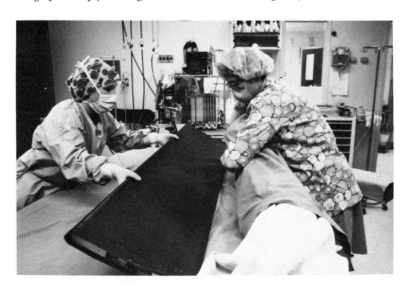

Brzenski, T. S. "Pacemaker: Pulse of life." *AORN J* 32:967, 1980.

Calvin, J. W. "Intraoperative pacemaker electrical testing." *Ann Thorac Surg* 26:165, 1978.

Campbell, E. E. "Modern trends in surgery for hearing." *Point View* 15:4, 1978 (Ethicon Inc.).

The Care & Handling of Surgical Instruments. Randolph, Mass.: Codman & Shurtleff, 1977.

Church, R., Hamlin, Wm. T. "Electrosurgery demands OR vigilance." *AORN J* 22:903, 1975.

Cloward, R. B. *Signature Series 3: Surgical Techniques for Lumbar Disc Lesions*. Randolph, Mass.: Codman & Shurtleff, 1975.

Cloward, R. B. *Signature Series 4: Ruptured Cervical Intervertebral Discs*. Randolph, Mass.: Codman & Shurtleff, 1975.

Coates, H. W., ed. *Care and Handling of Surgical Instruments*. Chicago: American V. Mueller, 1980.

Committee on Infection Control in Handling Endoscopic Equipment. "Guidelines for preparation of laparoscopic instrumentation." *AORN J* 32: 65, 1980.

Committee on Infection Control in Handling of Endoscopic Equipment. "Guidelines for cleaning and disinfection of flexible fiberoptic endoscopes (FFE) used in G.I. endoscopy." *AORN J* 28:907, 1978.

Eisenberg, M. E., Copass, M. K., Hallstrom, A. P., Blake, B., Bergner, L., Short, F. A., Cobb, L. A. "Treatment of out-of-hospital cardiac arrests with rapid defibrillation by emergency medical technicians." *N Engl J Med* 32:1379, 1980.

Ethicon. *Suture Use Manual: Use & Handling of Sutures & Needles*, 3rd ed. Somerville, N.J., 1981.

Ethicon. *Nursing Care of the Patient in the O.R.* Somerville, N.J., 1976.

Exy, G. A. "Advance in defibrillation." *Emerg Med* 12:72, 1980.

Frigitronics of Connecticut. N_2O *Cryosurgical System*. Shelton, Conn., 1981.

Gatch, G. "Cardiac arrest in the OR." *AORN J* 32:983, 1980.

Grubb, R. D., Ondov, G., and Bagley, L. *Operating Room Guidelines: An Illustrated Manual*. St. Louis: C. V. Mosby, 1979.

Gruendemann, B., Casterton, S., Hesterly, S., Minckley, B., and Shetler, M. *The Surgical Patient: Behavioral Concepts for the Operating Room Nurse*. St. Louis: C. V. Mosby, 1977.

Hoerenz, P. "The operative microscope." *J Microsurg* 1:364–369, 1980.

Kildea, J. "Mediastinoscopy in bronchogenic carcinoma." *AORN J* 33:57, 1981.

Liebermann, T. R., and Barnes, M. "Gastrointestinal fiberoptic endoscopy diagnostic and therapeutic aspects." *Surg Clin North Am* 59:787, 1979.

Maala, R. M. "Electrical hazards in the O.R. *D & G Gown Gloves* 1:1, 1976 (Davis & Geck American Cyanamide Co.).

McElmurry, M., and Byrd, D. "Surgical instruments: Manufacture and proper care." *AORN J* 19:1074, 1974.

Medtronic. *Pacing Your Heart*. Minneapolis, 1980.

Medtronic. *The Heart of the System*. Minneapolis, 1981.

Nadol, J. B., Jr. "Hearing loss as a surgical disease." *Surg Rounds* 2:42, 1978.

Olympus Corp of America. *Instructions for Olympus B.F. Bronchofiberscope*. New Hyde Park, N.Y., 1981.

Pawlowski, J. "Operative endoscopy: Challenge for OR nurse." *AORN J* 29:651, 1979.

Richards Manufacturing Co. *Otology Instrumentation Manual*. Memphis, 1981.

Richards Manufacturing Co. *An Introduction to Basic Microsurgical Procedures: Myringotomy Stapedectomy Tympanoplasty*. Memphis, 1976.

Rhodes, M. J., Gruendemann, B. J., and Ballinger, W. F. *Alexander's Care of the Patient in Surgery*, 6th ed. St. Louis: C. V. Mosby, 1978.

Stroumtsos, Oneta. *Perspective on Suture*. Davis & Geck, American Cyanamide Co., Pearl River, New York, 1978.

Surgical Products Division/3M. *Air Instrument System: Air & Battery Instruments*. St. Paul, 1981.

United States Surgical Corp. *Stapling Techniques: General Surgery*, 2nd ed. New York, 1981.

Ward, P., Berci, G., and Calcaterra, T. C. "Advances in endoscopic examination of the respiratory system." *Ann Otol Rhinol Laryngol* 83:754, 1974.

Ward, S. "Rigid endoscopy of the respiratory tract." *AORN J* 34:1058, 1981.

White, N. "O.R. nursing in otomicrosurgery." *AORN J* 22:889, 1975.

Orthopaedic Instruments & Procedures. Columbus: The Fred Schad Co., 1970.

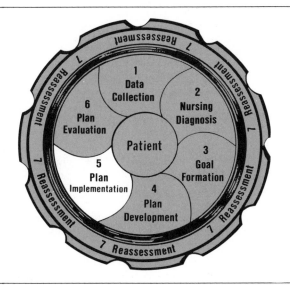

Reassessment
1 Data Collection
2 Nursing Diagnosis
6 Plan Evaluation
Patient
3 Goal Formation
5 Plan Implementation
4 Plan Development
Reassessment

The nurse assures an aseptic environment for the patient.

Maintaining Asepsis

As a patient advocate, an operating room nurse has as one of her most important functions establishing and maintaining asepsis during the intraoperative phase of surgery. It is imperative, therefore, that operating room nurses develop a *surgical conscience* that allows no compromises in the principles of asepsis and sterile technique. Anything less than strict attention to these principles increases the potential of postoperative infection.

Surgical Conscience

A surgical conscience means attention to aseptic principles during the perioperative period. It involves constant inspection, monitoring, and regulation of the surgical patient, environment, personnel, and equipment. The nurse anticipates the patient's and the surgical team's needs and gives unselfish, vigilant care to the patient.

A surgical conscience builds on the principles of asepsis, and can be considered fully developed when the operating room nurse's attention to sterile technique and aseptic practices becomes automatic. It requires awareness of what is occurring at all times during the intraoperative period, even when attention is directed to other activities.

Developing a surgical conscience requires:

1. Knowledge of principles of asepsis
2. Self-discipline in inspecting and regulating one's own hygiene, dress, and nursing practice, with attention to breaks in technique
3. Ability to anticipate the need for supplies and services based on knowledge of the patient, the procedure being performed, the preferences of the surgical team, and where and how to obtain necessary supplies
4. Good communication skills to determine the needs of patients and team members and identify and correct breaks in technique
5. Maturity to overcome personal preference and prejudice to provide optimum patient care, regardless of the surgical procedure, the patient's circumstances, or other surgical personnel.

As part of a surgical team, each member assumes not only individual responsibility but also responsibility for the surgical conscience of the group. Monitoring others' activities and calling attention to their errors should not be taken as personal affronts but as positive steps in providing optimal patient care. Correcting others or being corrected is often stressful for inexperienced operating room personnel and requires the development of communication and assertiveness skills as well as maturity (1).

The scope of a surgical conscience includes continuing evaluation of the surgical patient, environment, personnel, and equipment. Continuous, simultaneous attention to these four areas may be the hardest aspect of the surgical conscience to develop. It requires a broad knowledge base in anatomy and physiology, interpersonal relationships, and environmental safety. It relies on skilled observation using each of the senses. An operating room nurse with a well-developed surgical conscience has eyes that watch the minutest details of sterile supplies, surgical environment, and the patient; ears that detect slight voice inflections or sounds of malfunctioning equipment; a sense of smell to detect unusual odors; and an acute sense of touch to detect changes in a patient's responses. Operating room nurses also use equipment to monitor the patient, but it is frequently experience and the senses that signal the need for more in-depth investigation of a potential problem.

Aseptic Practice

Aseptic practices form the basis of a sound surgical conscience and operating room nursing. The guidelines are few, but knowledge of and adherence to them are essential to the safe practice of nursing in the operating room and will serve not only the novice but also the experienced nurse.

Aseptic practices are carried out during every phase of the perioperative role: preoperatively in establishing the aseptic environment and sterile field; intraoperatively in maintaining the sterile field and confining and containing contamination; and postoperatively in terminal cleaning of the room and sterilization of supplies.

Although serving as the foundation for safe patient care in the operating room, the techniques of asepsis are nonetheless appropriate for nurses in other areas. Applying these techniques will aid in dressing changes, catheter insertion and care, intravenous therapy, and other common nursing practices.

Why have we established guidelines for aseptic practices? Consider the many sources of wound contamination: shedding of resident and transient flora from the skin and hair of patients and operating room personnel; droplets expelled from the respiratory tract of patients and operating room personnel; inadvertent and unknowing use of unsterile equipment or supplies; airborne bacteria or particles; and endogenous bacteria from the patient's gastrointestinal tract or blood. Consider the cost to the patient of wound infection. Time and money are lost due to the increased length of hospital stay. Skin integrity is lost and there are possible threats to body image and even possible loss of life itself. Infection is costly to hospitals due to the need for increased staff and extended hospital stays. Because of the many sources of wound infection and the costs of treating it, each member of the operating room team must be aware of and practice good aseptic technique.

To better understand aseptic practices, a few terms must be defined:

- Asepsis: The condition of being free from disease-causing microorganisms.
- Aseptic technique: The methods used to maintain asepsis.
- Sterile: Free from microorganisms.
- Sterile field: Area immediately around the patient that has been prepared for a sterile procedure.
- Surgically clean: Cleaned mechanically but not sterile.
- Scrubbed and unscrubbed personnel: Scrubbed personnel include the surgeon and scrub nurse or technician and assisting physicians who are scrubbed, gowned, and gloved. Unscrubbed personnel include the anesthesiologist and circulating nurse, who wear surgical attire but are not gowned or gloved.

The overall goal in asepsis is to minimize contamination of the wound. The following guidelines to aseptic practice are well-accepted methods for minimizing the chances of contamination. In adhering to each practice, nurses should realize the purpose behind it. They should also realize that a break in aseptic technique will not automatically cause microbial contamination but only increase the probability of its occurring.

The Association of Operating Room Nurses has developed the following recommended practices for aseptic technique (2).

1. All items used within a sterile field should be sterile. Any items of questionable sterility should be considered unsterile. All items presented to the sterile field should be checked for proper packaging, processing, and handling. All packages should be checked for moisture, seal integrity, possible penetration of the sterile barrier (e.g., pinholes or tears), and the appearance of the sterilizer indicator. When items are delivered to the sterile field, the integrity of the contents and the sterile field must be maintained.

Packages should not delaminate during opening, should not reseal once opened, and must permit aseptic presentation of the contents to the sterile field. The inner edge of a peel package seal is considered the sterile boundary. If a dust cover is in place, it should be removed outside the operating room. Wrappers must be free of holes and should be memory free. When wrappers are opened they sometimes need to be flat. Once opened, wrappers are considered sterile to within 1 inch of the edge. When opening supplies wrapped in the central supply area, unscrubbed personnel should open the wrapper flap farthest away from them first and the nearest wrapper flap last (see Fig. 21.1). All wrapper tails should be secured when supplies are presented to the sterile field to prevent flipping of the wrapper (see Fig. 21.2). Scrubbed personnel opening wrapped supplies proceed in an opposite manner, opening the nearest wrapper flap first and the farthest flap last. All personnel should avoid undue handling and fanning of wrappers.

When dispensing sterile liquids, personnel should take care to prevent contents from splashing onto the sterile field or onto an unsterile area that might then drip onto the sterile field. Bottle contents should all be poured at one time or the unused portion discarded. Reuse of opened bottles can contaminate solutions, due to drops contacting unsterile areas and then running back over sterile bottle lips. Bottle caps should not be

Figure 21.1. Opening sterile supplies. Circulator opens flap farthest away first.

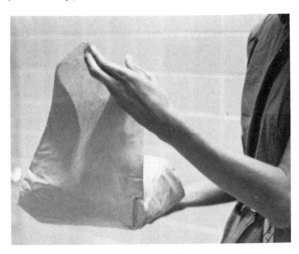

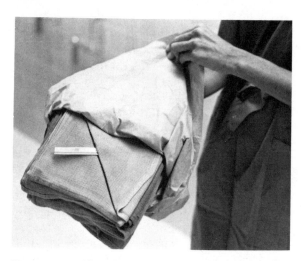

Figure 21.2. All wrapper tails are secured before presenting item to sterile field.

replaced, as the edges are considered unsterile once the container is opened.

Sterile items dropped on the floor should be considered unsterile. Any items of questionable sterility should be considered unsterile. The adage, "When in doubt, consider it unsterile," prevails when opening sterile supplies and maintaining the sterile field.

2. Gowns used by scrub persons should be sterile. Gowns worn by the surgical team are sterile before donning, and are considered sterile on the front from chest to table level and on the sleeves from the cuff to 2 inches above the elbow. Wraparound gowns are not considered sterile in the back, because it is not possible to keep a constant eye on that area. Cuffs of the gown, the neckline, shoulders, and underarm areas are also considered unsterile. Stockinette cuffs must be completely covered by gloves.

During the procedure, scrubbed team members must be alert so gown sterility at table level will be maintained during adjustments in table height. Scrubbed personnel should never lean or sit on unsterile areas. Sitting is allowed only when the entire procedure will be done in that position. Contamination of hands and arms may occur when they are lowered beyond waist level because they are out of sight.

3. Draped tables are considered sterile only at the table level. All drapes, supplies, and equipment extending over or dropping below table level must be considered unsterile because they are out of sight, and their sterility cannot be monitored. Before draping, tables must be checked to ensure they are clean and dry, and they must be monitored once the sterile field is established to prevent strike-through. Strike-through occurs when moisture soaks through unsterile layers to sterile layers, or vice versa.

4. Scrubbed personnel move only in the areas of similar preparation. All personnel moving within or around a sterile field should do so in a manner consistent with maintaining the sterility of that field. That is, scrubbed personnel only come in contact with and reach over sterile areas; unscrubbed personnel only come in contact with and reach over unsterile areas.

In delivering supplies to the sterile field, unscrubbed personnel must always be aware of the distance between themselves and the sterile field. Single-use transfer forceps may be used as an extension of the unsterile hand, ensuring a safe distance. Transfer forceps stored in solution should not be used because maintenance of sterility is questionable.

In pouring solutions, scrubbed personnel should hold sterile containers away from the sterile field or set them near the edge of the sterile field so unscrubbed personnel do not lean over the field while pouring. Unscrubbed personnel should maintain a distance between them and the sterile area. Unscrubbed persons should not pass between two sterile areas that are close together.

Scrubbed personnel must remain close to the sterile field and never turn their back to the field. When changing positions and passing other scrubbed personnel, they should turn face-to-face (see Fig. 21.3) or back-to-back (see Fig. 21.4). In draping unsterile areas, scrubbed personnel must drape those areas nearest to them first. This ensures that when they drape areas farther away, they will be leaning over a sterile field to do so.

A sterile field should be set up as closely as possible to the time of use. Once sterile sup-

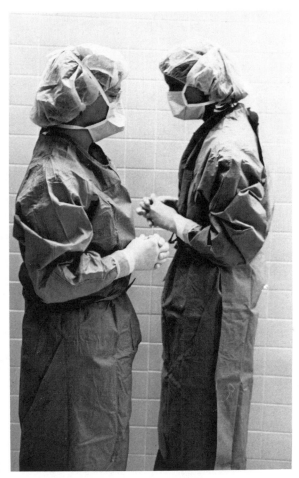

Figure 21.3. In keeping with the principle, sterile to sterile-unsterile to unsterile, scrubbed personnel pass face to face.

where sterile supplies have been opened, those supplies may only be used on that patient. In the event of case cancellation, supplies must be discarded to prevent cross-contamination.

The operating room setup is maintained until the patient leaves the room. This assures that if supplies are needed in an emergency, their integrity has been maintained, and the chance of contamination will be decreased.

To achieve the patient goal of freedom from infection, the OR nurse keeps microorganisms to a minimum. Hand-washing techniques, skin preparation, and other aseptic practices, and disinfection of grossly contaminated areas must be carried out with a knowledge of underlying principles.

Once the patient has been draped, the drapes must not be shifted or moved. Shifting or

Figure 21.4. Scrubbed personnel pass back to back.

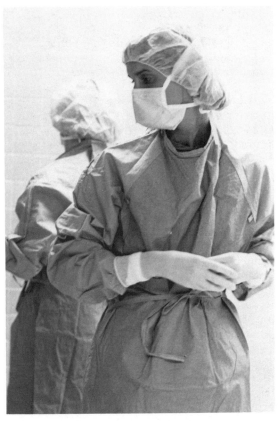

plies have been opened, they should not be left unattended because the chances of contamination are increased. The length of time sterile supplies can be opened and still be considered sterile depends on the type of procedure to be performed and the patient's status. Each institution must have an established policy regarding this practice; however, the practice of maintaining opened sterile supplies for more than one hour should be questioned.

Sterile supplies should never be opened and then covered, because it is virtually impossible to uncover the sterile field without contaminating it. Once a patient has entered a room moving the drapes contaminates the sterile field. Although the use of splash basins for rinsing and holding instruments is acceptable, precautions must be taken when they are used. Surgical team members using splash basins should do so in a manner that prevents contamination of the sterile field by water droplets. Use of splash basins to rinse powder from gloves is discouraged. But if a basin is used, that basin and its contents must be discarded immediately because it is a breeding ground for microorganisms.

Operating Room Attire

Operating room attire contributes to a safe environment and decreases the possibility of wound infection by minimizing exogenous contamination. Head and body coverings decrease the possibility of contamination due to natural shedding from the skin and hair of operating room personnel.

When personnel move from unrestricted to restricted areas of the surgical suite, they must change street clothes for proper operating room attire. The unrestricted area is around the central desk and the lounges. In the restricted area, which includes the operating rooms and hallways, dresses or suits, hair covers (caps or hoods), and shoe covers are required. Masks are also required in restricted areas. All personnel who enter the surgical suite must be appropriately attired, according to the guidelines of the institution.

Donning operating room attire proceeds from head to toe. The surgical cap or hood is the first item to be donned. This eliminates possible contamination of scrub clothes by falling hair. All hair should be covered and contained within the head covering (see Fig. 21.5). Materials used for caps and hoods should be lint free. Head coverings should be comfortable and allow for ventilation. Most are disposable, but nondisposable caps should be laundered in a facility used for laundering other hospital textiles. Personnel with facial hair should use a hood to cover all hair.

Scrub suits and dresses are available in many styles and qualities. Scrub suits, which

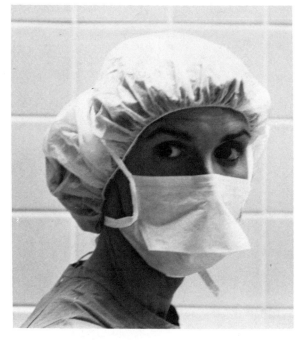

Figure 21.5. *The surgical cap should cover all hair and be of a style to keep the hair contained.*

are put on after covering the hair, are considered to be more effective barriers to contamination than scrub dresses. Scrub shirts should be secured at the waist or tucked into scrub pants to reduce shedding. Loose shirttails and baggy scrub clothing should be avoided. Scrub pants should have ankle closures and not be dragged on the floor when donned. The attire chosen depends on the policies of the institution and the extent to which they implement established standards.

Garments should fit the body closely and be comfortable and easy to don. They should also be designed so it is not necessary to step into the garment, drag it on the floor, or pull it over the head. Ideally scrub clothes should be laundered daily and remain clean and dry. They should be changed when soiled.

When wearing operating room apparel with short sleeves, unscrubbed operating room personnel should wear warm-up jackets with stockinette cuffs or unsterile long-sleeved gowns to avoid possible contamination by shedding from the arms. Warm-up jackets should remain snapped to prevent flapping of the jacket tails (see Fig. 21.6).

Shoe covers are then put on. Disposable shoe covers should completely cover the shoe, be antistatic if flammable anesthetics are used, and be changed between cases to avoid possible cross-contamination. In the interest of safety, clogs, sandals, and tennis shoes should not be worn in the operating room. A shoe that provides some protection from foot injury should be worn.

When personnel enter the restricted area of the surgical suite, masks remain in place while they are functioning in that area. Masks are essential in avoiding contamination by respiratory droplets from personnel to patient. Dis-

Figure 21.6. Unscrubbed personnel should wear warm-up jacket with stockinette cuffs on the sleeves and fasteners which keep jacket close to wearer's body.

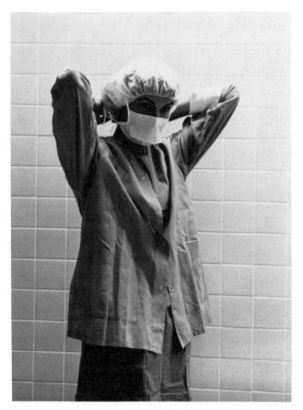

posable masks of high-filtration efficiency (95 percent or above) should be used. Cloth and gauze masks are unacceptable in the operating room environment because of their ineffective filtration and rapid wetting from expired moisture. (Cloth masks are made that meet filtration needs, but they are not readily available.)

Masks should cover both the nose and the mouth and venting at the sides should be minimized by proper positioning. Strings should be tied snugly and should not be crossed because this prevents the mask from conforming to the face (see Fig. 21.7).

Once a mask is taken off, it should be discarded. Masks are changed between procedures. Some disposable masks may be efficient for eight or more hours. When removing a mask, personnel should take care to avoid touching the mask itself. It should be removed by untying the strings or touching the elastic band only and disposed of properly. Good hand-washing technique must be carried out after removing the mask.

Operating room attire should not be worn outside of the surgical suite. If it is necessary to leave the suite, personnel can wear laboratory coats, but these are not an effective barrier to contamination. If they are worn, laboratory coats should be buttoned, long sleeved, and of an adequate length to cover the scrub suit to the knees. Ideally, they should be laundered after each use. Whether laboratory coats are worn, attire worn outside the suite should be changed upon returning. Since masks, caps, and shoe covers will have already been removed before leaving the suite, all the proper attire must be donned in the correct sequence.

Questions are often asked about jewelry, earrings, scissors, watches, and other accessories. Jewelry should not be worn in the operating room. The only exception is earrings for pierced ears if they are small studs and completely covered by the cap or hood. Other jewelry is inappropriate. Necklaces, rings, and watches are sources of contamination and difficult to keep clean. Wearing nail polish in the operating room suite is absolutely prohibited, because bacteria breeds in and around chipped polish and inhibits inspection for dirt under

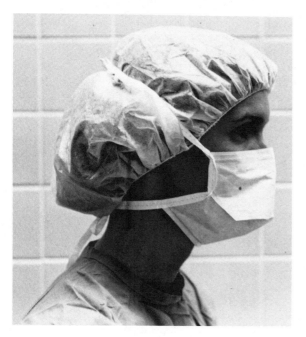

Figure 21.7. Masks must cover both the nose and the mouth. The sides should conform closely to the face to minimize venting.

titis should not scrub because of the high number of bacteria on the hands.

Upper respiratory and other infections should be carefully monitored. Personnel with untreated rhinorrhea or productive coughs should be restricted from scrubbing. If they do circulate, they should change masks frequently during the procedure. Personnel with infections should be cleared by a physician before they return to work.

Personal grooming is another aspect of controlling infections. Makeup should be used judiciously. Fingernails should be short, clean, and free of polish. Hair should also be clean. Daily attention to hygiene is important. Each institution should have an established policy regarding employee health and instances when work in the surgical suite is prohibited. Policies should also address when personnel with infections are permitted within the suite and the guidelines for any precautions.

and around nails. Scissors should be cleaned routinely. Whenever scissors are used in the operating room suite, they should be sterilized.

Each institution determines its own operating room apparel and standards according to constraints of finance, traffic patterns, and other factors. Within these constraints, each operating room suite maintains the highest standards possible.

Personal Health, Hygiene, and Grooming

Operating room personnel must be aware of possible contaminants they bring into the environment. Persons with draining wounds or other infections should not work in the operating room. Good hygiene practices, including daily bathing and frequent hair washing, will help minimize the number of pathogens brought into the operating room. The skin should be clean, with no open, draining wounds or infections. Personnel with hand wounds or derma-

Surgically Clean Skin

Skin preparation of the patient and operating room personnel is of equal importance. Surgically clean skin serves to prevent infection. Skin preparation of the patient includes the removal of hair and scrubbing of the incisional area. Skin preparation of operating room personnel includes good hand-washing techniques and surgical hand scrubs. The objectives of skin preparation include: removing skin oil, dirt, and microbial deposits; decreasing the microbial count as much as possible; and leaving a film of antimicrobial residue on the skin.

The skin is composed of two layers, the epidermis and the dermis. The dermis, or lower layer, contains sebaceous glands, connective tissue, hair follicles, and blood and lymph vessels. The epidermis, or outer layer, acts as a protective barrier and constantly sheds cells. Resident flora found in the dermis are shed by the body, with the movement of old cells and skin secretions from the dermal layer to the epidermal layer. Shedding of resident flora is a source of wound contamination. Transient flora that reside on the epidermis are usually only loosely attached to the skin surface and can be removd by cleansing the skin with soap or detergent.

Providing for surgically clean skin includes mechanical and chemical actions. The mechanical actions use friction to remove soil and the transient flora of the epidermis. The chemical actions reduce the flora. The chemical process of skin preparation uses antiseptic agents that meet criteria for effectiveness. They should be rapid-acting in reducing the microbial count and have a broad-spectrum effect. Antiseptic agents should be able to be applied quickly and maintain effectiveness for an extended period of time. They should be nonirritating and nonsensitizing. Alcohol, organic matter, soap, and detergents should not render such agents ineffective. Chlorhexidine, hexachlorophene, iodophors, and alcohols are recommended by the Centers for Disease Control (CDC) for hand-washing. For preparation of the operative site, the CDC recommends tincture of chlorhexidine, iodophors, and tincture of iodine. Alcohol as a single agent is only recommended for minor procedures such as inserting an intravenous device. The CDC does not recommend plain soap, aqueous quarternary ammonium compounds, or hexachlorophenes as single agents for operative site preparation.

Povidone-iodine solutions, or iodophors, are effective against Gram-positive and Gram-negative organisms. Iodophors are not as irritating as tincture of iodine solutions and have a persistent effect if not rinsed off. The chlorhexadine group is effective against Gram-positive and Gram-negative organisms and has a persistent effect.

Hexachlorophenes are most active against Gram-positive organisms and least active against fungi and Gram-negative organisms. Hexachlorophene has a long-lasting cumulative bacteriostatic effect, which makes it effective when used as a preoperative patient shower for several days preceding surgery or when used consistently by operating room personnel. It is soluble in alcohol, however, and washing with alcohol reduces its persistent action. Hexachlorophene can be toxic when absorbed from the skin. Although the CDC recommends it for hand-washing, it is not recommended for surgical site preparation and

should not be used for routine bathing of infants or by pregnant women.

Alcohol in a 70–90 percent solution is used as an antiseptic, but should not be applied to mucous membranes because it is inactivated by coagulating protein. Iodine compounds may be irritating for hand-washing but are excellent for surgical skin preparation.

Surgical Hand Scrub

The scrub itself differs among institutions, but within an institution, the scrub procedure should be the same for all personnel. It should be a written policy, available to everyone who scrubs within the operating room suite, and a part of the procedure manual.

All scrub personnel must meet certain criteria before beginning the surgical scrub. Nails must be short, clean, and free of polish. Hands and arms should be free of cuts and any other skin problems. The operating room cap should be in place, covering and containing all hair. The surgical mask should be properly positioned, tied securely, and venting minimized. Surgical attire should be donned, with ties and shirttails properly controlled.

There are two types of surgical hand scrubs, the timed scrub and the stroke-count scrub. Initial scrubbing procedures for both techniques are the same and proceed from hands to arms. Hands and arms are washed with the antimicrobial agent to remove transient flora and gross contamination. Nails are cleaned under running water, using disposable or metal nail cleaners. Wooden sticks are not used for this purpose. After rinsing, the selected scrub procedure is carried out, using either a terminally sterilized, nondisposable brush or a disposable sponge brush.

The timed scrub will usually take at least 5 minutes to complete. There is no significant reduction in microbial count with a 10-minute instead of a 5-minute scrub. Each anatomical area is scrubbed for a specified length of time, with special attention to the fingers and hands. Each aspect of the fingers, between digits, palms, and the back of the hand, must be subjected to light friction with sudsed antimicrobial agent (see Fig. 21.8). Once hands are scrubbed, the procedure is extended to arms, scrubbing with a circular motion to 2 inches above the elbow. Hands should be held higher than the elbow to allow water to run from the cleanest area down to the arm (see Fig. 21.9). Care should be taken during scrubbing to prevent water from splashing onto the scrub clothes. At the completion of the timed scrub, the hands and arms are rinsed. The water is turned off using a foot pedal or knee or elbow handle, being careful not to contaminate the hands. The brush is properly disposed of. With hands held higher than arms, the scrubbed person proceeds into the operating room.

The stroke-count scrub will also take about five minutes to complete. It differs from the timed scrub in that all aspects are scrubbed using a specific number of strokes rather than a specified length of time. There are a number of formulas for stroke-count scrubbing. A documented procedure should be specified for each institution. Rinsing, disposal of brushes,

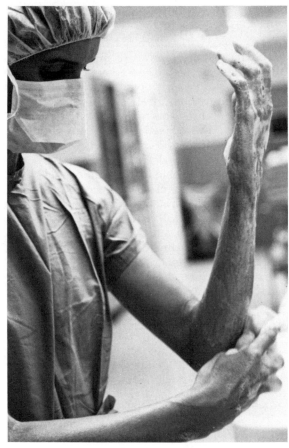

Figure 21.9. Keeping the hands elevated to allow water run off, the scrub proceeds in a circular motion to 2 inches above the elbow.

Figure 21.8. During the surgical scrub each aspect of the fingers, palms, back of the hand, and wrist are subject to light friction with a sudsed antimicrobial agent.

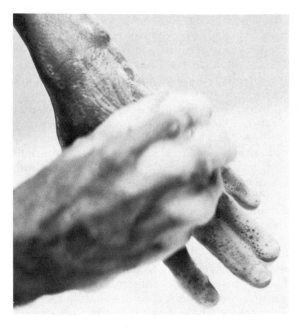

and entry into the operating room are the same as for the timed scrub procedure.

Rescrubbing procedures are the same as the initial method. Rescrubbing should last five minutes, because bacteria can multiply rapidly in the warm, moist environment of a gloved hand. A sterile towel is used for drying the hands. Towels should be removed from the sterile field carefully to avoid dripping water onto the field. Grasping the towel with one hand, the person lifts it from the sterile field and allows it to unfold to its full length. Ideally, the towel, gown, and gloves should be on a separate table from other supplies. Scrub personnel should lean slightly forward so the towel is hanging away from the body and will not contact the body or the scrub personnel's clothing. Hands must be dried thoroughly, using one hand with the towel to dry the opposite hand. Dry hands make gloving easier and prevent moisture strike-through to the gown sleeve. The towel is then advanced up the arm, drying each subsequent area with a rotating motion and taking care not to retrace an area. The towel is reversed, and the opposite hand and arm are completely dried in a similar manner. The towel is then discarded without manipulation (see Fig. 21.10).

Gowning and Gloving

Gloves and gowns donned by surgical personnel are barriers to the transfer of microorganisms from personnel to patient and vice versa. The materials used for gowns and drapes should have similar characteristics, whether reusable or disposable. Most important, the material must be an effective barrier to the transfer of microorganisms. It should prevent liquid penetration and must be resistant to abrasion. The material should also meet the safety guidelines of the National Fire Protection Standards and be lint free and porous, allowing steam penetration and eliminating excessive heat buildup. Finally, the material should be memory free and highly drapable.

Surgical gowns should be comfortable to wear, allowing ease of movement without being bulky or awkward. They should be wraparound with impervious material in the front from waist to shoulders and sleeves below the elbow. The stockinette cuffs should fit snugly. Surgical gloves are usually disposable. They are made of latex or neoprene rubber. Processing reusable gloves is difficult and time-consuming and may not be cost-effective. Gloves should meet the surgical glove standards of the American Society for Testing and Materials.

Scrubbed personnel who establish and organize the sterile field are responsible for gowning and gloving themselves with assistance from circulating personnel. Gowns and gloves for these initial scrubbed personnel are

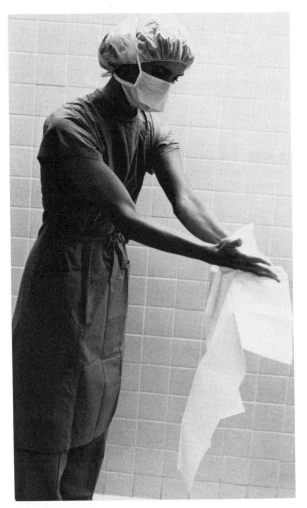

Figure 21.10. Drying of hands following scrub procedure. The towel is carefully removed from the sterile field to avoid dripping, the arms are fully extended to prevent touching of attire with the towel as drying of the first hand begins. The towel is reversed after first hand and arm are completely dried. Arms are dried with a rotating motion and care is taken not to retrace an area.

individually packaged to allow their gowning and gloving without water contamination of sterile packs. All gowns are packaged and folded inside-out. This allows scrubbed personnel to grasp the gown and put it on without contaminating the sterile front.

GOWNING

The gown should be grasped firmly at the neckline (see Fig. 21.11) and allowed to unfold completely (see Fig. 21.12). Keeping the hands on the inside of the gown, the person identifies the armholes and inserts both arms simultaneously (see Fig. 21.13). Haphazard donning of the gown may flip ties from sterile to unsterile areas. Next the circulator assists by pulling the gown up over the shoulders of the scrubbed person and securing it at the neck and waist (see Fig. 21.14). Unscrubbed personnel should only touch the unsterile inside of the gown.

If scrub personnel are using the closed-glove technique, they should not extend their hands through the cuff of the gown but should wait until gloves have been donned. With closed-glove technique, it may be necessary to don gloves before tying the back of the gown to allow enough arm length to manipulate gloves.

GLOVING

Closed and open gloving have been shown to be equally effective (3). The closed-glove technique begins with the hands remaining in the gown sleeves. The enclosed hand grasps the

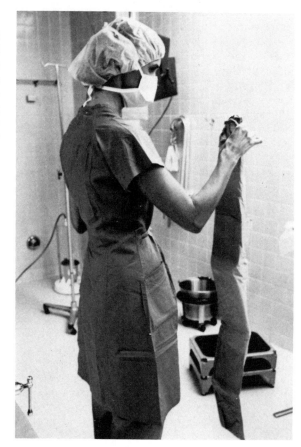

Figure 21.12. Allow complete unfolding without touching unsterile objects.

Figure 21.11. The gown is grasped firmly at the neckline.

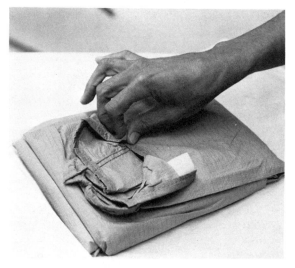

folded cuff of the glove. The glove is placed on the upturned, gown-enclosed hand, with glove fingers extending toward the body and the glove thumb on the appropriate side. The inferior glove cuff should be grasped by the enclosed thumb. Using the still-enclosed hand, the person stretches the glove up and over the stockinette cuff of the sleeve. The hand is then advanced through the cuff into the glove, being careful to keep the entire stockinette cuff enclosed in the glove. The other hand is gloved in a similar manner. Using the already gloved hand, the remaining glove is placed with fingers extended toward the body and the glove thumb to the right, on top of the upturned, enclosed hand (see Figs. 21.15–21.17).

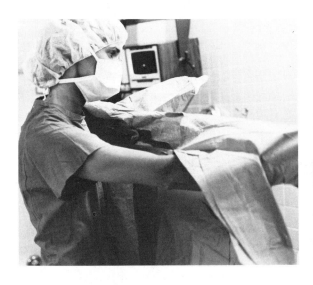

Figure 21.13. *Keeping the hands on the inside of the gown, the person identifies the armholes and inserts both arms simultaneously.*

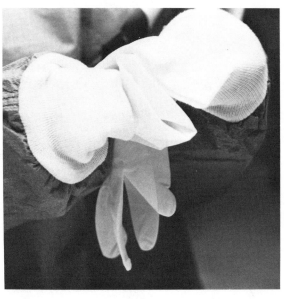

Figure 21.15. *Closed gloving technique begins with the hands remaining in the gown sleeves. The glove is grasped through the stockinette.*

Figure 21.16. *The cuff of the glove is stretched up and over the cuff of the sleeve.*

Figure 21.14. *The circulator assists by pulling the gown over the shoulders, securing it at the neck and waist, taking care not to touch any other outer areas.*

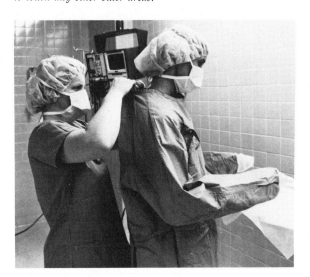

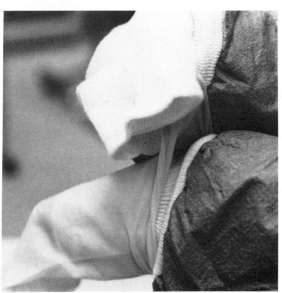

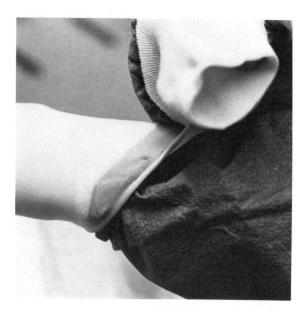

Figure 21.17. Care is taken to get the entire stockinette cuff enclosed in the glove.

When using the open-glove technique, the hands are extended through the cuffs of the sterile gown. The exposed hands should never come in contact with the glove exterior. The glove is grasped at the cuff, on the fold, by the opposing hand (see Fig. 21.18). The other hand is inserted into the glove without turning the cuff back (see Fig. 21.19). The gloved hand is then used to pick up the other glove, keeping the sterile glove under the cuff, glove to glove. The hand is inserted into the glove, and the cuff is then pulled up over the stockinette cuff to completely cover it. The hand can then be placed under the opposite cuff, glove to glove, and the cuff pulled up over the stockinette cuff of the sleeve.

To wrap the gown once gloving is completed, scrubbed personnel can use the prepackaged cards attached to disposable gowns or can attach a sterile instrument or glove wrapper to the end of the tie. Carefully handing the card or instrument to the circulator (see Fig. 21.20), the scrub person then pivots away from the circulator. The belt is then grasped and tied by the scrubbed member, and the circulator retains the card or instrument (see Fig. 21.21). If

other scrubbed personnel are present, they can assist but without the use of an instrument. They can grasp the tie with a sterile gloved hand.

Occasionally, the sterile gown will be contaminated before donning the gloves. When this happens, the scrub personnel should complete the gowning and gloving procedure using aseptic technique. Then the gown should be removed first, pulling the more contaminated upper aspect of the sleeve down over the arms and the still-gloved hands. The gloves protect the hands. The gloves should then be removed using a skin-to-skin, glove-to-glove technique. Or the circulator may remove the glove without touching the skin of hand or arm. If no further contamination occurs, the scrub personnel can then regown and reglove. If any contamination of the arms or hands occurs, however, the entire scrubbing procedure should be repeated, just as it would be if contamination occurred at any time during the initial scrub.

If a glove is contaminated after the initial donning, the open-glove technique should be

Figure 21.18. Open-glove technique. The right glove is grasped at the cuff, on the fold, by the left hand.

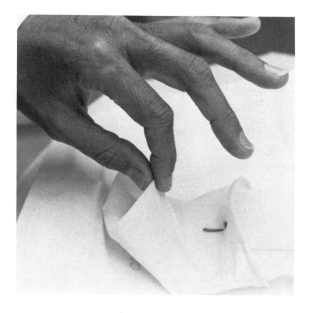

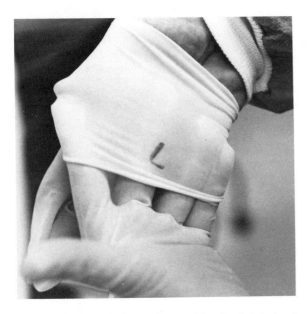

Figure 21.19. Open glove technique. The gloved right hand is used to pick up the left glove under the cuff, the left hand is inserted, and the glove cuff is pulled up over the sleeve stockinette.

used to prevent contamination during regloving unless both gown and glove are changed. The scrubbed personnel should be careful that the gown cuff does not extend down over the hand during the glove changes. This prevents contact of a clean area, the hand, by the more contaminated surface of the stockinette cuff edge. (Stockinette is a moisture collection area and not an effective microbial barrier. The cuff should be considered contaminated once the gloves are donned.)

At the termination of the surgical procedure, the gown and gloves should be removed; they should not be worn outside the operating room. Proper removal of the gown minimizes contamination of the clothes and arms of personnel. An unscrubbed person should untie the gown in the back. The scrub person then grasps the gown's shoulders on the outside and pulls them down over the arms, everting the sleeves in the process. The gown is pulled completely down over the hands, folded outside-in without undue handling, and discarded.

Gloves are then removed, again avoiding gross contamination by using a skin-to-skin, glove-to-glove technique. Gloves are discarded in the appropriate waste container.

Once the initial member of the team has scrubbed, gowned, and gloved, other personnel can be dressed similarly. Gowning others uses the same skills as gowning oneself but an opposite approach. The scrubbed team member passes a towel to a newly scrubbed member without touching her outstretched hands. The unfolded sterile towel should be held by the upper end and carefully laid over the unscrubbed team member's hand. She will then dry the hands and dispose of the towel. The scrubbed team member can then proceed in gowning others. The gown should be grasped at the neck and held away from the sterile field to unfold. The armholes are located and turned toward the newly scrubbed member. The scrubbed person's hands are positioned on the exterior of the gown at shoulder-level, with the neck area draped over the hands, acting as a cuff to protect the gloves from possible contamination (see Fig. 21.22). The gown is then placed on the outstretched hands of the team member. Scrubbed personnel then release the gown and allow the newly scrubbed member to advance hands and arms into the gown.

Figure 21.20. Scrubbed personnel hand the prepackaged card or a sterile instrument to the circulator who holds the apparatus securely.

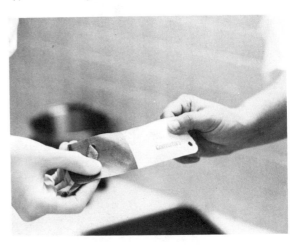

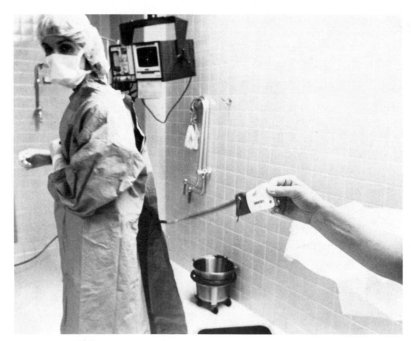

Figure 21.21. The scrub person pivots away from the circulator. The belt is then pulled free and tied while the circulator retains the card or instrument.

Figure 21.22. Gowning other team members. The gown is opened carefully, the scrubbed person's hands are positioned on the exterior of the gown at shoulder level, with the neck area draped over the hands, acting as a cuff to protect the gloves from possible contamination.

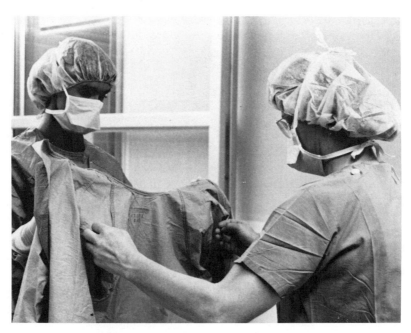

Once the gown is secured by circulating personnel, the newly scrubbed member is ready to don gloves. Hands should be extended through the gown cuff. Scrubbed personnel assist in gloving others. The sterile glove should be grasped under the everted cuff and turned with the palm facing the newly scrubbed member, glove thumb in opposition to their thumb. The cuff is stretched open, with special attention to keeping the sterile thumbs away from the glove interior (see Fig. 21.23). The newly gowned member then advances a hand into the glove, while a slight upward pressure is exerted by the scrubbed person (see Fig. 21.24). The cuff should be extended to cover the stockinette cuff entirely. The second glove is then donned in a similar manner.

If contamination occurs during the procedure, the glove should be removed without pulling the gown cuff down over the hand. A new glove is applied using the procedure described above or the open-glove technique.

Unscrubbed personnel can remove the gowns and gloves of others. After the gown is

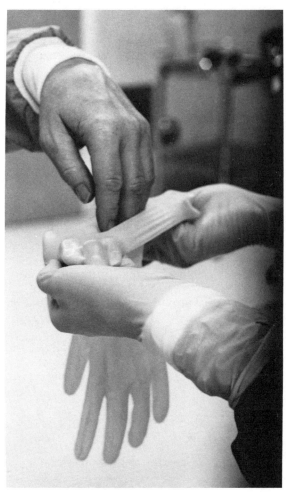

Figure 21.24. *The newly gowned member advances a hand into the glove, while a slight upward pressure is exerted by the scrubbed person.*

Figure 21.23. Gloving other team members. The cuff is stretched open, with special attention to keeping the sterile thumbs away from the glove interior.

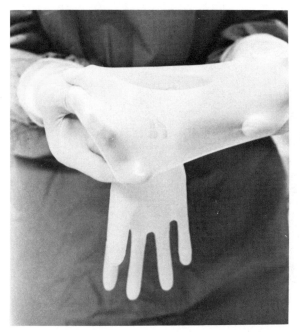

untied, the scrubbed personnel face the circulator. The gown shoulders are grasped by the unscrubbed person, who withdraws the gown, everting the sleeves, and pulling it completely off. Gloves can also be removed by unsterile personnel. Since no part of the scrubbed person's skin should be touched, the unscrubbed person grasps the previously sterile, external side of the glove and removes it in a smooth, single action. Regowning can then take place if necessary. Circulating nurses should wash their hands after touching others' gowns or gloves because these may be contaminated by the patient's microflora.

At the conclusion of gowning and gloving procedures or after glove changes, scrub personnel should remove the glove powder from newly donned gloves. Powder residue has been associated with granulomas and peritonitis. Glove powder can be removed by the use of moistened towels and sponges or splash basins. Whatevr method is used, the towel, sponge, or splash basin and its contents should be removed from the sterile field.

Patient's Skin Preparation

The boundaries of the skin area to be prepared will be identified by written policies of each institution and by surgeon's preferences. Generally, a wide area around the incision site will be prepared to provide a wide margin of safety during draping and in the event that incisions are extended.

After hair removal has been completed and immediately prior to draping, the patient's skin is scrubbed at and around the incision site

with an antiseptic agent such as povidone-iodine, chlorhexidine, or tincture of iodine.

Before beginning the prep, all equipment and supplies should be assembled on a sterile field. Most often, a small, movable table is used as a prep table. The prep set is disposable or nondisposable, depending upon the institution. It should include containers for holding the prep solutions, sponges for prepping, sterile gloves, and extra containers for depositing used sponges. Occasionally included are cotton applicators for cleaning out small areas, such as the umbilicus, ears, and nose. Solutions used vary depending on effectiveness, institutional preference, cost, and availability.

The circulating nurse or in a teaching hospital the resident or medical student is usually responsible for the skin preparation. This person assembles the supplies and proceeds with the scrub prep when agreeable to both surgeon and anesthetist. Circulating nurses should be aware of the activities of the anesthetist and should not proceed with the prep until the patient is fully anesthetized and the nurse's assistance is not immediately required by other team members (see Fig. 21.25). Preparation of

Figure 21.25. The circulator should be aware of the activities of the anesthesiologist and should not proceed with the prep until the patient is fully anesthetized.

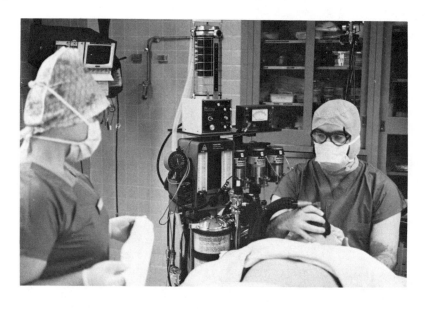

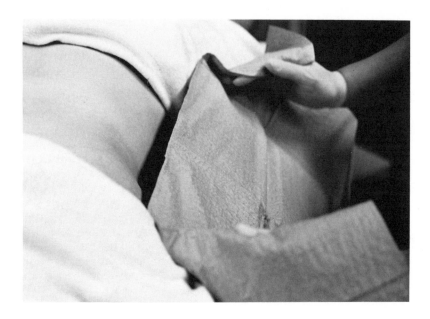

Figure 21.26. Place towels on either side of the area to be prepped. This prevents pooling of fluids and undue wetting of bed linens.

the incision site requires at least a five-minute scrub with an effective antimicrobial agent.

The procedure for doing the skin preparation is essentially the same, no matter what area of the body is to be prepped. First, sterile gloves are donned, and the prep set arranged for most efficient use. Sponges to be used should be folded if necessary and placed in appropriate containers to avoid undue handling later. Any draping with sterile towels should be done before scrubbing of the skin. This includes placing sterile towels on either side of the abdomen at the table's edge to prevent pooling of the antiseptic solution under the patient or placing sterile, impervious drapes under extremities to be prepped to avoid undue wetting of bed linens (see Fig. 21.26).

Prepping intact skin begins at the site of the incision. Using friction and an effective antimicrobial agent, the prep is extended in a circular motion away from the incision site as far as is necessary to ensure a wide margin of safety around the incision (see Figs. 21.27 and 21.28). Once the sponge has been used and the periphery prepped, that sponge should be dis-

Figure 21.27. The prep should be extended as far as is necessary to ensure a wide margin of safety around the incision.

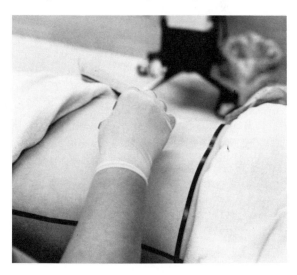

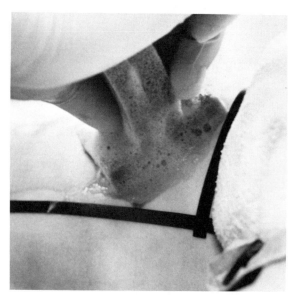

Figure 21.28. *The nurse begins the prep at the site of incision and works toward the periphery in a circular motion.*

operative field in accordance with institutional policy.

Occasionally, modifications of the prepping procedure will be used, usually when the prep area includes an open, drained wound or a body orifice. Modifications are based on the basic principle that washing should proceed from clean to dirty areas. The most contaminated area, whether or not it is the site of incision, should be scrubbed last. For instance, with colostomies, the operative area around the colostomy would be prepped first, the stoma itself would be prepped last, and then the sponge discarded. Vaginal preps should proceed from the mons and perineum to the vagina itself. The anus should be washed last. The umbilicus should be scrubbed just before disposal of the sponge.

carded in a manner that prevents strike-through. Subsequent sponges are used in the same manner, proceeding from the incision site to the periphery. Surgeon's preference dictates whether the prepped area will be dried. If drying of the incision site is requested, a sterile towel should be used and removed after blotting. The edges of the towel farthest away from the prepper should be grasped, and the towel should be lifted up and away from the skin, avoiding contamination of the area with the towel edges.

Once the prep has been carried out, sponges should be discarded in an appropriate manner, depending on the institution and its policy. Prep sponges should be of a different size and shape than those used during the operative procedure. This allows for a much easier sponge count during the procedure and avoids confusion as to what type sponges are to be counted. Sponges should be contained in a defined area until the end of the operative procedure. Prep solution, once used for prepping, should be considered contaminated and disposed of in the same manner as suction container contents or other liquid from the

Draping

Draping establishes a sterile field around the operative site. Isolating the operative field with drapes prevents cross-contamination from other unprepared body areas. Disposable or reusable woven sterile towels and sheets are used.

The characteristics of draping materials are the same as for OR apparel. Drapes must be resistant to moisture strike-through, safe, and easily drapable.

Reusable draping materials of 100 percent cotton treated with a fluid repellent and with a thread count of 288 per square inch have proven to be effective barriers to fluid and bacterial penetration. The textile threads must not be damaged by sharp objects, towel clips, or needles. If holes occur, heat-sealed fabric patches should be used. Reusable material is easily handled, memory free, and has excellent drapability, but it is more prone to shed lint particles than some nonwovens. Patches do not significantly inhibit sterilization in pre-vacuum or EO sterilizers (4).

Disposable drape materials are also resistant to the fluid and bacterial penetration. They are manufactured to meet a variety of draping specifications for special procedures. Disposables are soft and nonirritating. As with reusable drapes, care should be taken to prevent damage from sharp objects. Being compact, disposables take up less storage space, although a larger inventory may be needed than for reusables. Maintaining adequate supplies may be costly. Disposal according to community environmental standards is sometimes a problem.

Occasionally, plastic incisional drapes are used in conjunction with other draping materials. They decrease the need for skin clips, prevent the migration of microorganisms, stabilize other drapes, and isolate gross sources of contamination such as stomas and fistulas. Their use, which is controversial, depends on physician preference. If plastic incise drapes are not used properly, bacteria growth at the edges can be increased. Studies support both views.

When selecting draping materials, the most important factors are maintenance of sterility and cost-effectiveness. Packaging, presentation to the sterile field, and draping of the operative site should not compromise sterility. Cost should be studied in relation to the institutional setting, availability and need for supplies, and staff preferences. Materials should also be free of toxic agents or dyes.

During draping, the surgeon is responsible for delineating the area to be draped and the type of drapes to be used. The surgical team is responsible for maintaining asepsis during the procedure. Scrub personnel should be adept at handling drapes and draping the patient (see Figs. 21.29 and 21.30). Circulating nurses should be aware of the limits of the sterile field.

Many styles, shapes, and sizes of drapes are available. The draping described here is for general surgeries. After the sterile field has been established, draping materials should be collected and kept in a specific area of the table to avoid undue handling of the drapes and prevent undue disturbances of air currents or other sterile supplies. Sterile towels, placed with a folded edge toward the operative site, are used to outline the area. Towel clips, used to secure the drapes, should be considered contaminated at the point of entry and should not be repositioned. Two or four towels can be used for this purpose and should be secured to prevent displacement. A laparotomy sheet, often called a lap sheet, with a fenestration, or window, is placed on the operative site, slitside down. The sheet is then unfolded to cover the

Figure 21.29. Scrub personnel should know how to handle the drapes correctly.

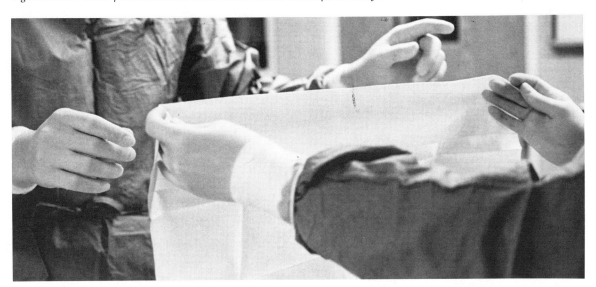

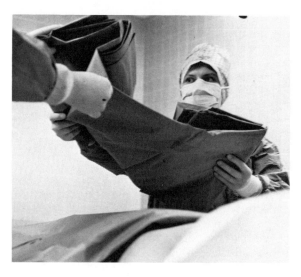

Figure 21.30. The drape is kept above patient level until being placed over the site of incision.

Drapes should be handled as little as possible. They should never be passed over an unsterile area or held below the waist, and during transfer from the sterile field to the patient, they should be held in a compact position, avoiding fanning or haphazard unfolding.

To avoid contamination, scrubbed personnel do not touch the patient's skin, and the gloved hands should always be protected by cuffing the draping material back over the hands.

Aseptic Practices during the Operative Procedure

During the procedure, the main aseptic goal is to maintain the integrity of the sterile field. The entire team is attentive to the activities of everyone else in the room, alert to breaks in technique, and quick to make corrections.

Once the skin has been incised, the knife used to make the skin incision and clamps used on the skin or subcutaneous tissue are frequently discarded. This is done because deep tissues could be contaminated by instruments that had been in contact with the patient's disinfected but unsterile skin. This practice has not been supported by current research.

Blood should be removed from instruments each time they are passed from the incision back to the Mayo stand. They can be wiped with damp sponges or towels or carefully submerged in sterile water. Blood remaining on the instruments can be a source of wound contamination and corrode the stainless steel finish. Blood can be difficult to remove during terminal cleaning.

Connecting ends of drill cords, electrosurgery cords, suction tubing, and the like, must be handed off the sterile field for attachment to their power source, using the principles of asepsis. The scrub personnel should extend enough length off the sterile field to allow the circulating nurse to connect the equipment without contaminating the field. Once connected, the cords should be secured and not be repositioned.

Once draped, tables should be considered sterile at table level only. Any suture, instruments, or cords that extend beyond the edge

patient entirely, with adequate length and width for draping the anesthesia screen and both arms (see Figs. 21.31 and 21.32). General dimensions of the lap sheet are 9 by 6 feet with a longitudinal fenestration 10 by 4 inches, located approximately 4 feet from the top. Standard-sized, single sheets, 9 by 6 feet and folded in half, can also be used for draping in conjunction with lap sheets to provide a larger sterile area.

Special procedures may require sheets with the fenestration elsewhere to expose the operative site. For instance, thyroid drape fenestrations are located closer to the head of the sheet and are transverse, whereas breast and chest drape fenestrations are larger and square. Perineal drapes, used for patients in the lithotomy position, may have two leggings located on either side of a fenestration. When in place, the drape will cover the patient's legs, abdomen, and the lower end of the operating room table. U-shaped split sheets are frequently used to drape extremities and are the same overall size as other lap sheets.

The incision site should be the only exposed area. All other unprepared areas of the patient must be covered by sterile drapes (see Fig. 21.33).

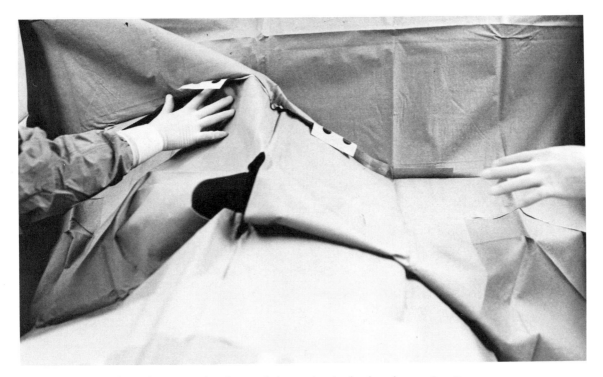

Figure 21.31. In abdominal surgery, a lap sheet, with fenestration, is placed on the operative site.

Figure 21.32. The sheet is unfolded completely to cover the patient.

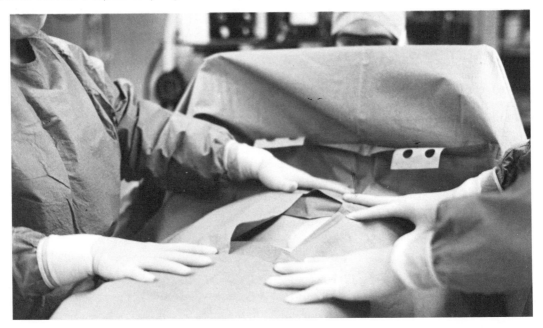

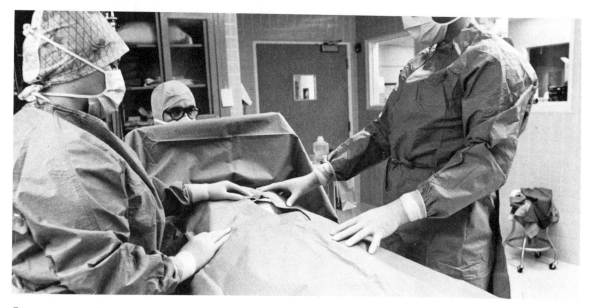

Figure 21.33. *All unprepared areas of the patient must be covered by sterile drapes.*

of the sterile field should be considered contaminated.

During the operative procedure, special equipment and supplies that cannot be sterilized are often used. Among these are microscopes, eyepieces, and magnets. The sterile field can be maintained by completely covering any extra equipment used within the field with sterile drapes.

Both the circulating nurse and scrubbed person must be attentive when solutions are poured for use during the procedure. Liquid containers should be set near the edge of the sterile field so the circulating nurse does not have to lean over the sterile field to present solutions. Light handles should not be used, because this requires the scrubbed person to reach above the level of the shoulders of the gown out of the line of sight. If lights are repositioned with blood- and serous-coated gloves, a residue is left on the light handles; when drying this can be a source of airborne contamination.

Needles and other sharp instruments used during the procedure can occasionally perforate the draping material, leading to contamination. Scrubbed personnel are responsible for avoiding such penetrations. If penetration takes place, the area should be isolated by covering with new draping material, and the penetrant discarded from the sterile field.

During the procedure, blood, other serous drainage, and irrigating solutions become sources of contamination if strike-through occurs. Once an area becomes wet, it must be considered contaminated. That area should be isolated, either by adding extra waterproof drapes or by redraping the area.

Once sponges become soiled, they should be discarded from the sterile field to avoid contamination, maintain clear visibility of the wound site, prevent an increase in the number of airborne contaminants, and assist the circulating nurse to confine and contain contamination.

During certain types of procedures when unsterile body cavities are opened, such as in vaginal closures during abdominal hysterectomies, bowel resections, and bronchus transections, some authorities believe extra care should be taken in handling of instruments. This practice dictates that once instruments have been in contact with a contaminated area, they are isolated and no longer used. This is the responsibility of the scrubbed surgical team, and they must pay strict attention to instrument handling.

Other authorities believe these precautions are necessary only for colon resections when the patient has not had a cleansing enema or gastrointestinal-specific antibiotics. Except in cases of ruptured viscus or unprepared large bowel, copious irrigation may have the same effect in limiting the spread of contaminants.

Instruments used for cancerous lesions may also be segregated, because they can be sources of "seeding" of malignant cells to other parts of the body.

Observers of the surgery can be a threat to the sterile field. Both new and veteran personnel may be eager to see surgical procedures being carried out. They must occasionally be reminded that they should not lean over the sterile field. This includes the anesthetist who leans over the anesthesia screen.

Another danger is insects. Once found, they should be removed, and any portion of the sterile field that might have been contaminated should be isolated. If there is doubt about whether an insect landed on a sterile field, it should be considered contaminated and either isolated or struck and set up again.

Occasionally, once drapes are positioned, the fenestration is found to be in the wrong position or too small for the incision to be made. Surgeons and other operating room personnel may be tempted to remedy the situation by cutting the drapes, a poor technique, that compromises the sterility of the field.

Other possible sources of contamination are perspiration, contact lenses, and loose hair that might fall into the sterile field. If perspiration becomes a problem, the scrubbed person should turn away from the sterile field to allow mopping of the damp area. Perspiration drops should not be allowed to fall onto the sterile field. Contact lenses worn by the surgical team must also be monitored. Loose hair should not be a problem, providing the

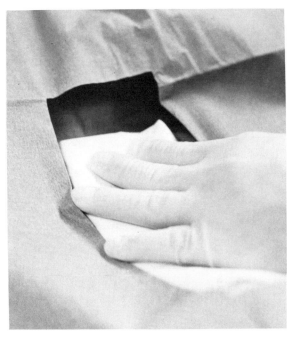

Figure 21.34. Sterile dressings are applied before removal of the drapes to avoid contamination of the incision.

surgical team has dressed appropriately before entering the surgical suite.

At the conclusion of the operative procedure and with closure of the incision, sterile dressings are usually applied. This should be done before removal of the drapes so the incisional area is not contaminated (see Fig. 21.34). The dressing is completed and secured by the circulating nurse or the ungloved surgeon after drape removal. Drapes should be removed in an orderly manner, and they should be disposed of in an appropriate container. Suction tubing or other drainage devices should be connected and secured to the patient.

The surgical team is the patient's advocate. Team members must be alert in establishing and maintaining asepsis. Each member of the surgical team should have developed a surgical conscience which will allow for no breaks in technique and no less than excellent practice during the intraoperative phase.

References

1. Gruendemann, B. J., Casterton, S., Hesterly, S., Menckley, B., and Shetler, M. *The Surgical Patient: Behavioral Concepts for the Operating Room*, 2nd ed. St. Louis: C. V. Mosby, 1979.
2. "Standards for basic aseptic technique." In *AORN Standards of Practice*. Denver: Association of Operating Room Nurses, 1978.
3. "Glove study shows both open and closed techniques appropriate." *AORN J* 34(September): 390, 1981.
4. Green, V. W., Borlung, G. M., and Nelson, E. "Effects of patching on sterilization of surgical textiles." *AORN J* 33(June):1249–1261, 1981.

Suggested Readings

Association of Operating Room Nurses. "Standards for surgical hand scrubs." *AORN J* 23(May): 976-977, 1976.

Centers for Disease Control. *Guidelines for Hospital Environmental Control, Antiseptics, Handwashing, and Handwashing Facilities*. Atlanta, February 1981.

Cruse, J. E., and Foord, R. "A five-year prospective study of 23,649 surgical wounds." *Arch Surg* 107(August):206, 1973.

Dineen, P. "An evaluation of the duration of the surgical scrub." *Surg Gyn Obstet* 129(December): 1181–1184, 1969.

"Proposed recommended practices for OR wearing apparel." *AORN J* 33(January):100–106, 1981.

"Proposed recommended practices for preoperative skin preparation of patients." *AORN J* 35(April): 918–923, 1982.

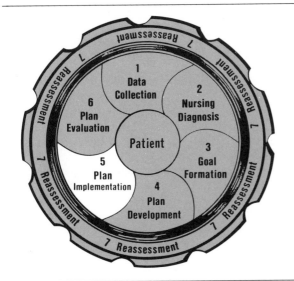

The nurse positions the patient.

Positioning the Patient

Perhaps the first responsibility of the nurse in the operating room is to recognize that knowledge regarding safe positioning of patients is dynamic and that constant new information must be added to basic knowledge not only of surgical patients but also of the physiological effects of posture in normal awake and disease states.

The ideal position is one that provides optimum exposure for the surgeon, the best airway and monitoring access for the anesthetist, and is physiologically safe for the patient. The basic components for safe positioning have been described as knowledge, forethought, teamwork, and housekeeping (1). Knowledge includes physiological consequences of positioning and individual patient limitations. Forethought involves understanding of the procedure and the problems of exposure for each member of the team and developing an appropriate plan. Teamwork means adequate communication and coordination as well as having sufficient personnel available when the positioning is done. Housekeeping is knowing the equipment needed and having it available and in working order.

Planning and preparation begin with the preoperative interview. From the patient history and interview the nurse determines any potential problems with the specific surgical position. Influencing the patient's ability to cope with the surgical position are factors such as age, weight, activity level, muscle tone, central or peripheral nerve dysfunction, metabolic function, and cardiopulmonary status as well as preexisting disorders such as arthritis, obesity, diabetes, or general debilitation. Nursing assessment during the interview includes, if possible, having the patient assume the position required during surgery. An example would be extension of the legs of an arthritic patient for lithotomy position. The limitations should be carefully described in the nursing care plan. Under anesthesia, a patient's limitations can easily be exceeded as the central nerve reflexes are obtunded and skeletal muscles, which normally provide support and safeguard, are relaxed.

Physiological Changes during Positioning

It is necessary to understand some of the changes in normal physiology that occur with position changes before application can be made to the anesthetized patient. Respiration, circulation, peripheral nerves and vessels, and skin pressure are the areas that pose the most problems and have been the most widely studied.

RESPIRATORY SYSTEM

Position influences respiration in several ways. First, the ventilation-perfusion ratio is disturbed. That is, the pulmonary capillary blood volume and consequently the amount of blood available for oxygenation are altered by gravity. At the same time, the inspired air in the lungs is redistributed, affecting the air available to oxygenate blood. For example, patients with unilateral lung disease have an increase in arterial oxygen pressure when lying with the "good lung down" because the best oxygenated lung also receives the greatest amount of blood (2).

Another position effect on respiration is that the compliance or stretchability of the lung tissue is decreased by ventilators or changes in blood volume, reducing the amount of air that can be taken in for gas exchange.

Perhaps the most significant factor affecting respiration is the mechanical restriction of lung expansion at the ribs or sternum and the reduced ability of the diaphragm to push down against abdominal retractors. Normally, the thoracic cage expands in all directions except posteriorly. Interference with any of these movements reduces respiratory function.

Preoperatively, the nurse can evaluate respiratory function by patient history. Such factors as smoking and obesity as well as preexisting pulmonary disease should alert the nurse to look further for medical evaluation of respiratory status. Arterial blood gases or pulmonary function tests can help the nurse determine that patient's ability to cope with transport as well as the surgical position. The nurse should also keep in mind that patients with reduced pulmonary function may suffer respiratory difficulties with heavy premedication and must be observed closely.

CIRCULATORY SYSTEM

Anesthesia causes circulatory changes. Whether general or regional anesthesia is used, peripheral blood vessels tend to dilate, resulting in a drop in blood pressure. The dilated vascular beds allow venous blood to pool in dependent areas, reducing the amount of blood returned to the heart and lungs for oxygenation and redistribution. Both general and spinal anesthesia obtund normal compensatory mechanisms for maintaining blood pressure. General anesthesia depresses the cerebral medulla, which normally maintains cardiac output and peripheral vascular constriction. Muscle relaxants used during general anesthesia reduce the milking action of normal muscle tone that aids in venous return. Reduced respiratory effort as well as ventilator-assisted positive respiration diminish the negative thoracic pressure that aids in pulling venous blood back to the heart. Spinal or epidural anesthesia directly blocks autonomic output from the spinal cord, bringing about extreme vasodilation and venous pooling below the areas of the block.

Any patient with poor cardiac status, hypovolemia, or arteriosclerotic vascular disease will be at greater risk under anesthesia in most positions. Again, the severely obese individual (100 pounds overweight) exhibits marked deviations from normal circulatory function even without the additional stress of anesthesia and compromising positions.

PERIPHERAL NERVES AND VESSELS

The most evident changes seen as a result of poor positioning are damage to peripheral nerves and vessels, usually due to direct mechanical pressure. The principle factor in nerve injuries is ischemia or inadequate blood supply to the nerve caused by stretching or compression. Pressure for even a few minutes can bring about impaired nerve function, resulting in sensory or motor loss, or both. Preexisting conditions such as alcoholism, diabetes, peripheral neuropathies, and hypothermia can contribute to nerve damage. Most postoperative palsies, however, are thought to result from malposition on the operating table. Generally, the longer the peripheral nerve and the more superficial its position, the greater the chance of injury. The most vulnerable time is during anesthesia when muscle tone is reduced. Damage to nerves and vessels is not usually discovered until recovery from anesthesia is complete and may be masked for days by postoperative sedation.

Peripheral vascular damage occurs with occlusion of the vessels. The most frequent cause is external pressure such as a tight restraint or crossed legs. Vessels may also occlude by hyperextending or twisting a limb, thereby obliterating flow by compressing the vessel against the body's bony structure. For example, one study showed that even in normal, awake people, 85 percent could obliterate a radial pulse by simply hyperabducting their arm over their head (3).

SKIN PRESSURE

Another important nursing responsibility often overlooked in operating rooms is skin pressure. Decubitus ulcers can develop as a consequence of poor positioning and poor protection during surgery. One study found a 13 percent incidence of pressure sores in patients having operations lasting longer than two hours (4). The highest incidence was in the elderly and in those in poor general condition. The critical factor in the formation of pressure sores is tissue perfusion. Pressure sores can develop if capillary pressure is lowered, as with low blood pressure; blood flow is obstructed by compression of vessels or torsion of tissue; or external pressure increases, as with a hard surface or tissue edema. Body weight is unevenly distributed when a person is lying on a hard surface. The concentration of weight is on the bony prominences and surrounding tissue. If blood pressure is normal, capillary pressure will remain in the range of 12–22 mm Hg. Therefore, if external pressures are higher than this, ischemia could result. With a lower blood pressure, even less pressure could produce ischemia. Also, duration rather than intensity is thought to be the more important factor. Healthy individuals can tolerate external pressures up to 100 mm Hg on bony prominences without tissue ischemia for short periods of time. Tourniquet pressures over nonbony portions of limbs are indeed much higher for even an hour or more. But low, constant pressures on bony prominences of even 70 mm Hg have been shown to cause microscopic changes in healthy individuals after two hours (5). Intermittent pressures of high intensity are also tolerated better than low, constant pressure. The significant factors in pressure sore information are a bony prominence and constant pressure. Patients with diabetes, peripheral vascular disease, debilitated states, or those who are hypotensive are particularly vulnerable.

Positions

SUPINE (DORSAL RECUMBENT)

The most common position, the supine position, is used for any anterior approach, such as abdominal surgery, most extremity procedures, some thoracic procedures, and head and neck surgery. Although the most common practice is to have the table flat, extending the patient's legs, back, and arms—the "lawn chair position"—has been advocated for all but abdominal surgeries because slight flexion of the knees reduces tension on the back (1). The head should be on a small pillow, flexing the neck slightly. Arms are either at the sides or extended on armboards (see Fig. 22.1).

The supine position is thought to be the least harmful. Significant physiological changes, however, have been measured. Vital capacity decreases almost 9.5 percent because of restricted posterolateral chest movement. A gallbladder rest archs the patient's back, and if it is up, vital capacity is reduced further to 13.5 percent due to additional diaphragmatic restriction. Tidal volume will decrease 14 percent from the upright position during anesthesia and as much as 24 percent with the gallbladder rest up (6). Without adequate respiratory assistance, a patient may easily become hypoxic when the gallbladder rest is used. An extended or elevated thorax position for upper abdominal surgery has been recommended instead of the gallbladder rest (7). Healthy individuals have been found to have much less adverse cardiovascular and respiratory effects with this position than with an extended gallbladder rest.

When supine, obese patients (100 percent over normal weight) have as much as 40–50 percent increase in the mechanical work of breathing. At the same time, oxygen consumption increases 11 percent (8). Therefore, supplemental oxygen should be considered in any obese patient who must remain supine for extended periods of time. If the patient is awake, respiration should be assessed periodically.

Circulatory changes in the supine position are usually less pronounced than in other positions. Both regional and general anesthesia, however, will decrease mean arterial pressure. Abdominal retractors, packs, or large intra-abdominal mass as in pregnancy can markedly obstruct venous return to the heart. A person with such a mass may become normotensive when placed in a left lateral position reducing the direct pressure on the vena cava.

Even in the supine position, obese patients are at greater risk of cardiovascular deficiencies. Blood volume in the heart and lungs is increased. Cardiac output increases as much as 35 percent over sitting, and pulmonary artery wedge pressure can increase 44 percent, presenting a risk of heart failure (9). Therefore, ongoing cardiac and blood pressure monitoring are necessary even in the awake obese patient.

As with all surgical positions, careful placement of extremities is important to prevent peripheral nerve and vessel damage. Damage is most likely to occur in areas exposed to hard surfaces or in misaligned limbs. Brachial plexus injury is considered the most common nerve injury. In the supine position, most patients with reported injuries had an arm extended. The extended arm must be kept at less than a 90-degree angle from the body. Having the head and neck turned in the opposite direction from the arm and extension and suspension of the arm straight from the wrist will also place undue pressure on the brachial plexus. Damage to the brachial plexus results in motor and sensory loss to the arm and shoulder girdle. Also, subclavian and axillary arteries may be compressed or occluded with hyperabduction of the arm. If the arm is abducted on an armboard, radial or brachial pulses should be checked periodically (see Fig. 22.2).

Figure 22.1. Supine (dorsal) position.

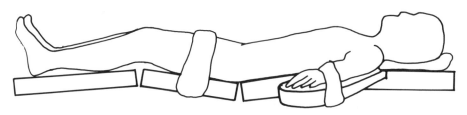

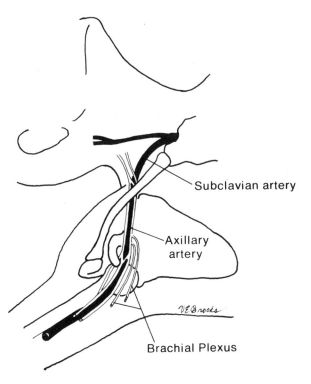

Subclavian artery

Axillary artery

V E Brooks

Brachial Plexus

Figure 22.2. Anatomical structure of the upper arm and shoulder.

Misplacement of the arm or compression against the side of the table can result in radial (wrist drop), median (ape hand), or ulnar nerve (claw hand) damage. Ulnar nerve paralysis has occurred in thin or emaciated patients because their elbow or arm was pressing against a hard surface (see Figs. 22.3 and 22.4).

The leg strap should be placed at least 2 inches above the knee. No direct pressure should be placed on the popliteal space as might be seen with a pillow and tight leg strap (see Fig. 22.5). Compression in this area can result in venous thrombosis. Although less common, tibial or sural nerve damage can occur and cause numbness on the plantar surface of the foot (see Fig. 22.6).

Skin pressure areas occur most frequently in the supine position. Underweight as well as obese individuals are vulnerable to pressure areas. Underweight individuals have greater intensities of pressure in smaller areas, while obese individuals have more extensive moderate pressure areas. Patients having surgery of two or more hours duration, or those who are diabetic, hypotensive, hypothermic, underweight, or obese, should have protective padding under heels, elbows, sacrum, and occiput. Sheepskin, foam rubber, or alternating pressure pads have been used successfully.

TRENDELENBURG'S POSITION

Used for lower abdominal surgery or whenever better visualization of abdominal organs is needed, as with the obese patient, Trendelenburg is a variant of the basic supine position, with the body tilted head down. The leg may be lowered parallel to the floor to maintain the position and to allow more room for the Mayo stand above the toes. Care must always be taken to prevent pressure on the toes once the position is attained. As in the supine position,

Figure 22.3. Anatomical structure of inner aspect of left arm.

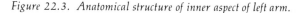

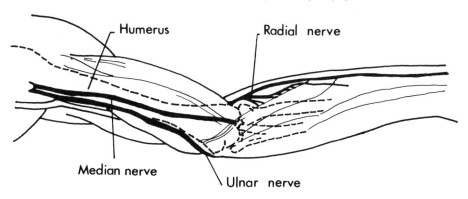

Humerus   Radial nerve

Median nerve   Ulnar nerve

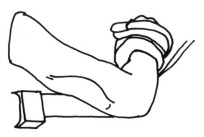

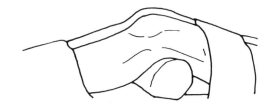

Figure 22.4. Nerve damage can occur when elbow is pressed against hard surface.

Figure 22.5. Pressure on popliteal space with a pillow under knees and a tight strap over thighs. This compression can cause venous thrombosis.

arms may be extended on armboards or tucked at the side, palm down or toward the body. Shoulder braces may be used for maintaining the position with extreme angles of Trendelenburg (see Fig. 22.7). However, if the shoulder brace is misplaced over soft tissue, the brachial plexus can be damaged. Other possible nerve and vessel injuries are similar to the basic supine.

Respiratory changes are more pronounced than in the supine position. Vital capacity falls 14.5 percent below that in sitting, and tidal volume decreases progressively with the degree of Trendelenburg. At 10 degrees, tidal volume has been measured to decrease 3 percent; at 20 to 30 degrees, it decreases 12 percent (6). Respiratory depression is due to limitation of

diaphragm expansion and maldistribution of blood to ventilation. The apex of the lung receives the greatest blood supply in this position but has less alveolar tissue than the base of the lung. In addition, the Trendelenburg position increases intrathoracic pressure, which could be undesirable in patients with cardiac decompensation or in those whom increased intracranial pressure may be hazardous.

REVERSE TRENDELENBURG

In the reverse Trendelenburg, another variation of the basic supine, the entire table is slanted feet down. For extreme angles, a padded foot board may be needed to support the patient's body. Reverse Trendelenburg is

Figure 22.6. Anatomical structure surrounding popliteal area. Specifically, the popliteal nerve and common peroneal nerve.

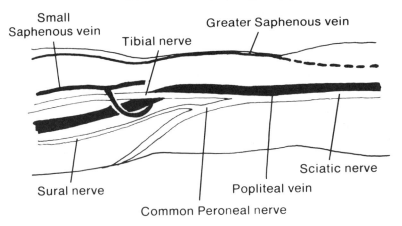

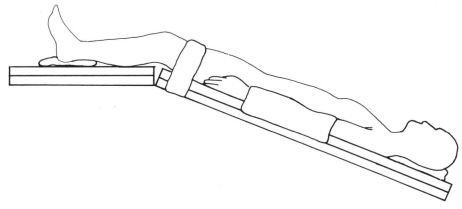

Figure 22.7. Trendelenburg's position.

used for head and neck surgery. A roll, bolster, or sandbag may be placed under the shoulders for better access and stabilization in neck surgeries, such as thyroid, radical neck, tracheostomies, or in jaw and mouth surgery. The head may be turned to one side in carotid surgery.

Respiratory and circulatory problems are nearly the opposite of the Trendelenburg position. Respiration is less affected, while circulation can be greatly compromised. There is only a 9 percent decrease in vital capacity from sitting (6). However, the reverse Trendelenburg position permits considerable peripheral pooling of as much as several hundred milliliters of blood in the lower extremities. As expected, mean arterial pressure decreases. Movements from both the Trendelenburg and the reverse Trendelenburg positions under anesthesia must be done slowly to allow the heart time to adjust to the great changes in blood volume.

LITHOTOMY POSITION

The lithotomy position is used for perineal surgery, including procedures on the vulva, vagina, prostate, and rectum. The second most common position used in surgery, the lithotomy position carries the potential for a variety of injuries (see Fig. 22.8).

Systemic changes that occur with this position can be significant. Respiratory effective-

Figure 22.8. Lithotomy position.

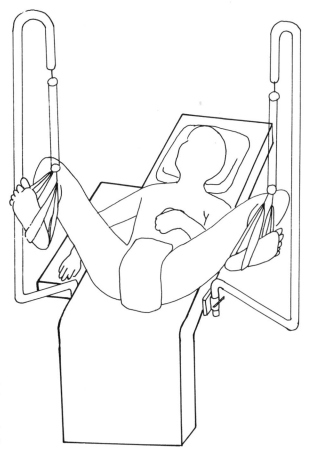

ness is reduced by marked restriction of diaphragmatic movement caused by increased abdominal pressure from the thighs. Pulmonary blood volume is increased, resulting in engorgement of lung tissue, reducing its compliance. Vital capacity decreases 18 percent and tidal volume 3 percent from sitting posture. With an addition of 10-degree Trendelenburg, tidal volume can decrease 14 percent (6). Circulatory pooling occurs in the lumbar region in the lithotomy position. Venous flow can be reduced by interference with lung expansion, which normally provides a negative "thoracic pump" aiding in venous return. When the legs are lowered, 500–600 ml of blood may drain into the legs from the trunk, resulting in severe hypotension. Elastic stockings may prevent some of this large influx by increasing venous pressure. Slow and smooth movement when lowering the legs is extremely important. The legs should be lowered over a period of not less than two minutes.

Special considerations are needed in preventing peripheral nerve damage in the lithotomy position. If the arms are allowed to remain at the sides, pressure injuries or even crushing injury to the hand can occur when the end of the table is raised or lowered. The hands should not extend beyond the break in the table. If the arms are placed at the patient's sides, then the arms should be crossed over the patient's chest prior to raising the end of

the table. The arms may be folded across the chest loosely at the beginning of the procedure and held by the patient's gown or a sheet. Respiratory effort is restricted, however, and ulnar nerve damage can result from pressure on the inner aspect of the elbow against the table. Armboards placed parallel against the table are ideal.

Placement of the legs in stirrups is extremely important. The buttocks must not extend beyond the break in the table or undue stress will be placed on the back as the legs are lowered. The need for realignment is minimized by having the patient position himself with buttocks just above the break in the table. Since most of the body weight rests on the sacrum, additional padding may be needed to prevent a pressure area. Two people should simultaneously raise the legs and place the feet in stirrups while supporting the lower leg. Hips should be symmetrical. Calves of the legs should be parallel to the table. If more abduction is needed for greater exposure, then flexion or external rotation should be done at the hip and not the knee. If the patient has had a prior hip pinning, total hip replacement, or is arthritic, the hip should be supported by one hand as the leg and foot are gently extended.

Damage can occur to the femoral and obturator nerves in the groin from undue pressure (see Fig. 22.9). Such an injury might be caused by misplacement of instruments. The

Figure 22.9. Location of the anatomical structures in order to prevent pressure on the groin and popliteal area. Pressure on the peroneal nerve has the potential of causing foot drop.

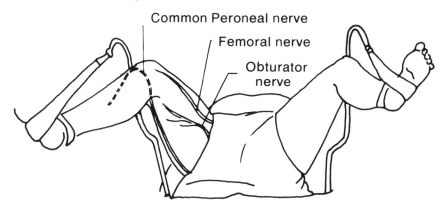

Common Peroneal nerve

Femoral nerve

Obturator nerve

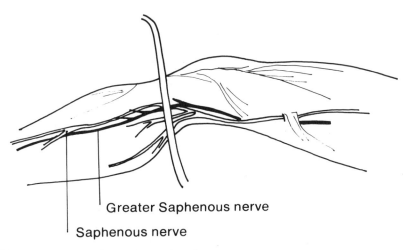

Greater Saphenous nerve

Saphenous nerve

Figure 22.10. Direct pressure causes damage to vessels and nerves.

obese patient is particularly at risk as extra effort is frequently needed for adequate retraction. Damage to the femoral or obturator nerve can result in sensory disturbances to the inner aspect of the leg and the abductor muscles of the inner thigh.

Unpadded or misplaced stirrups can damage the saphenous vessels and nerves on the medial aspect of the knee (see Figs. 22.10 and 22.11). The most prevalent problem, however, is peroneal nerve damage on the lateral aspect of the knee, which can produce foot drop. Stirrup holders should be placed well on the outside of the leg, allowing no contact between the leg and the holder. If necessary, additional foam padding around the knee may be used (see Fig. 22.9).

SITTING POSITION

This position is used primarily in neurosurgical procedures, such as posterior fossa craniotomies or posterior cervical spine procedures. Physiologically it is the best possible position for respiration. There is practically no abnormal restriction on chest expansion, but the sitting position can greatly compromise systemic circulation. Hypotension and loss of

Figure 22.11. The Saphenous vein and nerve.

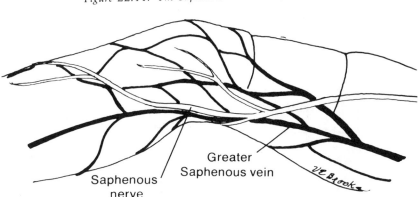

Saphenous nerve

Greater Saphenous vein

consciousness have occurred even in unanesthetized individuals when placed in sitting position from a supine position. Antigravity suits (G-suits) have been used to reduce venous pooling in the dependent legs. It is recommended that either a G-suit, elastic stocking, or preferably ace leg wraps to the groin be applied to all patients in this position. In addition, the craniotomy patient is at further risk to develop vascular air emboli, and a central venous pressure (CVP) monitor along with a precordial Doppler are almost always standard anesthesia equipment for such procedures.

In this position most of the body weight rests on the ischial tuberosities. Unless the table is well padded, skin pressure areas can develop here, as can sciatic nerve damage, particularly in thin or diabetic individuals. Supporting the feet at a near right-angle alignment to the legs will reduce sacral pressure as well as prevent foot injuries.

Placing the patient in the sitting position is a carefully planned step-by-step process. The novice is encouraged to do a simulated "dry-run" to gain confidence and familiarity with equipment prior to positioning the anesthetized patient. All equipment—head holder, pillows, tape—should be in the room before positioning is started. If an antigravity suit is used, it should be placed on the table prior to the patient. For cervical procedures, one or two pillows are placed on the thigh section of the table, which will help elevate the patient. In the final position, the patient's second or third thoracic vertebra are at the elevated table edge when the head platform is removed (10).

To put the patient in the sitting position, the nurse first loosens the thigh straps, then flexes the table fully and lowers one foot section at least 45 degrees. Slowly, he elevates the back section and at the same time tilts the table chassis in steep Trendelenburg. Foot section is kept horizontal. The patient's blood pressure is carefully monitored with each table manipulation, and the patient may require vasopressors before additional back elevation is added. The nurse continues to elevate the back section until the desired position is obtained with the patient's legs horizontal and at about the level of the heart.

The head portion of the table is removed as the head is manually supported. The head can be stabilized with a horseshoe headrest, or preferably better with a head holder or pin (Mayfield) holder. All head holder units can become partially or completely dislodged, causing either eye injury (more common with horseshoe holder) or neck injury. Scrupulous attention must be paid to head stabilization prior to draping. Arms are usually crossed in the patient's lap and secured with wide adhesive tape to the table frame. Elbows should be supported on pillows to prevent ulnar nerve damage (see Fig. 22.12).

Figure 22.12. Sitting position.

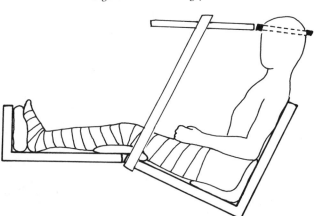

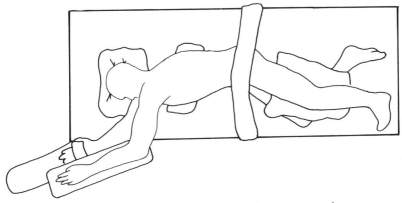

Figure 22.13. Lateral position for thoractomy procedures.

LATERAL POSITION

The lateral position is used for hip, thoracic, or kidney procedures. The patient is anesthetized while supine and then turned onto the un-affected side. Teamwork is essential as four people are needed for a smooth and gentle turn. The anesthetist guides the head and shoulders, one person is on each side, and one is at the feet. The break of the table should be at the level of the iliac crest instead of under the flank or lower ribs. The patient is first moved close to the edge of the table, keeping good alignment. The "down" arm is brought forward to reduce direct pressure, then the patient is gently turned with affected side up. The head should be neutral, and midline supported with a pillow and the back in straight alignment. A pillow is placed between the legs with the lower leg flexed to 90 degrees and the upper leg straight, or vice versa (see Fig. 22.13). Both feet should be flexed. For hip procedures, stabilization is maintained with a suction bean bag that is covered with a bath blanket or towel to reduce skin friction and pressure. For thoracotomy procedures, the back torso is stabilized with a sandbag or pillow at the back and in front of the chest. For kidney pro-cedures, the table is flexed with the patient's head and feet down. In addition, the table's "kidney rest" may be raised for better access. The upper arm is either supported with a raised armboard or several pillows (see

Fig. 22.14). An axillary roll should be under the "down" axilla with the lower shoulder forward. The down arm is slightly or fully flexed. Radial pulse should be checked often to ensure circulatory adequacy in the down arm. Wide adhesive tape is used over the hips and frequently over the shoulders to stabilize the position.

A simple lateral position reduces vital capacity 10 percent and tidal volume 8 percent. The kidney position decreases vital capacity 14.5 per-cent (6). This is due to restriction of chest expansion as well as a change in blood-to-gas exchange ratio in each lung.

Blood pools in dependent limbs. Blood pres-sure measurements are lower than the actual arterial pressure. The pressure in the upper arm is measured above the level of the heart, and in the down arm it is measured on a partially compressed axillary artery. Direct arterial pressure measurements, however, are known to drop. Eggers and coworkers (11) measured a 24 mm Hg drop in the left lateral position and a 33 mm Hg drop in the right lateral position. It is postulated that more obstruction to vena caval flow occurs on the right side, and there may also be actual inter-ference with heart action, that is, a possible shift in heart position.

Skin pressure areas can develop between the legs from the weight of the upper leg on the lower and may be minimized with proper placement of pillows. Pressure under the

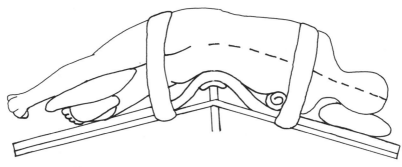

Figure 22.14. Lateral position for kidney procedures.

greater trochanter major of the femur has been measured as high as 110 mm Hg on standard operating room table pads (5).

Peripheral nerve injuries to the brachial plexus and the median, radial, and ulnar nerves can occur if the upper arm is not properly supported on the overhead armboard. The most common nerve damage with the lateral position is peroneal nerve damage from compression of the down knee against a hard surface. Extra padding should be provided under the down knee, particularly in thin individuals.

PRONE POSITION

The prone position is used for any procedure requiring a dorsal approach. It is used most often for spinal surgery, such as laminectomies or fusions. It may also be used for posterior cervical and occasionally for occipital procedures when a sitting position is not preferred. If the patient has had a recent spinal cord injury requiring immediate decompression or stabilization, special precautions are taken.

The patient is almost always anesthetized in the supine position, usually on the stretcher or bed and then turned prone onto the table. The anesthetist or anesthesiologist coordinates the turn because he is responsible for the head and airway management. Movements should not be made until the anesthetist is ready. One or two people (if the patient is large) stand on both sides of the patient on the outside of the stretcher and the table. It is preferable to have one person at the foot. The patient's arms are either straight down at the sides or straight above the head (usually for the awake patient). The patient is moved to the side of the stretcher and then, as the anesthetist holds the head, is gently rotated onto the side and then onto the abdomen. The team members on the opposite side of the stretcher receive the patient with their arms under the abdomen, chest, and shoulders. If the arms are to be placed on armboards, it is critical that the elbow be bent and the palm of the hand face inward before the arm is extended. Dislocations can very easily occur during this maneuver. If the patient has had a recent cervical trauma, then the head must remain in a neutral position throughout positioning. Traction may be needed prior to intubation or turning to stabilize the neck. An additional person must be available to assist anesthesia. If there is no recent cervical injury, slight flexion is preferred when moving the head.

Once the patient is prone, restriction on the chest and abdomen are reduced by either a preplaced laminectomy frame or body rolls extending from shoulders to iliac crest on either side (Fig. 22.15). Breasts should be free, and male genitalia protected by an additional towel or small pillow at the pubis. Feet should be supported at no less than a 45-degree angle to the legs by pillows or rolls under the anterior surface of the ankle with no pressure on the toes. With the head turned to one side, a head donut or small towel will help prevent pressure on the ear and eye.

Blood pressure always drops in the prone position. Eggers and coworkers (11) measured

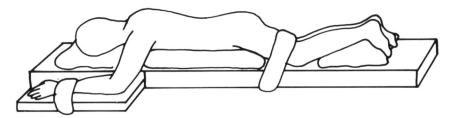

Figure 22.15. Prone position.

a 20 mm Hg drop in mean arterial pressure. With the use of chest rolls, however, mean arterial pressure was seen to drop less (15 mm Hg). Chest rolls or a laminectomy frame relieve the mechanical restriction on chest movement, which can reduce vital capacity 10 percent and tidal volume 11 percent (6). The improvement of respiratory effectiveness facilitates venous flow and assists blood pressure. Skin pressure areas are greatest on the chest, knees, and ankle, but occur on the shoulders and iliac crests in thin individuals. Because many procedures done in the prone position are of long duration, sheepskin or additional padding placed under these pressure areas is helpful.

JACKKNIFE OR KRASKE POSITION

A variation of the prone position, the jackknife position is used most frequently for proctological procedures. The patient is either anesthetized supine and turned prone or is placed in position before a caudal or hypobaric spinal anesthetic is administered. The hips are on a pillow or towel directly over the table break, and the table is flexed 90 degrees with the head and legs down. The patient's arms are on armboards with hands toward the head (see Fig. 22.16). The buttocks may be separated at the level of the anus on both sides with wide adhesive tape and secured to the table. The patient is taken out of the position by first flattening the table and then reversing the order of moving into the prone position. Arms are usually held over the head for turning.

The jackknife position has been described as the most pernicious of surgical positions. Both respiration and circulation can be most adversely affected. Vital capacity has been measured to reduce 12.5 percent due to restricted diaphragmatic movement and to increased blood volume in the lungs, reducing lung compliance (6). With blood pooling in both the chest and feet, mean arterial pressure drops

Figure 22.16. Jackknife or Kraske position.

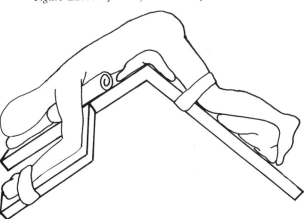

significantly. A most severe drop in blood pressure can occur when a lateral tilt is added to the jackknife. A 38 mm Hg drop has been recorded in a right lateral jackknife and a 27 mm Hg drop in a left lateral jackknife position. Although lateral tilt is not often used, the additive effect should be known (11). In addition to dependent pooling, venous return may also be seriously limited by mechanical obstruction at the point of the table break as well as by the reduced negative intrathoracic pressure. The slowed venous return of blood in combination with obtunded compensatory mechanisms by anesthesia can produce a decrease in stroke volume affecting cardiac output. A drop in blood pressure may be accompanied by bradycardia. Continuous cardiac and blood pressure monitoring is recommended even in patients under local anesthetic. An intravenous line should also be open. Blood pressure may be maintained with the use of fluid volume, and intravenous medications such as atropine may be needed.

Skin pressure areas are similar to those seen in the prone position, with greater pressure on the pubis at the table break if no protection is used.

References

1. Martin, J. "General requirements of safe positioning of the surgical patient." In *Positioning in Anesthesia and Surgery*, pp. 1–5. Philadelphia: W. B. Saunders, 1978.
2. Remolina, C., Khan, A. U., Santiago, T. V., and Edelman, N. H. "Positional hypoxemia in unilateral lung disease." *N Engl J Med* 26:304, 523–525, 1981.
3. Wright, Irving, "The neurovascular syndrome produced by hyperabducting the arms." *Am Heart J* 29(1):1–19, 1945.
4. Hicks, Dorothy. "An incidence study of pressure sores following surgery." *ANA Clin Sess*, 49–54, 1970.
5. Souther, Sherman, Carr, Stephen, and Vistnes, Lars. "Pressure tissue ischemia and operating table pads." *Arch Surg*, 107:544–547, 1973.
6. Little, David M. "Posture and anesthesia." *Can Anesthetist Soc J* 7(1):2–10, 1960.
7. Videbek, F. "Posture with elevated and extended thorax." *Acta Anesthes Scand* 24:458–461, 1980.
8. Alexander, James. "Obesity and the circulation." *Mod Conc Cardiovasc Dis* 32:799–803, 1963.
9. Alexander, James. "Obesity and cardiac performance." *Am J Cardiol* 14:860–865, 1964.
10. Martin, J. "The head-elevatal positions." In *Positioning in Anesthesia and Surgery*, pp. 44–79. Philadelphia: W. B. Saunders, 1978.
11. Eggers, G., DeGroot, William, and Tanner, Charles. "Hemodynamic changes associated with various surgical positions." *JAMA* 185:1–5, 1963.

Suggested Readings

Callahan, Robert, and Brown, Mark. "Positioning techniques in spinal surgery." *Clin Orthoped Related Res* 154:22–26, 1981.

Forsyth, William, Allen, Gerald, and Gaither, Everett. "An evaluation of cardiorespiratory effects of posture in the dental outpatient." *Oral Surg* 34(4):562–579, 1972.

Foster, Charlene, Mukai, Gail, Breckenridge, Flora, and Smith, Cheryl M. Jane. "Effects of surgical positioning." *AORN J* 30(2):219–232, 1979.

Horton, Jean Mary. "Anesthesia for surgery of the spine and spinal cord." *Int Anesthesiol Clin* 15(3):253–263, 1977.

Kaye, Michael, and Waxler, Richard. "Alteration, esophageal peristalsis by body position." *Dig Dis Sci* 26(10):897–890, 1981.

Kosiak, Michael. "Etiology of decubitus ulcers." *Arch Phys Med Rehab* 42:19–29, 1961.

Linden, Olgierd, Greenway, Robert, and Piazza, Janet. "Pressure distribution on the surface of the human body: 1. Evaluation in lying and sitting positions using a 'Bed of Springs and Nails'." *Arch Phys Med Rehab* 46:378–385, 1965.

Lipe, Hillary, and Mitchell, Pamela. "Positioning the patient with intracranial hypotension: How turning and head rotation affect the internal jugular vein." *Heart Lung* 9(6):1031–1036, 1980.

Nicholson, Morris, and Eversole, Orbon. "Nerve injuries incident to anesthesia and operation." *AORN J* 2(March-April):44–65, 1964.

Parks, Barbara. "Postoperative peripheral neuropathies." *Surgery* 74(3):248–357, 1973.

Paul, Douglas, Hoyt, John, and Boutros, Azmy. "Cardiovascular and respiratory changes in response to changes of posture in the very obese." *Anesthesiology* 45(1):73–78, 1976.

Smith, Robert A. "The prone position." In John Martin, ed. *Positioning in Anesthesia and Surgery*, pp. 32–43. Philadelphia: W. B. Saunders, 1978.

Wilbourn, Samuel. "Anesthetic considerations in urology." In John Martin, ed. *Positioning in Anesthesia and Surgery*, pp. 170–175. Philadelphia: W. B. Saunders, 1978.

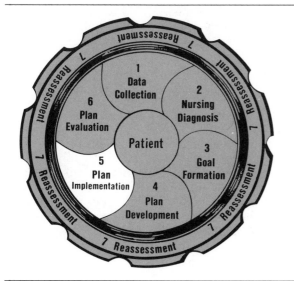

The nurse is responsible for sponge, needle, and instrument counts.

Performing Counts

Some 12 percent of all malpractice claims reported by one source involve foreign objects left in patients during surgery. The average settlement to patients from 1975 to 1978 was more than $18,000 for each such incident (1). Sponge, needle, and instrument counts help to prevent this problem. Sponge counts are well established, yet a number of hospitals still do not count needles and instruments. Some argue that needle and instrument counts are not justified. These three types of counts should be part of daily practice in every operating room. Some cases involving negligent counts are illustrated in Figs. 23.1–23.4.

Since 1976, the Association of Operating Room Nurses (AORN) has recommended that sponge, needle, and instrument counts be done for all procedures. The association considers this an optimal but achievable practice for all operating rooms. The introduction to the recommended practices states, "Every hospital and operating room should establish specific written policies and procedures for sponge, needle, and instrument counts which should define materials to be counted, the times when counts must be done, and the documentation required" (2:3-21). Major points for such a policy are then outlined.

Having a policy is the key to a successful count program. The policy should be developed

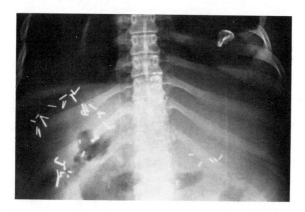

Figure 23.1. An x-ray of a patient who has had a gastroplasty with a sponge left in the gallbladder bed. The patient was brought back to surgery and the sponge removed. In this case, the circulating nurse did not follow the hospital procedure of bagging the laparotomy sponges in sets of 5 and the small sponges in groups of 10. Also, the scrub nurse and circulating nurse did not do a joint count. Rather, the circulating nurse had someone from the anesthesia department validate the count.

jointly by the medical and nursing staffs and approved by the hospital administration. It should become a part of the hospital's standard operating procedure. Once these ground rules have been established, every member of the OR team will know what is expected. The time for debate about counts is while the policy is being written, not during a case when the surgeon is ready to close the wound. When a hospital has a policy, operating room nurses as employees have an obligation to uphold it.

What should such a policy require? Sponge, needle, and instrument counting policies at the University of Colorado Hospital are based on the AORN recommended practices (see Fig. 23.5). Under such policies, the counts are carried out as indicated in the following sections.

Sponge Counts

1. Before surgery, the scrub person and circulating nurse count the sponges aloud.

Figure 23.2. This patient has had a cesarean section. The scrub nurse and circulating nurse did only one count and reported it as correct. The patient came back to the hospital six weeks after delivery with an abscess and complained of pain. Before the patient could be brought to surgery, the abscess broke.

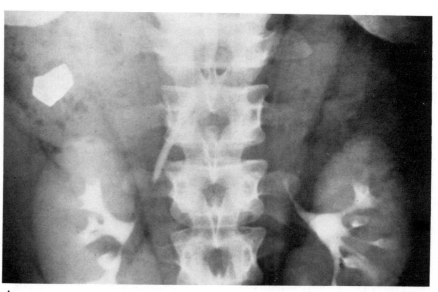

A

The scrub person should hold the sponges up off the table, and each sponge should be separated and checked closely by both persons. Both are responsible for verifying that all sponges have x-ray-detectable strips. The circulating nurse records the number and type of sponges in units of 5 or 10 on a count sheet or count board.

Nurses should never take for granted that the count on prepackaged sterilized sponges is accurate. If a package does not contain the right number of sponges, the sponges should be bagged, and the bag should be marked with the actual number, initialed, and isolated from the rest of the sponges. Some institutions require that inaccurately numbered sponges be returned immediately to central supply. It is unwise to attempt to compensate for an incorrectly numbered package during the case.

2. During surgery, the scrub nurse's responsibilities are as follows:

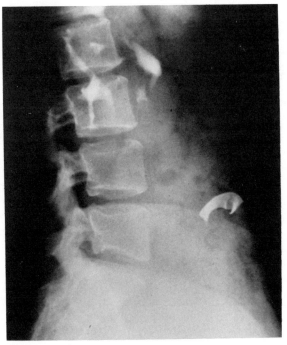

B

- She discards soiled 4-X-4 and laparotomy sponges into one kick basin lined with a plastic bag.
- She keeps small soiled sponges contained on the field, grouping them in fives or tens, according to the way they were originally packaged.
- She replaces 4 X 4s with laparotomy sponges as the body cavity is opened.
- She accounts for all free 4 X 4s or sponge sticks used.
- She notifies the circulating nurse if a 4 X 4 is to remain temporarily in the wound, such as when a sponge is placed in the vagina during a hysterectomy.

3. During surgery, the circulating nurse's responsibilities are as follows:

- She discards prep sponges into trash as the prep is being done to avoid mixing them with the counted sponges.
- She uses two plastic-lined kick buckets for handling sponges. The first is for soiled sponges thrown off the field by the scrub person, and the second is for counting. She takes sponges from the first bucket and lays them around the rim of the second bucket for counting. She weighs the sponges for blood loss as they are being transferred if the anesthesiologist requests.
- When a unit of 5 or 10 sponges is on the rim of the second bucket, she counts these aloud with the scrub person prior to bagging and checks for the x-ray detectable strip. The sponges are then placed in separate plastic bags and closed. Sponges are always handled with forceps or gloves, never with bare hands.
- She places bagged sponges away from sterile supplies in view of the anesthesiologist so that the anesthesiologist can estimate blood loss.
- She marks off a unit on the count sheet or board as each unit is bagged to keep the count current.

4. As wound closure begins, the scrub person and circulating nurse count aloud all sponges on the sterile field, the Mayo stand,

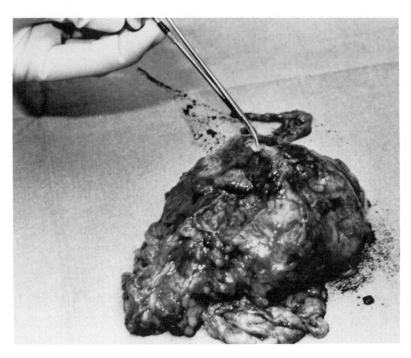

Figure 23.3. A laparotomy sponge one year after it has been left in a patient. The patient had had a cesarean section, with the sponge count reported as correct. This mass with the lap sponge was found by x-ray one year later when the patient came back to the hospital wanting to be sterilized.

and the back table. Then they count the sponges discarded in the kick buckets. The circulator should add the total of bagged sponges to the current total at this time to verify that all sponges are accounted for. The circulator reports the results to the surgeon.

5. As closure of the skin begins, the final count is done in the same manner, with the circulator reporting the results to the surgeon.

6. To prevent the possibility of sponges being left in the operating room, all 4-X-4 sponges are placed in the trash, and all laparotomy sponges are placed in the kick bucket's plastic bag, and the bag is closed and placed on top of the laundry hamper.

7. All linen and supplies are left in the OR until the patient leaves the room.

8. When the count is complete, the registered nurse who participated in the count must sign the operative record that the count

is correct. Many hospitals have both the scrub person and the circulating nurse sign the count record.

9. If a count is incorrect, the nurse notifies the surgeon immediately and initiates a search. If a sponge is not accounted for in the search, the nurse fills out an incident report and makes arrangements for an x-ray. If the surgeon refuses to have an x-ray taken, the nurse notifies the charge nurse and documents this on the incident report. She has the surgeon sign the incident report. Then she documents the event on the nurse's notes in the patient chart.

10. When a scrub person or circulator is relieved for any reason, the name of the relief person is added to the operative record, followed by the word *relief*. A complete count of sponges must be made between shift changes. If this is impossible because of the nature of

the case, attempts to do a count are documented on the operating room record.

Needle Count (Including Knife Blades and Other Small Objects)

1. Before surgery, the scrub person counts the total number of needles in the packs to be used, and the circulator records the number on a count sheet.

2. During surgery, as each needle package is opened, the scrub person verifies that it contains the correct number of needles. If the

Figure 23.4. A needle has been broken off during an anterior and posterior repair. Informed of the needle's location, the patient elected to have it left in rather than have surgery to retrieve it. One year later, the patient reported no ill effects.

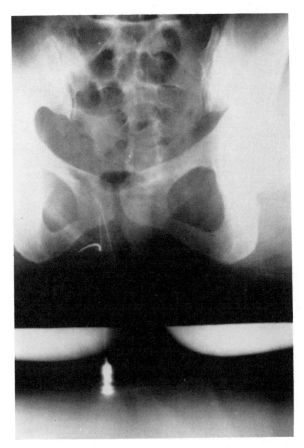

number is not correct, the package is handed to the circulator who isolates it from the field. She then subtracts the number from the count sheet.

3. Open needle packages are kept in a basin separate from other items to aid checking if a count is incorrect. The scrub person retains broken needles and blades in their entirety. If a needle or blade is flipped off the field, the circulator retrieves it and isolates it off the field. Used needles are kept on a needle disposal pad. When a pad is full, the scrub person may hand it to the circulator, who counts the needles on the pad, verifies the count with the scrub person, and subtracts it from the total remaining on the sterile field.

4. As with sponges, closing counts are taken when closure of the incision begins, and again when skin closure begins. Results are reported to the surgeon.

5. If a count is incorrect, the team follows the same procedure as for an incorrect sponge count. If the tally has too many needles, the scrub nurse hands the circulator the basin of open needle packages. The scrub person and circulator then count the unopened packages together. These two numbers plus the number of needles used should match the number recorded on the count sheet. The count is entered in the operative record and signed by the RN circulator. Used needles are disposed of properly to prevent injury to hospital personnel.

6. As with sponge counts, names of relief personnel are entered in the operative record.

Instrument Counts

1. Before surgery, the sterile instrument set is placed on the back table. The top rack of instruments is removed from the pan and placed on a rolled towel. Knife handles, towel clips, suction tips, tissue forceps, and sponge sticks are removed and placed on the back table.

2. The scrub nurse and circulator count the instruments. The circulator calls off the instruments from the count sheet. The scrub person points to each instrument and counts aloud.

Sponge count policies

- A sponge count will be taken on all operating procedures except cystoscopies, transurethral resection of the prostate, or when a particular surgeon has given the associate director of nursing service a written letter stating she does not want a count of sponges taken on her cases and she is assuming full responsibility for sponges used on her patients.
- Sponges are counted in the operating room by scrub and circulating personnel: (1) prior to the beginning of the operation; (2) as closure of the wound begins; and (3) as closure of the skin begins.
- The count is carried out audibly. The scrub person audibly counts the sponges on the sterile field. The circulating nurse audibly counts the sponges off the sterile field.
- Additional counts will be done before any part of a cavity or a cavity within a cavity is closed, as in a cesarean section, a gastrointestinal anastomosis, and the retroperitoneal space.
- Additional counts will be taken at any other time judged necessary, for example, if two incisions are made, as in a bilateral hernia repair.
- The count is recorded on the operating room counting sheet immediately after it is taken. Additional sponges added to the case are recorded.
- A registered nurse must participate in every count and sign the operative record accordingly.
- Incorrectly numbered packages of sponges are isolated. They are *not* removed from the room. These sponges should not be added to the count and should be labeled appropriately and initialed by the RN isolating them.
- Counts omitted due to an extreme patient emergency must be documented by the circulating nurse on the nurse's notes in the chart.
- All personnel must comply with the procedure of the hospital. If there is any deviation from this policy, the circulating nurse reports it to the operating room associate director of nursing service or to the head nurse, who documents it on the operating room record and initiates an incident report.
- Counted sponges are not taken from the operating room for any reason while a count is in effect.
- X-ray detectable sponges will not be used for dressings. All sponges are packaged in groups of 5 or 10, including dental rolls and cottonoids.
- Soiled sponges are handled as little as possible, using forceps or gloved hands if necessary.
- The ongoing tally is recorded on the count sheet.
- If a sponge cannot be located, an incident report will be filled out.
- When a sponge cannot be located, an x-ray will be taken before the patient leaves the operating room. If the surgeon refuses to have the x-ray taken in the operating room, this must always be documented on the incident report and signed by the surgeon. An incident report will be completed whether the x-ray is negative or reveals a sponge.

Needle and knife blade counting policies
Policies are the same as for counting sponges, with these additions:
- Needle and knife blade counts are done for all procedures.
- Scrub personnel count needles and blades continually during the procedure and should hand them to the surgeon only on an exchange basis.
- Needles broken during a procedure are accounted for in their entirety.
- Used needles are kept on a needle count pad to ensure their containment on the sterile field.

Instrument counts
Policies are the same as for counting sponges, with these differences:
- Instruments are counted on all surgical procedures when the abdominal, thoracic, pelvic, and retroperitoneal cavities are opened. This includes all hernia repairs.
- Standardization of instrument sets is established for ease in counting, based on the minimum number and types of instruments in the set.
- Instruments broken or disassembled during a procedure are accounted for in their entirety.

Figure 23.5. Sample policies for sponge, needle, and instrument counts. These policies are those of the operating room at the University of Colorado Hospital, Denver.

The circulator records the number on the count sheet.

3. During surgery, instruments added to the field are counted aloud by the scrub person, observed by the circulator, and recorded on the count sheet.

4. If an instrument falls off the sterile field, the circulator retrieves it, shows it to the scrub nurse, and isolates it from the field. Then she records it on the sheet as being off the field.

5. The closing count is taken when closure begins. Results are reported to the surgeon.

6. If the count is incorrect, personnel follow the same procedure as for incorrect sponge and needle counts.

The Nurse's Legal Responsibility

Counting is part of the professional nurse's responsibility for patient safety; moreover, it is an area of legal accountability. Nurses can no longer take the attitude that the surgeon bears total responsibility for their actions as "captain of the ship." Under this traditional operating room doctrine, nurses were considered "borrowed servants" during surgery. That is, while the operation was in progress, the surgeon was considered in command, and the nurses, though hospital employees, were temporarily under her sole authority. Recently, courts have recognized that nurses have independent areas of responsibility in the operating room. The captain-of-the-ship doctrine has weakened, especially in the area of counts. Nurses and hospitals are being held liable.

When a patient sues in a surgical case, a judge or jury will decide whether there has been negligence on the part of the personnel involved. In reaching a decision, they will examine what is considered to be the standard of care for hospitals and for the professions involved. One test of negligence is whether the professionals involved exercised the degree of care that other reasonable professionals would have exercised. The same would be considered for hospitals. When a foreign body is left in a patient, and the patient sues, the courts are likely to examine, first, whether the

hospital had a counting policy and, second, whether the nurses followed the policy. When negligence is found in this area, the hospital, not the surgeon, will probably be held liable as employer of the nurses whose duty is to execute a correct count.

A 1977 ruling by the Texas Supreme Court illustrates how the captain-of-the-ship doctrine is breaking down. The decision came in *Sparger* v *Worley Hospital et al Texas* (547 SW 2d 582). A sponge was left in a patient's abdominal cavity. The count, performed by the scrub nurse and circulating nurse, did not show a missing sponge. The nurses were employees of the hospital, not of the surgeon performing the operation. The hospital had written policies and procedures for the duties of the scrub nurse and circulator, which included sponge counts.

The trial court held that the hospital, as the nurses' employer, was liable, not the surgeon. The hospital appealed, saying the surgeon should be held responsible as captain of the ship. The state supreme court turned down the appeal, saying the doctrine was a false rule of law. The court found instead that, as hospital employees, the nurses were obligated to follow the institution's policies, which specified a sponge count (3). The decision, as William A. Regan points out, does not mean surgeons are never liable for the actions of nurses. When nurses are directly employed by the surgeon instead of the hospital, they still are considered "borrowed servants" (3). Nevertheless, the case did emphasize that nurses can be held liable for their own actions and that they do have a legal duty to follow hospital policy.

Professional standards are used by courts to measure whether personnel have been negligent. Standards provide a guideline for what is considered a reasonable degree of care within the field. The AORN-recommended practices for sponge, needle, and instrument counts, although voluntary, are considered the standard for when and how counts should be performed in the operating room. They are a way that operating room nurses indicate to society that they are self-regulating professionals. In turn, the recommended practices may be used

Figure 23.6. Instrument count sheet (permission given by University of Colorado Health Sciences Center).

INSTRUMENT COUNT SHEET OPERATING ROOM	NAME								
	DATE								
Instruments	First Count	Add	Off Field	FINAL		Needle	Umb Tape	Clips	Blades
Knife Handles									
Scissors									
Pickups									
Needleholders									
Mosquitoes - CVD									
Mosquitoes - ST									
Criles - CVD									
Criles - ST									
Crawfords									
Allis									
Kockers									
Peans									
Babcocks									
Penningtons									
Tonsils									
Rt. Angles									
Metal Suctions & Parts									
Sponge Sticks						Laps	Raytec	Peanuts	Cotton oids
Kidney Pedicle									
Lung Clamps									
Towel Clips									
Balfour Sidewall Blades & Screw									
G.I. SPECS									
Doyans ST & CVD Rubber Pieces									
Shoe Strings									
Colostomy Rod									
DeMartel Clamps & Pts.									
Allen Kochers									
Glassman Bowel Clamps									
Debakey Bowel Clamps									
G.B. INSTRUMENTS									
Dilators									
Probes									
Stone Forceps									
Trochar									
GYN SPECS									
Heaneys									
Tenaculums									
C.V. TRAY									
C.V. Clamps									
Bulldogs									
Rummel Tourniquet & rubber pieces									
Nerve Hook									
Freer Elevator									
Penfield									
Clip Appliers									
Chest Retractor & Parts									

by those who are attempting to determine whether nurses have met the expected standards of conduct.

Why Needle and Instrument Counts?

Nurses often ask if needle and instrument counts are necessary because some hospitals do not require them. Both, however, should be part of the routine in every operating room because of the principles of patient safety.

Some nurses object to needle counts because they are time-consuming and too complex. Hundreds of needles may be used on a case, and needle packages of different types do not contain a standard number of needles. These nurses believe the probability of an incorrect count is high, even though a needle may not, in fact, be missing (4). These objections, however, do not outweigh the merits of doing needle counts. The process need not be time-consuming, because the scrub person and circulator should be counting needles continuously throughout the case. A well-organized count, using the system described, should keep incorrect counts to a minimum.

Instrument counts are the most controversial. The principal argument is that the count may be too time-consuming, extending the time of the patient's anesthesia. Some argue that the incidence of instruments left in wounds is so rare that counts are not justified. The California Hospital Association is one group that takes this position, recommending that formal instrument counts not be done (5).

But what happens when an instrument remains in the body? In one case, a patient had had a cholecystectomy. The procedure was uneventful, but six days later, the bowel obstructed because a loop of the bowel had slipped through a ring of a Kelly clamp that had been left in the wound. The patient was taken back to surgery, given general anesthesia once again, and the clamp was removed. He died several weeks later of acute hepatitis. Given the seriousness of such an incident, developing an instrument count procedure is well worth it, even if such cases are uncommon.

As with other types of counts, organization and efficiency are the keys to preventing delays in cases. Instrument counts cannot be done properly until instrument sets are standardized. Mehaffy and Seawalt have described practical ways for instituting count procedures (6, 7). Generally, instrument sets should contain only the minimum number of instruments required for the typical case. Extra instruments that the surgeon requests can be counted and added separately. Having an instrument counting sheet such as that in Fig. 23.6 expedites the process. The circulating nurse need only write in the number of those instruments used on the case.

After instrument sets are standardized, instrument counting should not begin until the staff has had a chance to practice and become thoroughly familiar with the procedure. Mehaffy suggests that the staff visit other hospitals where instrument counts are done to see how they have mastered the process. She also suggests having the staff practice with mock setups, so they become accustomed to counting in the proper sequence. Nurses who have implemented their count system gradually and deliberately report that they do not have problems with delayed cases.

Some hospitals believe it is acceptable to take x-rays of every surgical patient rather than to perform counts. This is inappropriate, however, because counting can be done efficiently. It is not necessary or wise to expose patients to the extra radiation.

Nurses should not underestimate their role in developing count policies and carrying them out. Counts are not a trivial matter. They are a crucial aspect of assuring the patient's safety while she is under their care in the operating room. A well-developed hospital policy is the backbone of an enforceable and consistent counting system. If a hospital does not have a policy, one should be instituted. If a hospital does have a policy, the nurse should be aware that it is her legal and professional responsibility to abide by it.

References

1. *Malpractice Claims, Final Compilation*, vol. 2. Milwaukee: National Association of Insurance Commissioners, 1981.

2. Association of Operating Room Nurses. *AORN Standards of Practice: OR.* Denver, 1978.
3. Regan, W. A. "Texas court holds OR nurses agents of hospital." *AORN J* 26:458, 1977.
4. Hart, M. "To count or not to count." *AORN J* 3:775, 1980.
5. Ludlam, J. E., and Wright, J. N. "Formal instrument counts: Yes or no?" *Hosp Med Staff* 3:6, 1982.
6. Mehaffy, N. L. "Implementing counts in the OR." *AORN J* 25:1275, 1977.
7. Seawalt, S. "Eight steps to implementing a count system." *AORN J* 28:1098, 1978.

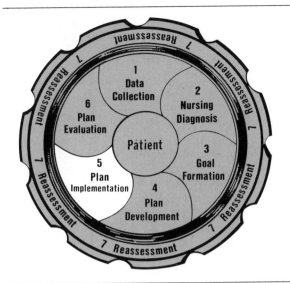

The nurse records and reports nursing care.

Documenting Patient Care

The care patients receive intraoperatively must be recorded to provide other members of the health care team with information about what care was given and the patient's response during surgery. This chapter examines documentation as a process that starts before admission and continues throughout the surgical patient's hospital stay. Documentation provides an ongoing picture of the patient as he progresses through his surgical experience. The rationale for communicating important information via hospital records and reports is discussed as well as the responsibilities involved in keeping an accurate picture of the patient on permanent file. The sources of data obtained, the types of information that should be retained, and how to record the data are included.

Documentation: A Process

A surgical patient's record begins at the physician's office or in the hospital clinic. The record is kept up to date by the physician and nurse, who record the patient's medical, social, and psychological status during his visits to the office. When the patient decides to have surgery, personnel at the office or clinic call the operating room to schedule the patient. This is usually the first contact with the hospital.

Data recorded in the OR scheduling book at the hospital include the patient's name, age, sex, surgical procedure, surgeon, and anesthesiologist. Other pertinent comments may also be written, such as weight, height, or physical disabilities. The data entered in the scheduling book for all patients are used to produce the surgery schedule. The surgery schedule is likely to be the first place the perioperative nurse will look in planning his preoperative assessment (see Chapter 6).

The patient's hospital record begins when he is admitted to the hospital. Admission data are obtained. This might be completing a nursing data base that includes information about the date, time, and mode of admission plus nursing observations and examination, habits of daily living, and a medical history. The nursing observation admission note might state under physical status and general appearance, "Elderly gentleman showing no signs of shortness of breath, slight edema in both ankles." Under emotional status and behavior the nurse might record, "Mild anxiety stated by patient. He does understand why he is hospitalized." Other chart forms might be the progress record for nurses and allied health personnel and the problem list. On the allied health record the nurse states mode of admission and begins identifying problems through the SOAP (subjective, objective, analysis, and planning) format or any format which is standard in the particular institution.

In some instances, patients will have had preadmission laboratory tests, radiological studies, or other diagnostic studies, and the data will be made available at admission.

When admitted, the patient is usually assigned a bed on a surgical unit. At this time, members of the health care team begin to record information on the patient record. Nurses on the surgical unit complete nursing interview forms with information about daily routines at home, allergies, likes and dislikes, and health problems, including present illness. A nursing history is taken covering such subjects as functional and dysfunctional health patterns (see Chapter 7). This nursing history is different from the medical history. The medical history includes the medical diagnosis, the physician's history and physical examination including history of the present illness, previous medical and surgical history, and findings of the physical and laboratory examinations. In contrast, the nursing history covers not only the patient's health problems but factors such as his emotional and social states, which may have a bearing on his surgery and recovery. A nursing history may be present in a variety of forms depending on the hospital. The nurse documents the patient's reason for being admitted to the hospital, the length of time he has had his current problem, previous hospitalizations and illnesses, observations of his condition, mental and emotional status, allergies, medications, and any prosthesis the patient might have. A review of systems, his health patterns, and a typical day profile may also be included, depending on hospital procedure.

Other documentation is added to the patient's record while he is on the unit. As evidence of the patient's informed consent to surgery, the surgical consent form is completed by the patient and surgeon and validated by the nurse. Physician's orders are in the record and provide data about the patient's diet, diagnostic tests, medications, and preoperative preparation required for his surgery. All information in the record is later used to evaluate the care provided and the effectiveness of care given. Each health team member has the responsibility for recording complete and accurate facts.

In performing the preoperative assessment, the perioperative nurse analyzes all the data obtained thus far. The data provide clues to what further information is needed from the patient during the assessment to complete a care plan that will meet the patient's individual needs. The intraoperative care plan is the major contribution the OR nurse makes to the patient's documentation because it describes the nursing diagnoses, goals, and activities to be carried out during surgery. On it, the nurse will note skin condition, neurological status, allergies, anxiety, emotional distress, physical disabilities, and preexisting disease processes. In some institutions, the form used for the care plan incorporates information about the patient's surgery, the patient's surgeon, procedure, previous surgery, preoperative diagnosis, and vital signs.

Consider, for example, a patient who is scheduled for implantation of a Harrington rod. The patient has a fracture at T_7-T_{12}. In addition, he is hypertensive and has chronic obstructive pulmonary disease, arthritis, and osteoporosis. Two potential problems the perioperative nurse has identified, carried through, and documented are illustrated in Table 24.1. Information for completing the intraoperative care plan is obtained from the unit nurses, the patient record, the patient, and family members.

The purpose of the care plan is to provide a guide for those involved in actually giving the care. Keep in mind (1) that the plan should be consistent with the overall medical regimen; (2) that human and material resources called for in the plan are available; (3) that the plan is based on the immediate needs of this patient; (4) that the plan reflects participation of the patient, family, and other members of the health care team; and (5) that the plan includes the nursing diagnosis, patient goals, and activities to meet the established goals. The format of the OR care plan should be as close as possible to the one used on the surgical unit so that all personnel will better understand the data. This will also aid in planning postoperative care and may help promote continuity of care.

During the patient's admission to the surgical unit, personnel review a preoperative checklist to verify that prerequisites have been met. This summary sheet is in addition to the care plan and is completed by nursing personnel on the unit and in the operating room. It assists the operating room nurse because data such as vital signs, allergies, information from the history, physical, and laboratory tests are in one place, so the nurse does not have to look on many forms to find all these data. In the operating room, other forms are introduced to document activities during surgery. The anesthesia record specifies the time anesthesia begins and ends, the operative procedure, preoperative and postoperative diagnoses, and a record of the anesthetic agents used and the patient's physiological response. Operating room nurses make their notes in another record, sometimes called the intraoperative nursing record. Focusing on nursing care given intraoperatively, this form may include sponge, needle, and instrument counts; grounding location for the electrosurgical unit; monitors used; tourniquet location, times, and pressure set; implants and lot numbers; dressings; drains; specimens; cultures; medications; patient position on the operating room table; and types of safety devices such as hand restraints, heel protectors, and a safety belt. The record usually allows space for nurses' comments. A third record, called the operative record, completed by the surgeon after the procedure, gives a detailed account of the operation. When the patient is transferred from the operating

Table 24.1. Information Documented on the Intraoperative Care Plan

Nursing Diagnosis	Goal	Plan	Implementation	Evaluation
1. Potential for respiratory problems 2° chronic COPD and emphysema.	1. The patient will maintain present respiratory status.	1. Explain coughing, deep breathing, give rationale for postop implementation.	1. Explained rationale and demonstrated exercises with patient.	1. Postop: Patient doing exercises with encouragement.
2. Potential for neuromuscular problems 2° to osteoporosis 2° to steroids and T_7-T_{12} fx	2. The patient will maintain current neuromuscular comfort.	2. Have several people available for positioning. Care when moving patient. Use padding.	2. Assistance available when moving. Foam padding used.	2. Postop: Patient not experiencing neuromuscular problems.

room to the recovery room, another record is initiated that documents the patient's condition during his emergence from the anesthetic.

With properly kept OR records, surgical unit personnel caring for the patient can readily determine what happened to him during the time he was away from the unit. They can see his physiological as well as emotional responses to the surgery. The intraoperative documentation of activities and patient responses shows a continuous picture of the patient's condition. Thus, there is no interruption in the documentation process while the patient is in surgery.

The perioperative nurse completes the documentation process when he does postoperative follow-up. Documentation includes observations of the wound site, evaluation of the patient's response to surgery, and the patient's perception of his care. The patient's and family's perception of care should be solicited in an effort to measure goal attainment from their point of view. The documentation process is congruent with the nursing process in that the patient record will depict application throughout. As the nurse from the operating room does the postoperative follow-up interview and evaluation of the patient, he records the patient's progress based on the preoperative nursing diagnosis and established goals. Documentation at this point reflects effectiveness of nursing care and the patient's response.

Unit nurses continue to document care throughout the patient's stay in the hospital. The final recording is the discharge summary, which includes plans for the patient at home. Plans for discharge start at admission and are considered throughout the patient's stay.

Approaches to Documentation

The documentation of nursing activities furnishes information about what the nurse does for the patient and about the patient's condition and response to care. Data are obtained and documented through observation, written records, and asking the patient about his perception of his care.

As a guide to observation, the nurse should:

1. Know what to look for when he observes and inspects the patient.
2. Conduct a systematic inspection.
3. Never jump to conclusions; he should ask himself what contributing factors might exist and what else could be going on.
4. Never make judgments based on preconceived ideas.
5. Examine his feelings about the patient and the patient's problems.
6. Use touch when appropriate during his observation and inspection.
7. Follow up on hunches; he should be certain that he has all the facts.
8. Continue to observe and inspect throughout the patient's hospital stay.
9. Identify the patient's problem first, then gather additional supporting data that will assist him in writing the care plan.
10. Understand why observing and inspecting is so important and how it relates to the total nursing process (1).

The patient's perception is as important as observation when documenting. He can furnish information about his physical and emotional condition that is available in no other way. Careful observation and questioning assist the nurse in gathering pertinent data. In evaluating care, for example, the nurse should ask simple questions such as, "Did your family know where to wait during your surgery?" "Did your doctor explain your surgery to you?" "Did anyone communicate to you the reason the surgery took longer than you expected?" The patient's and family's perceptions indicate their satisfaction with the care given. Each time the nurse visits the patient, he can obtain additional data for reporting the patient's response to his surgery on the nurse's notes, progress notes, or other forms in the patient record.

Written records or reports are the third method used for documentation. As discussed, the OR nurse bases his documentation on a variety of other written records, beginning with the surgery schedule and including notes from the unit nurse, physician, and other health team members. It is crucial as well that his documentation be in writing. The data must be put in writing for it to be communicated to other members of the health care team. Sharing information promotes continuity of care because at each stage of care, personnel will know what has been done before. They will not be planning care in a vacuum.

The perioperative nurse who records the facts in writing is also demonstrating accountability. Documented care is a legal record of the nurse's action and the patient's response to those actions. A written record can be compared with the institution's standards of practice to evaluate the quality of care (see Chapter 27). Still another reason for writing the information is so it can be retrieved for research and other uses, which will ultimately improve care.

Many nurses ask what they should record. In general, all basic facts are documented. Specifically, the nurse should write:

1. What he sees: bleeding, color, amount of fluid, type of drainage.
2. What he hears: chest rales, moaning, patient complaints.
3. What he smells: acetone breath, feces, malodorous drainage.
4. What he feels: body heat, distended stomach, motion at a fracture site.
5. What he does for the patient and the patient's response to treatment: after Demerol (meperidine hydrochloride) 100 mg is given for pain in the right ankle, the patient states he still has had no relief.
6. What he does to protect the patient: placed foam pads under heels, secured safety belt, placed on egg crate mattress.
7. What he did to the patient's private property to protect it from loss: gave hearing aid to wife, placed dentures in bedside stand (2).

Every hospital has its own format for charting. The format will vary depending on the philosophy of nursing and the methods chosen to record. Some methods of nursing documentation are source-oriented recording, problem-

oriented recording, the SOAP or SOAPIE format (see Fig. 24.1), baseline recording, and the APIE format.

SOURCE-ORIENTED RECORDING

Source-oriented recording is a description of what is happening to the patient in narrative format. It depicts a sequence of nursing activities performed and is done chronologically. The typical types of forms used with this type of documentation are operating room nurse's notes, surgery worksheets, flow sheets, and the operative record. For example, the operating room nurse's notes might say:

5/4/83   4:30 A.M.
Mr. Clark admitted to OR from unit. Placed in supine position on operating room table. Foam pads placed on both heels. Heels slightly reddened due to pressure of hard mattress.

K. Crawford, RN

PROBLEM-ORIENTED RECORDING

Problem-oriented medical records (POMR) is the most popular method used for recording. All the patient's problems are recorded and documentation is conducted to show the extent to which the problem is resolved (see Fig. 24.2). If this system is being used, it usually incorporates the nurse's notes, physician record, and other documentation by other members of the health care team. For example:

5/4/83   7:30 A.M.
1. Anxiety. Expresses fear of anesthesia. States, "I am afraid I will not wake up after my surgery." Eyes blinking, perspiring while expressing feelings. Continue to allow patient to express feelings. Encourage him to walk up and down the hall and see other patients who have had surgery.

K. Crawford, RN

SOAP AND APIE

Another type of recording is the SOAP or SOAPIE (subjective, objective, analysis, and planning). The IE stands for implementation and evaluation. Similar to this is the APIE (assessment, planning, implementation, and

DATE	TIME	PROB #	PHYS PROB #	PROBLEM TITLE AND S.O.A.P. FORMAT (S-Subjective O-Objective A-Analysis P-Plan)
9/9/81	1530			Admitted per ambulatory an elderly appearing gentleman.
		1		S: "I'm here to find out what's wrong with me."
				O: Admitted for surgical removal of recurrent carcinoma of (L) lateral tongue and alveolar ridge.
				A: Patient with jaw mass scheduled for surgery.
				P: ① Encourage patient to express concerns.
				② Explain hospital routines.
				③ Include family in information and instruction.
				④ Validate understanding of surgical procedure. L. Geringer, RN

Allied Health Personnel
PROGRESS RECORD

(Addressograph)

Figure 24.1. Illustration of SOAP charting format.

DATE	PROB #	PHYS PROB #	DATE OF ONSET	ACTIVE PROBLEMS	DATE RESOLVED	INACTIVE OR RESOLVED PROBLEMS
9/9/81	A-1		9/9/81	Mild anxiety related to		
	A-			jaw mass. L.G.		
	A-2		9/9/81	Lack of knowledge	9/9/81	
	A-			about surgical procedure L.G.		
	A-					7/6/78 Circulatory
	A-					problem due to
	A-					phlebitis
	A-					
	A-					
	A-					
	A-					
	A-					
	A-					
	A-					
	A-					
	A-					
	A-					
	A-					
	A-					

Name	Init.	Name	Init.	Name	Init.	Name	Init
L. Goeringer, R. L.G.							

PORTER MEMORIAL HOSPITAL
Denver, Colorado

(Addressograph)

Figure 24.2. Allied health personnel problem list illustrating the method in which patient problems are documented, the date resolved, and the status of the problems.

evaluation). Both approaches to documentation are a variation of the POMR method of recording. They both reflect the nursing process and provide a good framework for documentation. For example:

5/4/83   7:30 A.M.
A: Anxiety. Patient states he is afraid he will not wake up after surgery. Perspiring and blinking eyes excessively.
P. Encourage patient to express feelings of fear and walk in hall to observe postoperative patients.
I. Nurse from operating room talked with patient. Anesthesiologist reviewed type of anesthesia and explained what would happen during his anesthesia.
E: Patient states he is confident that he will return from the operating room.

Whatever the system, the general principles are the same. Documentation must include time and date care was given; the signature of the person giving or observing care; notations placed in chronological order; use of uniform abbreviations; and notes that are clear, concise, unambiguous, and accurate. Above all, notes must be legible. If a patient refuses treatment, the nurse has a responsibility to encourage compliance with the medical regimen. If he chooses not to have the treatment after the nurse has provided adequate rationale, the nurse has a responsibility to record what the patient refused and why he refused it (3).

The following dos and don'ts of charting for the perioperative nurse are taken from *Reporting and Documenting Patient Care: Operating Room* (4):

Dos: When charting patient care given in the operating room, the nurse should:

- Read previous nurse's notes before giving care
- Imprint name, identification number, date, and time on every sheet
- Always use ink for recording data
- Write legibly
- Use appropriate form for charting
- Describe symptoms or patient conditions accurately and completely

- Use patient's own words if possible
- Use acceptable hospital-approved abbreviations whenever possible
- Use concise, descriptive terms
- Be definite in descriptions and wording
- Begin each phrase with a capital
- Begin each new entry on a separate line
- Document need for nursing action
- Record all nursing care provided before, in the operating room, and afterward
- Sign the completed record

Don'ts: When documenting patient care given, the nurse in the operating room should not:

- Record without checking name on record
- Record on blank forms
- Use ordinary paper
- Use pencil
- Back-date entry
- Tamper with or add to previous charting
- Skip lines or leave spaces
- Erase
- Chart in advance of nursing actions
- Use broad, nonspecific terms (e.g., "good condition," "tolerated well")
- Use medical terminology unless absolutely sure of meaning
- Rely on memory, but should chart immediately
- Discard nurse's notes or records with errors, but should use specific error correction format
- Repeat in narrative what is recorded in other parts in chart
- Use imprecise terms (e.g., "appears to," "seems to," or "apparently")

Legal Protection

The patient care record is a legal document that may be used in case of a lawsuit. It will show the series of events leading up to the patient's complaint about care in the hospital and aid in determining if anyone is to blame. The courts may use the record to prove what information the staff had available in giving care. Records are also used to show if important information was transferred from one hospital department to another.

Good documentation provides protection both for the patient and nurse. Nurses can protect themselves by reporting specific facts and avoiding generalities. Instead of writing "Feet swollen," the nurse should write, "Feet swollen; warmth, color, and movement satisfactory." This makes it clear that the nurse is aware the swelling is not dangerous. Noting that the patient is in "good condition" could mean anything. Rather the nurse should ask, "What facts about the patient led me to the conclusion he was in good condition?"

The patient record should show continuity of care. Flow sheets depict all activities, the times each activity is performed, and the patient's response on an ongoing basis.

Each hospital should have a written policy and procedure for documenting care. The policy will vary from institution to institution but should include what to do when:

- The nurse cannot reach the doctor when needed, and how and where this action should be recorded.
- What and where to report when the nurse has given a medication or fluids inappropriate for a patient.
- What to do when the doctor gives an oral order or unclear written order not to resuscitate a terminally ill patient.
- When and where to record when a patient refuses his medication or other prescribed treatment.
- What to do when the nurse believes standing orders are no longer valid for the medication or treatment being given.

A rule of thumb is that the nurse's documentation should reflect that he followed the established hospital policy and what the result was. This should be documented in proper time sequence.

Another way to protect himself legally is to chart at various times throughout the patient's stay or the shift he is working. Chronological entries show the nurse has recorded care and patient responses while care is being given. In the operating room, if the care is long, the nurse should chart his ongoing monitoring of physiological responses to surgery, position on the operating room table, and other nursing measures. His full name—not just an initial—should be placed on each form he records on. If he has made an entry on any form in the patient record, and he wishes to erase it, he should simply put one line through it. The nurse should not try to scratch out the entire notation, and should not try to cover up his mistakes or those of another person.

The focus of documentation should be on communicating important data about the patient from one member of the health care team to another. If the nurse describes what he did and how the patient responded as objectively as possible, his documentation will be accurate and complete.

The purpose of documenting patient care is to provide a complete picture of the patient from the time he decides to have surgery until he is discharged from the hospital. Every member of the team—surgical unit nurse, perioperative nurse, surgeon, and others—has the same goal: returning the patient to his normal level of functioning. They cooperate through the documentation process.

References

1. Robinson, J., ed. *Documenting Patient Care Responsibly*. Nursing Skillbook Series. Horsham, Penn.: 58 Intermed Communications, 1978.
2. Kerr, A. "Nurse's notes: Making them more meaningful." *Nurs 72* (September):2, 1972.
3. Eggland, E. T. "Charting: How and why to document your care daily—and fully." *Nurs 80* 10 (February):38–43, 1980.
4. Manuel, B. J. *Reporting and Documenting Patient Care: OR MILs*. Denver: Association of Operating Room Nurses, 1980.

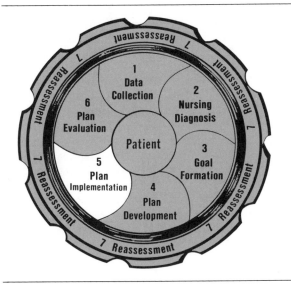

The nurse watches over the patient's emergence from anesthesia.

Immediate Postoperative Care

In the immediate postoperative recovery phase, the patient presents nurses with multifaceted challenges that require clinical expertise, perception, and effective measures to assure the patient's return to previous homeostasis. The patient who has undergone an anesthetic, regardless of the surgical procedure, deserves the optimum environment and trained personnel provided by a recovery room. Recovery room nursing includes the ability and knowledge to assist the patient in the transition from the operative phase. This is best approached through the nursing process.

Care of the patient in the recovery room starts even before the patient has surgery. Although recovery room nurses do not usually interview patients on the unit, they can take advantage of the information gathered by other members of the health care team. To obtain an overview of the patient's status, the recovery room nurse may consult the preoperative assessment, laboratory data, nursing and medical history, documentation of previous admission, and nursing flow sheets. This information is available in the patient's chart. The recovery room nurse can also review the OR nurse's patient care plan which is in the room where surgery will be done. If she has questions, she can consult with the perioperative nurse who interviewed the patient. If during the surgical procedure additional information or equipment not previously planned is needed, the perioperative nurse communicates this to the recovery room nurse. From the data obtained, the recovery room nurse can determine if there are patient characteristics or potential complications that will require additional staffing or special equipment. An elderly orthopedic patient, for instance, might require additional staff to help move him, or a patient with a history of cardiac arrhythmias will need a monitor. Complete information and a data base on the patient are also necessary when implementing certain treatments in the recovery room. For example, a history of any drug allergy is essential before administering drugs in the recovery room.

Some individuals may need special consideration in the recovery room. Children or teenagers may need to be segregated to protect them from exposure to other patients. Conscious patients who have had local or spinal anesthesia are aware of their surroundings and may also need to be separated from other patients. Patients with massive infections such as dehiscence due to wound infection, with peritonitis, or with infectious diseases such as tuberculosis may need to be isolated or segregated. Patients with some radiation implants should also be separated from other patients. Patients with known psychological disturbances may also need special consideration.

The recovery room nurse also needs to look at the total surgical schedule for the day in terms of providing adequate staffing and sufficient equipment and planning for discharge of patients to provide bed space for the arrival of new patients.

Assessment

When the patient is brought to the recovery room, the surgical team provides relevant data to the recovery room nurse. This includes the patient's medical history, psychological and sociological status, drug allergies or abuse, physical disabilities, and the presence of any prosthesis. The operation and its rationale are usually described. The surgical team's report, including that of the anesthesiologist and the operating room nurse, to the recovery room nurse, describes the anesthetic agent, narcotics, and muscle relaxants administered, as well as any reversal agents or antibiotics. The anesthesiologist gives a report of colloid, crystalloid, and blood administration so that the recovery room nurse is apprised of the patient's fluid and electrolyte balance. The operating room nurse discusses any complications the patient had during the surgical procedure. For example, if a patient undergoes an excessive blood volume loss intraoperatively, she will require replacement therapy consisting of blood, blood products, colloids, or crystalloids. The recovery room nurse must be alerted at the onset of the recovery phase so she may assess the cardiovascular status while the patient recovers.

As soon as the patient arrives, the recovery room nurse's first concern is to assess the patient's total status. The nurse determines temperature, heart rate and rhythm, and respiratory status. With some intraoperative anesthetic agents, heart rate may be increased and blood pressure decreased. Respiratory depression may also occur as a result of anesthesia. Because the operating room is cool, the patient may be hypothermic in the recovery room. If the abdominal cavity is irrigated or the wound is open for hours, these also contribute to hypothermia. This will require the application of warm blankets, aquathermia and temperature monitoring to ensure protection against cardiac arrhythmias and further complications.

The patient arrives in the recovery room usually asleep or reacting to oral commands. Patients can usually breathe without assistance of a breathing bag or mechanical ventilation. Over the course of an hour, most patients return to an oriented state with a tendency to fall into sleep and are arousable upon either oral or tactile stimulation.

In assessing the respiratory status, the nurse checks the rate of respirations per minute, depth of respiration, symmetry of chest expansion and excursion, breath sounds, color, mucous membranes, presence of stridor, air hunger, presence of mechanical airway (nasal, oral, endotracheal tube), and airway patency. She will assess the need for position changes of jaw, head, and neck to facilitate adequate respiratory exchange (see Fig. 25.1). Anesthetic agents may need to be reversed, and the nurse can discuss this with the anesthesiologist who makes a clinical decision. The nurse assesses respiratory status concurrently with muscle function. She would check muscle functions such as hand grasping on command and the patient's ability to perform a head lift from a

Figure 25.1. When the patient is admitted to the recovery room, the perioperative nurse reports the status of the patient, the type and extent of the surgical procedure, and other information pertinent to care in the recovery room.

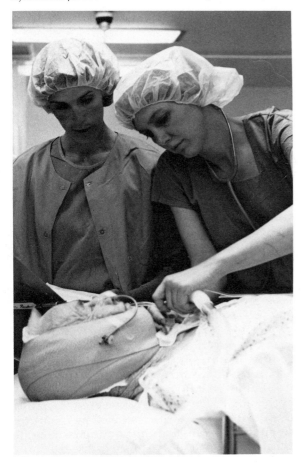

supine position, unless the surgical procedure (e.g., cervical laminectomy) contraindicates this movement.

In assessing cardiac function, the recovery room nurse determines the arterial blood pressure value through invasive or noninvasive arterial monitoring. The recovery room nurse ascertains these values at least every 15 minutes throughout the postanesthetic recovery phase. The recovery room nurse reports these initial clinical parameters, which establish the patient's level of stability, to the nurse anesthetist or anesthesiologist.

After establishing vital signs and giving the initial report, the nurse determines the patient's status through observation. She observes the patient's level of consciousness. This varies from a state of unconsciousness to wakefulness, depending on the type of anesthesia administered. Pupillary response is noted. Muscular strength is determined to aid the nurse's assessment of muscle relaxant reversal. She continues to monitor the respiratory and cardiovascular status.

Assessing skin integrity, she looks for the presence of rash, petechiae, abrasions, and burns. A rash may indicate drug sensitivity or allergy, while a burn may indicate an electrical cautery grounding pad burn. She checks circulation to the patient's extremities.

While checking dressings and surgical incisions, the nurse looks for hemorrhaging and hematomas. She maintains the sterility of dressings. Drains are checked to assure minimal postoperative bleeding. Suction to drains is established if ordered. The amount of drainage is continuously monitored and documented on the recovery room record. The nurse also assesses the patient's need for warmth. Adequate body warmth speeds recovery because it increases metabolism, thereby enhancing circulation and respiratory capabilities. Patients are better able to breathe deeply and expel inhalation agents. Postoperative shivering, however, may be an effect of certain inhalation anesthetic agents and not an indication of a hypothermic state. The nurse encourages frequent deep breathing, and may order oxygen therapy or an intravenous narcotic.

Postoperative pain is common in the recovery room since incised and traumatized tissues mean severed or damaged pain-stimulating nerve fibers. In the postanesthetic patient, pain affects respiratory, cardiac, and endocrine systems.

Assessment of pain involves a number of factors. Patients will begin to experience pain before consciousness is fully regained. Cues relating to pain may also be signs of other complications. Restlessness, for instance, may be one of the initial signs of hypoxia as well as a symptom of pain. Increased or decreased blood pressure and pulse may be signs of pain and compromised cardiac status or incipient shock. Table 25.1 cites the cues pertinent to the above nursing diagnosis in the conscious patient. Vasovagal responses such as a transient rise in blood pressure and pulse followed by decrease in blood pressure may be among the first signs of pain noted in the patient emerging from anesthesia. Pain is a personal experience and believed to be an interaction between physiological and psychological factors. Assessment of pain is, therefore, complicated by the psychological component. Fear and expectation of pain affect an individual's response. People who live with chronic pain seem to have a higher tolerance for acute pain. Cultural ways of expressing pain may determine the patient's response, and cultural patterns of pain relief vary. The patient's expectation, fear, experience with pain, and ways of coping with pain should be assessed during the preoperative interview by the OR nurse.

Severity of pain is a factor to consider. Since pain is a personal experience, the nurse cannot know how intense pain is for another. Experience, both personal and in caring for patients with pain, enables a nurse to estimate severity and empathize more readily. Severity can be related to the type of surgery as well as to anticipation and fear of pain. For example, rectal and knee surgery seem to create intense pain rather quickly.

The type of anesthetic agent is also a factor in pain. Balanced anesthesia that combines narcotic analgesics with inhalation agents and muscle relaxants is commonly used. The type of analgesic used, its short- and long-term effects, and whether a reversing agent has been administered at the conclusion of surgery have a bearing on the presence of pain. Patients given spinal anesthesia may not require analgesics during their stay in the recovery area because motor control may be restored before pain sensation returns. It is common practice to administer intravenous narcotic analgesics in the immediate postoperative phase in order to expedite relief of pain as well as minimize respiratory depression. Intramuscular administration may initially be given in divided doses again to ensure respiratory integrity.

Table 25.1. Alteration in Comfort: Pain.

Etiology	Defining Characteristics	
	Subjective	Objective
Injuring agents Biological Chemical Physical Psychological	communication (verbal or coded) of pain describers	guarding behavior, protective self-focusing narrowed focus (altered time perception, withdrawal from social contact, impaired thought processes) distraction behavior (crying, moaning, pacing, seeking out other people or activities, restlessness) facial mask of pain (eyes lack luster, "beaten look," fixed or scattered movement, grimace) alteration in muscle tone (may span from listlessness to rigid) autonomic responses not seen in chronic stable pain (diaphoresis, blood pressure and pulse rate change, pupillary dilitation, increased or decreased respiratory rate)

Reprinted with permission from *Classification of Nursing Diagnoses*, Edited by M. Kim and D. Moritz copyright © 1982 by McGraw-Hill, p. 285.

The nurse anticipates pain management by obtaining data related to analgesic allergies. Opium derivatives and meperidine are commonly used analgesics in the recovery area, although some of the newer synthetic narcotics are also used. Data related to such allergies may not be easy to elicit because patients are not always aware of an allergy.

Finally, the nurse should be aware of factors that will affect pain management during recovery. The patient's body weight is one. The robust muscular patient who weighs 220 pounds requires a larger amount of medication than a small-framed, fragile patient who only weighs 99 pounds. Age is also important. Children and younger persons are more sensitive to pain than the elderly, and this must be considered in relation to other physiological responses that affect pain thresholds.

The surgical procedure itself will influence pain management. Incisions that cut through highly vascular areas with many nerve endings cause more pain. After an abdominal hysterectomy, for instance, the patient experiences pain associated with the skin incision, muscle and nerves cut transversely, retracted tissue and manipulated organs. Less pain would ordinarily be experienced by the patient with cranial surgery, where pain is associated with the skin incision and swelling of brain tissue. Patients having cranial and thoracic surgery are often denied analgesics until stabilization of the respective systems has been fully accomplished. Pain management for individuals with a history of substance abuse, particularly alcohol and narcotics, necessitates adaptations.

Since the patient's condition is continually changing, the nurse monitors and records patient data a minimum of every 15 minutes. The postanesthetic recovery nurse should be continually aware of the clinical manifestations of the patient's response to anesthesia and surgery. A recovery room scoring system is helpful in assessing the patient when she is admitted to the recovery room, when her status changes, and when discharged (see Fig. 25.2A,B,C, and D). The scoring method includes level of consciousness, muscular response, cardiovascular status, respiratory status, and skin color. The assessment phase continues throughout the patient's stay in the recovery room until she returns to comfort, orientation to surroundings, adequate normal temperature range, adequate respiratory integrity, and cardiovascular stability.

Planning

The goals for nursing care of the postanesthetic patient are derived from data obtained when the patient is admitted to the recovery room as well as preadmission data. An example of a goal for an asthmatic pediatric patient might be: "Minimal postanesthetic wheezing." The nurse would assess breath sounds carefully through auscultation to detect postanesthetic wheezing.

In determining goals, the nurse reviews the patient's cardiovascular, pulmonary, renal, integumentary, neurological, and psychological functions through clinical observations and data base and history gathering. The nurse considers the type of surgery, duration of the anesthesia, type of anesthetic and drugs used. She also notes the patient's age, preoperative physical status, level of orientation, and medical history. She will be aware of psychological and social implications of surgery and anesthesia for the patient. For example, the recovery room nurse would be attuned to the psychological implications and needs manifested by a woman entering the recovery room after a D and C for incomplete abortion.

The patient care plan is based on nursing diagnoses. As she administers care, the nurse continually observes and analyzes the patient's changing condition. During the recovery period, nursing diagnoses may change rapidly, and all phases of the nursing process may take place simultaneously. For example, a patient might be stable on admission to the recovery room, but may suddenly begin to exhibit signs of dyspnea, cyanosis, and decreased chest expansion. Airway obstruction is suspected. The nurse quickly changes the position of the head and neck to facilitate breathing. She notes that the patient's chest expansion, color, and expired airflow have returned to normal and no further action is needed. The nursing diagnosis might

VITAL SIGN RECORD

TIME

220 · 200 · 180 · 160 · 140 · 120 · 100 · 80 · 60 · 40 · P · R

POST ANESTHESIA RECOVERY SCORE

Able to Deep Breath &/Or Cough	=2
Asleep - Adequate Airway	=1
Dyspnea or Limited Breathing or Apneic	=0
BP + 20% of Preanesthetic Level Pre-Op	=2
BP + 20%-30% of Preanesthetic Level BP	=1
BP + 50% of Preanesthetic Level	=0
Oriented and/or Awake	=2
Arousable on Calling	=1
Non-Responsive	=0
Normal Skin Color	=2
Pale, Dusky, Blotchy, Other	=1
Cyanotic	=0
Moving Extremities- 3 or 4	=2
If Chronic Deficit- 1 or 2	=1
Explain	=0
Post Anesthesia	
Score Upon Transfer TOTALS	

MEDICATIONS AND TREATMENTS

HOUR

TOTAL IV in OR:
Crystalloid _____ cc
Blood _____ cc
Colloid _____ cc

IV INFUSING:
Crystalloid _____ cc
Blood _____ cc
Colloid _____ cc

TOTAL INTAKE OR and RR
Crystalloid _____ cc
P.O. _____ cc
Blood _____ cc
Colloid _____ cc

IV Added In RR

Output EBL: OR _____ cc
Urine: OR _____ cc RR
NG: OR _____ cc RR
Emesis: OR _____ cc RR
Other: OR _____ cc RR

TOTAL OUTPUT OR _____ cc RR

Type of Airway _____   Time Out _____
O₂ Not Given O₂ TIME STARTED TIME DC'D O₂ Liters/Min. _____ Temp. _____

Surgical Procedure:

Anesthetic Agent:

Angiocath Gauge:

HOUR NOTES

Pertinent Health Information

Allergies

Report Given To:
Accompanied by: _____
Discharge Time _____ To _____ (Responsible Person)
Mode of Discharge
Discharge Nurse
Post-Op Instructions

RECOVERY ROOM RECORD

PORTER MEMORIAL HOSPITAL

7211-023-81C

A

Figure 25.2. A. Nursing postanesthesia assessment record; B. Anesthesia record; C. Anesthesia standing orders; D. Example of special procedures record for recovery room. Reprinted with permission of Porter Memorial Hospital, Denver.

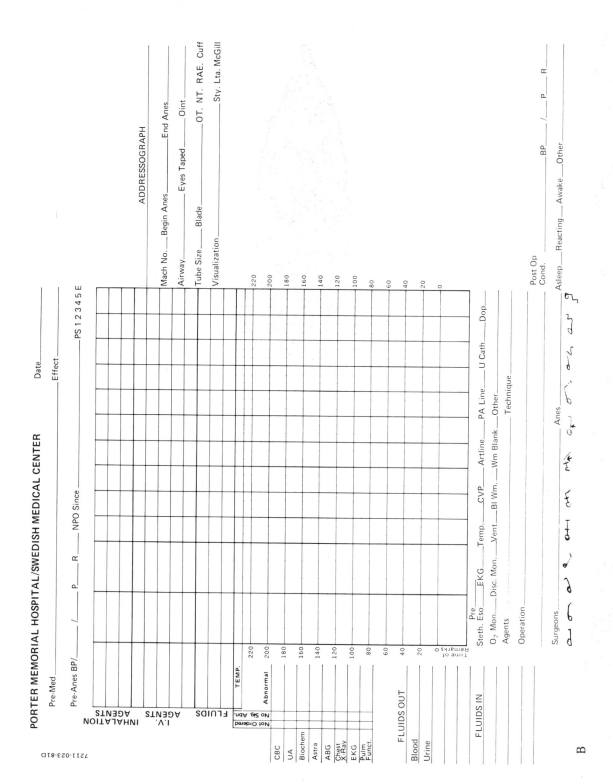

PORTER MEMORIAL HOSPITAL/SWEDISH MEDICAL CENTER

Date ___

Pre-Med ___ Effect ___

Pre-Anes BP/ ___ / ___ P ___ R ___ NPO Since ___ PS 1 2 3 4 5 E

ADDRESSOGRAPH

Mach No. ___ Begin Anes ___ End Anes ___
Airway ___ Eyes Taped ___ Oint ___
Tube Size ___ Blade ___ OT. NT. RAE. Cuff
Visualization ___ Sty. Lta. McGill

TEMP.

	Abnormal	No Sig. Abn.	Not Ordered
CBC			
UA			
Biochem			
Astra			
ABG			
Chest X-Ray			
EKG			
Pulm Funct.			

INHALATION AGENTS
I.V. AGENTS
FLUIDS

220 200 180 160 140 120 100 80 60 40 20 0
Time of Remarks 0

FLUIDS OUT
Blood ___
Urine ___

FLUIDS IN

Pre
Steth. Eso ___ EKG ___ Temp. ___ CVP ___ Artline ___ PA Line ___ U Cath ___ Dop. ___
O₂ Mon. ___ Disc. Mon. ___ Vent ___ Bl Wm. ___ Wm Blank ___ Other ___
Agents ___ Technique ___
Operation ___

Surgeons ___ Anes ___

Post Op
Cond. ___ BP ___ / ___ P ___ R ___
Asleep ___ Reacting ___ Awake ___ Other ___

7211-023-81D

B

477

ANESTHESIOLOGIST ORDERS	NOTES/ALLERGIES
ANESTHESIA ORDERS FOR RECOVERY	POST ANESTHESIA EVALUATION
Date	
Time	Date _____ Time _____
	Awareness _____
IV Orders	Respiratory System _____
_____ 1000 cc Dextrose 5% in Water	Circulatory System _____
_____ 1000 cc Dextrose 5% in Lactated Ringers	Complications and Treatment _____
_____ 1000 cc Lactated Ringers	
_____ 1000 cc Dextrose 5% in .2 Normal Saline	
_____ 1000 cc Dextrose 5% in .45 Normal Saline	
_____ 500 cc Normal serum albumin (Human) 5% usp (Plasbumin 5%)	
_____ 500 cc Dextrose 5% in Water	
_____ 500 cc Dextrose in Lactated Ringers	
_____ 250 cc Normal serum albumin (Human) 5% USP (Plasbumin 5%)	

MEDICATIONS FOR RECOVERY ROOM USE ONLY

_____ Narcan _____ mg IV if narcotized _____ May repeat as necessary x _____

_____ Antilirium _____ cc IV if patient unruly, or overly sedated.

_____ May repeat as necessary x _____

_____ Atropine _____ mg IV for bradycardia less than _____

_____ Morphine _____ mg IV q̄ 5-10 min. up to _____ mg

_____ Demerol _____ mg IV every 5 to 10 minutes up to _____ mg

_____ Nisentil _____ mg IV PRN x _____

_____ Ephedrine _____ mg IV _____ May repeat x _____

_____ Tensilon _____ mg IV _____ May repeat x _____

_____ Robinul _____ mg IV _____ May repeat x _____

_____ Dopram _____ cc IV _____ May repeat x _____

_____ Inapsine _____ cc IV for nausea.

MISCELLANEOUS

_____ K—Pad PRN

_____ K +

_____ Continue O$_2$ at _____ liters/min.

_____ ANESTHESIOLOGIST _____ ANESTHESIOLOGIST

C

Figure 25.2. (Continued)

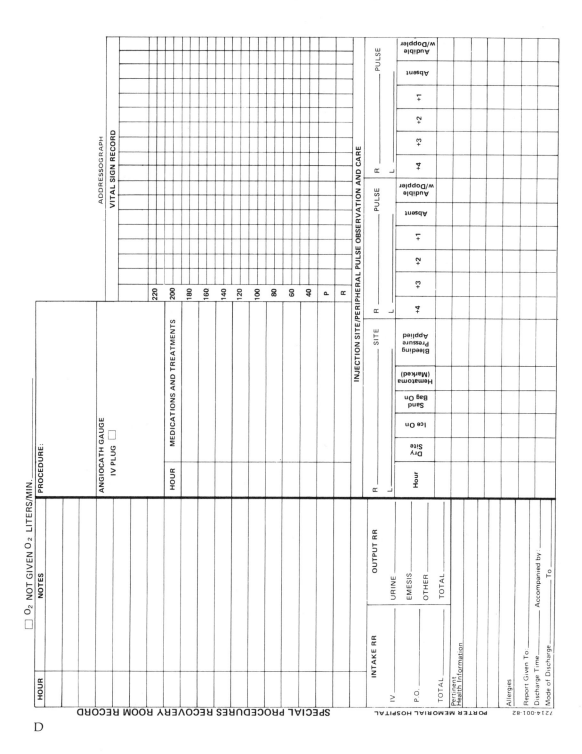

SPECIAL PROCEDURES RECOVERY ROOM RECORD   PORTER MEMORIAL HOSPITAL   7214-001-82

D

479

be stated as, "Ineffective airway clearance related to pharyngeal obstruction."

Goals for the postanesthetic patient must always include respiratory and cardiovascular maintenance or improvement, the stabilization of fluid and electrolyte balance, protection from infection, management of pain and nausea, environmental safety, privacy, and emotional support.

Implementation

The implementation of the goals for the postanesthetic patient is multidisciplinary and requires scientific knowledge, clinical skill, and decision making based on assessment and planning.

The nurse administers drugs, obtains radiographic films and laboratory reports as ordered by the physician, and institutes treatments according to procedures. For example, orthopedic patients may require ice and elevation of the operative extremity and site to reduce edema and tissue trauma. For a patient with a gastric procedure, the nurse may aspirate gastric contents postoperatively to decompress the stomach or intestine to rest the operated sites and promote the healing of delicate tissue where sutured.

RESPIRATORY

Respiratory care is essential because narcotics and anesthetic agents induce respiratory depression. Anesthesia may paralyze the natural physiological response to ventilate properly. Barbiturates, narcotics, muscle relaxants, and inhalation anesthetic agents reduce the natural ability of the respiratory center of the brain and respiratory muscles, causing respiratory depression. The nurse needs to ascertain the need for administration of reversal drugs such as atropine and neostigmine.

Signs of respiratory distress include decreased breath sounds, respiratory rate, and depth of respiration; crowing or stridor; pallor of the skin or cyanosis; restlessness; and increased pulse rate. The nurse determines vital signs and investigates the etiology of the symptoms through observation and arterial blood gas determinations. For airway obstruction due to narcotic depression, the nurse changes the jaw, head, and neck position and maintains it manually through extension and subluxation. The position recommended is at the head of the bed above the patient with each forefinger maintaining the chin and each fourth finger placed in the notches at the angle of the jaw. Pressure applied at the notch of the angle of the jaw stimulates the vagus nerve causing deep respiratory exchange (see Fig. 25.3). Figure 25.4 depicts an alternative method for increasing the airway space. This technique is invaluable to recovery room nurses. If the airway is obstructed by secretions, the nurse may use suctioning techniques (see Fig. 25.5). This is accomplished with a size 10 or 14 French catheter inserted either through the nares into the trachea or through the mouth into the pharynx to remove secretions. The nurse may need to insert either a nasal or oral airway to provide adequate ventilation. At this point, the nurse must also question the need for reversal of agents used intraoperatively and communicate with the anesthesiologist.

Oxygen is administered by cannula, catheter, mist, or mechanical ventilator via endotracheal tube. The nurse observes the effectiveness of the oxygen administration. It may be necessary to obtain arterial blood gas

Figure 25.3. Elevation of mandible. Approach from head of patient. Head should be pulled back as above. Fourth finger at notch of mandible. Forefinger on side of mandible.

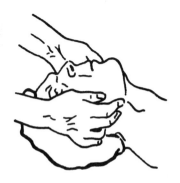

J. NAZARIO

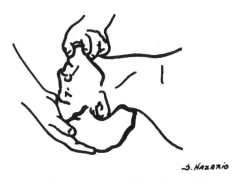

Figure 25.4. *Elevation of mandible. Approach from side of patient. A combination of backward head tilt and anterior mandibular displacement is most effective to relieve airway obstruction.*

values to provide more data in assuring that the patient is getting proper oxygenation. If a mechanical ventilator is used the nurse may need to make adjustments in oxygen concentrations, tidal volume, and rate.

The nurse should continually monitor the unconscious patient to prevent aspiration of mucus or gastric secretions. Proper anatomical body positioning affords maximum respiratory function and protects the surgical site. Proper positioning depends upon the type of surgical intervention. In any case, it is important that the body be positioned so the surgical site is protected and splinted and chest expansion is maximized.

Applying the "stir-up" routine, the nurse uses frequent talks to the patient to arouse her. She also encourages the patient to cough and deep breathe and exercise her arms and legs. Control of postoperative pain facilitates these measures. The regimen prevents patchy atelectasis and speeds alveolar reexpansion as well as enhances circulatory function. As the lungs excrete the inhalation agents, active pulmonary expansion affords faster recovery from their effects.

If an endotracheal tube is present, it must be secured with tape to stabilize it for the patient's comfort, to prevent skin breakdown, and to secure proper placement. The nurse keeps the tube patent by suctioning. Patient position changes may cause displacement of the tube. A well-positioned tube may enter a bronchus

if the patient's head is turned or moved, resulting in absence of ventilation in the contralateral lung. Shift of the carina during Trendelenburg positioning can also cause the tube to slip into a main stem bronchus. Thus the nurse may need to determine the tube's placement by radiography. Auscultation of the chest for clarity and symmetry of breath sounds is necessary.

If extubation is indicated, the nurse must first determine tidal volume, rate, and depth of respiration; color of patient with attention given to mucous membranes and nailbeds; blood gas values, if necessary; muscular response; and level of consciousness. Before extubation, thorough suctioning is required

Figure 25.5. *The recovery room nurse is removing secretions with a catheter through the tracheostomy tube.*

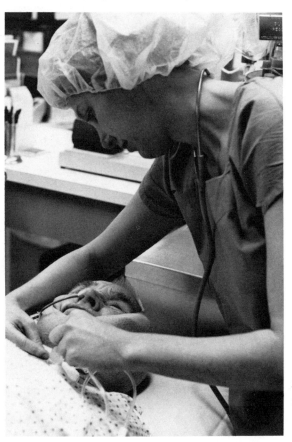

followed by cuff deflation of the tube. Removal of the tube with cuff inflated will traumatize tracheal tissue, which could produce future airway obstruction. Deep breathing is encouraged. Since the patient is probably awake and feeling the discomfort of the tube, the nurse must offer oral and tactile reassurance. She then extubates the patient as the patient inspires her breath and provides supplemental oxygen following tube removal. She then needs to observe and document the effects of extubation, carefully assessing and evaluating the patient's color, respiratory rate and depth, breath sounds on auscultation, chest expansion, and level of consciousness. Any deviation from the patient's preextubation status must be diagnosed—for example, hypoxia secondary to inadequate ventilation.

Postanesthetic laryngeal spasm requires immediate diagnosis and emergency treatment. The anesthesiologist must be notified at once. Laryngeal spasm, which closes the larynx, is characterized by inadequate pulmonary exchange, gasping upper airway noises, loss of skin color, and hypoxemia. It may be secondary to edema, postsurgical trauma, and endotracheal irritation. Laryngeal spasm may occur from secretions irritating the vocal cord tissue or pharynx. The treatment is airway management and ventilation with Ambu breathing bag via mask assistance. If this fails to relieve the patient, the nurse may administer intravenous succinylcholine to relax the larynx, which is in spasm. It may be necessary to insert an endotracheal tube. Throughout the duration of the laryngeal spasm, ventilatory assistance is needed to provide adequate tissue oxygenation. The nurse must observe the patient closely until the patient's respiratory integrity is restored. Emergency resuscitation equipment must be available at all times.

Treatment of postoperative nausea and vomiting is important in recovery room care. When nausea occurs, the nurse must first prevent the patient from aspirating vomitus into the airway. The nurse immediately suctions the patient's mouth, turns the patient's head to the side, and places the patient on her side. With ear procedures and others where nausea is likely, the patient should be positioned on her side when she arrives in the recovery room. The nurse should make sure that her airway is patent. In treating the patient for nausea and vomiting, the nurse may give the patient oxygen or antiemetics either intravenously (the faster route) or intramuscularly. She can encourage deep breathing exercise, and provide splinting of the surgical site and emotional support to lessen the discomfort of postoperative nausea.

CARDIAC

The nurse evaluates cardiac status continuously throughout the recovery phase. She interprets arterial blood pressure values. She assesses pulse regularity, rate, and rhythm. A cardiac monitor may be used during the course of the immediate recovery phase to observe and treat arrhythmias. The cardiovascular status of the postanesthetic patient requires careful management. Cardiovascular status is determined by the patient's vital signs, which are taken every 15 minutes until they are stable.

The patient's heart rate should be in the range of 60 to 110 and should be compared with the preoperative record. If the pulse rate rises above 110, reasons for the increase should be determined. The heart rate is expected to be somewhat faster during the immediate postoperative period than in the patient's baseline assessment. Peripheral pulses should be taken to ascertain the circulatory status in all extremities. These include the axillary, brachial, radial, femoral, popliteal, and dorsalis pedis pulses. Adequate fluid and electrolyte balance is necessary to maintain heart action and to assure satisfactory pulse rate and circulatory status.

Systolic blood pressure should be no less than 90 mm Hg and no more than 150–160 mm Hg. Diastolic pressure should not fall below 50 or be higher than 90. It is important for the nurse to compare current blood pressure with the patient's preoperative blood pressure. Changes in blood pressure reading may be more significant than a consistent high or low reading. A consistent dropping of 10 mm Hg from 130 to 140 mm Hg systolic pressure with each blood pressure check may indicate impending problems more than a stable systolic pressure of 90 mm Hg. General anesthetic drugs lower blood pressure, especially agents such as enflurane, halothane, and methoxyflurane. Other causes of hypotension include hemorrhage, impaired venous return to the heart as in mechanical ventilation (positive pressure breathing), and pooling of blood in the extremities caused by paralysis of sympathetic innervation to arterioles (1). Any one of these factors affects the patient's circulatory status.

Hypotension, a rapid weak thready pulse, cool moist skin, and decreased level of consciousness are symptoms of shock, which may be due to cardiac insufficiency or hypovolemia. Shock is an ever-present threat from hypovolemia, which may be due to excessive blood and tissue fluid loss during the intraoperative period or hemorrhage in the immediate postoperative period. The nurse must be alert for symptoms of hemorrhage because decreased blood flow may damage vital organs such as the brain, heart, and kidneys. Blood viscosity increases when blood and fluid are lost, creating a potential for thrombus formation.

The postanesthetic patient's blood pressure may be elevated for several reasons, such as anxiety or the intraoperative administration of drugs such as epinephrine, which is used in some ear, nose, and throat procedures. Labile hypertension may occur in specific procedures, such as carotid endarterectomy. Hypertension may develop as a reaction to increased PCO_2, hypervolemia, intense pain, or shivering. The nurse and physician need to determine the cause of the hypertension and actions to be taken. Administration of a sedative or an antihypertensive drug may be prescribed. Other measures may include administering oxygen, reducing infusion flow rate, or applying blankets. The physician and the nurse may determine that the elevated blood pressure will be self-limiting. The recovery room nurse obtains, interprets, and records blood pressure values as well as treatment modalities and their effects.

The patient's temperature is expected to be lower during the immediate postoperative period. Warm blankets are applied until body temperature approaches a normal range. Afterward it rises to about 100°F, or 38°C. Malignant hyperthermia is a critical complication that commences during the operative period when the patient receives general anesthesia. Body temperature may rise to 108°F or more. Hypothermia measures and administration of dantrolene are instituted immediately. In the recovery room, special nursing care includes close monitoring of vital signs and continuing hypothermic measures and drug therapy.

The recovery room nurse must recognize the signs and symptoms of shock. If signs of shock are evident, immediate action is indicated. Hypotension, diaphoresis, decreased level of consciousness, increased heart rate, oliguria, cardiac arrhythmia arrest, or respiratory distress are signs of shock. The nurse must act quickly in any type of shock to maintain and support cardiovascular and respiratory functions in an effort to reduce hypoxemic states of the cardiac, renal, and central nervous systems. The nurse initially increases the fluid administration rate, starts oxygen therapy if not in progress, places pillows under both legs of the patient, and notifies the anesthesiologist and surgeon of the complicating symptoms. Further treatment includes cardiac monitoring, frequent blood pressure taking, and continuous observation of the patient until the etiology of the symptoms can be determined and medical treatment instituted. Medical treatment may include elastic hose to prevent venous stasis and pooling of blood, insertion of a central venous pressure (CVP) line, and restoration of blood pressure by a lidocaine or dopamine drip. Bicarbonate may be ordered to combat metabolic acidosis. Nursing measures, including constant observation of the patient, are necessary to prevent complications from the medical therapy instituted.

Cardiac arrhythmias may be caused by hypoxia, drugs, hypovolemia stress, imbalanced electrolytes, and hypothermia or hyperthermia. Arrhythmias are identified by the nurse on auscultation or by cardiac monitoring. Appropriate measures may include antiarrhythmic medications, electrolyte administration, or cardiopulmonary resuscitation.

URINARY OUTPUT

The amount of urinary output indicates the adequacy of circulating fluids, renal function, and cardiac output. Blood pressure must be sufficient to maintain hydrostatic pressure within the kidneys. The adequacy of renal function is directly related to the preservation of fluid and electrolyte balance. If the patient has an indwelling catheter, the nurse can easily measure output. The patient should not leave the operating room until a urine output of at least 30 ml/hour has been noted. If the patient does not have an indwelling catheter, orders are usually written to catheterize the patient every 8 to 10 hours as necessary. This will be done after the patient has been discharged from the recovery room. Patients without indwelling catheters must be carefully watched for urinary bladder distention. Such distention may cause restlessness as the patient emerges from general anesthesia. If spinal anesthesia was used, cord innervation to the urinary bladder may be blocked. The bladder can become seriously distended as a result of the combination of nerve blockade and intravenous fluid administration.

Inadequate output may indicate hypovolemia, electrolyte imbalance, or impending shock. Output may be low because of renal tubular damage from severe hypotension, hypoxia, or hypovolemia during the operative period. Or the cause may be a severe stress response that increases release of the antidiuretic hormone. This response can occur from the general anesthetic itself. Blood transfusion incompatibilities may cause severe oliguria because of associated tubular necrosis. Fluids must be restricted if the cause of oliguria or anuria is determined to be tubular damage. Adequate urine output may be restored in 3–5 days if the damage is not severe, but adequate renal function may not be restored for 10–21 days after severe tubular necrosis (2).

FLUID REPLACEMENT

The main goals for parenteral fluid therapy in the recovery room are: (1) to correct past deficits, (2) to replace concurrent losses such as from drainage or nasogastric tubes, and (3) to maintain satisfactory blood pressure and urine output. Fluids are given at a rate to maintain sufficient blood pressure, but the potential for overload should not be overlooked.

The amount of fluid replacement is determined by the amount of body surface area. The anesthesiologist calculates this from tables based on height and weight measurements. Accurate intake and output are one method to assess fluid balance. Central venous pressure (CVP) monitoring is another method for patients who have this type of monitoring. Overloading the circulatory system causes a rise in the CVP reading from the baseline. Conversely, inadequate circulatory volume causes the CVP reading to fall from the patient's baseline (3).

The physician orders the rate of flow or the amount of fluid to be given per hour or over an eight-hour period. The nurse calculates the rate of flow. First, she must know the drop size of the commercial infusion set being used. The usual infusion rate is 3 ml/minute and is rarely more than 4 ml/minute. If cardiac or renal function is impaired, the rate is kept at 2 ml/minute or less. Fast infusion rates cause circulatory overload because there is not enough time for circulating fluids to diffuse into the extracellular tissue fluid compartments. Pulmonary edema is likely to develop.

Plasma expanders such as plasmanate, dextran 40, dextran 70, albumin (salt poor or regular), or blood transfusion may be necessary if the patient has had excessive fluid or blood loss during surgery or postoperative hemorrhaging. Dextran has an advantage over plasma in that it does not need to be refrigerated, but it may cause allergic reactions manifested by hives, itching, bronchospasm, wheezing respirations, tightness of chest, angioedema, and anaphylaxis. Cases of renal shutdown have also been reported. These reactions usually develop during the first 30 minutes, but absence of early allergic signs does not negate the necessity of continual observation.

Dextran 70 increases clotting time because it decreases platelet adhesiveness. Its anticoagulant effect is equivalent to dicumarol in preventing thrombosis following major pelvic surgery or femoral neck fractures. The usual rate of infusion is 20–40 ml/minute, but this rate may be increased if there is severe hypovolemia. Slower rates are less likely to produce allergic reactions (4).

Plasma may be frozen up to one year. It should be used within two hours after thawing. Because blood cells and antibodies are washed away in the preparation of plasma, it does not cause allergic reactions.

Whole blood is another volume expander used to replace blood loss. Blood transfusions predispose the patient to reactions such as headache, chills, fever, flushing, feeling of tight restricting chest pain, dyspnea, nausea, hypotension, itching, rash, or unexplained bleeding from the lysis of blood cells. Severe reactions cause the urine to become dark due to the breakdown of red cells. Also, the patient's serum bilirubin level rises, and anemia may ensue.

Observation for signs of reactions to blood transfusions is an important nursing function. Most reactions occur within the first 20–30 minutes after starting the transfusion. This is the critical period. After this initial period, however, reactions may still occur, and the nurse's responsibility for continuing surveillance does not decrease.

There may be problems with transfusing blood that has been refrigerated or frozen. Blood should be warmed to room temperature before administration. Otherwise the patient will have unnecessary discomfort, and it may be difficult to differentiate chilling from the onset of reactions. Care must be exercised in warming blood because a temperature above 98.6°F, or 37°C, will destroy cells. The rate of flow is begun slowly at 2–3 ml/minute for the first 50–100 ml of each unit of blood. Then if no indications of incompatibility are detected, the rate is adjusted to 5–10 ml/minute. The flow is usually maintained at a slower rate for the elderly and for those with cardiac decompensation. There are emergency situations, however, when it is necessary to infuse the blood rapidly. This can be accomplished by placing a cuff around the plastic container of blood. The cuff is inflated to create the amount of pressure needed to achieve the desired

infusion rate. The use of a mechanical blood warming device should also be installed.

If the patient still is partially anesthetized, hypotension and tachycardia may be the first manifestations of transfusion reaction that the nurse can detect. The blood transfusion must be stopped at the first indication of untoward reaction. The nurse must monitor urinary output because of the possibility of impaired kidney function due to hemolyzed blood cells. Severe hypotension also decreases renal blood flow and the filtration process necessary to produce urine.

Medications such as bicarbonate are given as ordered to combat acidosis that may develop because of transfusion reaction. Vasopressors are given to increase blood pressure. Other drugs may be ordered to produce diuresis. Antihistamines are ordered if the allergic reaction is not severe, and the physician may decide to continue the transfusion at a slower flow rate if receiving the blood is crucial to the patient's recovery. This requires constant monitoring for detection of more severe reactions. Steroids may be ordered for severe allergic reactions.

PAIN MANAGEMENT

One of the most crucial functions of the recovery room nurse is management of postoperative pain. Once the nurse has diagnosed the presence of pain, a decision must be made regarding what can be done to alleviate it. If the patient is still emerging from anesthesia, the nurse considers whether the progress of the patient toward consciousness will be impeded by an analgesic. The status of cardiac and respiratory systems is of concern. The anesthetic agents used and the reversal of these may also be a factor.

Analgesia may be indicated. Usually, the anesthesiologist provides standing medication orders. In many instances the nurse may determine the route. In the absence of orders or protocols, the nurse cannot decide on the specific drug nor can she specify the amount. The anesthesiologist or surgeon must be consulted since these are medical decisions. The nurse contributes important data in the decision-making process. Postponing relief and inadequate dosage of analgesic can initiate an escalating pain experience where severe pain is relieved for short time periods, but then reaches a second peak of severe intensity. The cycle begins again to reach a higher third peak. Fear of pain increases in such patients. Pain has a retarding effect on the surgical patient's recovery (see Fig. 25.6). When to give an analgesic is usually determined by the nurse. Judicious control for the patient's benefit is important, since the patient has no control over this aspect of pain relief.

Before administering any palliative medications for pain, the nurse must establish the clinical signs and symptoms for the anesthetic agents and drugs administered. For example, if fentanyl, a potent narcotic, is given intraoperatively, the nurse must ascertain when the patient received it so as not to incur unnecessary respiratory depression. She also needs to determine if the patient has any allergies to narcotic analgesics.

In conjunction with the anesthesiologist, the nurse may administer intravenous or intramuscular analgesics to provide comfort for the patient. Careful monitoring of the patient's respiratory and cardiovascular status is essential after narcotic analgesic administration.

Analgesics may be given intravenously or intramuscularly in the recovery room. The most direct route that gets the analgesic into the blood stream the fastest is preferred. If cardiac and respiratory stability have been obtained, the intramuscular route can be used, but the drug cannot be reversed if the status of the systems change. The use of the intramuscular route is contraindicated in patients who have only tenuous cardiac and respiratory stability. Poor circulatory status causes minimal absorption of the drug. Although slight improvements increase absorption, the patient may receive a sufficient bolus into the blood to negate the improvement, which further depresses circulation and cellular respiration.

The intravenous route is safest and preferred because it provides almost immediate relief. Frequently used narcotics such as morphine and Demerol are administered intravenously.

If necessary, reversal of intravenous drugs can be accomplished rapidly by the same route.

If the alleviation of pain by analgesics must be postponed, other measures are indicated. The nurse can help the patient change position and provide additional support for the operative area. Backrubs may relax tense muscles and provide some relief. If the patient is conscious, refocusing attention through conversation may help. Mental concentration on other matters can be encouraged. Stroking the skin in certain areas may distract attention if it is not offensive to the patient and may have pain-relieving effects. Through sensitive communication, including touch and oral reassurance, the nurse can provide emotional support.

One of the newest developments in the management of postoperative pain is the electronic pain stimulator. This battery-powered device controls pain by delivering continuous electrical stimulation to the incision site. Adhesive strips are placed on both sides of the incision and connected to the device by small wires. The device may be instituted in the recovery room; however, narcotics may still be administered as an adjunct therapy immediately postoperatively. The device is particularly helpful as the patient regains full consciousness in the following days of the postoperative course. The benefit for the patient is an increased comfort level by alleviating pain and a decreased need for postoperative analgesics. The decrease in postoperative pain can also decrease the length of stay in the hospital. If pain is controlled, the patient is more likely to ambulate, cough, deep breathe, and undertake other activities that return her to recovery in a shorter time.

GENERAL

Each surgical procedure requires execution of specialized measures by the recovery room nurse. The nurse must acquire knowledge of possible complications and outcomes for specific operations. For example, vascular surgery requires the recovery room nurse to concentrate particularly on the extremity or extremities that may be affected postoperatively. She

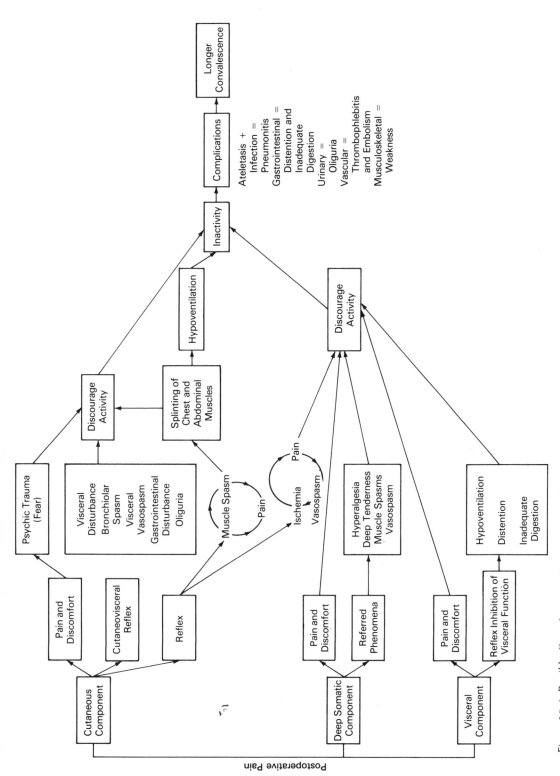

Figure 25.6 Possible effects of postoperative pain. Reprinted with permission from The Management of Pain, *by J. J. Bonica, p. 1241. Copyright © 1953 by Lea & Febiger.*

reports any loss of color, decreased temperature, absence of peripheral pulses, and loss of movement or sensation as potential for an undesirable surgical outcome. The recovery room nurse monitors the affected extremity by palpation, observation, and Doppler, if available, and documents findings on the recovery room record.

Particular attention must be given to any tissue invaded by the surgical procedure because of the potential for hemorrhage. An extremely vascular area such as the breast has the potential for hemorrhage postoperatively. For example, the recovery room nurse must check the dressings for untoward amounts of drainage throughout the duration of the recovery process. If bleeding is suspected, the recovery room nurse must remove the dressing and inspect the surgical site. If a hematoma is forming, the surgeon must be notified to ascertain whether the patient should return to surgery to stop the bleeding.

The nurse must be in constant attendance with any pediatric patient recovering from surgery and anesthesia. The pediatric patient demands intensive observation of the respiratory system during the immediate postoperative phase as well as precautions to protect the child during a restless emergence from anesthesia. Emotional support of children depends on a knowledge of growth and development. Such knowledge is essential, particularly in postanesthetic recovery areas that prohibit attendance of a parent.

Each patient is a special entity in the recovery room regardless of the procedure. The nurse must be a specialist in many areas in order to perform effectively.

DISCHARGE FROM RECOVERY ROOM

The nurse bases discharge from the postanesthetic area on the accomplishment of the goals she has established. The minimum expected outcomes for the patient to return to the unit are: vital sign stability, normal thermic state, orientation to surroundings, absence of surgical and anesthetic complications, a minimum of pain and nausea, controlled wound drainage, adequate urine output (20 to 30 cc/hour), fluid and electrolyte balance, and adequate pulmonary exchange. The patient's recovery room score should be high on the discharge scale if one is used, unless limited by preoperative conditions. Figure 25.7 gives a sample of discharge criteria. The patient should also be able to summon help if needed. If the patient is to go home following a short-stay surgery, such as a D and C, the patient must be fully awake and demonstrate the ability to take nourishment by mouth and ambulate as well as meet those criteria identified for a patient staying in the hospital. Without approved discharge protocols, the anesthesiologist must be apprised of her patient's condition and approve discharge of the patient from the recovery room.

When the patient is discharged from the recovery room, the nurse gives the unit nurse or primary nurse a report including the type of surgery and anesthesia; blood loss; crystalloid, blood component, and colloid administration; medication administration; vital signs, measurable and nonmeasurable outputs; and any complications. The nurse makes sure that the patient's family or significant others are informed of the transfer and the patient's condition.

Evaluation

At the time of transfer to the postoperative unit, the recovery room nurse documents the patient's progress on the record. The progress reported should indicate the extent to which the patient goals were met. When planning the immediate postoperative care, the recovery room nurse considers data obtained from the perioperative nurse as well as the patient care plan. She then sets forth goals for the patient during recovery along with an individualized plan to be implemented during the patient's stay in the recovery room. To complete the nursing process, an evaluation of the patient's goal attainment plus measurement of the effectiveness of nursing care is essential.

The discharge criteria score used just prior to transfer to the postoperative unit is one method of evaluating attainment of patient

Figure 25.7. Wohrle discharge criteria scoring system. Printed with permission of Carmen Wohrle, RN, MSN, assistant director of nursing/critical care areas, Deaconess Hospital, Spokane, Wa.

Level of Consciousness
1. Infant awake (cries; has startle reflex; moves freely). — 2
2. Adult awake (answers simple questions; follows two-step commands). — 2
3. Patient very sleepy (requires light tactile or verbal stimulation to arouse; attempts to follow commands; falls back to sleep easily). — 1
4. Patient requires deep painful stimuli to awaken; does not respond to other stimuli. — 0

Circulatory Status
1. Urinary output:
   1 cc/kg/hour. — 2
   0.5 cc/kg/hour. — 1
   Less than 0.5 cc/kg/hour. — 0
2. Capillary activity:
   Capillary beds bilaterally are equally pink, warm, blanche rapidly. — 2
   Capillary beds are not equal in response or blanche sluggishly, skin cool. — 1
   Capillary beds fail to blanche, skin cold and pale in appearance. — 0
3. Dressings:
   Dressing did not require reinforcement; no evidence of bright red bleeding within last hour. — 2
   Dressing required reinforcement due to serosanguinous drainage within last hour. — 1
   New bright red bleeding noticed on dressing within last 15 minutes. — 0
4. Vital signs stable × 30 minutes
   Systolic blood pressure:
   ± 10 mm Hg of preop value. — 2
   ± 20 mm Hg of preop value. — 1
   ± greater than 20 mm Hg of preop value. — 0
   Pulse:
   ± 20/min of preop rate. — 2
   ± 30/min of preop rate. — 1
   ± greater than 30/min of preop rate. — 0
   Respirations:
   ± 5/min of preop rate. — 2
   ± greater than 5/min of preop rate. — 0
   Temperature:
   ± 1 degree of oral/rectal preop temp. — 2
   ± 2 degrees of oral/rectal preop temp. — 1
   ± greater than 2 degrees oral/rectal preop temp. — 0
5. Drains, tubes:
   Tubes are patent with less than 100 cc/hour drainage; no presence of bright red bleeding in last hour. — 2
   Drainage in excess of 100 cc/hour but not bright red. — 1
   Bright red bleeding within last hour. — 0
6. Edema:
   Edema of extremities, sacrum, and surgical site not in excess of initial postop assessment. — 2
   Edema in excess of initial assessment but no moist basilar lung rales auscultated. — 1
   Edema in excess of initial assessment and rales developing in lung bases. — 0

Airway Patency
1. Airway assistance:
   Requires no airway assistance. — 2
   Requires oral/nasal airway or chin lift. — 1
   Requires endotracheal tube. — 0
2. Breath sounds (auscultation):
   Bilateral exchange with no abnormal breath sounds. — 2
   Bilateral exchange with rhonchi and/or faint rales. — 1
   Absent or diminished breath sounds in any part of lungs and/or coarse rales; wheezes; stridor — 0
3. Able to cough and swallow on command. — 2
   Requires external tracheal irritation to cough; drooling. — 1
   Requires suctioning and side-lying position. — 0

4. Has not retched or gagged; no nausea; or had emesis within last 30 minutes.	2
Required antiemetic within the last 30 minutes.	1
Has vomited within last 30 minutes.	1
5. Has had no bright red bleeding from nose or throat in last hour.	2
Has had copious dark bloody secretions requiring suctioning in last 30 minutes.	1
Is having bright red bleeding or copious dark secretions requiring suctioning in last 15 minutes.	0

Figure 25.7. (Continued)

goals. If the score is at an acceptable level, the patient's vital signs should be stabilized, she should have regained a level of consciousness that would allow her to call for assistance if necessary, and her dressings should be dry and intact. The predetermined goals have been attained.

Other ways of evaluating patient care in the recovery room are by implementing quality assurance activities that review and evaluate care provided the patient during her stay in the recovery room.

Observation and assessment of nursing responsibilities and practices are done to determine effectiveness. Some of the factors affecting patient welfare and safety that can be measured include: the patient is warm and comfortable; siderails are up and safety strap or restraints have been applied, if needed; measures have been taken to control nausea and vomiting; respiratory integrity has been maintained by positioning of jaw, head, neck, and body; stir-up regime has been implemented; and measures have been taken to control postoperative pain.

Other nursing activities observed for evaluation purposes are wound site observation, oxygen therapy, parenteral therapy, fluid output, and special procedures.

Records and reports are another way to evaluate care given. The patient care record can be reviewed to determine such things as the completion of the anesthesia record and flow sheets. Are they labeled and signed, and do they have the needed data? Are orders completed and signed? Are allergies documented on the recovery room record? Are all portions of the recovery room record completed according to criteria for documentation? The patient care plan should also be reviewed to determine if realistic goals were established and if the

prescribed plan of care was implemented. Medication documentation, another component of the patient record, should be reviewed for accuracy related to time, dosage, and route of administration. The progress notes should indicate the patient's responses to narcotics, barbiturates, and reversal agents. The patient observation index used throughout the patient's stay in the recovery room should show evidence of constant patient monitoring. This should include admission criteria and scoring, ongoing monitoring, and discharge criteria. The parenteral fluid record should include the date, time, and solutions used.

The recovery room environment should be reviewed on an ongoing basis. Is the environment clean and orderly? Are the fire alarms and exits accessible? Are unused equipment and supplies stored in designated areas and is soiled linen contained and confined? Other areas of concern are emergency equipment, its function, and accessibility.

Standards of care for the recovery room provide another avenue for evaluating the care patients receive in the immediate postoperative period. The format for most standards include the patient's potential or actual problem, expected outcome, time frames, and nursing orders. A comparison of the nursing orders prescribed in the standards with those on the patient care plan should reveal consistency. To demonstrate professional as well as legal accountability, the recovery room nurse must implement the standards of care established by the institution.

A review of care can be done through a peer review process where colleagues evaluate each other's practices. This may be a structured formal process where specific criteria have been established for evaluating care given or it may be an informal process.

References

1. Hercules, P. L. "Nursing in the postoperative care unit: A review. Part 2: Other complications." *AORN J* 28(December):1049–52, 1978.
2. Sabiston, D. C., ed. *Davis-Christopher Textbook of Surgery*, 12th ed. Philadelphia: W. B. Saunders, 1981.
3. Luckmann, J., and Sorensen, K. C. *Medical-Surgical Nursing: A Psychophysiological Approach*, 2nd ed. Philadelphia: W. B. Saunders, 1980.
4. Hoover, J. E., ed. *Remington's Pharmaceutical Sciences*. Easton, Penn.: Mack Publishing Co., 1975.

V

Evaluating
Perioperative
Patient Care

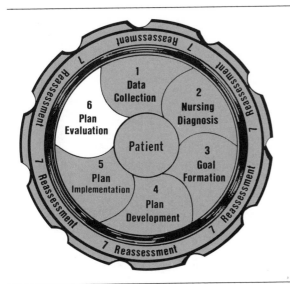

The degree of goal achievement is determined.

Evaluating Goal Attainment

Evaluation is a process for determining worth, value, or effectiveness. To make an evaluation, the evaluator assesses data and compares the findings to established criteria (1,2).

Evaluation is the final or fourth phase of the nursing process (see Fig. 26.1). It follows implementation of the nursing actions identified in the patient care plan and reflects how the patient responds to those actions (3). As the final component of the patient care plan, it allows the nurse to make an objective and measurable judgment regarding the resolution of the problem or the patient's progress toward achieving his goal. It indicates the completion of one cycle of interventions and may begin another one based on current data and changing patient responses. Evaluation is a continuous process.

Standard VI in the *Standards of Perioperative Nursing Practice* applies to evaluation (see Figs. 26.1 and 26.2). The standard states that the "plan for nursing care is evaluated" (4). The standard refers the nurse back to the goals at the beginning of the nursing process. Thus, the standards reflect a continuum of nursing care.

The patient care plan forms the framework for evaluation. It clearly states the patient's problem, the established goals, the planned intervention, and the criteria for measuring

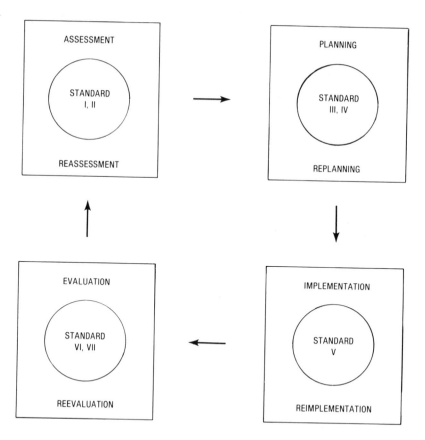

Figure 26.1. As a part of the nursing process, evaluation marks the completion of one cycle of interventions and the beginning of another. Evaluation leads to reassessment, replanning, reimplementation, and reevaluation. The phases of the nursing process correlate with the Standards of Perioperative Nursing Practice.

goal achievement. The plan is designed to encompass the nurse's intellectual, interpersonal, and technical interactions with the patient (see Fig. 26.3) (2).

Steps in the Evaluation Process

Evaluation consists of three steps: (1) selection of criteria for judging goal attainment, (2) collection of data, and (3) comparison of data with the criteria to determine whether goals have been attained. The process requires ongoing assessment of the patient during and following nursing interventions (5).

SELECTION OF CRITERIA

Criteria are supporting evidence the nurse uses to determine whether a goal has been achieved. A criterion states a desired or normal condition to compare with the actual condition. Outcome criteria are used to evaluate the nursing interventions selected to assist the patient in achieving a goal.

The outcome criteria should be individualized for each patient, specific, and measurable. For example, one criterion for blood pressure might state, "48 hours postoperatively, the patient's systolic pressure is no greater than plus or minus 20 mm Hg, compared with the

Standard VI: The Plan for Nursing Care Is Evaluated.

Interpretive Statement
Evaluation is a process the operating room nurse uses to determine the degree of goal attainment. The evaluation is continuous and is based on the nurse's observations and the individual's responses to the nursing interventions. The operating room nurse reviews each of the formulated goals to determine the results of the individual's care. The results of the nursing actions are then compared to the desired goals to determine the degree of goal attainment. The individual, significant others, and health personnel contribute to the evaluation of goal attainment. The data collected from these sources reflect the outcomes of nursing activities.

Criteria
1. The degree of goal achievement is communicated by the operating room nurse to the individual, significant others, and health personnel.
2. The results of nursing actions are documented by written records, observations of nursing practice, and/or confirmation by the individual or significant others.

Figure 26.2. Standard VI of the Standards of Perioperative Nursing Practice. *The plan for nursing care is evaluated.*

preoperative value." The criterion would not have been individualized or realistic if it had stated, "48 hours postoperatively, the systolic pressure is no greater than 120 mm Hg," because this is an average value for middle-aged adults.

Criteria can be stated in many ways. They can be stated as signs and symptoms, data from diagnostic or laboratory tests, statements from the patient, or patient responses. Figure 26.4 shows examples of ways in which criteria can be stated.

The number of criteria for each goal varies. The criteria should be sufficient in number and precise enough to measure change in the patient's status. For example, two patients may undergo the same surgical procedure, such as a bowel resection, but not follow the same postoperative regimen. The first patient may have a nasogastric tube following sur-

Figure 26.3. Depicts the nurse following through to evaluate patient's ability to attain goals.

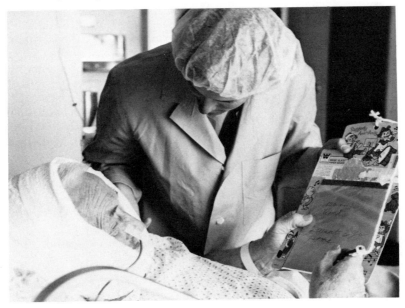

Goal:	The patient will demonstrate adequate pulmonary ventilation throughout a surgical procedure performed under local anesthesia.

Criteria	Source of Data
No rales or rhonchi heard on chest auscultation.	signs and symptoms
A $PaCO_2$ which is consistent with patient's preoperative value of 40 mm Hg.	laboratory data
No abnormalities identified on preoperative x-ray.	diagnostic data
No flaring of nostrils or facial grimacing.	expressions
Compliance with deep breathing instructions when requested.	demonstration

Figure 26.4. Examples of criteria statements. Criteria can be stated in a variety of ways as a value for measuring patient outcome.

gery, but the second may not. A goal for both patients may be the same, but the outcome criteria would indicate different measurements for evaluation. A goal applicable to both patients might be, "The patient demonstrates no evidence of fluid and electrolyte imbalance." Criteria for the first patient might include, "No loss of electrolytes through drainage from the nasogastric tube." This would not be a criterion for the second patient because he has no nasogastric tube.

The criteria specify when a patient is expected to reach a goal. Each goal statement should indicate whether the goal is immediate, intermediate, or long term. Immediate and intermediate goals usually have a specific interval for checking the patient's progress. Long-term goals may not include a final date and may not be measurable until after the patient is discharged to the home or community. If the goal statement is, "The patient's skin integrity is maintained," a criterion for immediate evaluation could read, "No evidence of lost sponges after wound closure." An intermediate evaluation criterion is, "No evidence of wound dehiscence within 48 hours after surgery." Long-term evaluation is indicated with, "Evidence of intact skin and closure after removal of suture from incision site." Regard-

less of the time and conditions identified in the goal statement and outcome criteria, nursing activities must be appropriate to the goal so evaluation can be done and a judgment made (6).

COLLECTION OF DATA

In the evaluation process, the nurse gathers data identified in the criteria. This is an assessment of the patient during or after the implementation of the nursing activities in the patient care plan.

The nurse must gather and report data in a manner that will allow quantitative and qualitative measurement. The measurement should be reliable so each observer following the patient's plan of care will record the data consistently (5). For example, one goal statement with outcome criteria might read:

- Goal: The patient will be free from injury caused by improper safety measures during intraoperative period.
- Criteria:
  1. The skin is free from abrasions.
  2. There is no edema from positioning devices.
  3. There are no fractures or dislocated bones.

In this example, each nurse following the plan of care would collect the same data. Each nurse would assess the patient's skin for abrasions, the tissue for edema caused by positioning devices, and the bony structure for dislocations. Data gathered by two or more nurses could be compared because the same criteria were used. The criteria are individualized for the patient. The third criterion regarding "no fractures or dislocated bones" would not be valid for measurement purposes if the procedure included fractured or dislocated bones.

COMPARISON OF DATA

The final step of the evaluation process requires the nurse to compare the data to the criteria. This comparison enables the nurse to determine the degree of goal attainment and record it as a problem that is either resolved or needs further action (5).

The nurse can use a variety of methods to determine relationships between the criteria and patient responses. The criterion itself identifies the means for gathering the data; e.g., "No rales or rhonchi heard on chest auscultation." Methods for data collection include observation of signs and symptoms; review of laboratory and diagnostic data; intervention with technical skills or teaching techniques; or use of interpersonal skills through communication with the patient, family, or significant others. For example, in evaluating a patient's response during local anesthesia, a nurse might ask the following questions (see Fig. 26.4):

1. Were rales or rhonchi auscultated during the surgical procedure?
2. If arterial blood gases were drawn during the procedure, what was the relationship of the drawn value to that of the preoperative value of 40 mm Hg?
3. Did the preoperative x-ray reveal any abnormalities in the lung field?
4. Did the patient complain of any shortness of breath during the procedure?
5. Did the patient flare his nostrils or grimace?
6. Did the patient take deep breaths when instructed during the procedure?

One tool used in evaluation is the patient outcome scale, which requires assigning a numerical value. An example is the Glasgow Coma Scale, an assessment tool that numerically describes the level of consciousness. It is a means for a quick and accurate evaluation of the patient's neurological status, as noted in eyes open, verbal responses, and motor responses. The patient's responses in these categories are objectively scored and plotted on a graph. The scale is becoming widely used for admitting and discharging patients from neurological units and postoperative care units (7). The OR nurse could adapt the Glasgow Coma Scale for intraoperative patient care by using it to determine the patient's level of consciousness and as a principal component of preoperative assessment and postoperative evaluation data.

Other assessment tools include those which evaluate patient outcome according to patient classification scales or level of activity. Another tool that uses a numerical rating scale on which to chart the patient's progress toward goal attainment is discussed by Inzer and Aspinall in *Nursing Outlook* (8).

As the nurse compares the data with the patient's response to the criteria, a judgment can be made regarding goal attainment, the validity of the nursing activities, or the circumstances under which the activities were performed. A relationship can be defined among the goal, the nursing action, and the evaluation. Results may be any one or a combination of the following (3):

1. The patient's response was as expected, and the problem was resolved. There is no need for further nursing actions, and those used were appropriate.
2. The patient's response indicated that the entire problem was not resolved. Evidence indicated that immediate goals were achieved, but intermediate and long-range goals were not. Complete problem resolution may be slow, and nursing actions should be directed at solving intermediate and long-range goals. Reevaluation will be necessary.
3. The patient's response revealed little evidence that the problem is being resolved. Immediate intervention and long-range goals were not reached and, in some instances, not even approached. Reassessment and replanning are needed.
4. The patient's response indicated that new problems exist. Assessment and planning for the new problem must be coordinated with the planning for the previous problems. Evaluation will follow implementation for new problems.

When the nurse puts the evaluation data into one of these categories, he then examines factors that may have affected the evaluation process. These may include internal or external factors that control or alter the patient's response to the nursing actions. These might be economic (low income), cultural (adherence to a vegetarian diet), sociological (no family or friends), and religious aspects of the patient's lifestyle (refusal of blood), or physical or psychosocial factors external to the patient's environment. The effect of these factors on the patient or the surroundings where the nursing actions took place may directly correlate with the patient's response to nursing intervention (5).

Once the nurse has analyzed evaluation data and considered the influencing factors, he plans further actions appropriate to the situation. Further action includes reassessment, replanning, changes in implementation, and reevaluation.

For example, in Fig. 26.4, the patient underwent a surgical procedure under local anesthesia. The goal statement was that the patient demonstrate adequate pulmonary ventilation throughout the surgical procedure while a local anesthetic was administered. A criterion for the goal was, "No statements of shortness of breath." If at some time during the procedure, the patient complained of shortness of breath, the criterion would not have been met, and the nurse would reassess the data, reevaluate the goal, and alter the plan of care to assist the patient toward adequate pulmonary ventilation. Once the new plan is implemented, evaluation is again determined based on reassessment of the data on hand.

Reassessment

Reassessment, a necessary sequel to evaluation, is Standard VII of the *Standards of Perioperative Nursing Practice* (see Fig. 26.5). It involves reassessing the patient's health status, reconsidering the identified problems, resetting goals, and reorganizing the care plan (4). The new plan is activated, evaluated, and judged again based on the patient's changing needs. Thus, the nursing process continues with the changes in the patient's status until his problems are resolved.

Documentation

Throughout implementation of the patient care plan and as the nurse evaluates the data, the patient's response is recorded in the patient record. Intraoperatively the operating room nurse's notes are used for recording care. The record is then used for validation of nursing actions and continuity of care. By evaluating and recording nursing actions and patient outcomes, the nurse establishes accountability for care given. As a part of the patient record, the notes show a patient-

Figure 26.5. Standard VII of the Standards of Perioperative Nursing Practice. *Reassessment is a necessary sequel to the evaluation phase of the nursing process.*

Standard VII: Reassessment of the Individual, Reconsideration of Nursing Diagnosis, Resetting of Goals, and Modification and Implementation of the Nursing Care Plan Are a Continuous Process.

Interpretive Statement
Reassessment allows the operating room nurse to critically examine the total process from which the planned and delivered nursing interventions are derived. Implementation of the nursing process establishes a feedback to the nurse that facilitates the review of individual professional practice. The steps of the nursing process are taken concurrently and recurrently. New data and/or the degree of goal achievement are assessed and used to reconsider the nursing diagnoses, goals for individual, and plan of care. Reassessment allows the dynamics of nursing to operate in an open system whereby modification of the plan of care can be made as changes occur in the individual's internal and external environment.

Criteria
1. Review or revision of the plan of care is documented by written records, observations of patient responses, and the perception of the individual or significant others.
2. Status of the plan of care is communicated to appropriate others.

oriented plan of care. If the nurse does not record his actions or the patient's response, measurement of goal attainment becomes very difficult. Documentation, its purposes and uses, is discussed in greater detail in Chapter 4.

Intraoperative nursing records are a recent addition to the patient record. The value of recording nursing care provided during the intraoperative period has become apparent for legal purposes and as a method for evaluating the quality of care provided. Figure 26.6 is an illustration of an intraoperative nursing record that incorporates the patient goals and has identified criteria for measuring achievement. One of the goal statements is, "Patient's skin at site will be surgically clean." The evaluation criteria used by this hospital to measure extent of goal achievement is:

1. Was the operative site free from excess hair?
2. Was the skin free from razor nicks?
3. Was site cleaned from incisional area to periphery?

The three goals and criteria used on the form illustrated can be adapted to any intraoperative record. The criteria could also be used in the form of a review and evaluation tool constructed for quality assurance purposes.

This chapter demonstrates how to measure the effectiveness of nursing care and the patient's response to that care. It shows how to use a goal statement as a desired patient outcome and how to develop criteria that can be used to evaluate the individual's care. The actual results of care are then compared to the goals. From this, the degree of goal attainment is measured. All persons who are involved in the care—the patient, health personnel, and family—contribute to evaluation of the goal attainment.

Evaluation is not confined to the fourth step of the nursing process but, like the other three components, is recurrent and cyclical. It is the thread that ties patient care together. Just as goals tell us where we are going, evaluation tells us if we arrived at our destination. Without evaluation to judge the effectiveness of

care, nursing care may not improve, and the patient's progress may remain at a standstill. Evaluation is essential (see Fig. 26.7).

Patient Situation

When evaluating the patient care plan, the nurse compares the desired outcome criteria with the patient's actual response to care. The guide for measurement is the preoperative goal statements given in the patient care plan (see Figs. 26.8 and 26.9). We formulate the goals for Mr. Fischer in Chapter 8. Here we evaluate success in meeting the goals.

One nursing diagnosis was a communication problem related to an altered airway, wired jaw, and tongue resection. The goal to alleviate the problem was that Mr. Fischer would be able to communicate postoperatively. Criteria that could be used to evaluate the effectiveness of nursing care might be:

1. Was Mr. Fischer able to communicate with the magic slate board? Factors influencing the attainment of this criterion would be his level of consciousness postoperatively; his ability to see, which would probably mean using his glasses; his orientation to time and space; and his physical strength. Could he hold the magic slate board, and were his hands steady enough to write legibly? The nursing record indicated Mr. Fischer was able to use the magic slate board to communicate his needs on the second postoperative day.
2. Was Mr. Fischer able to use the nurse call bell? Factors that might influence this criterion could be his level of consciousness, his orientation to time and space, and the availability of the bell within reach. Mr. Fischer was not confused, was awake the morning after his surgery, and did not have any problems with using the nurse call bell. The bell was within his reach at all times when personnel were not at his bedside. This was documented in the patient care plan.
3. Did Mr. Fischer use the finger code for yes and no questions?
4. Did he respond on the telephone by tapping once for yes and twice for no in response to questions?

Criteria that can be used to measure Mr. Fischer's goal of understanding his perioperative care prior to administration of preoperative medication might be:

THE METHODIST HOSPITAL
TOTAL HEALTH CARE CENTER
INTRAOPERATIVE NURSING RECORD

DATE	O. R. NO.

R N S	CIRCULATING	SCRUB	OTHER

TIME	ARRIVAL	AM ☐ PM ☐	ANESTHESIA	AM ☐ PM ☐	DEPARTURE	AM ☐ PM ☐

PRE-OPERATIVE DIAGNOSIS

OPERATIVE PROCEDURE

POST-OPERATIVE DIAGNOSIS

SURGEON	ASSISTANT

OTHER TEAM MEMBER

ANESTHESIA	GENERAL ☐	LOCAL ☐	ANESTHESIOLOGIST	CRNA

NURSE/PATIENT GOALS

I. THE PATIENT'S SKIN AT SITE WILL BE SURGICALLY CLEAN

   A. PREOPERATIVE SHAVE _____
                     AREA   NAME OF INDIVIDUAL INITIATING SHAVE

   B. SKIN PREP _____
                SOLUTION   SITE AND AREA

II. THE PATIENT WILL BE FREE FROM ADVERSE EFFECTS OF LACK OF SAFETY & PROTECTION

   A. IDENTIFICATION MEASURES: BY DR. _____ AT _____ AM ☐ PM ☐

      IDENTIFICATION BAND CHECKED FOR: NAME ☐   HOSPITAL NUMBER ☐   PATIENT STATED OWN NAME ☐

      PHYSICIAN'S NAME ☐   PROCEDURE ☐   OPERATIVE PERMIT CHECKED WITH: PATIENT'S STATEMENT ☐

      SCHEDULE ☐   PATIENT'S NAME CHECKED WITH SCHEDULE ☐

   B. POSITION   SUPINE ☐   PRONE ☐   LITHOTOMY ☐   LATERAL ☐R ☐L

      OTHER _____

   C. PROTECTION   HEEL ☐R ☐L   ELBOW ☐R ☐L   SAFETY STRAP ☐R ☐L   ARMS SECURED AT SIDE ☐R ☐L

      ARMS EXTENDED ☐R ☐L   INFLATABLE BEAN BAG ☐

      OTHER _____

   D. COUNTS   INDICATED ☐   NOT INDICATED ☐

	FINAL COUNTS		INCORRECT
OPENING COUNTS _____	SPONGES 4 x 4	☐	☐
	LAP SQUARES	☐	☐
CLOSING COUNTS _____	DISSECTORS	☐	☐
	BRONCHOSCOPY	☐	☐
	NEEDLES	☐	☐
MEASURES TAKEN TO LOCATE INCORRECT COUNTS	INJECTION NEEDLES	☐	☐
	BLADES	☐	☐
	INSTRUMENTS	☐	☐
	OTHER	☐	☐

Figure 26.6. Intraoperative nursing record. By recording nursing actions, the nurse becomes accountable for actions and demonstrates responsibility in patient involvement.

502 *V. Evaluating Perioperative Patient Care*

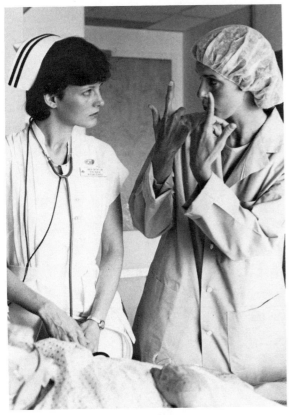

Figure 26.7. The unit nurse and perioperative nurse evaluate Mr. Fischer postoperatively.

1. Asks questions about his impending surgery.
2. Describes in own words effect of surgery.
3. Expresses feelings of concern and fears regarding body image.
4. Demonstrates turning, coughing, and deep breathing exercises.
5. Tells family where waiting room is located.

Another goal pertained to intraoperative care. Mr. Fischer would be free from neuromuscular complications 24 hours postoperatively. Because of the nature and length of the surgical procedure, the potential for damage to the neuromuscular system was greater than usual. Mr. Fischer was in the operating room approximately 12 hours. Criteria used to measure extent of goal attainment might include, but not be limited to:

1. No tingling sensation
2. No numbness
3. No edema in lower extremities
4. No cramping
5. No pain or aches in joints
6. No swelling in joints
7. Flexion and extension of extremities
8. Abduction and adduction of extremities
9. No weakness
10. No stiffness

Mr. Fischer had denied any limitations of range of motion during the preoperative assessment. This was the baseline for comparing the patient's response postoperatively. The nurse had observed during the physical assessment that he had trace edema bilaterally in the lower extremities. No other significant findings were recorded on the patient care plan. Postoperatively, the patient record indicated that on the first and second postoperative day, there was no evidence of edema. However, beginning on the third postoperative day, trace edema was noted and recorded. Its presence was documented throughout the remainder of the hospital stay.

Observations by physicians and nurses indicate all the criteria were met. The edema was present upon admission to the hospital; it was not a negative response to care given. In evaluation, any baseline established on admission should be noted in the record as well as the patient's present status.

Another of Mr. Fischer's problems was respiratory. Because he would have a tracheostomy, hemiglossectomy, and jaw-wiring, the goal was that his alternative airway be patent until the tracheostomy was closed (see Fig. 26.10). Criteria for evaluating continued patency of the tracheostomy tube are:

1. Presence of bilateral breath sounds without rales
2. No gurgling or bubbling of mucus in trachea
3. Absence of crowing respirations
4. Absence of straining on inspiration

In evaluation of the above criteria, the nurse noted that Mr. Fischer had some difficulty immediately postoperatively coughing up mucus from his trachea. He was suctioned frequently, and moderate amounts of secretions were obtained. He was taught to use the suction and was able to cough and suction himself when necessary. The record indicated that all the criteria were met; thus, the alternative airway was maintained until the tracheostomy was closed.

Mr. Fischer had a potential for respiratory problems due to his history of bronchitis, smoking, and

INTRAOPERATIVE PATIENT CARE PLAN

Mr. Ralph Fischer

NURSING DIAGNOSIS	GOAL	PLAN	IMPLEMENTATION	EVALUATION
PREOPERATIVE Knowledge, lack of external resources (people or material)	Patient will verbalize understanding of his perioperative care prior to administration of preoperative medications.	Provide explanations regarding each phase of perioperative period. 1. Preop: NPO, preop meds, IV line, shave, antiseptic scrub, where family could wait, approximate length of surgery, etc. 2. Intraop: EKG, BP, Foley catheter, possible blood transfusions, drains, jaw wiring, trach, etc. 3. Postop: ICU, possible ventilator, frequent suctioning, turning, respiratory therapy, pain meds, dressing change, etc.	• Specific information provided regarding the events surrounding the surgical procedure • Explanations given regarding expectations of the patient and family • Encouraged to express fears and anxieties • Patient explained his understanding of the surgical procedure and anesthesia. • Preoperative instruction regarding postop care: 1–coughing, deep breathing, turning 2–pain 3–drains and tubes 4–IV 5–possible ventilator • Patient demonstrated turning, coughing and deep breathing exercises.	The patient verbalizes understanding of his perioperative care prior to administration of preoperative medications 1. Asks questions about his impending surgery 2. Describes in own words effect of surgery 3. Expresses feelings of concern and fears regarding body image 4. Demonstrates turning, coughing, and deep breathing exercises 5. Tells family where waiting room is located.
Communication, impaired verbal due to required anatomical resection, jaw wiring, tracheostomy.	Patient will be able to communicate postoperatively.	1. Teach patient to use magic slate and nurses call bell 2. Teach patient hand signals (one finger-yes, two fingers-no) 3. Ask patient yes and no questions whenever possible 4. Teach patient to communicate on phone by tapping on mouth piece.	• Nurse conducted preoperative assessment • Rapport was established with patient and wife • Patient taught how to use alternative methods of communicating • Patient and wife return demonstrated use of fingers and phone messages.	The patient was able to communicate postoperatively 1. Write words on magic slate 2. Push nurse call bell 3. Use one finger for yes responses 4. Use two fingers for no responses 5. Tap on mouth piece of phone to respond yes or no to direct questions.
INTRAOPERATIVE Potential for neuromuscular damage due to required positioning and length of surgical procedure.	Patient will be free from neuromuscular complications 24 hours postoperatively.	1. Question patient preop re: any ROM limitations or neurosensory problems. 2. Use positional devices on OR table to prevent pressure over bony prominences (i.e. flotation order mattress, egg crate, etc.) 3. Place foam pads on heels and elbows and consider foam ring under buttocks 4. Have rolled towel available for affected shoulder (prn) 5. Check with anesthesiologist and/or surgeon re: padding desired head and neck 6. Check with anesthesiologist and/or surgeon re: flexion of table or placement of blanket under popliteal space to lessen strain to lower back 7. After preliminary positioning ask patient about his level of comfort and adjust accordingly. 8. Prior to RR transfer check bony prominences and buttocks for discoloration document findings and communicate abnormal findings to RR	Operating Room: 1. Patient denied ROM limitations preoperatively. 2. Patient placed in supine position with egg crate mattress. 3. Foam pads on both elbows and heels. 4. Rolled towel placed under shoulder. 5. Head and neck slightly extended. 6. O.R. table flexed to lessen strain on lower back during procedure. 7. Patient states he is comfortable. 8. Physical assessment when transferring to recovery room revealed no evidence of pressure areas or impaired skin integrity.	The patient was free of neuromuscular complications 24 hours postoperatively 1. No tingling sensation 2. No numbness 3. No edema 4. No cramping 5. No pain or ache in joints 6. No swelling in joints 7. Flexion and extension of extremities 8. Abduction and adduction of extremities 9. No weakness 10. No stiffness

Figure 26.8. Intraoperative patient care plan including preoperative and intraoperative nursing diagnoses, goals, plan, implementation, and evaluation for Mr. Fischer.

INTRAOPERATIVE PATIENT CARE PLAN
Mr. Ralph Fischer

NURSING DIAGNOSIS	GOAL	PLAN	IMPLEMENTATION	EVALUATION
POSTOPERATIVE				
Respiratory: Alteration in airway (tracheostomy, hemiglossectomy, mandibular fixation.)	Patient will have patent alternative airway until tracheostomy is closed.	1. Intraop: have ABG kits available 2. Check with surgeon re: type and size of tracheostomy tube. 3. Notify recovery room if ventilator necessary 4. Have ambu bag and oxygen tank ready on patient bed prior to transport 5. If jaw wired, have wire cutters available for recovery room.	Operating Room: 1. Blood drawn for ABG and sent to lab. 2. Silastic tracheostomy tube size #7 inserted. Recovery Room: 3. Placed on ventilator per ET tube at 50% FiO_2, 1000 tidal volume, rate 12. 4. Ambu bag at bedside. 5. Wire cutters at bedside.	The patient's alternative airway was patent until tracheostomy closed 1. Presence of bilateral breath sounds 2. No gurgling or bubbling of mucus in trachea 3. Absence of crowing respirations 4. Absence of straining on inspiration
Increased risk for postop complications due to: 1. History of bronchitis 2. History of smoking 3. Exposure to environmental irritants	Patient will be free of respiratory complications 48 hours postop. 1. Infection 2. Atelectasis 3. Aspiration	1. Preoperatively teach respiratory exercises (coughing, deep breathing, turning). Have patient return demonstrate and state rationale. 2. Discuss altered breathing pattern via tracheostomy 3. Explain need for frequent suctioning 4. Due to increased risk of aspiration elevate head of bed per physician's orders and monitor closely for signs of respiratory distress during transport. 5. Monitor nasogastric tube for patency and return of gastric secretions.	Note: 1. Preoperatively the nurse conducted an assessment and taught the patient return demonstration. 2. (see Implementation Problem #1) 3. (see Implementation Problem #1) 4. Head of bed elevated immediately postop and until patient returned to nursing unit. Postop Unit: 1. Nasogastric tube to gravity drainage with scant amount of light green drainage. 2. Complaining of nausea and NG tube being uncomfortable. 3. Patient vomiting and aspirated secretions into lungs. 4. Physician notified.	The patient was free of respiratory complications 48 hours postoperatively 1. Presence of bilateral breath sounds 2. Free of rales or wheezes 3. Scattered ronchi for 8 days post-op. 4. Nonproductive cough. 5. Low grade temperature for 3 days. 6. Free of chest pain. 7. Sputum questionable for pseudo-monas and Escherichia coli.

Figure 26.9. Intraoperative patient care plan including postoperative nursing diagnosis, goals, plan, implementation, and evaluation for Mr. Fischer.

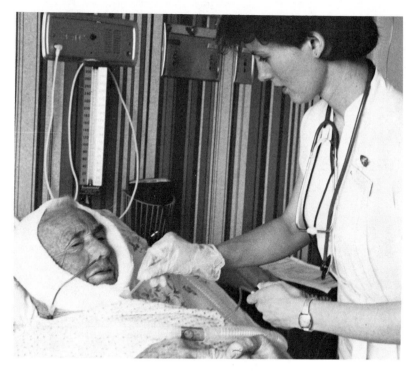

Figure 26.10. Evaluation of patent alternative airway.

exposure to environmental irritants. The goal was to prevent respiratory complications 48 hours postoperatively. Complications anticipated were infection, atelectasis, and aspiration. The criteria were:

1. Presence of bilateral breath sounds
2. Free of rales or wheezes
3. Free of rhonchi
4. Nonproductive cough
5. Temperature same as preoperative baseline
6. Free of chest pain

Mr. Fischer aspirated gastric contents on the second day postoperatively. When reviewing the patient record to measure goal attainment, the nurse found the following information:

1. There was questionable right lower lobe atelectasis on the second postoperative day.

2. Mr. Fischer had scattered rhonchi for eight days postoperatively.
3. No rales or wheezes were present except on the fourth postoperative day when a few wheezes were detected in the right lower lung base.
4. The third day postoperatively, x-rays showed slight fluffy infiltrate in the right lower lobe.
5. Sputum was questionable for *Pseudomonas* and *Escherichia coli*. (Antibiotics were ordered specifically for these organisms.)
6. Mr. Fischer ran a low-grade temperature for three days postoperatively.

Comparison of these data with the criteria indicates the goal was not met because Mr. Fischer developed respiratory complications due to the aspiration of gastric contents, which were present for eight days postoperatively. The aspiration was due to vomiting created by gastric distention secondary to a nonfunctioning nasogastric tube.

References

1. Luker, K. A. "An overview of evaluation research in nursing." *J Adv Nurs* 6(March):98, 1981.
2. Redman, B. K. *The Process of Patient Teaching in Nursing*, 4th ed. St. Louis: C. V. Mosby, 1980.
3. Yura, H., and Walsh, M. B. *The Nursing Process*, 3rd ed. New York: Appleton-Century-Crofts, 1978.
4. *Standards of Perioperative Nursing Practice*. Kansas City: American Nurses' Association and the Association of Operating Room Nurses, 1982.
5. Little, D. E., and Carnevali, D. L. *Nursing Care Planning*, 2nd ed. Philadelphia: W. B. Saunders, 1976.
6. Manuel, B. J. *MIL's*TM *The Nursing Process Series, V: Evaluation*. Denver: Association of Operating Room Nurses, 1979.
7. Jones, Cathy. "Glascow coma scale." *Am J Nurs* 79:1151, 1979.
8. Inzer, F., and Aspinall, M. J. "Evaluating patient outcomes." *Nurs Outlook* 29(March):78, 1981.

Suggested Readings

Association of Operating Room Nurses. "Operating room nursing: perioperative role." *AORN J* 27:1156, 1978.

Block, D. "Interrelated issues in evaluation and evaluation research." *Nurs Res* 29(March–April):69, 1980.

Bower, F. L. *The Process of Planning Nursing Care*, 2nd ed. St. Louis: C. V. Mosby, 1977.

Davis, D. L., Kneedler, J. A., and Manuel, B. J. *MIL's*TM *The Nursing Process Series, II: Assessment*. Denver: Association of Operating Room Nurses, 1979.

Gallant, B. W., and McLane, A. M. "Outcome criteria: A process for validation at the unit level." *J Nurs Admin* 9:14, 1979.

Given, B., Given, C. W., and Simoni, L. E. "Relationships of process of care to patient outcomes." *Nurs Res* 28(March–April):85, 1979.

Kneedler, J. A. *MIL's*TM *The Nursing Process Series, VI: Implementation of Standards of Nursing Practice: OR*. Denver: Association of Operating Room Nurses, 1979.

Kneedler, J. A., Reed, E. A., Manuel, B. J., and Fehlau, M. J. "From standards into practice." *AORN J* 28:603, 1978.

McGilloway, F. A. "The nursing process: A problem-solving approach to patient care." *Int J Nurs Stud* 17:79, 1980.

McKeehan, K. M. *Continuing Care*. St. Louis: C. V. Mosby, 1981.

Manuel, B. J. *MIL's*TM *Reporting and Documenting Patient Care: OR*. Denver: Association of Operating Room Nurses, 1980.

Manuel, B. J. *MIL's*TM *The Nursing Process Series, I: An Overview*. Denver: Association of Operating Room Nurses, 1979.

Manuel, B. J. *MIL's*TM *The Nursing Process Series, III: Planning*. Denver: Association of Operating Room Nurses, 1979.

Mayers, M. G. *A Systematic Approach to the Nursing Care Plan*. New York: Appleton-Century-Crofts, 1978.

Mayers, M. G., Norby, R. B., and Watson, A. B. *Quality Assurance for Patient Care: Nursing Perspectives*. New York: Appleton-Century-Crofts, 1977.

Prescott, P. A. "Cost-effectiveness: Tool or trap?" *Nurs Outlook* 27(November):722, 1979.

Ramey, I. G. "Setting nursing standards and evaluating care." *J Nurs Admin* 3 (May-June):27, 1973.

Stevens, B. J. *The Nurse as Executive*, 1st ed. Wakefield, Mass.: Contemporary Publishing, 1975.

"The relationship of nursing process and patient outcome." *J Nurs Admin* 6(November):18, 1976.

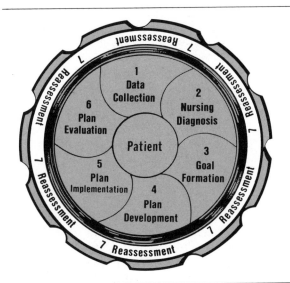

1 Data Collection
2 Nursing Diagnosis
3 Goal Formation
4 Plan Development
5 Plan Implementation
6 Plan Evaluation
Patient
7 Reassessment

Nursing activities and patient responses are evaluated.

27

Measuring the Effectiveness of Nursing Care

What does quality assurance mean and what is its importance to patients having surgery? *Quality* is a class, kind, or grade of something, in this case, patient care. The quality of care is a continuum that ranges from poor to excellent. *Quality assurance*, then, is generally defined as, "To make good or excellence certain." A hospital quality assurance program is established to make sure that excellence in health care is provided to each patient. The program has two distinct components:

1. Obtaining measurements and determining the degree to which standards are met
2. Making changes based on the information obtained from the measurements

The intent is to improve the total effort of all members of the health care team and, indirectly, to have more satisfied patients.

Why the Current Emphasis on Quality Assurance?

Health care today is complex. Most people rely not on a small town family doctor as their parents did, but on medical specialists and large hospitals or medical centers. Rapid tech-

509

nological advancements and increases in medical knowledge have contributed to this change.

The way health care is paid for adds to its complexity. Most people do not pay all their doctor and hospital bills directly. Instead a large part of their bills is paid by third parties—insurance companies or the government through Medicare and Medicaid. Because these third-party payers spend billions of dollars each year in health expenses, they are naturally concerned about how their money is used. Their concern has intensified in recent years as health costs have risen faster than inflation. The government particularly has been exerting great pressure on hospitals to contain costs, account for how the money is spent, and provide a means of measuring the quality of the services provided.

Emphasis on quality assurance also comes from the Joint Commission on Accreditation of Hospitals (JCAH), the independent voluntary agency that evaluates most of the nation's hospitals. JCAH requires each institution to establish a hospital-wide program for ongoing review and evaluation of patient care. As part of this program, the nursing administration usually has a comprehensive quality assurance system for all nursing units including the operating room. In addition, nurses may participate on interdisciplinary quality assurance committees.

Nursing has been a leader in quality assurance. The American Nurses' Association (ANA) has had a long-standing commitment to the quality of patient care. In 1966, the association established the Division on Nursing Practice and assigned it to develop standards of nursing practice that would be appropriate for all professional nurses. These standards were made available in 1973. Because they were general guidelines for all nursing practice, the standards also became a means for determining the quality of nursing care. They became a model that hospital nursing departments as well as individual nurses could follow in determining standards for their own practice.

When the federal government authorized professional standards' review organizations as its quality assurance system in 1972, ANA prepared *Guidelines for Review of Nursing Care at the Local Level* (1). This manual provided an educational tool to help registered nurses develop a system for evaluating the quality of nursing care. The volume included a nursing model for quality assurance that could be applied in any health care setting. Sample sets of outcome criteria were provided to assist nurses involved in establishing such criteria in their practice setting. Simultaneously, the JCAH developed audit methodology to assist hospitals to review and evaluate patient care objectively. In 1974, JCAH specified the number of audits to be performed. This was a controversial way to monitor quality because audits measure patient outcomes through retrospective chart review. The validity of these data was questionable. Many patient records had limited information. Hospitals attempted to meet JCAH requirements, but survey findings could not show that patient care had improved to the extent anticipated.

In 1979, the numerical requirement for audits was eliminated, and a new quality assurance standard was designed to help health professionals develop a more comprehensive approach to quality assurance activities. The emphasis now is on a coordinated, hospital-wide quality assurance program with flexibility in the approaches used to identify, assess, and resolve problems. The focus is on identifying problems whose resolution will have a significant impact on patient care. A problem that might be identified relates to environmental control of temperature and humidity that impacts potential for infection. JCAH is discouraging the use of quality assurance studies only for the purpose of documenting high-quality care (2). Therefore a review of care while the patient is still hospitalized and the solution of identified problems have become more important in relation to measuring the effectiveness of care given.

Quality Assurance for Nursing

Under the current JCAH quality assurance standard, each hospital department is responsible for putting together a plan that will be usable for them and fit into the hospital-wide program. Nursing asked itself what quality assurance programs should include. Those who were attempting to establish quality assurance programs for nursing were confused by terminology being used in different ways. What were utilization review, peer review, structure, outcomes, and standards? How did all of these fit together? Norma Lang put the pieces together and proposed the first nursing quality assurance model (3). Her model includes five components:

1. Formation of values
2. Establishment of outcome, process, and structure standards and criteria for nursing care
3. Assessment of the degree of discrepancy between established standards and criteria and the current level of nursing practice

4. Selection and implementation of an alternate nursing practice to correct the discrepancy
5. Improvement of nursing practice

ANA's Congress for Nursing Practice adopted the model as the official ANA model for quality assurance (see Fig. 27.1).

As the model shows, each component is applied in sequence. Although the model is circular, it logically begins with the identification of values. Standards and criteria should reflect these values. Once standards are developed, methods for measuring care are determined and implemented. When data are retrieved, interpretations are made, and alternative actions prescribed and chosen. Once the action is taken, follow-up is done, and evaluation becomes an ongoing process.

Figure 27.1. ANA quality assurance model. From Plan for Implementation of the Standards of Nursing, *published by the American Nurses' Association. Reprinted with permission of ANA.*

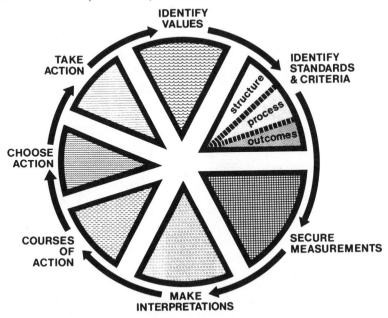

QUALITY ASSURANCE MODEL

Identifying Values

Exploring society's values for health care is important because these expectations influence services available. Consumers of health care in turn are susceptible to advancements in technology and economic and social changes. Their beliefs expand, broaden, and change.

Nurses' beliefs about nursing practice change with education and research. Professional values influence care provided, and the institution has a philosophy that affects how care is given. In addition, each nurse has her own set of values derived from a philosophy of life, cultural or ethnic background, and self-concept. Values are not constant. That is why the quality assurance model is circular. Values must be reexamined regularly.

Examples of values to consider prior to establishing standards might be:

there may be any number of criteria for judging nursing care.

Standards can be statements of what should be done (such as the ANA-AORN *Standards of Perioperative Nursing Care*) or as numerical goals. Numerical values in a criterion are used to determine the extent to which the criterion should be met. An example of such a criterion is, "The patient will be free of infection at discharge—100 percent." Certain guidelines are followed in the development of standards. Standards are (1) established by authority, opinion, or general consensus; (2) an agreed-upon level of excellence or an established norm; (3) based upon appropriate knowledge; (4) broad in scope; (5) subject to continued evaluation and revision; (6) a reflection of the state of the art.

When writing criteria to measure a standard, the following points should be kept in mind.

Person(s)	Value Held	Interpretation
Patient	Individual with knowledge and skill	Competent physicians and nurses to provide care.
Hospital	Quality care	Set high-level standards for the institution.
Nursing service	Health	Return patient to optimal level of wellness.
Operating room	Safety	Maintain a safe environment for the surgical patient.
Perioperative nurse	Uniqueness and individuality	Provide a supportive environment to enhance emotional stability.

Identifying Standards and Criteria

After exploring values and establishing a philosophy of care, the next step is developing standards. *Standard* is defined by Ramey as a model or example established by authority, custom, or general consent (4). A standard may also be defined as something used by general agreement to determine whether a thing is as it should be—an agreed-upon level of excellence; an established norm (5). Standards serve as models to guide practice. The criteria that accompany each nursing standard are measurable statements and reflect the intent of the standard. For each standard,

A criterion is:

- R: realistic or reasonable
- U: useable
- M: measurable
- B: behaviorally stated
- A: achievable or attainable

BASIC ELEMENTS OF STANDARDS

Standards have common elements that help make them acceptable to the health care team. First, OR nursing standards should be based on the voluntary agreement of the nurses in the operating room. They as a group must believe they should and can attain the level prescribed by the standards. The standards should be approved by all providing care, making them consensus standards.

Standards should be based on reliable scientific data, not guesswork. For example, a standard stating, "The patient has little or no pain three days postoperatively," is normal for patients having a total hip replacement. A standard establishes an essential condition or limitation for safe care. For instance, it is important for patients to know about their medications before discharge. If a standard states patients must know the side effects of their medications, then the nurse has a responsibility to instruct patients and evaluate whether they know the side effects.

Standards should reflect the state of the art, rather than pushing nurses beyond what is currently an acceptable level of performance. It is easy for a group of nurses, an institution, or an agency to set standards beyond existing practice because they want nurses to grow and move toward excellence. This intention is commendable, but it does not reflect reality. Standards should be consistent with current knowledge and technology.

TYPES OF STANDARDS AND CRITERIA

Standard statements about nursing care can be expressed in terms of structure, process, or outcome. *Structure* standards and criteria describe the purpose of the hospital, its legal authority, organizational characteristics, fiscal resources, qualifications of health professionals and other workers, and physical facilities and equipment, plus its status relating to accreditation, licensure, and certification or registration. Typical structure standards that cover the hospital, specifically the operating room, are: (1) JCAH standards for accreditation, (2) AORN *Standards of Administrative Nursing Practice* (6), and (3) hospital policy and procedure manuals. Examples of structure standards that might be used in hospital operating rooms are:

- Staffing requirements: A registered nurse shall circulate for each patient in surgery.

- Environment: A safe environment shall be established and monitored on an ongoing basis.
- Counts: Sponges, needles, and instruments shall be counted on all surgical procedures.
- Education: A minimum of 15 hours of continuing education is required of each nurse every year.

Criteria used to measure the above structure standard for counts could be:

1. All sponges, needles, and instruments are counted and recorded prior to beginning the operative procedure.
2. All sponges, needles, and instruments are counted and recorded before closure begins.
3. All sponges, needles, and instruments are counted and recorded when skin closure is started.

Process standards and criteria relate to activities nurses perform, including interactions with patients, other nurses, other health team members, and patients and significant others. Process standards also evaluate the extent to which nursing objectives have been reached, the skill with which nurses carry out nursing care, and appropriate utilization of material and human resources. Examples of process standards available as guides to nursing are: (1) ANA *Medical/Surgical Standards of Practice* (7), (2) ANA-AORN *Standards of Perioperative Nursing* (8), (3) *Slater Nursing Competencies Rating Scale* (9), (4) *Quality Patient Care Scale* (10), (5) *The Nursing Audit: Self Regulation in Nursing Standards* (11), and hospital standards of care.

Specific process standards for one institution might be:

Standard: The nurse shall complete a preoperative assessment on all patients having local anesthesia.

Criteria:
1. The nurse interviews the patient preoperatively.
2. The nurse reviews the patient chart prior to surgery.
3. The nurse gathers information about the

patient from the patient's family and members of the health care team.

4. The nurse records information pertinent to surgical procedure on patient record and nursing care plan.

Standard: The nurse shall admit all patients to the operating room suite.
Criteria:
1. The nurse introduces self to patient.
2. The nurse identifies patient by asking patient to state name, surgeon, and operation.
3. The nurse checks patient's name against identification bracelet and chart.
4. The nurse checks chart for allergies, accuracy of consent forms, and diagnostic tests.
5. The nurse transfers patient to designated operating room.

Outcome standards and criteria pertain to the end result of nursing care, a demonstrated measureable change in the patient's health state. Patient outcomes are probably the most important indicator of quality care. The critical question is, What happens to the patient as a result of what nurses do or do not do?

Of all the types of standards, outcome standards are the most practical and easiest to develop and measure. This is because most of the outcomes included in standards are already being used by nurses as goals in their nursing care plans. Although nurses may differ in the actions they use to achieve the result, the outcome criteria specify only the patient behaviors that come from good nursing care. Outcome standards available to use as models include: (1) *Outcome Standards for Cancer Nursing Practice* (12), (2) *The Relationship between OR Nursing Activities and Patient Outcomes: An AORN-WICHE Report* (13), and "Guidelines for OR Outcome Audit" (14).

An example of an operating room outcome standard and criteria might be:

Standard: The patient achieves optimal preoperative health status.
Criteria:
1. The patient will describe the nature of her surgery in own words.

2. The patient will demonstrate deep breathing and coughing exercise.
3. The patient's respiration rate is 12–22/minute.
4. The patient's lungs are clear (free of rales and rhonchi).

Standard: The patient demonstrates management of anxiety immediately prior to induction.
Criteria:
1. The patient is lying quietly.
2. The patient's facial expressions are relaxed.
3. The patient states a feeling of security.

Nurses involved in planning a quality assurance program must decide the type of standard and criteria they will use. This will be based on what they are attempting to measure. As demonstrated, it is easy to establish patient outcomes because the nurse already does it in the nursing process when she formulates goals and puts them on the patient care plan. Process standards are more complex because of the wide range of nursing activities that can be used. Structure standards are also complex but are required in some instances by voluntary and governmental approval bodies.

Measuring Standard and Criteria Achievement

Methods for measuring the attainment of standards include review and evaluation, the problem-focused approach to quality assurance, peer review, performance evaluation, and audits. Currently, the Joint Commission on Accreditation of Hospitals advocates what it calls reviews and evaluations. Essentially they are audits used on an ongoing basis to screen components of care such as infections, the unit environment, resource utilization, nursing care, and patient responses. A systematic approach to review and evaluation should be established based on the volume and impact of service on direct patient care. Reviews and evaluations are a means of identifying problems that require further investigation. The evaluation focuses on the actual nursing care provided, not only on how well it has been documented as in retrospective chart review (see Fig. 27.2). The review is done on a selected patient still in the hospital and focuses on no more than the past 48 hours. An example of indicators that might be used for the operating room are: (1) administration of medication, (2) patient satisfaction, (3) admission of patient to operating room, (4) patient teaching, and (5) monitoring devices.

For example, to obtain the measurement for patient teaching, the review and evaluation form would ask for responses to the following:

1. Inclusion of teaching objectives in patient care plan
2. Utilization of perioperative teaching records
3. Documentation of patient's response to teaching

The new JCAH quality assurance standard requires a problem-focused approach to measure effectiveness of patient care. The hospital identifies patient care problems that affect patient care directly or indirectly and works to resolve them. The steps in the problem-solving process are:

1. Identifying problems
2. Determining priorities for problem assessment and problem resolution
3. Establishing clinically valid criteria and selecting appropriate assessment methods
4. Establishing causes of problems most amenable to correction and planning and implementing corrective actions
5. Evaluating and monitoring problem resolution

The success of this approach in evaluating the quality of care depends on the resolution of the identified problems and the continued efforts to measure the overall effectiveness of the solution. A problem-focused summary used in the operating room is shown in Fig. 27.3.

Peer review is another method used to measure quality of patient care. Nurses with the same role expectations and job descriptions examine care provided by colleagues. These peers identify strengths and weaknesses in other nurses' practice and assume the responsibility for improvement of patient care.

Nurses have developed a variety of peer review tools for evaluating care provided to patients having surgery. The Association of Operating Room Nurses has published *Peer Review for Nursing Practice: OR* (15), which provides guidelines for OR peer groups who are developing instruments to measure the quality of care given by individual nurses. The major categories which can be used for evaluation purposes are: (1) physiological, (2) psychosocial, (3) accountability, (4) skills, and (5) personal qualities.

A more recent AORN publication, *Developing Basic Competencies for Perioperative Nursing* (16), outlines 25 basic competencies an operating room nurse can be expected to have after 6–12 months experience. The competencies can be used as a foundation for objective peer review or for performance appraisal. The competencies are categorized into: (1) physiological and psychosocial statements, (2) skills statements, (3) professional characteristics statements, and (4) accountability statements.

Performance appraisal is still another means for measuring the quality of care patients receive. Supervisory and management personnel can identify problems in patient care as they evaluate a nurse's level of performance.

Even though the JCAH no longer has specific requirements for audits, there are still times when an audit study may be appropriate. The audit tool will probably take the same format as the screening device which we called review and evaluation earlier in this chapter.

Whatever quality assurance method is chosen, its purposes are to identify strengths and deficiencies in care given during the perioperative period and to determine whether records reflect the care given. Through quality assurance, the nurse can identify problems that directly and indirectly affect the quality of care and report findings and make recommendations to the hospital administration. Finally, the nurse can make an assessment of whether nursing care has improved when changes have been instituted.

ADMISSION OF PATIENT TO OPERATING ROOM

	YES	NO	N/A
1. Secretary checks pre-op check list for evidence of completion			
2. Secretary checks operative permit and appropriate consents			
3. Secretary communicates any discrepancy to Charge Nurse			
4. Circulating Nurse:			
a. introduces self to patient			
b. identifies patient by asking patient to state name, surgeon and operation			
c. checks patient's name against identification bracelet and chart			
d. checks chart for:			
1) accuracy of consents			
2) lab and EKG results			
3) allergies.			
e. notifies anesthesiologist/surgeon of abnormalities			
f. transfers patient to designated operative room by			
1) providing reassurance			
2) lowers side rails, unwraps outer blanket prior to entrance to the operative room table			
3) aligns, stabilizes gurney during transfer to operating room table			
4) applies safety strap properly			

COMMENTS: _____

Figure 27.2. One segment of a Patient Care Review and Evaluation Record for Nursing Service Quality Assurance. Used with permission of Porter Memorial Hospital, Denver.

Figure 27.3. Quality assurance problem: Solution summary report. Used with permission of Porter Memorial Hospital, Denver.

PROBLEM/SOLUTION SUMMARY REPORT

DEPARTMENT/COMMITTEE _____ OPERATING ROOM_____

PROBLEM IDENTIFIED BY _____ KAREN BALES, R.N., STAFF NURSE_____

ROUTED TO ____ CYNTHIA MORRIS, R.N., CHARGE NURSE_____ DATE _6/7/82_____

ROUTED TO _____ DATE _____

1. PROBLEM: Currently there is a lack of qualified staff to transport patients to and from surgery.

2. IDENTIFICATION: Initially the problem was identified by observation of performance and delay in transporting patients. This was followed up with an audit based on the existing Policy and Procedure.

3. ASSESSMENT: Hospital Policy and Procedure #153.006--Transportation of Patients to and from Surgery.

4. CAUSE OF PROBLEM: Audit revealed existing policy was unrealistic, nurses were not communicating essential information to recovery room personnel, inadequate staff in recovery room to provide safe transportation to unit and unit nurses not present when patient taken or returned from surgery.

5. ACTION TO SOLVE PROBLEM:
   A) Policy and Procedure for transportation was revised and unrealistic problems deleted.
   B) Audit tool revised into four categories:
      1) Transportation
      2) Admission of patient to O.R.
      3) Transportation of patient from O.R. to Recovery Room
      4) Transporting patient from Recovery Room to unit
   C) Staff inservice was held to discuss the identified problem and corrective action.
   D) Unit nurses involved in revising portions of policy affecting the unit.
   E) Inservice for transportation orderlies to review revised Policy and Procedure and their role.

6. MONITORING THE PROBLEM AFTER ACTION INITIATED: Reauditing is being done every three months in each of the four categories for a period of six months. Then the routine review and evaluations will be done on an ongoing basis. Periodic observation checks will be done to evaluate how transportation is being done and monitor communications.

7. SOLUTION: Problem is solved for the present with input from unit nurses, transportation orderlies, Recovery Room and O.R. nurses.

DATE: __7/5/82___

Methods of Data Collection

Valid and reliable means of gathering information to measure the quality of care in the operating room include direct observation of patients, interviews, questionnaires, performance observation, and review of the patient record.

In direct observation of patients, someone familiar with the evaluation criteria examines the patient to determine the outcome of care given. The evaluator assumes a nonparticipative role and does not get involved in providing care unless absolutely necessary. For example, the evaluator would observe the patient's skin for pressure points or reddened areas. Upon the patient's admission to the operating room, the evaluator would observe whether the patient is comfortable and seemingly managing her fear and anxiety. In the operating room, the evaluator would observe the environment and room setup to determine the nurse's ability to organize necessary supplies and equipment.

The interview is another means of obtaining data. The evaluator can talk with the patient, family, or any member of the health care team to validate the care received. Questions the evaluator might ask a patient are: (1) Were you told where your family might wait during your operation? (2) Did you know you would have pain postoperatively? Questions the evaluator might ask nurses in an interview would be: (1) Did you explain the operating room environment to the patient? (2) Did you assess the patient's level of anxiety related to his surgery?

A written questionnaire is another way of assessing the patient's satisfaction with her care or determining her knowledge level and compliance with treatment. Questions might be: (1) Were you comfortable and warm during transfer to the operating room? (2) Was the waiting area quiet? (3) Were you given an explanation when someone approached you to do a procedure? If constructed in a way that produces meaningful data, questionnaires can provide helpful information.

Performance observation is the process of examining the care provided by nurses while the care is being given. The evaluator observes the nurse to identify strengths and weaknesses in an effort to improve the quality of nursing performance. The evaluator again must be familiar with the procedures and standards of performance the hospital has established. The evaluator observes whether: (1) the nurse communicates pertinent information about the surgical procedure to the recovery room nurse, (2) the nurse explains to the patient what she is going to do prior to beginning the procedure, (3) the nurse performs a sponge, needle, and instrument count according to established procedure.

The patient record is used to compare actual care to established levels of care. The hospital's established standards of practice become the yardstick for measuring the quality of care. The record can be used at two different times—concurrently and retrospectively. A concurrent record review is done while the patient is still in the hospital. For example, an evaluator checks the patient's record to determine if the nurse documented that she gave the patient an opportunity to discuss her fear of mutilation due to radical neck dissection prior to going to the operating room. The record should also indicate such items as placement of the electrosurgical grounding pad and positioning.

A retrospective review is done after the patient is discharged. The same data described above should be present in the record. If care is documented, as it should be, it will be available for review either during the patient's stay or after discharge.

All these methods can be used separately or in combination.

INTERPRETING DATA

Data obtained with these measurement tools are used to make interpretations about strengths and weaknesses in nursing care. The standards and criteria become the guidelines for review. When comparisons between the established standards and actual practice reveal a difference, this is interpreted as either a strength or a deficiency. The staff will benefit from knowing their care has improved or that it was good in the beginning. Identifying positive areas increases job satisfaction and enhances morale. Staff are also reminded of their responsibilities for caring, comforting, and individualizing care.

Deficiencies usually occur because of noncompliance, not a lack of knowledge or skills. It is important to analyze deficiencies to determine how to best correct the problem. Questions to ask about a deficiency are, "Why is it important?" and "Would there be serious consequences if nothing were done about it?" Sources of weakness can be traced to a group, individuals, or sometimes, the institution. Group deficiencies might be noncompliance with instrument counts or lack of documentation, whereas individual deficiencies could be breaks in aseptic technique or continued noncompliance with the policy for disposing of specimens. Institutional deficiencies might be a lack of medical resources or inadequate facilities.

There are three reasons for deficiencies which must be considered when determining courses of action: lack of knowledge, inadequate skills, and nonperformance. Knowledge deficiencies arise either when nurses have not learned a subject thoroughly or fail to apply what they have learned. Skills also may not have been adequately taught or used enough for the nurses to become proficient. Performance deficiencies are the most difficult to manage. To improve performance, managers need to focus on the desired performance and what is hindering it. When desired performance occurs, it should be rewarded.

Choices of Action

The choice of corrective action will relate directly to the deficiencies identified. Emphasis is on actions that will improve patient care through expanding knowledge, skills, and performance. Continuing education, inservice, meetings, peer pressure, environmental changes, administrative changes, self-initiated change, research, and reward or punitive action are all methods of correcting deficiencies.

Continuing education and inservice meetings are planned education activities designed to promote nurses' clinical competency. For example, if the deficiency found is lack of knowledge about how to develop nursing care plans, the nurse could plan educational programs to assist other nurses in learning the components of the care plan. On the other hand, planned inservice sessions may be the way to correct deficiencies in positioning patients on the operating table. Although inservice and continuing education are effective ways to correct deficiencies, the deficiency must be monitored to determine whether further education has helped.

Peer pressure is another method that can be effective in correcting deficiencies. Nurses look to their peers for reinforcement and support. Discrepancies in practice can be brought to the group, the operating room staff, which then assumes responsibility for determining actions to be taken and changes required. If the group is cohesive, harmonious, and can communicate easily, the pressure they create will improve patient care. Consider the following example: A nurse has accompanied the patient and anesthesiologist to the recovery room after surgery. The anesthesiologist is busy giving her report. The nurse from the operating room is in a hurry or a little shy, and she does not want to interrupt the anesthesiologist or take an assertive role. Consequently, she leaves without communicating any nursing information to the recovery room nurse. When the deficiency is found that not all nurses are communicating essential data to recovery room personnel, a discussion ensues among the OR staff. The group as a whole decides they must all be more assertive because they have an obligation to the patient. They decide that they will observe each other daily and give positive or negative feedback on whether they communicate essential data to the recovery room nurses.

If deficiencies are continually found in physical facilities, efforts need to be made to change those conditions. An example might be adding a storage room to get equipment out of the corridors for safety reasons or building a holding area where patients can be monitored prior to admission to the operating room.

Some deficiencies may require changes in administrative policies and procedures or other components of the administrative structure. For instance, a review and evaluation may identify the problem that the staff is not doing the surgical scrub properly. Further investigation shows the department policy for scrubbing needs updating. Scientific evidence is found to support the change to a new procedure, and a new written procedure is issued.

Clinical research is an important ally for the manager in correcting deficiencies. She should be alert for research reports that provide the answers to operating room practice questions, such as the value of preoperative shaving or the barrier qualities of drapes. Nurses are gradually building a scientific base for their practice. Putting research findings into practice will further this effort.

Individual members of the staff can help in the change process. As they gain knowledge and skills, they can inspire and assist others to improve the way they practice. Achievements by staff members should be recognized and rewarded and opportunities to share their new knowledge with others should be available. This improves practice and builds morale. Nurses respond to recognition and appreciation. Posting staff achievements in a central location or pointing out staff improvements at inservice meetings is helpful.

It is far more effective to correct deficiencies through positive reinforcement than through punishment. When all else fails, punishment may be the only recourse, but it should be considered as a last resort. If discipline is necessary, the punishment should be selected carefully because it may have a serious effect not only on the staff member involved but on the rest of the staff as well.

In taking any of these actions to improve practice, it should be remembered that results count. The actions should be followed through and monitored. A target date should be set for reevaluating the action taken and determining objectively whether the change sought has occurred.

The ANA quality assurance model is cyclical. Quality assurance efforts do not end with the evaluation of the effects of actions taken. All the steps in the process—reviewing values, changing standards and criteria, updating measurement tools, and evaluating quality of care—should become a continual activity in the operating room.

References

1. *Guidelines for Review of Nursing Care at the Local Level.* Washington, D.C.: U.S. Department of Health, Education and Welfare, 1976.
2. Kaplan, K. O., and Hopkins, J. M. *The QA Guide: A Resource for Hospital Quality Assurance.* Chicago: Joint Commission on Accreditation of Hospitals, 1980.
3. Lang, N. M. "Quality assurance in nursing." *AORN J* 22:180–186, 1975.
4. Ramey, K. B. "Setting nursing standards and evaluating care." *J Nurs Admin* 3(May–June): 27–35, 1973.
5. *Plan for Implementation of the Standards of Nursing Practice.* Kansas City: American Nurses' Association, 1975.
6. Association of Operating Room Nurses. "Standards of administrative nursing practice." *AORN J* 23(June):1202–1208, 1976.
7. *Medical-Surgical Standards of Nursing Practice.* Kansas City: American Nurses' Association, 1973.
8. *Standards of Perioperative Nursing Practice.* Kansas City: American Nurses' Association and Association of Operating Room Nurses, 1982.
9. Wandelt, M. A., and Stewart, D. S. *Slater Nursing Competencies Rating Scale.* New York: Appleton-Century-Crofts, 1975.
10. Wandelt, M. A., and Ager, J. *Quality Patient Care Scale.* New York: Appleton-Century-Crofts, 1974.
11. Phaneuf, M. C. *The Nursing Audit: Self Regulation in Nursing Practice.* New York: Appleton-Century-Crofts, 1976.
12. *Outcome Standards for Cancer Nursing Practice.* Kansas City: American Nurses' Association, 1979.
13. *The Relationship between OR Nursing Activities and Patient Outcomes: AORN-WICHE Report.* Denver: Association of Operating Room Nurses, 1978.
14. "Guidelines for OR outcome audit." *AORN J* 27:219, 1978.
15. *Peer Review for Nursing Practice: OR.* Denver: Association of Operating Room Nurses, 1977.
16. Ad hoc committee on basic competencies. "Developing basic competencies for perioperative nursing." *AORN J* 35:871–884, 1982.

Index